Endocrinology: A Clinician's Handbook

Endocrinology: A Clinician's Handbook

Edited by Donovan Douglas

hayle medical

New York

Hayle Medical,
750 Third Avenue, 9th Floor,
New York, NY 10017, USA

Visit us on the World Wide Web at:
www.haylemedical.com

ISBN: 978-1-63241-598-1

Cataloging-in-Publication Data

Endocrinology : a clinician's handbook / edited by Donovan Douglas.
 p. cm.
Includes bibliographical references and index.
ISBN 978-1-63241-598-1
1. Endocrinology. 2. Internal medicine. 3. Hormones. 4. Clinical medicine.
I. Douglas, Donovan.
RC648 .E53 2019
616.4--dc23

Table of Contents

Preface

Endocrinology is a branch of medicine that is concerned with the study of the endocrine system, its associated diseases and hormonal secretions such as insulin, thyroid hormone and growth hormone. Hormones are classified into the classes of amines, steroids, and peptides and proteins. A number of endocrine feedback mechanisms are integral to the working of the endocrine system. These act in such a way that one feedback mechanism controls the release or action of another hormone. Some endocrine diseases are hypothyroidism, diabetes mellitus and metabolic syndrome, among others. Most of such disorders require lifelong care. The diagnosis of endocrine disorders is performed by laboratory techniques especially through inhibition/suppression testing or excitation/stimulation testing. Different approaches, evaluations, methodologies and advanced studies on endocrinology have been included in this book. There has been rapid progress in the understanding of endocrine disorders, their diagnostic techniques and treatments, which have been included in this extensive book. It is an essential guide for both academicians and those who wish to pursue this discipline further.

After months of intensive research and writing, this book is the end result of all who devoted their time and efforts in the initiation and progress of this book. It will surely be a source of reference in enhancing the required knowledge of the new developments in the area. During the course of developing this book, certain measures such as accuracy, authenticity and research focused analytical studies were given preference in order to produce a comprehensive book in the area of study.

This book would not have been possible without the efforts of the authors and the publisher. I extend my sincere thanks to them. Secondly, I express my gratitude to my family and well-wishers. And most importantly, I thank my students for constantly expressing their willingness and curiosity in enhancing their knowledge in the field, which encourages me to take up further research projects for the advancement of the area.

Editor

Rare Skeletal Complications in the Setting of Primary Hyperparathyroidism

Nikos Sabanis,[1] **Eleni Gavriilaki,**[2] **Eleni Paschou,**[3] **Asterios Kalaitzoglou,**[2]
Dimitrios Papanikolaou,[4] **Pinelopi Ioannidou,**[4] **and Sotirios Vasileiou**[1]

[1]*Department of Nephrology, General Hospital of Pella, 58200 Edessa, Greece*
[2]*Medical School, Aristotle University of Thessaloniki, 54124 Thessaloniki, Greece*
[3]*Department of General Practice & Family Medicine, General Hospital of Pella, 58200 Edessa, Greece*
[4]*Department of General Surgery, General Hospital of Pella, 58200 Edessa, Greece*

Correspondence should be addressed to Eleni Paschou; el_paschou@yahoo.gr

Academic Editor: Yuji Moriwaki

Parathyroid carcinoma represents an extremely rare neoplasm with diverse clinical manifestations which vary from asymptomatic patients to severe complications of hypercalcemia or parathyrotoxicosis while skeletal involvement is rather common. Herein we aimed at presenting a unique case of a young patient with rare aggressive skeletal complications of parathyroid cancer that initially were misdiagnosed. Ossification of the cervical ligamentum flavum and skull tumor illustrates erosive bonny lesions of hyperparathyroidism that in association with previous medical history of recurrent nephrolithiasis and biochemical findings guide the diagnosis. We suggest that increased awareness and holistic approach are needed in order to recognize and further investigate signs and symptoms of hyperparathyroidism.

1. Introduction

Parathyroid carcinoma represents an extremely rare neoplastic entity, accounting for approximately 1% of primary hyperparathyroidism (HPT). Although hormonally functional tumors are observed in the majority of cases, clinical manifestations of parathyroid carcinoma can vary from none (asymptomatic patients) to severe complications of hypercalcemia or parathyrotoxicosis. Thus, its diagnosis remains a challenge for the clinicians and is primarily based on laboratory and imaging testing [1].

Herein we aimed at presenting a unique case of a young patient with severe complications of parathyroid cancer and briefly reviewing the relevant literature.

2. Case Report

A 45-year-old, Greek, Caucasian, male patient presented to the Emergency Department due to severe, colicky pain in the left pleura reflected to ipsilateral lower abdomen quadrant accompanied by nausea and vomiting. His personal medical history included recurrent episodes of nephrolithiasis, laminectomy in the cervical spine due to ossification of the cervical ligamentum flavum in C2-C3 and C4-C5 without signs of myelopathy two years ago, and surgical resection of a giant cell tumor of the skull one year ago. No familial history of multigland disease or evidence of hypercalcemia in his relatives was recorded.

Based on the clinical examination and renal ultrasonography the patient was diagnosed with another episode of nephrolithiasis without evidence of obstructive uropathy. Beyond that, however, laboratory testing revealed findings of primary hyperparathyroidism (serum calcium 16.0 mmol/L with normal values 8.0–10.4 mmol/L, phosphorus 1.46 mg/dL with normal values 2.5–5.9 mg/dL, parathyroid hormone 8560.0 pg/mL with normal values 8.0–76.0 pg/mL, and urine calcium levels 1260 mg/24 h). It is noteworthy that, on admittance, biochemical testing revealed also acute kidney injury (serum creatinine levels 1.76 mg/dL with normal range

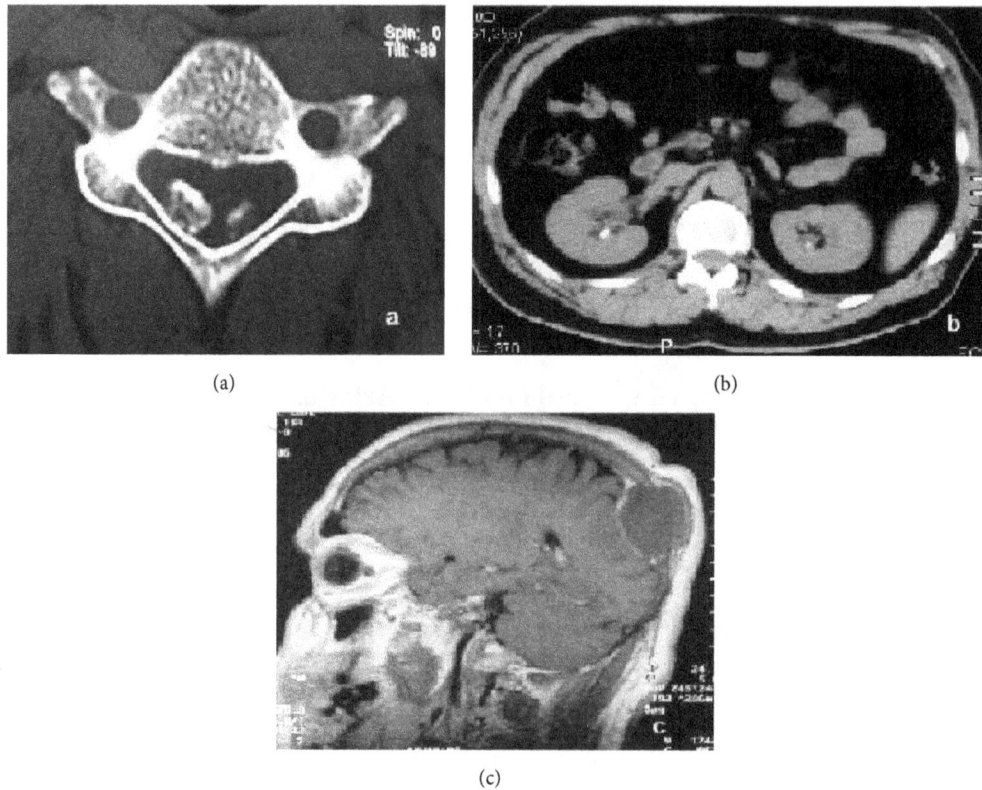

(a)

(b)

(c)

FIGURE 1: A 45-year-old man with parathyroid carcinoma: (a) ossification of the cervical ligamentum flavum in C2-C3 and C4-C5 without signs of myelopathy. (b) Nephrolithiasis in both kidneys and (c) left parietal bone tumor (5.5 × 3.2 × 4.4 cm) from Magnetic Resonance Imaging scan.

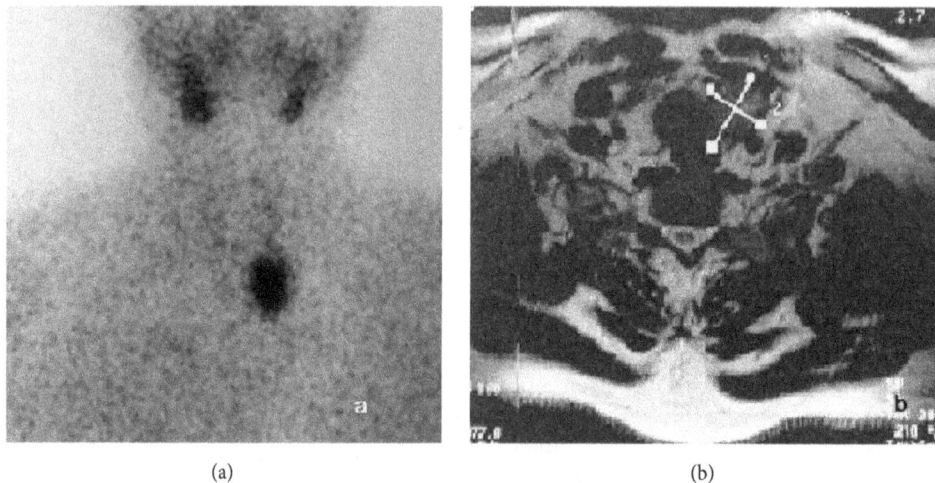

(a)

(b)

FIGURE 2: A 45-year-old man with parathyroid carcinoma: (a) Technetium-99m Sestamibi scan and (b) Magnetic Resonance Imaging scan showing the parathyroid tumor.

0.5–0.9 mg/dL). Thus, the patient was hospitalized for further diagnostic procedures.

During his hospitalization the patient's history and medical records were carefully reviewed. As shown in Figure 1, the patient had been suffering from misdiagnosed complications of hyperparathyroidism for the last two years. Based on his history, neck ultrasound and Technetium-99m Sestamibi scan were performed revealing a parathyroid tumor, as shown in Figure 2. Thorax and abdomen Computed Tomography were performed revealing no further pathological findings as well as neck Magnetic Resonance Imaging. No genetic testing was performed, in spite of the young age of the patient, because of the absence of familial history of multigland disease as well as clinical and imaging findings compatible to an inherited form of hyperparathyroidism [2]. Due to the persistently high serum calcium and parathyroid hormone levels, the high alkaline phosphatase levels (440.0 IU/L with normal values 38.0–155.0 IU/L), and the late complications of hyperparathyroidism, surgical excision of the tumor was scheduled. Meanwhile, the patient was treated with intravenous administration of normal saline 0.9% and renal adapted dosage of zoledronic acid (3 mg, MDRD eGFR = 52 mL/min/1.73 m^2). As a result, preoperative serum calcium and creatinine levels were improved. According to the histopathology the tumor was identified as parathyroid carcinoma and total surgical excision was achieved.

After surgery serum calcium and phosphorus levels were closely monitored in order to prevent potential hungry bone syndrome. The clinical course was uneventful and the patient remains on a regular follow-up program with no signs of recurrence or metastasis one year after the excision.

3. Discussion

In our case report we describe the coexistence of rare late complications of hyperparathyroidism, such as recurrent nephrolithiasis, ossification of the cervical ligamentum flavum, and skull brown tumor which had not been adequately investigated at their onset.

The clinical appearance of parathyroid carcinoma is diverse and not pathognomic. Skeletal involvement is rather common in parathyroid carcinoma (22–91%) [3]. It primarily includes diffuse osteopenia, osteoporosis, or pathological fractures as well as osteitis fibrosa cystic, subperiosteal bone resorption and absence of the lamina dura. Brown tumors had been extensively described as radiological features in 4.5–24% of patients with primary hyperparathyroidism [4, 5]. These erosive osseous lesions are observed in the setting of osteitis fibrosa cystic due to rapid osteoclastic activity. In the past decades, brown tumors were considered prominent manifestations of primary hyperparathyroidism [6, 7] or severe secondary hyperparathyroidism in hemodialysis patients [8]. Furthermore, ossification of the cervical ligamentum flavum has mainly been correlated to mechanical stress, growth factors, and trauma in exceptional limited case reports in Caucasian people [9].

Our patient had a medical history of atypical skeletal complications of hyperparathyroidism which had not been elucidated properly: a skull brown tumor, ossification of the cervical ligamentum flavum, and ligament calcification of the knee joint. Thus, he experienced two surgical operations. The histopathology of the skull brown tumor was initially misdiagnosed as a giant cell tumor of the bone and the previous medical history had been ignored. Of note, such misdiagnoses are also evident in the recent literature [10–12] but no previous report of ossification of the cervical ligamentum flavum in patient with hyperparathyroidism of any cause has been reported.

With regard to the renal manifestations of severe hyperparathyroidism we observed a history of recurrent episodes of nephrolithiasis in the context of excessive hypercalciuria. Silverberg et al. refer that calcium stone disease remains the most common clinical manifestation of primary hyperparathyroidism, ranging between 15 and 20% in most series. About 3% of patients with stone disease have primary hyperparathyroidism, and about 10% of patients with primary hyperparathyroidism present with recurrent calcium stone disease [13].

Beyond the high index of clinical suspicion, our patient presented also with extremely increased calcium, parathyroid hormone, and alkaline phosphatase levels. Therefore, the recommended imaging approach for the diagnosis of parathyroid cancer, which combines Technetium-99m Sestamibi scan and a neck ultrasound [1], proved to be important. Thorax, neck, and abdomen Computed Tomography as well as Magnetic Resonance Imaging scans were also advisable and were performed in order to exclude metastatic lesions due to the observed severe clinical manifestations. Complete tumor resection was achieved as confirmed by the histopathology. Normalization of calcium and parathyroid hormone levels was observed postoperatively without hungry bone syndrome appearance, persisting one year after initial surgery. Taking into consideration the high recurrence (more than 50%) and metastatic rate of the disease (approximately 25%) [1], long-term regular follow-up visits should be performed.

4. Conclusions

Parathyroid carcinoma is a rare neoplasm with diverse clinical manifestations. Since the patients are often referred to primary care physicians, general surgeons, orthopedic surgeons, or neurosurgeons for their initial symptoms, increased vigilance is needed in order to recognize and further investigate signs or symptoms mimicking those observed in hyperparathyroidism.

References

[1] C. H. Wei and A. Harari, "Parathyroid carcinoma: update and guidelines for management," *Current Treatment Options in Oncology*, vol. 13, no. 1, pp. 11–23, 2012.

[2] R. Eastell, M. L. Brandi, A. G. Costa, P. D'Amour, D. M. Shoback, and R. V. Thakker, "Diagnosis of asymptomatic primary hyperparathyroidism: proceedings of the fourth international workshop," *Journal of Clinical Endocrinology and Metabolism*, vol. 99, no. 10, pp. 3570–3579, 2014.

[3] E. Shane, "Clinical review 122: parathyroid carcinoma," *Journal of Clinical Endocrinology and Metabolism*, vol. 86, no. 2, pp. 485–493, 2001.

[4] J. S. Keyser and G. N. Postma, "Brown tumor of the mandible," *American Journal of Otolaryngology: Head and Neck Medicine and Surgery*, vol. 17, no. 6, pp. 407–410, 1996.

[5] P. Polat, M. Kantarc, F. Alper, M. Koruyucu, S. Suma, and O. Onbaş, "The spectrum of radiographic findings in primary

hyperparathyroidism," *Clinical Imaging*, vol. 26, no. 3, pp. 197–205, 2002.

[6] M. D. Walker, M. Rubin, and S. J. Silverberg, "Nontraditional manifestations of primary hyperparathyroidism," *Journal of Clinical Densitometry*, vol. 16, no. 1, pp. 40–47, 2013.

[7] D. Radulescu, B. Chis, V. Donca, and V. Munteanu, "Brown tumors of the femur and pelvis secondary to a parathyroid carcinoma. Report of one case," *Revista Medica de Chile*, vol. 142, no. 7, pp. 919–923, 2014.

[8] H. Tayfun, O. Metin, S. Hakan, B. Zafer, and A. Vardar, "Brown tumor as an unusual but preventable cause of spinal cord compression: case report and review of the literature," *Asian Journal of Neurosurgery*, vol. 9, no. 1, pp. 40–44, 2014.

[9] G. Fotakopoulos, G. A. Alexiou, E. Mihos, and S. Voulgaris, "Ossification of the ligamentum flavum in cervical and thoracic spine. Report of three cases," *Acta Neurologica Belgica*, vol. 110, no. 2, pp. 186–189, 2010.

[10] L. Vera, M. Dolcino, M. Mora et al., "Primary hyperparathyroidism diagnosed after surgical ablation of a costal mass mistaken for giant-cell bone tumor: a case report," *Journal of Medical Case Reports*, vol. 5, article 596, 2011.

[11] H. Resic, F. Masnic, N. Kukavica, and G. Spasovski, "Unusual clinical presentation of brown tumor in hemodialysis patients: two case reports," *International Urology and Nephrology*, vol. 43, no. 2, pp. 575–580, 2011.

[12] G. K. Gedik, O. Ata, P. Karabagli, and O. Sari, "Differential diagnosis between secondary and tertiary hyperparathyroidism in a case of a giant-cell and brown tumor containing mass. Findings by ^{99m}Tc-MDP, ^{18}F-FDG PET/CT and ^{99m}Tc-MIBI scans," *Hellenic Journal of Nuclear Medicine*, vol. 17, no. 3, pp. 214–217, 2014.

[13] S. J. Silverberg, B. L. Clarke, M. Peacock et al., "Current issues in the presentation of asymptomatic primary hyperparathyroidism: proceedings of the fourth International workshop," *The Journal of Clinical Endocrinology & Metabolism*, vol. 99, no. 10, pp. 3580–3594, 2014.

Pheochromocytoma in Congenital Cyanotic Heart Disease

Carmen Aresta,[1,2] Gianfranco Butera,[3] Antonietta Tufano,[2] Giorgia Grassi,[1,2] Livio Luzi ⓘD,[1,2] and Stefano Benedini ⓘD[1,2]

[1]Department of Biomedical Sciences for Health, Università degli Studi di Milano, Milan, Italy
[2]Endocrinology Unit, IRCCS Policlinico San Donato, San Donato M.se (MI), Italy
[3]Department of Congenital Cardiology and Cardiac Surgery, IRCCS Policlinico San Donato, San Donato Milanese (MI), Italy

Correspondence should be addressed to Stefano Benedini; stefano.benedini@unimi.it

Academic Editor: Carlo Capella

Studies on genome-wide transcription patterns have shown that many genetic alterations implicated in pheochromocytoma-paraganglioma (P-PGL) syndromes cluster in a common cellular pathway leading to aberrant activation of molecular response to hypoxia in normoxic conditions (the pseudohypoxia hypothesis). Several cases of P-PGL have been reported in patients with cyanotic congenital heart disease (CCHD). Patients affected with CCHD have an increased likelihood of P-PGL compared to those affected with noncyanotic congenital heart disease. One widely supported hypothesis is that chronic hypoxia represents the determining factor supporting this increased risk. We report the case of a 23-old woman affected with congenital tricuspid atresia surgically by the Fontan procedure. The patient was admitted to hospital with hypertensive crisis and dyspnea. Chest computed tomography revealed, incidentally, a 6-cm mass in the left adrenal lodge. Increased levels of noradrenaline (NA) and its metabolites were detected (plasma NA 5003.7 pg/ml, n.v.<480; urinary NA 1059.5 μg/24 h, n.v.<85.5; urinary metanephrine 489 μg/24 h, n.v.<320). The patient did not report any additional symptom related to catecholamine excess. The left adrenal tumor showed abnormal accumulation when 131I-metaiodobenzylguanidine scintigraphy was performed. A 18F-fluorodeoxyglucose positron emission tomography showed no significant metabolic activity in the left adrenal gland but intense uptake in the supra- and subdiaphragmatic brown adipose tissue, probably due to noradrenergic-stimulated glucose uptake. The patient underwent left open adrenalectomy after preconditioning with α- and β-blockers and histopathological examination confirmed the diagnosis of pheochromocytoma (Ki-67<5%). Screening for germline mutations did not show any genes mutation (investigated mutations: RET, TMEM127, MAX, SDHD, SDHC, SDHB, SDHAF2, SDHA, and VHL). Clinicians should consider P-PGL when an unexplained clinical deterioration occurs in CCHD patients, even in the absence of typical paroxysmal symptoms.

1. Introduction

Congenital heart disease (CHD) is a group of developmental abnormalities of the heart and great vessels whose incidence has considerably increased in the last decades. Cyanotic congenital heart disease (CCHD) represents a severe subset of CHD often characterized by neonatal systemic hypoxia. In CCHD a right to left shunt is observed and it results in deoxygenated blood entering the oxygenated limb of the vascular circuit. CCHD affects 1/1000 live newborns and represents approximately 10% of all CHD [1]. Early surgical treatment allows in most cases the reduction or elimination of chronic hypoxia.

Numerous case of congenital heart defects can cause Eisenmenger syndrome, including atrial septal defects [2], ventricular septal defects, patent ductus arteriosus, and more complex types of cyanotic heart disease. All these cardiovascular alterations can lead to a more or less evident cyanosis with potential effects favoring the development of chromaffin cell alterations.

Pheochromocytoma and paraganglioma (P-PGL) are catecholamine-secreting tumors, which respectively arise from chromaffin cells of the adrenal medulla and the sympathetic ganglia. P-PGL are rare tumors representing about 5% of incidentally discovered adrenal masses [3]. Up to 35-40% of patients have disease-causing germline

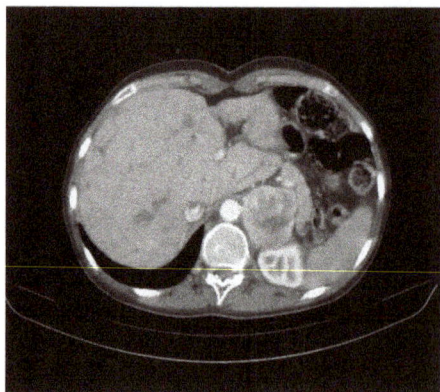

FIGURE 1: **Abdominal CT scan**: presence of a big mass in the left adrenal lodge (6-cm mass).

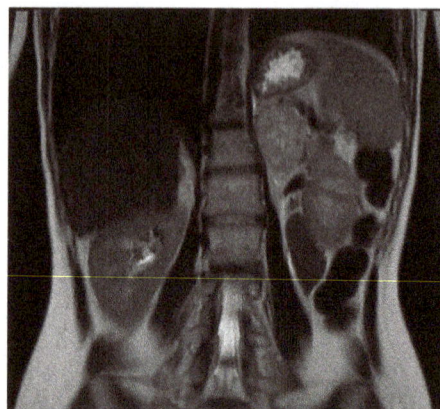

FIGURE 2: **Abdominal MRI scan**: presence of a big heterogeneous adrenal lesion, with hyperintense spots due to hematic content.

mutations [4] and the likelihood increases in young patients.

The coexistence of CHD and P-PGL has already been reported in previous studies and a causal link between the two conditions has been postulated [5, 6].

2. Case Presentation

We describe the case of a 23-year-old Caucasian female affected with congenital tricuspid atresia and intact ventricular septum. She had a history of palliative surgery since first days of life but her percutaneous oxygen saturation (SpO2) level remained around 80% even though a Fontan procedure was performed at 12 years of age. Persistent desaturation was related to the presence of venous collaterals between the Fontan circulation and left atrium.

The patient admitted to Policlinico San Donato (San Donato Milanese, Italy) for hypertensive crisis, worsening dyspnea, and hemoptysis. There was no family history of relevant morbidities. On examination, her height was 175 cm, weight was 64 kg (BMI 17.7 Kg/m2), blood pressure (BP) was 160/85 mmHg, and SpO2 was 81% (room air). Electrocardiogram (ECG) showed sinus tachycardia (heart rate 101 beats/min), first-degree atrioventricular block (PR 220 msec), and right bundle branch block (QRS 140 msec). Chest computed tomography (CT) (Figure 1) incidentally detected a 6-cm mass in the left adrenal lodge.

The presence of a heterogeneous adrenal lesion, with hyperintense spots due to hematic content, was confirmed by abdominal magnetic resonance imaging (MRI) (Figure 2).

Laboratory tests revealed increased levels of noradrenaline (NA) and its metabolites [plasma NA 5003.7 pg/ml, n.v. < 480 pg/ml; urinary NA 1059.5 μg/24 h, n.v. < 85.5 μg/24 h; urinary metanephrine 489 μg/24 h, n.v. < 320 μg/24 h; plasma adrenaline (A) 100 pg/ml, n.v. 20-190 pg/ml; urinary A 15 μg/24 h, n.v. 1.7-22.4 μg/24 h]. The patient reported no typical paroxysmal symptoms of catecholamine excess. Echocardiographic evaluation showed slight left atrial and ventricular enlargement, mild to moderate mitral regurgitation, and preserved systolic function (ejection fraction 65%).

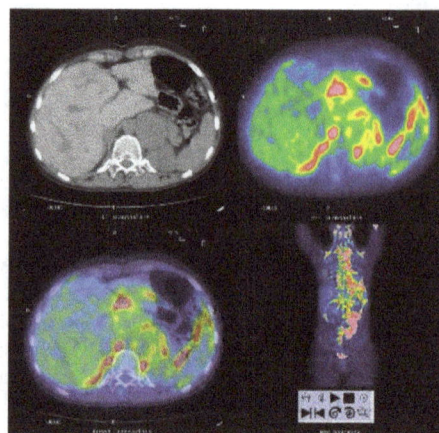

FIGURE 3: **Body 18F-fluorodeoxyglucose positron emission tomography scan**: no significant metabolic activity in the adrenal mass but intense uptake in supra- and subdiaphragmatic brown adipose tissue.

The diagnosis of pheochromocytoma was confirmed by 123I-metaiodobenzylguanidine (123I-MIBG) scintigraphy showing abnormal accumulation of radioactive tracer in the left adrenal gland. A 18F-fluorodeoxyglucose positron emission tomography (18F-FDG-PET) performed in order to exclude any extra-adrenal uptake: no significant metabolic activity in the adrenal mass but intense uptake in supra- and subdiaphragmatic brown adipose tissue was detected, likely due to noradrenergic-stimulated glucose uptake (Figure 3).

The patient underwent open left adrenalectomy after preconditioning with α-blockers (doxazosin) and, then, β-blockers (bisoprolol). Postoperative course was complicated by anemia due to hematoma formation in the left hypochondrium. Histopathological examination confirmed the diagnosis of pheochromocytoma with large hemorrhagic areas and scarce necrosis. No capsular or lymphovascular invasion was found. Immunohistochemistry revealed diffuse expression of chromogranin A, synaptophysin and neuron specific enolase, and S100 staining in sustentacular cells; Ki-67 was <5%. The P-PGL susceptibility genes VHL, RET, SDHA,

SDHAF2, SDHB, SDHC, SDHD, MAX, and TMEM127 were analyzed for germline mutations and large deletions, via direct sequencing and multiplex ligation-dependent probe amplification methods; RET was only analyzed by direct sequencing. No aberration was found in these genes. Twelve months after surgery patient's BP and heart rate were under control and urinary NA and metanephrine levels were within the normal range. Plasma NA levels remained slightly increased (715 pg/ml n.v. 70-480), consistent with the hemodynamic changes in Fontan circulation [7].

3. Discussion

We present a case of pheochromocytoma in a young patient affected with congenital tricuspid atresia treated by Fontan surgery. Several cases of cooccurrence of pheochromocytoma and CCHD have been described in the literature [5]. It has been hypothesized that chronic hypoxia plays a fundamental role in these cases. In the last decades much evidence has been gathered supporting the role of hypoxia in P-PGL tumorigenesis. In 1973 Saldana et al. [8] documented a higher prevalence of carotid body paraganglioma in Peruvian adults living at high altitude in the Andes compared with those living at sea level, suggesting a link with chronic hypoxia. Glomus cells of the carotid body, such as chromaffin cells of fetal adrenal medulla, are specialized in sensing local oxygen tension in mammals [9] and can undergo anatomical changes if exposed to chronic hypoxia [10]. The hypoxia hypothesis has subsequently been supported since the 2000s by the discovery of the molecular basis of hereditary P-PGL. In fact a number of genes implicated in P-PGL syndromes, including succinate dehydrogenase (SDHx), von Hippel-Lindau (VHL), and hypoxia induced-factor 2A (HIF2A) genes, cluster in a common molecular pathway leading to the abnormal activation and stabilization of hypoxia-inducible factors (HIFs) in normoxic condition. This dysregulated accumulation of HIFs induces a number of downstream genes involved in angiogenesis, tumor growth, apoptosis, and energy metabolism. These findings have led to the hypothesis that chronic exposure to hypoxia in CCHD patients may increase the risk of developing P-PGL. In a recent letter to editor of New England Journal of Medicine Vaidya and colleagues report the identification of gain-of-function somatic mutations of EPAS1, which encodes for HIF-2α, in pheochromocytomas and paragangliomas in four of five patients who presented with cyanotic congenital heart disease. The authors concluded that the EPAS1 mutations endow chromaffin cells exposed to chronic hypoxia amplified the ability of development of the oncogenic properties of HIF-2α [11].

Opotowky et al. [12] showed that patients with CCHD have a greater risk of developing P-PGL [(odds ratio (OR) 6.0] whereas the OR in those with non-cyanotic CHD did not differ from that seen in patients without CHD. The same authors also pointed out that pheochromocytomas in CCHD patients share a number of clinical and biochemical features with pseudohypoxic PPGL syndromes, such as young age of onset, multiple tumors, and noradrenergic phenotype, suggesting a common pathogenetic molecular pathway. Unfortunately, in this case report, a complete assessment of all currently known genes involved in P-PGL syndrome has not been performed.

This case displays an exclusive noradrenergic phenotype and a young age of onset, suggestive of pseudohypoxic pheochromocytoma-paraganglioma syndromes [4]. The patient, although treated immediately after birth, had sustained prolonged cyanotic episodes in her life. Therefore, in the light of the above, the cooccurrence of CCHD (as well as in other numerous case of congenital heart defects that can cause cyanosis) and P-PGL in this patient could be explained by exposure to chronic hypoxia. This hypothesis was further supported by the absence of specific genetic background, often detectable in P-PGL young patients.

In conclusion, the combination of cyanotic congenital heart disease with P-PGL is uncommon but clinically relevant. The diagnosis of pheochromocytoma can be difficult in this clinical setting, as catecholamine excess symptoms (palpitations, arrhythmias, fatigue, dyspnea, and orthostatic hypotension) overlap with CCHD complications. Clinicians should consider P-PGL as a possible and potentially curable cause of otherwise unexplained clinical deterioration (in this case a slight hypertensive crisis and worsening dyspnea) in CCHD patients, even in the absence of typical paroxysmal symptoms.

References

[1] J. I. E. Hoffman and S. Kaplan, "The incidence of congenital heart disease," *Journal of the American College of Cardiology*, vol. 39, no. 12, pp. 1890–1900, 2002.

[2] V. Thakran and A. Gupta, "Cyanosis in a patient with atrial septal defect," *Journal of the Practice of Cardiovascular Sciences*, vol. 1, no. 1, pp. 74-75, 2015.

[3] F. Mantero, M. Terzolo, G. Arnaldi et al., "A survey on adrenal incidentaloma in Italy," *The Journal of Clinical Endocrinology & Metabolism*, vol. 85, no. 2, pp. 637–644, 2000.

[4] H. Q. Rana, I. R. Rainville, and A. Vaidya, "Genetic testing in the clinical care of patients with pheochromocytoma and paraganglioma," *Current Opinion in Endocrinology, Diabetes and Obesity*, vol. 21, no. 3, pp. 166–176, 2014.

[5] T. Kim, H. K. Yang, H. Jang, S. Yoo, K. Khalili, and T. K. Kim, "Abdominal imaging findings in adult patients with Fontan circulation," *Insights into Imaging*, vol. 9, no. 3, pp. 357–367, 2018.

[6] M. K. Song, G. B. Kim, E. J. Bae et al., "Pheochromocytoma and paraganglioma in Fontan patients: Common more than expected," *Congenital Heart Disease*, vol. 13, no. 4, pp. 608–616, 2018.

[7] A. P. Bolger, R. Sharma, W. Li et al., "Neurohormonal activation and the chronic heart failure syndrome in adults with congenital heart disease," *Circulation*, vol. 106, no. 1, pp. 92–99, 2002.

[8] M. J. Saldana, L. E. Salem, and R. Travezan, "High altitude hypoxia and chemodectomas," *Human Pathology*, vol. 4, no. 2, pp. 251–263, 1973.

[9] J. Favier and A.-P. Gimenez-Roqueplo, "Pheochromocytomas: the (pseudo)-hypoxia hypothesis," *Best Practice & Research Clinical Endocrinology & Metabolism*, vol. 24, no. 6, pp. 957–968, 2010.

[10] J. Arias-Stella, "Human carotid body at high altitudes," *American Journal of Pathology*, vol. 55, p. 82a, 1969.

Coexistence of GH-Producing Pituitary Macroadenoma and Meningioma in a Patient with Multiple Endocrine Neoplasia Type 1 with Hyperglycemia and Ketosis as First Clinical Sign

A. Herrero-Ruiz,[1,2] **H. S. Villanueva-Alvarado,**[1] **J. J. Corrales-Hernández,**[1,2,3]
C. Higueruela-Mínguez,[1] **J. Feito-Pérez,**[4] **and J. M. Recio-Cordova**[1,2]

[1]*Service of Endocrinology and Nutrition, University Clinical Hospital of Salamanca, Paseo de San Vicente No. 58, 37007 Salamanca, Spain*
[2]*Department of Medicine, University of Salamanca, Campus Miguel de Unamuno, s/n, 37007 Salamanca, Spain*
[3]*Cancer Research Institute (IBMCC-CSIC/USAL) and Institute for Biomedical Research, University of Salamanca, Salamanca, Spain*
[4]*Service of Anatomic Pathology, University Clinical Hospital of Salamanca, Paseo de San Vicente No. 58, 37007 Salamanca, Spain*

Correspondence should be addressed to A. Herrero-Ruiz; aherreror@saludcastillayleon.es

Academic Editor: Lucy Mastrandrea

We present the clinical case of a patient who was admitted with an onset of diabetes mellitus (DM) with associated ketosis and whose clinical, hormonal, and radiological evolution revealed the presence of primary hyperparathyroidism, pancreatic neuroendocrine tumor, and GH-producing pituitary macroadenoma in the context of multiple endocrine neoplasia type 1 (MEN1). DM is relatively common in cases of acromegaly, but it is not generally associated with ketosis. Simultaneously, the patient presented a meningioma, which is associated with pituitary macroadenoma only in extremely rare cases.

1. Introduction

Multiple endocrine neoplasia type 1 (MEN1) is an autosomal dominant syndrome characterized by the combined appearance of tumors in the parathyroid glands, pancreas islet cells, and the anterior pituitary. This type of syndromes is known to be associated with the secretion of a wide range of hormones which are often responsible for alterations in the glucose metabolism. However, the presence of diabetic ketosis and/or ketoacidosis is a rare clinical situation, with very few cases reported so far. Also, and in an even less common case, the patient simultaneously presented a GH-producing pituitary macroadenoma and a meningioma, a combination which is extremely rare.

2. Case Report

We present the clinical case of a 35-year-old woman with a history of Chagas disease who was admitted in the Unit of Endocrinology with hyperglycemia and ketosis in the context of onset of DM with weakness, polydipsia, and polyuria of 4 months of evolution, together with a weight loss of 10 kg over the last 6 months. Also, she presented amenorrhea for 4 months and hyperhidrosis. The examination revealed a slight prognathism, growth of acral parts of the body, and grade 1 goiter with a 2-cm left thyroid nodule.

The analysis showed glucose 248 mg/dL, HbA1c 14.6%, calcium 11.3 mg/dL, phosphorus 2.3 mg/dL, and urine calcium 513 mg/24 h. Given the initial findings, the study was expanded to include a hormone profile test (Table 1), a thyroid ultrasound (28 × 16-mm mixed nodule in the left lobe and 1.2 × 0.9 cm hypoechoic nodule in the right infrathyroid region, which suggests an enlarged parathyroid gland), and an ultrasound-guided fine-needle aspiration (UGFNA) of the left thyroid nodule compatible with benign follicular nodule.

The endocrine study confirmed the clinical suspicion of primary hyperparathyroidism and GH hypersecretion. The parathyroid SPECT/CT was compatible with right

TABLE 1: Hormone measurements in plasma.

Hormone	Value	Normal range
TSH (μUI/mL)	4.7	0.27–4.2
Free T4 (ng/dL)	1.1	0.82–1.78
FSH (mUI/mL)	3.3	3.5–12.5
LH (mUI/mL)	1.9	2.4–12.6
Estradiol (pg/mL)	<5	12.5–166
Prolactin (ng/mL)	59.2	4.79–23.3
GH (ng/mL)	48.1	0–8
IGF1 (ng/mL)	702	109–284
Cortisol (μg/dL)	10.5	2.69–18
PTH (pg/mL)	203.4	11–67

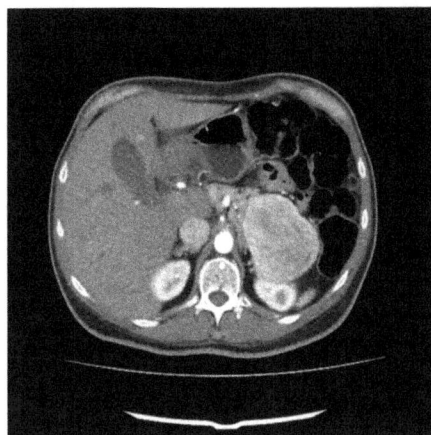

FIGURE 2: (CT) tail of pancreas with hypervascular heterogeneous and well-defined mass with lobulated edges measuring 6.8 × 7.7 × 6.4 cm.

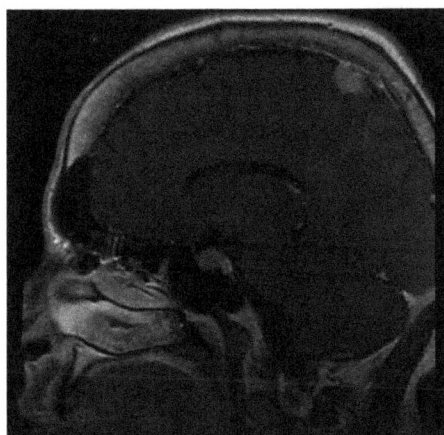

FIGURE 1: (NMR) pituitary macroadenoma and left superior parietal extra-axial lesion compatible with meningioma.

parathyroid adenoma. A nuclear magnetic resonance (NMR) revealed a pituitary macroadenoma of 20 × 13 × 15 mm which spread to the right cavernous sinus, with displacement of the optic chiasm, and a left superior extra-axial parietal lesion of 20 × 20 × 12 mm which suggested a meningioma (Figure 1).

Given these findings and the clinical suspicion of MEN1, the study was completed with a CT scan of the neck, chest, abdomen, and pelvis, which showed a hypervascular heterogeneous mass with lobulated and well-defined edges of 6.8 × 7.7 × 6.4 cm in the tail of pancreas, plus another mass of similar characteristics of 6 × 4.2 cm in the uncinate process and at least three more pancreatic focal lesions of less than 1 cm on the head and neck of pancreas (Figure 2). In the liver there were several hypervascular lesions in segments II and III, of 0.9 cm, compatible with metastatic involvement. Tumor markers revealed increased levels of somatostatin (30.9 pmol/L), pancreatic polypeptide (>200 pmol/L), and calcitonin (9.6 pg/mL), with normal levels of chromogranin A, gastrin, glucagon, and vasoactive intestinal polypeptide.

A somatostatin receptor scintigraphy (OctreoScan) was performed showing a pathological deposit in the tail of pancreas which suggested a tumor with expression of somatostatin receptors and also at the upper left parietal level, which was caused by a meningioma (Figure 3). The endoscopic ultrasound-guided fine-needle aspiration biopsy of the mass in the pancreas was compatible with a neuroendocrine tumor (NET). A genetic study confirmed the clinical suspicion of MEN1. The patient was a heterozygous carrier of the pathogenic change c.1378C>T (p. Arg460*).

The patient started treatment with high doses of basal-bolus insulin therapy, somatostatin analogs, and cinacalcet. Afterwards, cabergoline was added due to the persistence of high levels of IGF1. The pituitary macroadenoma was resected through a transnasal transsphenoidal and the IGF1 levels went back to normal, with octreotide treatment. The anatomic pathology revealed a pituitary somatotroph adenoma (densely granulated) and the immunohistochemical study: CAM 5.2 (+++), GH (+++), p53 (−), and MIB-1 <1%. An abdominal NMR was performed to control the evolution of her condition, and it still showed two heterogeneous lesions on the head and tail of pancreas, of 5.5 × 4.5 × 4 cm and 6 × 7.5 × 8 cm, respectively, contrast-enhanced and with well-defined edges. Also, the liver had normal size, morphology, and intensity, and the image did not reveal the lesions described in the CT scan image.

After an assessment by an interdisciplinary board, the patient underwent total pancreaticoduodenectomy, cholecystectomy, and splenectomy. The anatomical pathology showed 7 well-differentiated (G1) NETs in the pancreas, 1 well-differentiated NET (G1) in the pylorus of <0.5 cm, 14 lymph nodes in the tail of pancreas with no sign of malignancy, and 2 lymph nodes with NET metastasis out of 12 isolated nodes on the head of pancreas (pT2N1). All the tumors expressed chromogranin A and synaptophysin, with proliferation mediated by Ki67 <1%, except for the node found in the neck of pancreas, in which it reached 2-3%. Also, 2 out of the 7 tumors were intensely positive for glucagon (100%) (Figure 4), and an additional node in the body of pancreas was positive for calcitonin (70%), with positive isolated cells for glucagon and somatostatin (<2%).

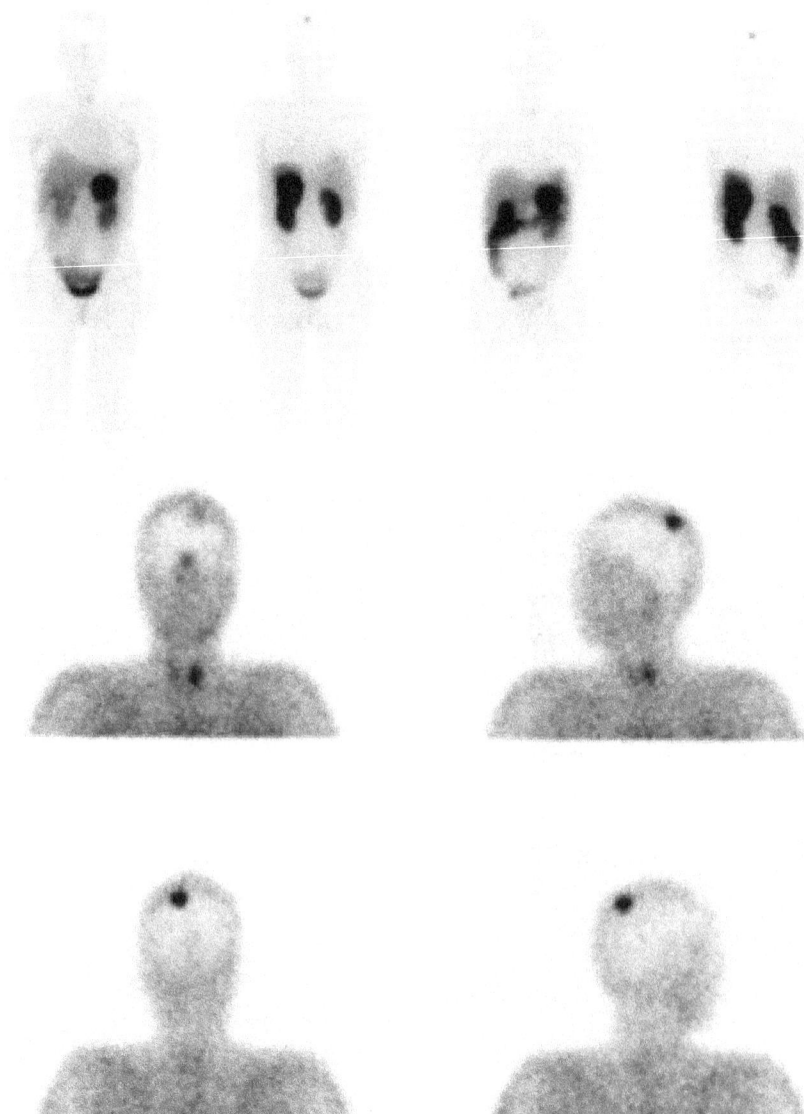

FIGURE 3: OctreoScan showing a pathological deposit at the upper left parietal level caused by meningioma and in the tail of pancreas.

3. Discussion

We present the case of a patient with MEN1 with some peculiar features.

(1) DM with ketosis as its first manifestation: alterations in the metabolism of glucose are a common characteristic in acromegaly, with a described prevalence of DM ranging from 19 to 56% [1–3]. However, these alterations are generally due to the insulin resistance caused by an excess of GH and IGF1, with an increase of gluconeogenesis and a decrease of peripheral glucose uptake [4, 5], and it typically does not show a tendency to ketosis, with only 11 cases of ketoacidosis having been described as the first sign of acromegaly [4]. Some authors have analyzed the factors which may predispose to alterations in the glucose metabolism of these patients, and they are related to the levels of IGF1 [1], GH [6], age, body mass index, arterial hypertension, and time of evolution of the disease [2, 3, 6]. In our case, hyperprolactinemia, due

to the compression of the pituitary stalk, may have also contributed to the alteration in glucose metabolism through an increase in insulin resistance. Some of the mechanisms suggested to explain this include a decrease in insulin receptors and/or deficiencies at a postreceptor level [4]. McCallum et al. identified an increased prevalence of diabetes and glucose intolerance in patients with MEN1, and several theories have been put forward in which adiponectin and enteropancreatic markers might be involved, or the MEN1 gene, which may cause a predisposition to this resistance [7]. On the other hand, primary hyperparathyroidism has also been associated with an increase in insulin resistance and DM [7]. Therefore, there are several underlying mechanisms which may have contributed to the atypical clinical presentation of our patient.

(2) Another peculiar trait in our case is the concomitant presence of a pituitary tumor and meningioma, because this is a rare clinical situation, with only 33 cases described [8, 9].

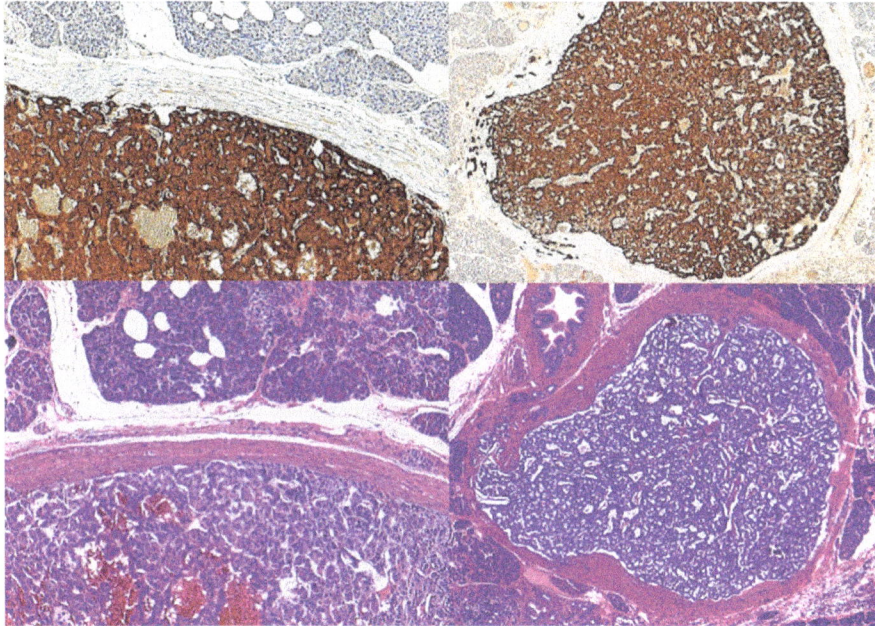

FIGURE 4: Immunohistochemistry with positive cells for glucagon.

Meningiomas represent 15–25% of all intracranial neoplasms, with an annual incidence of 6 per 100.000 people [8–11]. Radiotherapy is known to play a role in the appearance of intracranial tumors, but in cases such as ours, without prior exposition to radiotherapy, the origin is still unclear. Some authors suggest that it may happen by sheer chance, whereas others describe theories that may explain this association [8, 10]. Suzuki et al. suggest an involvement of the activation of signaling pathways for the receptor tyrosine kinases [12], and Friend et al. showed that meningioma may express GH and IGF1 receptors [13]. Although there are cases described in the literature of an association of meningioma with functioning and nonfunctioning pituitary adenomas, in the case of functioning adenomas, GH-producing varieties seem to predominate [9, 10, 14]. It remains to be seen whether GH itself or an overexpression of IGF1 receptors in these tumors induces a transformation into a meningioma. On the other hand, Asgharian et al. proved in a prospective study of 74 patients with MEN1 that 8% of the patients developed meningioma after 18 years of follow-up, and it is believed that the alterations in the MEN1 gene may have participated in its pathogenesis [15].

Authors' Contributions

Dr. Herrero-Ruiz collected data, analyzed all patient data, wrote the final paper, and intervened in the care of the patient; Dr. Villanueva-Alvarado collected data, analyzed all patient data, wrote the first draft, and intervened in the care of the patient; Dr. Corrales-Hernández, Dr. Higueruela-Mínguez, and Dr. Feito-Pérez intervened in the care of the patient; Dr. Recio-Cordova intervened in the care and follow-up of the patient.

References

[1] O. Alexopoulou, M. Bex, P. Kamenicky, A. B. Mvoula, P. Chanson, and D. Maiter, "Prevalence and risk factors of impaired glucose tolerance and diabetes mellitus at diagnosis of acromegaly: A study in 148 patients," *The Pituitary Society*, vol. 17, no. 1, pp. 81–89, 2014.

[2] E. Resmini, F. Minuto, A. Colao, and D. Ferone, "Secondary diabetes associated with principal endocrinopathies: the impact of new treatment modalities," *Acta Diabetologica*, vol. 46, no. 2, pp. 85–95, 2009.

[3] S. Fieffe, I. Morange, P. Petrossians et al., "Diabetes in acromegaly, prevalence, risk factors, and evolution: data from the French Acromegaly Registry," *European Journal of Endocrinology*, vol. 164, no. 6, pp. 877–884, 2011.

[4] M. Carrasco de la Fuente, O. González-Albarrán, G. Pérez López, and M. Cano Megías, "Diabetic ketoacidosis as the first manifestation of a mixed growth hormone and prolactin-secreting tumor," *Endocrinología y Nutrición*, vol. 57, no. 10, pp. 507–509, 2010.

[5] C. Galesanu, C. Buzduga, A. Florescu, and L. Moisii, "Diabetes mellitus, chronic complication in patients with acromegaly: case report and review of the literature," *Rev Med Chir Soc Med Nat Iasi*, vol. 119, no. 1, pp. 92–96, 2015.

[6] J. D. N. Nabarro, "Acromegaly," *Clinical Endocrinology (Oxf)*, vol. 26, no. 4, pp. 481–512, 1987.

[7] R. W. McCallum, V. Parameswaran, and J. R. Burgess, "Multiple endocrine neoplasia type 1 (MEN 1) is associated with an increased prevalence of diabetes mellitus and impaired fasting glucose," *Clinical Endocrinology*, vol. 65, no. 2, pp. 163–168, 2006.

[8] D. Moncet and G. B. Isaac, "Simultaneous association of pituitary adenoma and meningioma: report of three cases," *Revista Argentina de Endocrinología y Metabolismo*, vol. 52, pp. 29–34, 2015.

[9] F. Ruiz-Juretschke, B. Iza, E. Scola-Pliego, D. Poletti, and E. Salinero, "Coincidental pituitary adenoma and planum sphenoidale meningioma mimicking a single tumor," *Endocrinología y Nutrición*, vol. 62, no. 6, pp. 292–294, 2015.

[10] S. Mortazavi, A. Shirani M, S. Saeedinia, R. Sanjari, H. Hanif, and A. Amirjamshidi, "Coexisting pituitary adenoma and suprasellar meningioma: a coincidence or causation effect? report of two cases and review of literature," *IrJNS*, vol. 1, 43, no. 1, p. 46.

[11] L. Curto, S. Squadrito, B. Almoto et al., "MRI finding of simultaneous coexistence of growth hormone-secreting pituitary adenoma with intracranial meningioma and carotid artery aneurysms: report of a case," *The Pituitary Society*, vol. 10, no. 3, pp. 299–305, 2007.

[12] K. Suzuki, H. Momota, A. Tonooka et al., "Glioblastoma simultaneously present with adjacent meningioma: Case report and review of the literature," *Journal of Neuro-Oncology*, vol. 99, no. 1, pp. 147–153, 2010.

[13] K. E. Friend, R. Radinsky, and I. E. McCutcheon, "Growth hormone receptor expression and function in meningiomas: Effect of a specific receptor antagonist," *Journal of Neurosurgery*, vol. 91, no. 1, pp. 93–99, 1999.

[14] S. Cannavò, L. Curtò, R. Fazio et al., "Coexistence of growth hormone-secreting pituitary adenoma and intracranial meningioma: A case report and review of the literature," *Journal of Endocrinological Investigation*, vol. 16, no. 9, pp. 703–708, 1993.

[15] B. Asgharian, Y.-J. Chen, N. J. Patronas et al., "Meningiomas May Be a Component Tumor of Multiple Endocrine Neoplasia Type 1," *Clinical Cancer Research*, vol. 10, no. 3, pp. 869–880, 2004.

4

Clinical Phenotype in a Toddler with a Novel Heterozygous Mutation of the Vitamin D Receptor

Preneet Cheema Brar,[1] Elena Dingle,[1] John Pappas,[2] and Manish Raisingani[1]

[1]Department of Pediatrics, Division of Pediatric Endocrinology and Diabetes, New York University School of Medicine, New York, NY, USA
[2]Department of Pediatrics, Clinical Genetics Services, New York University School of Medicine, New York, NY, USA

Correspondence should be addressed to Preneet Cheema Brar; preneet.brar@nyumc.org

Academic Editor: Mihail A. Boyanov

We present the clinical phenotype of a toddler who presented with vitamin D-resistant rickets, with one of the highest initial levels of alkaline phosphatase and parathyroid hormone (PTH) levels reported in the literature. The toddler had novel compound heterozygous mutations in the ligand-binding site of the vitamin D receptor and had an excellent response to calcitriol (1,25(OH)2D).

1. Background

Hereditary vitamin D-resistant rickets (HVDRR) is an autosomal recessive disease caused by abnormality of the vitamin D receptor (VDR). Homozygous or compound heterozygous mutations of this gene result in the inability of VDR to regulate target genes even in the abundance of 1,25-dihydroxyvitamin D (1,25(OH)2D3) which results in compensatory hyperparathyroidism with hypocalcaemia, hypophosphatemia, and osteopenia [1, 2].

Though true prevalence is not well established, there are no gender differences in the incidence, with reported cases being in consanguineous families from the Mediterranean and Middle East regions [3, 4].

There are two main functional domains in the VDR protein: DNA-binding domain (DBD) and ligand-binding domain (LBD). Mutations in the DBD prevent the VDR from binding to vitamin D response elements (VDREs) in target genes causing absolute resistance to 1,25(OH)2D resulting in a more severe clinical phenotype. Mutations in the LBD prevent binding of VDR to 1,25(OH)2D or interfere with VDR signaling [5, 6]. Alopecia is a specific clinical manifestation of HVDRR and is usually associated with DBD mutations, though it is seen in some cases. In this report, we describe clinical manifestation of the two compound heterozygous mutations in the DBD and LBD domains, respectively.

2. Case Report

We present a 19-month-old Hispanic female toddler with poor interval growth. Though she was meeting her developmental milestones, her height and weight were below the third percentile with weight of 8.7 kg (<3%) and height of 75 cm (2%). She was a full-term, spontaneous vaginal delivery without complications during labor or pregnancy. She was the product of nonconsanguineous marriage. She was on no medications; there were no other siblings with failure to thrive. There was no history of malabsorptive conditions.

Her review of systems is negative for emesis, diarrhea, fever, appetite changes, swallowing abnormalities, respiratory symptoms, apnea, repeated acute illnesses, or frequent injuries. Her physical exam is significant for an alert, playful, developmentally appropriate child, small for her age. Her head/neck, cardiac, respiratory, gastrointestinal, genitourinary, musculoskeletal, and neurological exams were within normal limits. She had no evidence of dysmorphism and had no alopecia on exam. The laboratory testing at baseline included calcium of 7.6 mg/dl (8–10.4), alkaline phosphatase

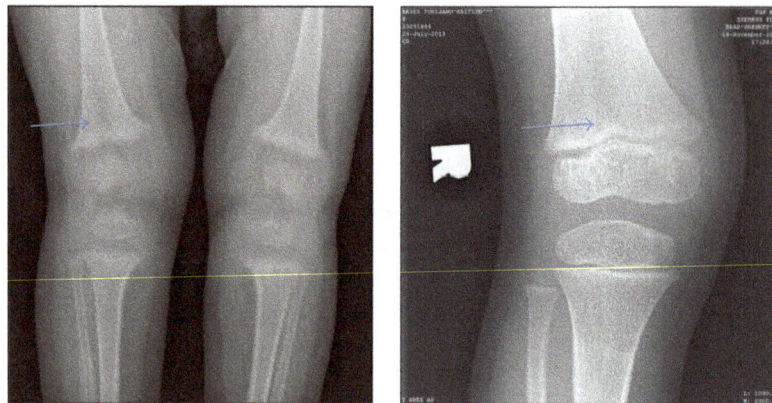

(a) Radiograph of the knees at initial presentation. AP radiograph of both knees. There is widening of the physes above the knee with splaying and fraying of the metaphyses. No fracture or dislocation is seen. Bones appear demineralized. Impression: findings compatible with rickets. The blue arrow points at the fraying at the end of the bones

(b) Radiograph of the knee after RX at the age of 3 years. AP radiograph of the right knee. Healed rickets. Bones appear demineralized. No fractures or dislocation is seen. The blue arrow points at the fraying at the end of the bones

FIGURE 1

of 2023 IU/L (25–100 adult reference in our lab, with 80% bone isoenzyme), PTH of 1115 pg/ml (14–72), phosphorus of 2.9 mg/dl (2.7–4.5), 25-OH vitamin D3 of 14.2 ng/ml (30–100), and 1,25(OH)2 vitamin D3 of 505 pg/ml (19–79). The skeletal survey: Figure 1(a) shows metaphyseal fraying and cupping of the distal femur, proximal tibia, and fibula consistent with rickets. Figure 1(b) shows healing rickets. The toddler was started on 4000 IU of ergocalciferol daily and 3 ml of calcium glubionate TID (200 mg/day; 23 mg/kg/day). 10 days later, her calcium went down to 7.3, and she received IV calcium (6 ml q6h, 64 mg/kg/day). Her calcium normalized within 48 hours and she was continued on 64 mg/kg/day of oral calcium and ergocalciferol dose of 2000 IU daily. Her calcium level was fluctuating between 7.7 and 8.3 (Table 1). At 21.5 months of age, she was started on calcitriol 0.5 mcg BID as we suspected resistant rickets. Calcitriol was gradually increased up to the current dose of 8 mcg BID. Her PTH and alkaline phosphatase were gradually trending down (Table 1). After 6 months of treatment on 8 mcg BID of calcitriol and 150–200 mg/day of elemental calcium, she had a PTH of 300 pg/ml and calcium of 8.7 mg/dl and had early radiological signs of healing rickets and clinical improvement in gait. Calcium treatment was finally stopped at 29 months of age with healing of rickets (Table 1).

3. Genetic Analysis

Genomic DNA was isolated from peripheral blood samples of the patient. The VDR gene was amplified by polymerase chain reaction (PCR) and all exons of the coding region of the VDR gene were directly sequenced at the Baylor Miraca Genetics Laboratories. Direct sequence analysis of PCR products was performed in both forward and reverse directions using automated fluorescence dideoxy sequencing methods. There

were two compound heterozygous mutations found in this patient. One of them was a heterogenous missense mutation of Arg274 (Arg274His) in exon 9 which changed the codon for arginine to histidine at amino acid 274. The second mutation was a heterogenous missense mutation of Arg73 (Arg73Glu) in exon 5 which changed the codon for arginine to glutamine at amino acid 73. The sequence analysis also identified benign sequence variants: homozygous c.2T>C (p.M1T) polymorphism in exon 4 and c.1056T>C (p.I352I) variant in exon 11. Both parents were asymptomatic though parental analysis of the VDR sequence will be performed.

4. Discussion

Our toddler had a remarkable response to calcitriol, despite having one of the highest initial PTH (1115.4 pg/ml) and alkaline phosphatase (2023 IU/L) levels reported. Sequence analysis of the toddler's DNA revealed two compound heterozygous mutations in the VDR gene.

The clinical severity in case of LBD mutations depends on the affinity of VDR and varies from reduced affinity to 1,25(OH)2D3 to a total absence of binding to 1,25(OH)2D3. Amino acids 123–427 constitute the VDR LBD with R274 being the ligand-binding site located in helix H5 that makes contact with the 1α-hydroxyl group of 1,25(OH)2D3 [7]. Mutant R274H is similar to mutant R274L and is characterized by 100-fold less responsiveness to 1,25(OH)2D3 compared to the wild-type VDR [3, 4]. All previously reported patients with R274H and R274L were from Middle Eastern countries. Later, two case presentations of the homozygous mutant R274H were reported by Aljubeh et al. [4]. The clinical manifestation of these two patients with HVDRR was much more severe compared to our toddler. Both patients developed respiratory complications with one of them requiring

TABLE 1: Metabolic parameters on diagnosis and during RX.

Time after diagnosis (weeks)	Calcium (mg/dl)	Alkaline phosphatase (IU/L)	25-OH vitamin D2 (ng/ml)	1,25(OH) vitamin D3 (pg/ml)	PTH (pg/ml)	Calcium/creatinine ratio (urine)
Baseline	7.6	2023	14	505	1115	0.15
2 weeks	7.3	1579	31	901	764	0.06
1 month	7.8	1708	20	784	924	0.31
1.5 months	7.7	1879	44	1165	866	0.29
2 months	7.9	1579	36	901	901	ND
3 months	7.9	1686	40	959	959	0.12
4 months	8.8	1343	44	2064	437	0.17
5 months	8.2	848	41	1300	536	0.3
8 months	8.7	705	33	>600	300	ND
10 months	9.5	662	36	>600	147	ND
12 months	9.5	441	58	>600	210	ND
16 months	9.4	287	45	>600	76	0.06
21 months	9.7	180	43	>600	35	0.06

Metabolic parameters (reference values): calcium = 8–10.4 mg/dl; alkaline phosphatase = 25–100 IU/L (adult reference in our lab, with 80% bone isoenzyme); PTH = 14–72 pg/ml; 25-OH vitamin D2 = 30–100 ng/ml; 1,25(OH) vitamin D3 = 19–79 pg/ml. ND: not done.

oxygen supplementation. The first patient was initially started on oral calcium at the dose of 500–600 mg/kg/day with a poor response. Both of them required high doses of IV calcium infusions (90–200 mg/kg/day) for at least three months. Our toddler had a heterozygous mutation of R274H which could explain her less severe presentation, although she had 10 times higher level of PTH and two times higher level of alkaline phosphatase compared to the two cases reported by Aljubeh et al. [4]

Our case has compound heterozygosity for the Arg274His and the Arg73Glu. The residue Arg73 is located at the tip of the second zinc finger of the intracellular vitamin D receptor and it is conserved in evolution. Hughes et al. (1988) reported on two sisters from consanguineous heterozygous and asymptomatic parents of a black Haitian origin. The described mutation resulted in an Arg70Gly substitution and a decreased affinity for DNA. The reported mutation is actually Arg73Gln (R73Q) based on corrected sequencing. In the functional cDNA analysis, Hughes et al. found decreased affinity of the expressed VDR mutant to 1,25(OH)2D3. Arginine at this position is critical for the interaction of receptor with DNA. The toddler in our case report had a compound heterozygous mutation that could explain her mild symptoms of HVDRR.

The cornerstone of treatment in HDVRR is to overcome the absent or reduced affinity of the ligand 1,25(OH)2D3 for the VDR using available formulations of 1,25(OH)2D3. In the previous report by Aljubeh et al., the dose of calcitriol was 10–15 mcg/day [4] in addition to 150–600 mg/kg/day of IV elemental calcium. Our patient has sustained normal serum calcium on much higher calcitriol treatment (24 mcg/day) without the need for oral elemental calcium. As long as the urine is being monitored for hypercalciuria, normalization of the PTH is the mainstay of treatment. Healing of the rickets has been observed in some children with discontinuation of

all therapy. This resolution of HDVRR may be the result of VDR-independent pathways of calcium absorption in the gut combined with effects of estrogens during puberty through upregulation of calcium transport protein 1 channels (CaT1) [8].

5. Conclusion

Our case illustrates compound heterozygous mutations in the VDR both in the hormone-binding and in the nuclear-binding site with a less severe presentation of rickets and a quick response to treatment with calcitriol and a short-term calcium requirement, despite having one of the highest initial PTH and alkaline phosphatase levels reported.

References

[1] P. J. Malloy, J. W. Pike, and D. Feldman, "The vitamin D receptor and the syndrome of hereditary 1,25-dihydroxyvitamin D-resistant rickets," Endocrine Reviews, vol. 20, no. 2, pp. 156–188, 1999.

[2] D. Feldman and P. J Malloy, "Mutations in the vitamin D receptor and hereditary vitamin D-resistant," BoneKEy Reports, vol. 3, 2014.

[3] K. Kristjansson, A. R. Rut, M. Hewison, J. L. H. O'Riordan, and M. R. Hughes, "Two mutations in the hormone binding domain of the vitamin D receptor cause tissue resistance to 1,25 dihydroxyvitamin D3," Journal of Clinical Investigation, vol. 92, no. 1, pp. 12–16, 1993.

[4] J. M. Aljubeh, J. Wang, S. S. Al-Remeithi, P. J. Malloy, and D. Feldman, "Report of two unrelated patients with hereditary vitamin D resistant rickets due to the same novel mutation in the vitamin D receptor," *Journal of Pediatric Endocrinology and Metabolism*, vol. 24, no. 9-10, pp. 793–799, 2011.

[5] N. S. Ma, P. J. Malloy, P. Pitukcheewanont, D. Dreimane, M. E. Geffner, and D. Feldman, "Hereditary vitamin D resistant rickets: Identification of a novel splice site mutation in the vitamin D receptor gene and successful treatment with oral calcium therapy," *Bone*, vol. 45, no. 4, pp. 743–746, 2009.

[6] P. J. Malloy and D. Feldman, "Molecular defects in the vitamin D receptor associated with hereditary 1,25-dihydroxyvitamin D resistant rickets," in *Vitamin D: Physiology, Molecular Biology, and Clinical Applications*, M. F. Holick, Ed., pp. 691–714, Humana Press, NJ, USA, 2010.

[7] N. Rochel, J. M. Wurtz, A. Mitschler, B. Klaholz, and D. Moras, "The crystal structure of the nuclear receptor for vitamin D bound to its natural ligand," *Molecular Cell*, vol. 5, no. 1, pp. 173–179, 2000.

[8] S. J. Van Cromphaut, K. Rummens, I. Stockmans et al., "Intestinal Calcium Transporter Genes Are Upregulated by Estrogens and the Reproductive Cycle Through Vitamin D Receptor-Independent Mechanisms," *Journal of Bone and Mineral Research*, vol. 18, no. 10, pp. 1725–1736, 2003.

5

Coexistence of Primary Hyperaldosteronism and Graves' Disease, a Rare Combination of Endocrine Disorders: Is It beyond a Coincidence —A Case Report and Review of the Literature

S. S. C. Gunatilake and U. Bulugahapitiya

Department of Endocrinology, Colombo South Teaching Hospital, Kalubowila, Sri Lanka

Correspondence should be addressed to S. S. C. Gunatilake; sonaligunatilake@gmail.com

Academic Editor: Toshihiro Kita

Background. Primary hyperaldosteronism is a known cause for secondary hypertension. In addition to its effect on blood pressure, aldosterone exhibits proinflammatory actions and plays a role in immunomodulation/development of autoimmunity. Recent researches also suggest significant thyroid dysfunction among patients with hyperaldosteronism, but exact causal relationship is not established. Autoimmune hyperthyroidism (Graves' disease) and primary hyperaldosteronism rarely coexist but underlying mechanisms associating the two are still unclear. *Case Presentation.* A 32-year-old Sri Lankan female was evaluated for new onset hypertension in association with hypokalemia. She also had features of hyperthyroidism together with high TSH receptor antibodies suggestive of Graves' disease. On evaluation of persistent hypokalemia and hypertension, primary hyperaldosteronism due to right-sided adrenal adenoma was diagnosed. She was rendered euthyroid with antithyroid drugs followed by right-sided adrenalectomy. Antithyroid drugs were continued up to 12 months, after which the patient entered remission of Graves' disease. *Conclusion.* Autoimmune hyperthyroidism and primary hyperaldosteronism rarely coexist and this case report adds to the limited number of cases documented in the literature. Underlying mechanism associating the two is still unclear but possibilities of autoimmune mechanisms and autoantibodies warrant further evaluation and research.

1. Background

Primary hyperaldosteronism (PA) is a leading endocrine cause for secondary hypertension, particularly in resistant hypertension [1, 2]. In addition to the hypertensive effect by aldosterone, it also exhibits proinflammatory actions on different organ systems, particularly cardiovascular system [3, 4]. Recent studies have demonstrated role of aldosterone on immunomodulation together with its effects on adaptive immune system, suggesting the possible link with development of autoimmune disorders [5]. Graves' disease is an autoimmune disease involving the thyroid gland resulting in thyrotoxicosis secondary to thyroid receptor autoantibodies. It accounts for up to 60–80% of all causes of thyrotoxicosis worldwide [6, 7]. There is a paucity of literature detailing any association between PA and Graves' disease. We report a

case of PA due to adrenocortical adenoma (Conn's syndrome) coexisting with Graves' disease in the same patient and review the available literature in view of identifying possible associations.

2. Case Presentation

A 32-year-old Sri Lankan female was referred to endocrine unit for further evaluation and management of hypertension and hypokalemia.

She was diagnosed to have hypertension while evaluating for persistent headache 4 months before. She was on three antihypertensive medications at the time of presentation but had poor blood pressure control. She also had non-specific body aches and intermittent muscle cramps for the past 2 months following which a biochemical evaluation

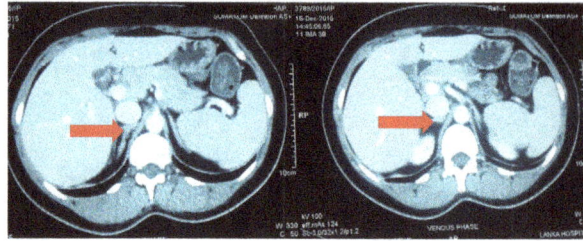

FIGURE 1: Contrast enhanced CT abdomen showing right-sided adrenal adenoma (red arrow).

revealed persistent hypokalemia. She also had palpitation and sweating with associated heat intolerance, recent weight loss, and increased bowel openings. She did not have any virilizing features. She was not on diuretics or any long-term medications except three antihypertensive medications. None of her immediate family members had hypertension, strokes, or sudden deaths at younger age.

On examination, she was averagely built with a BMI of $23 \, kg/m^2$. There was a small diffusely enlarged goiter (grade II) without any tenderness. A bruit was audible over the goiter and no cervical lymphadenopathy was detected. Her eyes were normal including eye movements and vision. There were fine tremors in the fingers with sweaty palms. No characteristic features of Cushing's syndrome were identified. Peripheral pulses were normal without a radio femoral delay. Her pulse rate was 110 beats/minute and blood pressure was 140/100 mmHg while on antihypertensive therapy, without a postural drop. There was no cardiomegaly or any murmurs. Abdominal examination revealed no ballotable masses or renal bruits.

Investigations revealed serum potassium, 2.1 mmol/L (3.5–5); spot urinary K, 46 mmol/L (normal < 20); and an arterial pH, 7.48 with bicarbonate of 28 mEq/L. Her serum magnesium level was 1.6 mg/dL (1.7–2.2 mg/dL). In the background of unremarkable physical findings in a patient with hypertension, hypokalemia, high urine potassium excretion, and metabolic alkalosis, possibility of primary hyperaldosteronism was considered. Aldosterone : renin ratio (ARR) was measured after correcting the potassium value and adjusting the interfering medications. Plasma renin activity was 0.15 ng/mL/hr (1.31–3.95) with serum aldosterone 20.6 ng/dL (1–16). ARR was 137 [ng/dL]/[ng/ml/hr] (<20) which is very high, suggesting PA. Intravenous saline infusion test as the test for confirmation of PA revealed basal plasma aldosterone level, 14.30 ng/dL, and postsaline loaded aldosterone level, 13.80 ng/dL (<10). Nonsuppressed aldosterone levels confirmed PA. A contrast enhanced computed tomography (CT) of abdomen according to the adrenal protocol showed a right-sided homogenously dense (density of 9.5 Hounsfield Units {HU}) adrenal lesion measuring 1.6 × 1.3 × 0.8 cm with an absolute washout of 67% confirming benign nature of the lipid rich adrenal adenoma (Figure 1).

Evaluation of the thyroid status revealed evidence of hyperthyroidism: TSH < 0.01 μIU/mL (0.27–4.0), free T4—4.60 ng/dL (0.7–1.9), and free T3—7.36 pg/mL (2–4.4). Ultrasound scan of the thyroid showed diffusely enlarged gland with increased echo pattern and vascularity on Doppler studies, compatible with Graves' disease. TSH receptor antibodies were positive (52 U/L).

Her renal function tests were normal. In addition, she had suppressed cortisol on overnight dexamethasone suppression test and normal 24-hour urinary vanillyl mandelic acid levels on two occasions.

Presence of hyperaldosteronism together with a right-sided adrenal adenoma was consistent with Conn's syndrome in this 32-year-old lady. In addition, there was evidence of coexisting Graves' thyrotoxicosis. Thyrotoxicosis was managed with antithyroid drugs (Carbimazole) according to the titration regimen and once patient rendered euthyroid while on carbimazole, laparoscopic right adrenalectomy was performed. Following the surgery, potassium was 4.4 mmol/l and blood pressure was 130/80 mmHg without medication. Postoperative aldosterone done 3 weeks after the surgery was normal (aldosterone, 4.40 ng/dL), confirming the correct diagnosis of aldosterone secreting adenoma and complete removal of the tumor. Histology revealed adrenocortical adenoma. Antithyroid medications were titrated and discontinued after 12 months following which patient achieved remission of Graves' disease.

3. Discussion and Review of Literature

Primary aldosteronism is now considered one of the common causes of secondary hypertension. Cross-sectional and prospective studies report PA in >5% and possibly >10% of hypertensive patients, both in general and in specialty settings [1, 2, 8, 9]. It is an important diagnosis as PA has higher cardiovascular morbidity and mortality than age- and sex-matched patients with essential hypertension with the same degree of blood pressure elevation [10]. These effects may be mediated at least in part by mineralocorticoid receptors in the heart and blood vessels which will enhance impaired endothelial function via reduced glucose 6-phosphate dehydrogenase activity [11, 12].

Aldosterone, in addition to its hypertensive effect, has shown to result in cardiovascular disease by promoting an inflammatory state that is enhanced by T cell immunity, thus establishing its role in the immune system. Aldosterone promotes inflammation characterized by vascular infiltration of immune cells, proinflammatory cytokine production (e.g., TNF α), and reactive oxidative stress. Further, it can promote $CD4^+$ T cell activation and Th17 polarization suggesting that it plays a role in the adaptive immune system and could contribute to the onset of autoimmunity [3–5, 13]. Herrada et al. had observed aldosterone enhancing the occurrence of autoimmune encephalomyelitis in mice studies, giving further proof. Molina-Garrido et al. had reported a case of primary hyperaldosteronism in whom vitiligo vulgaris and symptomless autoimmune hypothyroidism were identified [14]. Further, proinflammatory actions induced by aldosterone contributing to chronic inflammatory autoimmune diseases was elaborated and reported by Suh et al., describing coexistence of primary aldosteronism with ankylosing spondylitis in a 59-year-old female [15]. This is also supported by the observations by Bendtzen et al. [16], where spironolactone (aldosterone receptor antagonist) reduced tumor necrosis factor-α and interferon-γ production in patients with rheumatoid and juvenile idiopathic arthritis, thus reducing the inflammation. Therefore, aldosterone may play a significant role in development and progression of autoimmune diseases.

There is emerging evidence of stimulating autoantibodies against angiotensin II type I receptor (AT-1R) which had been isolated from patients with PA [17]. Kem et al. found the prevalence of such antibodies is 31% in patients with PA [18]. 92% of the patients with hyperaldosteronism secondary to primary adrenal adenoma had autoantibodies against AT-1R in one study [19], whereas Li et al. demonstrated a 46% prevalence [20]. AT-1R antibodies may chronically stimulate the zona glomerulosa resulting in hyperproliferative state, which can lead to somatic gain of function mutation, leading to aldosterone producing adenomas. Bilateral adrenal hyperplasia also showed AT-1R antibody positivity in 75% of the patients [20]. These findings support an underlying autoantibody medicated mechanism for PA.

Thyroid dysfunction is a common endocrine disease worldwide. Apart from the direct manifestations due to changes in the thyroid hormone levels, it is associated with several cardiovascular effects. TSH level is found to positively correlate with lipid abnormalities, atherosclerotic disease, diastolic hypertension, and endothelial dysfunction in hypothyroid patients [21]. Suppressed TSH levels are correlated with hypertension, atrial fibrillation, endothelial dysfunction, myocardial infarction, and heart failure in patients with thyrotoxicosis [22]. Graves' thyrotoxicosis is the commonest among all causes of spontaneous thyrotoxicosis. Although B and T lymphocyte-mediated autoimmunity are known to be directed at different antigens in Graves' disease, TSH receptor appears the primary antigenic site, resulting in hyperthyroidism. Main pathogenic mechanism is through stimulatory TSH receptor autoantibodies (TRAb) causing endogenous overproduction of thyroxin hormone.

Although concurrent presence of hyperaldosteronism and thyroid disorders could be a chance occurrence due to relatively high prevalence, presence of a direct association had been discussed for several decades although exact causal relationship is not yet established. A study conducted by Armanini et al. [23] looked into the thyroid abnormalities among 40 patients with PA, secondary to both idiopathic bilateral adrenal hyperplasia (IHA) and unilateral adrenocortical adenoma. It showed that ultrasonographic thyroid abnormalities were present in 60% of the patients with PA compared to 27% in normal controls ($p < 0.0001$).

Prevalence of multinodular goiter was significantly higher compared to the controls in the same cohort. In a study done on 188 patients with PA and hypertension, Turchi et al. demonstrated that higher prevalence of ultrasonographic alterations in patients with PA compared to patients with essential hypertension (66% versus 46%, $p < 0.05$) without any significant difference in thyroid function tests [24]. High prevalence of thyroid dysfunction was also observed by Santori et al. among patients with PA {28.6% of patients with PA compared to 16% in patients with essential hypertension (chi^2 = 0.012)} [25]. The above observations have led to the hypothesis of a common pathogenic mechanisms such as imbalance/interplay between various growth factors and/or inflammatory cytokines, although exact mechanism is not yet identified.

Considering the association of aldosterone with autoimmune disease development, spectrum of autoimmune thyroid disorders could also be considered as associations although a definitive autoimmune syndrome or a cluster is not described. Tanaka et al. had described a 43-year-old lady with combined PA and Cushing's syndrome complicated with Hashimoto' thyroiditis [26]. Krysiak and Okopien [27] described a 36-year-old lady in whom there was primary aldosteronism due to left-sided adrenal adenoma which exacerbated the course of autoimmune thyroid disease (Hashimoto's thyroiditis). The same authors have also noted the elevated proinflammatory cytokines (TNF α, interleukin 2, and interferon-γ) have reduced after adrenalectomy, which in turn resulted in improvement of thyroid functions and reduction in thyroid autoimmunity in Hashimoto's thyroiditis. An observational study by Sabbadin et al. [28] revealed that the prevalence of anti-thyroid antibodies was significantly higher in PA than in controls (31.5% versus 7.8%) and greater in PA due to adrenal adenomas than IHA (33.3% versus 29.4%). These studies clearly demonstrate the association of aldosterone and thyroid autoimmunity.

Literature on association between PA and thyrotoxicosis is limited. Medline search since 1960 using the terms "primary hyperaldosteronism", "bilateral adrenal hyperplasia", "Conn's syndrome", "hyperthyroidism", "thyrotoxicosis" "Graves' disease" and "goiter" was performed. Only seven case reports with a title suggesting an association between primary hyperaldosteronism and thyrotoxicosis were found [29–35], but of which no abstract was available in three of the articles (Table 1). Larouche et al. had described a 29-year-old lady in whom there was coexisting primary hyperaldosteronism due to the fact that IHA and Graves' disease were diagnosed, highlighting that PA may be associated with autoimmune hyperthyroidism [32]. Anaforoğlu et al. describe a 51-year-old lady who presented with hypokalemic paralysis precipitated by coexisting left-sided aldosterone secreting adenoma and toxic nodular goiter [33], while Yokota et al. reported a case of PA due to left-sided adrenal adenoma coexisting with Graves' thyrotoxicosis resulting in hypokalemic paralysis, highlighting rarity of the association and importance of diagnosis [34]. A 43-year-old lady with hypokalemia paralysis precipitated by underlying hyperaldosteronism due to left-sided Conn's adenoma and hyperthyroidism was described by Kuo et al. [35] emphasizing the mutual

TABLE 1: Reported cases on hyperthyroidism and hyperaldosteronism.

Authors	Year	Patient	Presentation	Thyroid status	Hyperaldosteronism	Other associations
Bru et al.	1963	N/A	N/A	Hyperthyroidism	Hyperaldosteronism	—
Kijima and Sasaoka	1983	N/A	Hypokalemic paralysis	Hyperthyroidism	IHA	—
Iacovlev et al.	1994	N/A	N/A	Hyperthyroidism due to diffuse toxic goiter? Graves' disease	Conn's adenoma	—
Larouche et al.	2015	29 y old female	Psychosis following radioactive therapy for Graves' thyrotoxicosis	Graves' disease	IHA	—
Anaforoğlu et al.	2009	51 y old female	Hypokalemic paralysis	Toxic nodular goiter	Conn's adenoma	Subclinical Cushing's syndrome
Yokota et al.	1991	35 y old male	Hypokalemic paralysis	Graves' disease	Conn's adenoma	—
Kuo et al.	2009	43 y old female	Hypokalemic paralysis	Hyperthyroidism (exact cause not documented)	Conn's adenoma	—

interaction between PA and thyrotoxicosis giving rise to fatal clinical manifestations. Yet, the findings of involvement of stimulatory autoantibodies in both Graves' disease (TRAb) and PA (antibodies against AT-1R) as elaborated earlier in the discussion point out to a definitive autoimmune association in both conditions.

In addition to above observations of coexistence of PA and thyrotoxicosis, thyrotoxicosis itself is a trigger for secondary hyperaldosteronism. Numerous researches have evaluated the state of aldosterone levels in patients with hyperthyroidism and effects of thyroid hormones on synthesis and secretion of renin-angiotensin system [36–40]. They have found an increase in renin and aldosterone levels in thyrotoxic patients compared to euthyroid and hypothyroid patients. This led to the finding of regulation of aldosterone secretion by thyrotoxic state, probably in the form of secondary hyperaldosteronism. Suggested mechanisms are intensified beta-adrenergic activity of the nervous system and increased catecholamine production participated in increase in the mineralocorticoid function of the adrenal glands during thyrotoxicosis and upregulation of renin-angiotensin-aldosterone system [41]. This again highlights the close relationship between the two hormones, thyroxin and aldosterone.

The index case in the current case report gives further evidence of simultaneous presence of Conn's syndrome resulting in PA and Graves' thyrotoxicosis. Although TRAb was performed, AR-1R was not performed due to unavailability. Arterial venous sampling of the adrenal lesions for lateralization was not performed in our patient and surgery was considered directly according to the current available guidelines as it was a small lesion (<2 cm) and patient

was under the age of 40 years. Normalization of blood pressure and ARR after the surgery further confirms that PA is due to the adrenal adenoma. Patient had achieved remission of thyrotoxicosis in 12 months after the onset of Graves' disease, much earlier than usually the expected 18-month period. Whether correction of hyperaldosteronism has contributed to the early remission is not clear. Degree of hyperaldosteronism altering the course of autoimmune disease as previously shown by Krysiak and Okopien in relation to Hashimoto's thyroiditis and its application in the course of Graves' disease needs further research.

4. Conclusion

In the background of paucity of cases detailing association between the PA and autoimmune thyroid disease, especially Graves' disease, index case illustrates the coexistence of PA in the form of Conn's adenoma and Graves' disease, adding to the limited number of cases described in the literature. It is not certain if the association is incidental, yet the clear association of hyperaldosteronism with autoimmune diseases and detection of stimulatory autoantibodies warrants further evaluation/research for the causal relationship and effect on the progression of the disease and associations, which would in turn aid in the evaluation and management of such autoimmune diseases.

Abbreviations

ARR: Aldosterone renin ratio
AT-1R: Angiotensin II type I receptor
BMI: Body mass index

CT:　　Computed tomogram
IHA:　　Idiopathic hyperaldosteronism
HU:　　Hounsfield Units
PA:　　Primary hyperaldosteronism
TRAb:　　Thyroid stimulating hormone receptor
　　　　antibodies
TNF α:　　Tumor necrosis factor alpha
TSH:　　Thyroid stimulating hormone.

Disclosure

U. Bulugahapitiya (MBBS, MD, FRCP, FCCP, FACE) is a Consultant Endocrinologist and S. S. C. Gunatilake (MBBS, MD, MRCP) is a Senior Registrar in Endocrinology, affiliated to to Colombo South Teaching Hospital, Kalubowila, Sri Lanka.

Authors' Contributions

U. Bulugahapitiya conducted the clinical diagnosis and supervised the manuscript drafting. S. S. C. Gunatilake drafted the first manuscript, reviewed the literature, and was involved in direct management of the patient. All authors read and approved the final manuscript.

Acknowledgments

The authors acknowledge the contribution of staff of Chemical Pathology Department and Surgical Professorial Unit, Colombo South Teaching Hospital, Sri Lanka, for the support provided in the process of diagnosis and management of this patient.

References

[1] J. W. Funder, R. M. Carey, F. Mantero et al., "The management of primary aldosteronism: case detection, diagnosis, and treatment: an endocrine society clinical practice guideline," *The Journal of Clinical Endocrinology & Metabolism*, vol. 101, no. 5, pp. 1889–1916, 2016.

[2] V. M. Montori, G. L. Schwartz, A. B. Chapman, E. Boerwinkle, and S. T. Turner, "Validity of the aldosterone-renin ratio used to screen for primary aldosteronism," *Mayo Clinic Proceedings*, vol. 76, no. 9, pp. 877–882, 2001.

[3] T. Yoshimoto and Y. Hirata, "Aldosterone as a cardiovascular risk hormone," *Endocrine Journal*, vol. 54, no. 3, pp. 359–370, 2007.

[4] P. Mulatero, S. Monticone, C. Bertello et al., "Evaluation of primary aldosteronism," *Current Opinion in Endocrinology, Diabetes and Obesity*, vol. 17, no. 3, pp. 188–193, 2010.

[5] A. A. Herrada, F. J. Contreras, N. P. Marini et al., "Aldosterone promotes autoimmune damage by enhancing Th17-mediated immunity," *The Journal of Immunology*, vol. 184, no. 1, pp. 191–202, 2010.

[6] Yeung, S. J. Graves Disease. (2016, July 16). Retrieved December 13, 2016, from http://emedicine.medscape.com/article/120619-overview.

[7] M. P. J. Vanderpump, "The epidemiology of thyroid disease," *British Medical Bulletin*, vol. 99, no. 1, pp. 39–51, 2011.

[8] A. Hannemann, M. Bidlingmaier, N. Friedrich et al., "Screening for primary aldosteronism in hypertensive subjects: Results from two German epidemiological studies," *European Journal of Endocrinology*, vol. 167, no. 1, pp. 7–15, 2012.

[9] G. P. Rossi, G. Bernini, C. Caliumi et al., "A prospective study of the prevalence of primary aldosteronism in 1,125 hypertensive patients," *Journal of the American College of Cardiology*, vol. 48, no. 11, pp. 2293–2300, 2006.

[10] P. Milliez, X. Girerd, P.-F. Plouin, J. Blacher, M. E. Safar, and J.-J. Mourad, "Evidence for an increased rate of cardiovascular events in patients with primary aldosteronism," *Journal of the American College of Cardiology*, vol. 45, no. 8, pp. 1243–1248, 2005.

[11] I. Z. Jaffe and M. E. Mendelsohn, "Angiotensin II and aldosterone regulate gene transcription via functional mineralocortocoid receptors in human coronary artery smooth muscle cells," *Circulation Research*, vol. 96, no. 6, pp. 643–650, 2005.

[12] J. A. Leopold, A. Dam, B. A. Maron et al., "Aldosterone impairs vascular reactivity by decreasing glucose-6-phosphate dehydrogenase activity," *Nature Medicine*, vol. 13, no. 2, pp. 189–197, 2007.

[13] A. A. Herrada, C. Campino, C. A. Amador, L. F. Michea, C. E. Fardella, and A. M. Kalergis, "Aldosterone as a modulator of immunity: implications in the organ damage," *Journal of Hypertension*, vol. 29, no. 9, pp. 1684–1692, 2011.

[14] M. J. Molina-Garrido, R. Enríquez, A. Mora-Rufete, A. E. Sirvent, and C. Guillen-Ponce, "Primary hyperaldosteronism associated with vitiligo vulgaris and autoimmune hypothyroidism," *The American Journal of the Medical Sciences*, vol. 333, no. 3, pp. 178–180, 2007.

[15] Y. S. Suh, H.-O. Kim, Y.-H. Cheon, W. Jo, J. Hong, and S.-I. Lee, "Ankylosing spondylitis associated with primary aldosteronism in a middle-aged woman," *Korean Journal of Internal Medicine*, vol. 32, no. 2, pp. 374–377, 2017.

[16] K. Bendtzen, P. R. Hansen, K. Rieneck et al., "Spironolactone inhibits production of proinflammatory cytokines, including tumour necrosis factor-alpha and interferon-gamma and has potential in the treatment of arthritis," *Clinical & Experimental Immunology*, vol. 134, no. 1, pp. 151–158, 2003.

[17] T. A. Williams, P. Mulatero, M. Bidlingmaier, F. Beuschlein, and M. Reincke, "Genetic and Potential Autoimmune Triggers of Primary Aldosteronism," *Hypertension*, vol. 66, no. 2, pp. 248–253, 2015.

[18] D. C. Kem, H. Li, C. Velarde-Miranda et al., "Autoimmune mechanisms activating the angiotensin AT1 receptor in 'primary' aldosteronism," *The Journal of Clinical Endocrinology & Metabolism*, vol. 99, no. 5, pp. 1790–1797, 2014.

[19] G. Rossitto, G. Regolisti, E. Rossi et al., "Elevation of angiotensin-II type-1-receptor autoantibodies titer in primary aldosteronism as a result of aldosterone-producing adenoma," *Hypertension*, vol. 61, no. 2, pp. 526–533, 2013.

[20] H. Li, X. Yu, M. V. Cicala et al., "Prevalence of angiotensin II type 1 receptor (AT1R)-activating autoantibodies in primary aldosteronism," *Journal of the American Society of Hypertension*, vol. 9, no. 1, pp. 15–20, 2015.

[21] X. Sun, Y. Sun, W.-C. Li et al., "Association of thyroid-stimulating hormone and cardiovascular risk factors," *Internal Medicine*, vol. 54, no. 20, pp. 2537–2544, 2015.

[22] S. Ertek and A. F. Cicero, "Hyperthyroidism and cardiovascular complications: a narrative review on the basis of pathophysiology," *Archives of Medical Science*, vol. 9, no. 5, pp. 944–952, 2013.

[23] D. Armanini, D. Nacamulli, C. Scaroni et al., "High Prevalence of Thyroid Ultrasonographic Abnormalities in Primary Aldosteronism," *Endocrine Journal*, vol. 22, no. 2, pp. 155–159, 2003.

[24] F. Turchi, V. Ronconi, V. Di Tizio, M. Boscaro, and G. Giacchetti, "Blood pressure, thyroid-stimulating hormone, and thyroid disease prevalence in primary aldosteronism and essential hypertension," *American Journal of Hypertension*, vol. 24, no. 12, pp. 1274–1279, 2011.

[25] C. Santori, C. Di Veroli, F. Di Lazzaro et al., "High prevalence of thyroid disfunction in primary hyperaldosteronism," *Recenti Progressi in Medicina*, vol. 96, no. 7-8, pp. 352–356, 2005.

[26] M. Tanaka, M. Izeki, Y. Miyazaki et al., "Combined primary aldosteronism and Cushing's syndrome due to a single adrenocortical adenoma complicated by Hashimoto's thyroiditis," *Internal Medicine*, vol. 41, no. 11, pp. 967–971, 2002.

[27] R. Krysiak and B. Okopien, "Coexistence of primary aldosteronism and Hashimoto's thyroiditis," *Rheumatology International*, vol. 32, no. 8, pp. 2561–2563, 2012.

[28] C. Sabbadin, C. Mian, D. Nacamulli et al., "Association of primary aldosteronism with chronic thyroiditis," in *Proceedings of the Endocrine Society's 95th Annual Meeting and Expo*, vol. 55 of *Presentation number SUN 446*, pp. 303–306, San Francisco, Calif, USA, June, 2013.

[29] Y. Kijima and T. Sasaoka, "Hypokalemic paralysis in a case with hyperthyroidism and idiopathic hyperaldosteronism," *Nihon Naika Gakkai Zasshi*, vol. 72, no. 11, pp. 1583–1590, 1983.

[30] V. A. Iacovlev, S. B. Shustov, and K. IuSh, "A case of Conn's syndrome combined with diffuse toxic goiter," *Probl Endokrinol (Mosk)*, vol. 40, no. 4, pp. 38-39, 1994.

[31] A. Bru, P. Dardenne, L. Douste-Blazy, P. Pinel, J. Planques, and J. R. Saint-Marc, "Hyperaldosteronemia and associated hyperthyroidism," *Ann Endocrinol (Paris)*, vol. 24, pp. 84–92, 1963.

[32] V. Larouche, L. Snell, and D. V. Morris, "Iatrogenic myxoedema madness following radioactive iodine ablation for Graves' disease, with a concurrent diagnosis of primary hyperaldosteronism," *Endocrinology, Diabetes & Metabolism Case Reports*, vol. 2015, Article ID 150087, 2015.

[33] I. Anaforoğlu, A. Şimşek, and E. Algün, "Conn's syndrome, subclinical cushing's syndrome and thyrotoxicosis presenting as hypokalemic periodic paralysis: a case report," *Turkish Journal of Endocrinology and Metabolism*, p. 13, 2009.

[34] N. Yokota, T. Uchida, A. Sasaki et al., "Thyrotoxic periodic paralysis complicated with primary aldosteronism.," *Japanese Journal of Medicine*, vol. 30, no. 3, pp. 219–223, 1991.

[35] C.-C. Kuo, W.-S. Yang, V.-C. Wu, C.-W. Tsai, W. J. Wang, and K.-D. Wu, "Hypokalemic paralysis: The interplay between primary aldosteronism and hyperthyroidism," *European Journal of Clinical Investigation*, vol. 39, no. 8, pp. 738-739, 2009.

[36] L. V. Rybina and E. S. Natarov Rom-Bugoslavskaia, "Regulation of aldosterone secretion in patients with thyrotoxicosis. I. role of the renin-angiotensin system and corticotropin in the development of secondary hyperaldosteronism in patients with thyrotoxicosis," *Probl Endokrinol (Mosk)*, vol. 29, no. 2, pp. 24–30, 1983.

[37] D. Koev, "State of the renin-angiotensin system in thyrotoxicosis," *Probl Endokrinol (Mosk)*, vol. 21, no. 3, pp. 16–21, 1975.

[38] T. P. Bezverkhaia, "Hyperaldosteronism in thyrotoxicosis," *Probl Endokrinol (Mosk)*, vol. 21, no. 5, pp. 26–29, 1975.

[39] B. J. Asmah, W. M. Wan Nazaimoon, K. Norazmi, T. T. Tan, and B. A. K. Khalid, "Plasma Renin and Aldosterone in Thyroid Diseases," *Hormone and Metabolic Research*, vol. 29, no. 11, pp. 580–583, 1997.

[40] F. Vargas, I. Rodríguez-Gómez, P. Vargas-Tendero, E. Jimenez, and M. Montiel, "The renin-angiotensin system in thyroid disorders and its role in cardiovascular and renal manifestations," *Journal of Endocrinology*, vol. 213, no. 1, pp. 25–36, 2012.

[41] C. W. Park, Y. S. Shin, S. J. Ahn et al., "Thyroxine treatment induces upregulation of renin-angiotensin-aldosterone system due to decreasing effective plasma volume in patients with primary myxoedema," *Nephrology Dialysis Transplantation*, vol. 16, no. 9, pp. 1799–1806, 2001.

6

Extreme and Cyclical Blood Pressure Elevation in a Pheochromocytoma Hypertensive Crisis

V. Larouche ⓘ,[1] **N. Garfield,**[2] **and E. Mitmaker**[3]

[1]*Adult Endocrinology and Metabolism Training Program, McGill University, Montréal, QC, Canada*
[2]*Division of Endocrinology, McGill University Health Centre, Montréal, QC, Canada*
[3]*Division of General Surgery, McGill University Health Centre, Montréal, QC, Canada*

Correspondence should be addressed to V. Larouche; vincent.larouche@mail.mcgill.ca

Academic Editor: Toshihiro Kita

Pheochromocytomas are rare adrenal neoplasms characterized by excess secretion of catecholamines. We describe the case of a 65-year-old man, known for hypertension, with no family history of hereditary pheochromocytoma syndromes. He reported a two-year history of flushing, systolic blood pressure surges to 200 mmHg, headaches, tremors, and syncope. His initial workup revealed elevated 24h urine catecholamines and metanephrines. An adrenal MRI in March 2017 showed a large 7.6 cm heterogeneous right adrenal lesion. Given orthostatic hypotension, his final preoperative dose was limited to a low dose of terazosin and metoprolol. In the operating room, shortly after intubation and Foley insertion, his blood pressure rose to 350 mmHg. Surgery was cancelled and he was admitted to the intensive care unit, where intravenous phentolamine, nitroprusside, and nicardipine were started. His systolic blood pressure would oscillate between 60 mmHg and 350 mmHg at 2-3 minutes' intervals. After 3 days, he was weaned off intravenous medications. His oral medications were uptitrated to high doses of phenoxybenzamine, metoprolol, and nifedipine. Three weeks later, he underwent successful open right adrenalectomy. This case outlines the importance of preoperative preparation of pheochromocytomas and raises the question if phenoxybenzamine is the alpha-blocker of choice for larger tumours with significant hormonal secretion.

1. Introduction

Catecholamine-secreting tumours that arise from chromaffin cells of the adrenal medulla and the sympathetic ganglia are referred to as pheochromocytomas and paragangliomas. Their annual incidence is 0.8 per 100,000 person-years. They are most common in the fourth to fifth decade and are equally common in men and women. The classic triad of symptoms consists of episodic headaches, sweating, and tachycardia. Most patients do not have the three classic symptoms. The diagnosis of pheochromocytoma is made based upon biochemical confirmation of catecholamine hypersecretion with 24h urine collection of metanephrines or plasma-free metanephrines followed by imaging studies such as CT Scan or MRI of the adrenals and possibly functional imaging with nuclear medicine modalities. The mainstay of management of pheochromocytoma is surgical excision of the tumour with careful preoperative preparation which includes volume expansion, alpha-adrenergic blockade first, followed by beta-adrenergic blockade. This case highlights the rare event of an extreme and cyclical blood pressure pattern in the context of a pheochromocytoma hypertensive crisis.

2. Case Presentation

We report the case of a 65-year-old man known for hypertension, cholelithiasis, and panic disorder with no personal or family history of pheochromocytoma, paraganglioma, Multiple Endocrine Neoplasia Type 2 syndrome, Von Hippel Lindau syndrome, Neurofibromatosis Type 1, or Succinyl Dehydrogenase mutations. He is a past smoker who quit 5 years prior to presentation and cumulated a 20-pack-year smoking history with no history of dyslipidemia or diabetes. The patient described a two-year history of frequent episodes of flushing, diaphoresis, systolic blood pressure surges up to 200 mmHg, loss of vision, headaches, palpitations, and

TABLE 1: Biochemical investigation.

24h urine collection for Metanephrines and Catecholamines	2016-12-26	2017-03-28	2017-07-13 (2 weeks post-op)	2017-10-12 (3 months post-op)	Normal Range
Epinephrine	219	642	Undet.	Undet.	0-110 nmol/d
Norepinephrine	782	1246	504	336	0-480 nmol/d
Dopamine	1368	1626	2519	1904	0-2620 nmol/d
Metanephrines	1718	3118	1869	Undet.	0-275 nmol/d
Normetanephrines	3478	5762	291	160	0-240 nmol/d

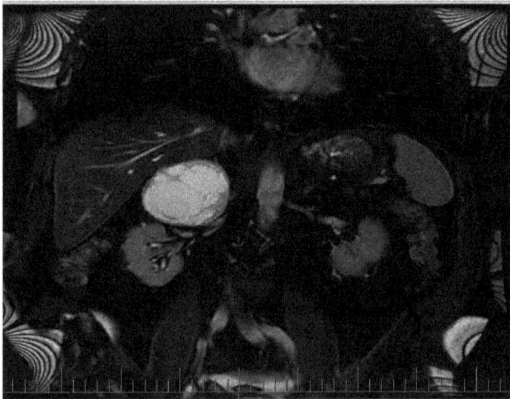

FIGURE 1: MRI adrenals.

tremors. He also complained of more frequent episodes of presyncope up to 6 times a day in the few weeks prior to seeking medical attention. The patient denied pallor, weight loss, weakness, or abdominal pain. His blood pressure was episodically elevated with only a moderately elevated baseline blood pressure. His only antihypertensive therapy at his first visit to our Endocrinology clinic was terazosin 1 mg once daily with only partial relief of his paroxysmal symptoms.

The patient was initially diagnosed with panic disorder and treated with cognitive-behavioural therapy. On physical exam, the patient's weight was 92 kg, his height was 1.77 m, and his BMI was 29.4 kg/m2. His blood pressure was 168/100 mmHg; his heart rate was regular between 90 and 100 bpm. His abdominal exam, however, revealed an obese nontender abdomen with a palpable right-sided suprarenal mass of 6-7 cm diameter, which was soft and mobile.

Two 24h urine collections for metanephrines and catecholamines were performed (c.f. Table 1) and confirmed hypersecretion. No plasma aldosterone or renin levels were drawn, and no Cushing syndrome screening test was performed.

An MRI of the adrenals (c.f. Figure 1) reported a large right adrenal mass measuring 7.6 x 7.6 x 7.2 cm with T2 hyperintensity centrally and no loss of signal in T1. It was reported as highly suspicious for pheochromocytoma with a normal left adrenal gland, liver, and pancreas and no evidence of metastasis. Of note, the patient was not known for any underlying cardiac arrhythmia and had a normal

baseline electrocardiogram in sinus rhythm at 95 bpm. No echocardiogram was ordered preoperatively.

The patient was referred to a urologist at an academic centre. He was then seen by Endocrinology one month prior to surgery. At his first visit to our clinic, he was counselled to have a high-salt diet and oral hydration was encouraged. The dose of terazosin was increased to 1 mg po bid x 1 week and then 2 mg po bid. Chromogranin A was elevated: 274 ng/mL (N < 82 ng/mL). An MIBG Scan was ordered, but the radiotracer was unavailable.

The patient was closely followed up by phone every week. Terazosin was increased to 2 mg po bid and metoprolol was added and increased to a maximal dose of 25 mg tid until he demonstrated orthostatic hypotension. The patient was admitted one day prior to surgery with a well-controlled blood pressure of 112/70 mmHg.

In the operating room, shortly after intubation and Foley catheter insertion and prior to surgical incision, the patient's blood pressure rose to 350/180 mmHg without improvement despite intravenous phentolamine boluses. Given the inability to control the patient's labile blood pressure, a decision was made to abort the operation and transfer the patient to the intensive care unit while remaining intubated.

In the intensive care unit, the patient required massive doses of intravenous phentolamine, nitroprusside, and nicardipine as well as intravenous hydration, as these are the main options for management of a pheochromocytoma hypertensive crisis as per current clinical practice guidelines [1]. Interestingly, his blood pressure would oscillate between 60/34 and 350/186 mmHg within a matter of 2-3 minutes in a cyclical pattern (c.f. Figure 2). A nasogastric tube was inserted, and the patient was started on phenoxybenzamine per tube. After 72 hours in ICU, he was weaned off intravenous antihypertensives and sedatives and extubated.

He was transferred back to the surgical ward, while gradually having his blood pressure medications uptitrated to phenoxybenzamine 120 mg po bid, metoprolol 100 mg po bid, and nifedipine XL 60 mg once daily. His blood pressure was then well controlled. The patient underwent successful open right adrenalectomy three weeks later. He was hypotensive intraoperatively, requiring vasopressors. He had an uncomplicated postoperative course.

Further investigations in hospital during his stay included free plasma normetanephrine 14.44 nmol/L (N<1.2 nmol/L) and metanephrine 6.09 nmol/L (N< 0.48 nmol/L), a negative

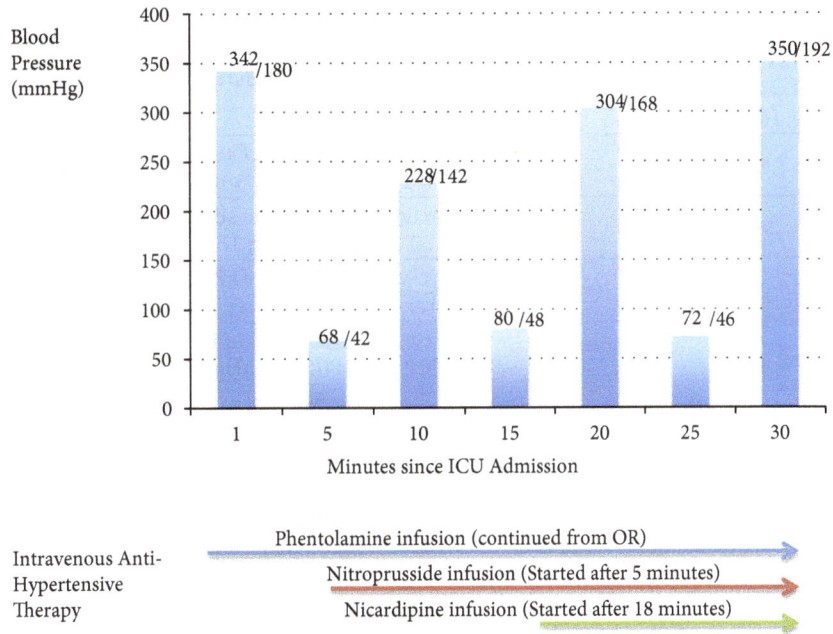

FIGURE 2: Blood pressure after admission to ICU.

cerebral CT scan, and an Octreoscan showing no site of extra-adrenal uptake. An Octreoscan was performed as a surrogate functional imaging modality given the unavailability of MIBG (recommended functional imaging modality) radiotracer at our centre around the time of this patient's admission. Pathology confirmed an 8 cm right adrenal pheochromocytoma without angioinvasion, extra-adrenal extension, or necrosis.

One month postoperatively, the patient was seen in the Endocrinology clinic and reported feeling overall well with no documented hypertension. He stopped all antihypertensive medications and had no palpitations, diaphoresis, flushing, headaches, or other symptoms of catecholamine excess. His 24h urine metanephrines and catecholamines normalized during follow-up (c.f. Table 1). The patient has not undergone genetic analysis during follow-up.

Unfortunately, the patient sustained a ST-elevation myocardial infarction three months postoperatively, requiring urgent percutaneous coronary intervention and stent placement. Unfortunately, he was treated at another hospital and results from his coronary angiogram were not available to authors. He survived this acute cardiac event and continues to be followed closely by Cardiology. His longstanding elevated blood pressure secondary to his pheochromocytoma and his prior smoking history were significant risk factors for his myocardial infarction.

3. Discussion

In summary, our patient is a 65-year-old man who developed a hypertensive crisis with extreme and cyclical blood pressure due to insufficient preoperative alpha- and beta-blockade in planning for an open adrenalectomy to resect a 7.6 cm right adrenal pheochromocytoma.

A Medline search from 1980 until now using the keywords "pheochromocytoma", "cyclic", "blood pressure", and "hypertension" revealed 8 similar cases of pheochromocytoma with recurrent oscillations between hypertension and hypotension.

As outlined in Table 2, Ganguly and colleagues [2] described a 67-year-old man with a 6 cm right-sided pheochromocytoma admitted to the coronary care unit with chest pain, adrenergic symptoms, bradycardia, and a systolic blood pressure varying between 60 and 240 mmHg every 5-10 minutes. Similarly, Guzik and colleagues [3] described a 52-year-old woman with a 10 cm right adrenal pheochromocytoma, norepinephrine predominant, who presented with cyclical blood pressure elevation up to 316 mmHg and decreased down to 50 mmHg.

Furthermore, Kobal and colleagues [4] reported the case of a 52-year-old woman with a 2.5 cm right adrenal pheochromocytoma, metanephrine predominant, who presented to the emergency room with an 8-hour history of chest and abdominal pain. She also had significant systolic blood pressure surges, up to 265 mmHg and down to 30 mmHg. Ionescu and colleagues [5] described a 47-year-old woman with a 4.2 cm right-sided adrenal pheochromocytoma, epinephrine predominant, who developed rapid oscillations between hypertension (BP up to 344/170 mmHg) and hypotension (BP down to 52/34 mmHg) every 14 minutes in an electrophysiological study for palpitations, triggered by anesthetic agents.

Jindal and colleagues [6] reported the case of a 55-year-old man with a 5.2 cm right adrenal pheochromocytoma, multihormone secreting, who presented with cyclical blood pressure variations from 80/55 mmHg to 190/99 mmHg in the context of Takotsubo cardiomyopathy. Along the same lines, Murai and colleagues [7] described a 42-year-old man with a 4.2 cm right-sided pheochromocytoma, secreting mostly

TABLE 2: Summary of similar cases.

Ref.	Age	Sex	Maximal Diameter (cm)	Side	Predominant Hormone	Blood Pressure Pattern	Clinical outcome
[1]	67	M	6.0	R	-	Cyclical Oscillations of sBP between 60-240 mmHg every 5-10 minutes	Successful right adrenalectomy.
[2]	52	F	10.0	R	NE	Cyclical Oscillations of sBP between 50-316 mmHg every 17 minutes	N/A
[3]	52	F	2.5	R	MN	Cyclical Oscillations of sBP between 30 and 265 mmHg every 15 minutes	Successful open right adrenalectomy.
[4]	47	F	4.2	R	EPI	Cyclical oscillations of BP from 52/34 to 344/170 mmHg every 14 minutes.	Successful open right adrenalectomy.
[5]	55	M	5.2	R	EPI/NE/DO	Cyclical oscillations of BP from 80/55 to 190/99 mmHg every 30 minutes	Successful open right adrenalectomy.
[6]	42	M	4.2	R	EPI/NE	Cyclical oscillations of BP from 70/50 to 160/100 mmHg every 15 minutes	Successful open right adrenalectomy.
[7]	69	M	-	R	NE	Cyclical oscillations of BP every 9-13 minutes	N/A
[8]	18	M	-	-	NE	Cyclical oscillations of BP every 3 minutes	N/A

norepinephrine and epinephrine, who presented with acute chest pain and blood pressure readings varying between 70/50 mmHg and 160/100 mmHg at 15 minutes' intervals.

Oishi and colleagues [8] reported a 69-year-old man with a right adrenal pheochromocytoma, norepinephrine predominant, who presented with blood pressure fluctuations in 9-13 minutes' cycles. Moreover, Wenting and colleagues [9] reported an 18-year-old man with a norepinephrine predominant pheochromocytoma whose blood pressure varied by amplitudes up to 80 mmHg at three minutes' intervals during intra-arterial pressure monitoring.

Overall, cases included 5 males and 3 females aged 18-69, all with right-sided adrenal pheochromocytomas (when side mentioned) with a largest diameter between 2.5 and 10 cm, mostly epinephrine or norepinephrine predominant. [2–9]. For those cases where the outcome was described, all patients had a successful adrenalectomy. For those cases where the surgical approach was detailed, all surgeries were open as opposed to laparoscopic. Open approach is generally recommended for hemodynamically unstable patients. The patient described herein had a similar clinical presentation as the other reported cases.

In this case, our patient was preoperatively prepared with small doses of alpha-blockade and beta-blockade as per current guidelines [1]. Dose increase was limited by orthostatic hypotension. In retrospect, he was inadequately blocked and possibly volume contracted, as he developed a hypertensive crisis with cyclical blood pressure changes after anesthetic induction and Foley catheter insertion. Selective alpha-blockers are commonly used, as the nonselective alpha-blocker phenoxybenzamine, which remains the gold standard, is not easily accessible in Canada.

Few studies have compared nonselective versus selective alpha-blockers for preoperative management of pheochromocytoma. Both Zhu et al. [10] and Weingarten et al. [11] showed that preoperative preparation with selective alpha-blocker leads to higher intraoperative systolic BP but less arterial BP fluctuation compared to phenoxybenzamine. No clear size cut-off has been identified as a factor to choose nonselective over selective alpha-blocker.

Interestingly enough, Groeben et al. [12] conducted an observational case series where they compared haemodynamic conditions and perioperative complications of 110 patients with pheochromocytoma who receive preoperative alpha-blockade to 166 patients who did not. Their data showed a slightly lower mean maximal systolic arterial pressure (17 mmHg, p = 0.024) in those who received preoperative alpha-blockade with no difference in the incidence of excessive hypertensive episodes or major complications. Further studies are needed to identify the optimal preoperative pharmacological regimen for individual cases of pheochromocytoma.

4. Learning Points

(i) Preoperative preparation with alpha-blockers first and then with beta-blockers, when preparing a patient for an adrenalectomy due to a pheochromocytoma, is of utmost importance in order to decrease the risk of intraoperative hemodynamic instability.

(ii) As per current guidelines, the nonselective alpha-blocker phenoxybenzamine remains the gold standard for preoperative preparation of a pheochromocytoma resection. However, no clear size cut-off or hormone level has been established in literature to guide clinicians to choose phenoxybenzamine over selective alpha-blockers.

(iii) Pheochromocytoma hypertensive crisis is a medical emergency requiring intensive care unit admission and prompt management of the blood pressure with intravenous antihypertensives and fluid repletion.

(iv) In catecholamine-mediated hypertensive crises, the blood pressure elevation can be extreme and cyclical in nature, varying between hypertensive surges and hypotensive episodes, therefore representing a clinical challenge.

References

[1] J. W. M. Lenders, Q.-Y. Duh, and G. Eisenhofer, "Pheochromocytoma and paraganglioma : an endocrine society clinical practice guideline," *The Journal of Clinical Endocrinology & Metabolism*, vol. 99, no. 6, pp. 1915–1942, 2014.

[2] A. Ganguly, C. E. Grim, M. H. Weinberger, and D. P. Henry, "Rapid cyclic fluctuations of blood pressure associated with an adrenal pheochromocytoma," *Hypertension*, vol. 6, no. 2, pp. 281–284, 1984.

[3] P. Guzik, A. Wykretowicz, I. K. H. Wesseling, and H. Wysocki, "Adrenal pheochromocytoma associated with dramatic cyclic hemodynamic fluctuations," *International Journal of Cardiology*, vol. 103, no. 3, pp. 351–353, 2005.

[4] S. L. Kobal, E. Paran, A. Jamali, S. Mizrahi, R. J. Siegel, and J. Leor, "Pheochromocytoma: cyclic attacks of hypertension alternating with hypotension," *Nature Clinical Practice Cardiovascular Medicine*, vol. 5, no. 1, pp. 53–57, 2008.

[5] C. N. Ionescu, O. V. Sakharova, M. D. Harwood, E. A. Caracciolo, M. H. Schoenfeld, and T. J. Donohue, "Cyclic Rapid Fluctuation of Hypertension and Hypotension in Pheochromocytoma," *The Journal of Clinical Hypertension*, vol. 10, no. 12, pp. 936–940, 2008.

[6] V. Jindal, M. L. Baker, A. Aryangat, S. D. Wittlin, J. D. Bisognano, and H. S. Richter, "Pheochromocytoma: Presenting with regular cyclic blood pressure and inverted Takotsubo cardiomyopathy," *The Journal of Clinical Hypertension*, vol. 11, no. 2, pp. 81–86, 2009.

[7] K. Murai, K. Hirota, T. Niskikimi et al., "Pheochromocytoma with Electrocardiographic Change Mimicking Angina Pectoris, and Cyclic Change in Direct Arterial Pressure—A Case Report," *Angiology*, vol. 42, no. 2, pp. 157–161, 1991.

[8] S. Oishi, M. Sasaki, M. Ohno, T. Umeda, and T. Sato, "Periodic Fluctuation of Blood Pressure and Its Management in a Patient with Pheochromocytoma Case Report and Review of the Literature," *Japanese Heart Journal*, vol. 29, no. 3, pp. 389–399, 1988.

[9] G. J. Wenting, A. J. Man in't Veld, F. Boomsma, and M. A. Schalekamp, "Cyclic blood pressure changes in a patient with a pheochromocytoma: role of a central oscillator?" *Journal of Hypertension Suppl*, vol. 3, no. 3, pp. S347–S349, 1985.

[10] Y. Zhu, H.-C. He, T.-W. Su et al., "Selective α 1-adrenoceptor antagonist (controlled release tablets) in preoperative management of pheochromocytoma," *Endocrine Journal*, vol. 38, no. 2, pp. 254–259, 2010.

[11] T. N. Weingarten, J. P. Cata, J. F. O'Hara et al., "Comparison of two preoperative medical management strategies for laparoscopic resection of pheochromocytoma," *Urology*, vol. 76, pp. 508–511, 2010.

[12] H. Groeben, B. J. Nottebaum, P. F. Alesina, A. Traut, H. P. Neumann, and M. K. Walz, "Perioperative α-receptor blockade in phaeochromocytoma surgery: An observational case series," *British Journal of Anaesthesia*, vol. 118, no. 2, pp. 182–189, 2017.

7

Mifepristone Accelerates HPA Axis Recovery in Secondary Adrenal Insufficiency

Pejman Cohan

Specialized Endocrine Care Center, 150 North Robertson Boulevard, Suite 210, Beverly Hills, CA 90211, USA

Correspondence should be addressed to Pejman Cohan; pcohan@mednet.ucla.edu

Academic Editor: Hidetoshi Ikeda

Context. Transient secondary adrenal insufficiency (SAI) is an expected complication following successful adenomectomy of ACTH-secreting pituitary adenomas or unilateral adrenalectomy for cortisol-secreting adrenal adenomas. To date, no pharmacological therapy has been shown to hasten recovery of the hypothalamic-pituitary-adrenal (HPA) axis in this clinical scenario. *Case Description.* A 33-year-old woman underwent uncomplicated unilateral adrenalectomy for a 3.7 cm cortisol-secreting adrenal adenoma. Postoperatively, she developed SAI and was placed on hydrocortisone 15 mg/day, given in divided doses. In the ensuing six years, the patient's HPA axis failed to recover and she remained corticosteroid-dependent. Quarterly biochemical testing (after withholding hydrocortisone for 18 hours) consistently yielded undetectable serum cortisol and subnormal plasma ACTH levels. While she was on hydrocortisone 15 mg/day, mifepristone was initiated and gradually titrated to a maintenance dose of 600 mg/day after 5 months. Rapid recovery of the HPA axis was subsequently noted with ACTH rising into the supranormal range at 4 months followed by a subsequent rise in cortisol levels into the normal range. After 6 months, the dose of hydrocortisone and mifepristone was lowered and both were ultimately stopped after 8 months. The HPA axis remains normal after an additional 16 months of follow-up. *Conclusion.* Mifepristone successfully restored the HPA axis in a woman with prolonged secondary adrenal insufficiency (SAI) after adrenalectomy for Cushing's syndrome (CS).

1. Introduction

Secondary adrenal insufficiency (SAI) invariably develops following successful adenomectomy of ACTH-secreting pituitary adenomas or unilateral adrenalectomy for cortisol-secreting adrenal adenomas. The abrupt postsurgical transition from a state of cortisol excess to SAI often leads to unpleasant symptoms of cortisol withdrawal including fatigue, nausea, and body aches. During this time, glucocorticoid replacement therapy is often mandatory, particularly during stressful situations. The subsequent recovery of the HPA axis is highly variable and may be influenced by factors such as the duration and severity of preexisting hypercortisolemia, and the dose of glucocorticoid replacement, as well as the underlying etiology of Cushing's syndrome (CS). In a recent retrospective analysis of 230 patients with CS, the median time to HPA axis recovery was 2.5 years, 1.4 years, and 0.6 years for unilateral adrenal, pituitary, and ectopic

CS, respectively [1]. Other than physiological glucocorticoid replacement therapy and time, no other treatment has been demonstrated to accelerate the recovery of the HPA axis.

Resumption of normal hypothalamic CRH production appears to be the critical step in HPA axis recovery [2]. As is axiomatic of all endocrine feedback loops, it follows that any treatment that interrupts cortisol negative feedback at the hypothalamic level leads to secondary rises in ACTH and cortisol. Mifepristone is a competitive antagonist of the human glucocorticoid receptor (GR) with an affinity approximately 18 times higher than endogenous cortisol [3]. When administered to healthy human volunteers, mifepristone results in significant dose-dependent increases in plasma ACTH and cortisol levels [4], an effect that is unaccompanied by clinical signs or symptoms of adrenal insufficiency [5]. Mifepristone (Korlym®) is FDA-approved for the treatment of hyperglycemia associated with CS but has never been studied as a treatment to aid HPA axis recovery [6].

TABLE 1: Time course of HPA axis recovery after initiation of mifepristone.

Month	0	1	3	4	5	6	8	10	11
Mife. dose (mg)	0	150 TIW	300 TIW	300 daily	600 daily	600 daily	300 TIW	0	0
HC dose (mg)	15	15	15	15	15	10	0	0	0
ACTH (pg/mL)	5	15	18	60	78	173	126	26	45
Cortisol (μg/dL)	<1	<1	<1	3.6	4.6	10.5	13.6	13.5	15.3
DHEA (ng/mL)	<0.05	<0.05	<0.05	<0.05	<0.05	<0.05	<0.05	<0.05	0.053

Mife.: mifepristone; HC: hydrocortisone; ACTH: adrenocorticotropic hormone; DHEA: dehydroepiandrosterone; TIW: three times per week.

Herein, I report a case of woman in whom the addition of mifepristone expedited the recovery of the HPA axis after six years of unsuccessful glucocorticoid replacement therapy.

2. Case Report

At age 20, the patient presented with depression for which she was placed on psychotropic medications. At age 28, she developed progressive malaise, 25-pound weight gain, muscle weakness, easing bruising, hypertension, and foot stress fracture. At age 31, DEXA bone density scan disclosed a T-score of -3.4 at the lumbar spine and -3.1 at the hip. Further testing for secondary causes of osteoporosis included 24-hour urinary free cortisol which was markedly elevated at 499 mcg/day (range 10–80 mcg/day). Plasma ACTH level was undetectable. Adrenal imaging revealed a right adrenal mass. At age 33, she underwent uncomplicated right laparoscopic adrenalectomy and histopathology confirmed a 3.7 cm adrenocortical adenoma. Postoperatively, the patient was placed on hydrocortisone replacement, initially at a dose of 40 mg/day given in divided doses and gradually tapered to 30 mg/day over the following several months. One year after her adrenalectomy, her body mass index was 20.4 kg/m^2, and her hydrocortisone had been further tapered to 15 mg daily, which remained her maintenance dose.

During the ensuing six years after her adrenalectomy, the patient generally felt unwell with symptoms of episodic nausea, headaches, lightheadedness, mood swings, and generalized weakness. Attempts to lower the dose of hydrocortisone below 15 mg/day were not tolerated by the patient. Quarterly biochemical testing (after withholding hydrocortisone for 18 hours) consistently yielded undetectable serum cortisol and subnormal plasma ACTH levels. During this 6-year period, she had one pregnancy, occurring 3 years after adrenalectomy and progressing to full-term delivery of a healthy boy. She had two other hospitalizations (separated by 4 years) for near-syncope, malaise, nausea, and vomiting (but without hypoglycemia or hypotension). Both episodes were treated with 48 hours of stress-doses of steroids and intravenous saline, followed by improvement of her symptoms and subsequent tapering of corticosteroids back to a replacement dose of hydrocortisone 15 mg/day.

The failure of the HPA axis to recover six years after adrenalectomy (despite physiological steroid dosing) prompted magnetic resonance imaging of the sella to rule out structural abnormalities of the hypothalamus, infundibulum, and pituitary. This MRI was unremarkable. Other pituitary hormones were also normal. After a detailed discussion of risk and benefit, mifepristone (Korlym) 150 mg every other day was initiated and her dose of hydrocortisone 15 mg/day was continued. Over the subsequent five months, the dose of mifepristone was gradually escalated to 300 mg every other day and then 300 mg daily and finally maintained at 600 mg daily. During this time, rapid recovery of the HPA axis was noted (initially with a rise in ACTH into the supranormal range 4 months after starting mifepristone, followed by a subsequent rise in cortisol levels). After 6 months, the dose of hydrocortisone and mifepristone was lowered and both were ultimately stopped after 8 months. The HPA axis remains normal after an additional 16 months of follow-up. Table 1 summarizes recovery of the HPA axis after initiation of mifepristone.

The patient tolerated mifepristone remarkably well with the only side effects being amenorrhea and pruritus (she had a preexisting history of idiopathic urticaria). The pruritus was tolerable and managed with over-the-counter antihistamines. At no point during treatment with mifepristone did the patient develop signs or symptoms of adrenal insufficiency. Her menses returned 3 weeks after discontinuation of mifepristone. The HPA axis remains normal after an additional 16 months of follow-up, during which the patient reported marked improvements in sense of well-being and quality of life.

3. Discussion

Cushing's syndrome remains one of the most challenging conditions in clinical medicine. Even after accurate diagnosis of hypercortisolemia and tumor localization, successful tumor removal invariably heralds a period of secondary adrenal insufficiency, which renders the patient glucocorticoid-dependent and may take months to years to recover. In a series of 323 patients who underwent successful selective adenomectomies for Cushing's disease, Flitsch et al. reported that 11% remained hypocortisolemic beyond 3 years [7]. In this series, those patients requiring long-term corticosteroid replacement exhibited larger amounts of Crooke's cells in the nonadenomatous pituitary tissue, suggesting that the severity of cortisol excess may be an important determinant in the recovery of the HPA axis. With regard to adrenal Cushing's syndrome, HPA axis recovery time of up to 12 years has been reported in the literature [8]. During this recovery, although the physical and metabolic manifestations of CS gradually regress, sense of well-being and quality of life remain compromised, presumably due to symptoms of cortisol withdrawal and the inherent shortcomings of adrenal replacement therapy.

In the case reported here, the patient's HPA axis showed no sign whatsoever of recovery over a 6-year period after unilateral adrenalectomy. The prolonged suppression of the HPA axis could not be explained by other factors: (1) the patient's maintenance dose of hydrocortisone was limited to only 15 mg/day; (2) stress-dosing of hydrocortisone was limited to only a handful of episodes meriting the stress-dose; (3) the patient was not treated with other glucocorticoids (i.e., transdermal, inhaled, intranasal, intra-articular, or parenteral) or other medications or supplements that could suppress the HPA axis; and (4) cranial MRI did not disclose structural abnormalities of the pituitary and hypothalamus. Even during pregnancy—a state of HPA axis activation—this patient continued to have an undetectable a.m. cortisol level. Only after adding mifepristone, did the HPA axis show signs of improvement. Based on mifepristone's mechanism of action and evidence that resumption of normal hypothalamic CRH activity appears to be the rate-limiting step in HPA axis recovery [2], I propose that central glucocorticoid receptor (GR) blockade deprived the hypothalamus from GR activity, thereby stimulating the CRH-producing neurons of the hypothalamus. Indeed, it has been previously shown that even a single 100 mg dose of mifepristone enhances the ACTH response to CRH in normal volunteers [9]. In this patient, the initial rise of ACTH into the supranormal range followed by the subsequent normalization of cortisol some 2 months later provides indirect support for this hypothesis.

One can argue that simply lowering the dose of hydrocortisone could have yielded similar results. However, innumerable attempts to taper the dose of hydrocortisone below 15 mg/day (even by 2.5 mg increments) failed due to intolerable symptoms of profound fatigue, nausea, and arthralgia. It is therefore noteworthy that the patient did not exhibit signs or symptoms of adrenal insufficiency during the treatment with mifepristone. One explanation may be that mifepristone was introduced gradually starting with a low dose of only 150 mg thrice weekly, while simultaneously maintaining the patient on hydrocortisone replacement. The positive modulatory effects of mifepristone on stress-sensitive regions of the central nervous system (prefrontal cortex and ventral subiculum) may be another potential explanation [10]. Regardless of the possible mechanism/s, this report suggests a differential response when net glucocorticoid exposure is reduced by introducing a GU receptor antagonist as compared to just lowering the dose of steroid replacement.

Although this patient tolerated mifepristone remarkably well, the potential adverse effects of mifepristone deserve mention, particularly for women of reproductive age [11, 12]. Since mifepristone is also a progesterone receptor antagonist, thickening of the endometrial lining can develop, sometimes leading to abnormal vaginal bleeding. The antiprogestational effects will lead to termination of pregnancy. Therefore, pregnancy must be excluded prior to initiation of mifepristone and prevented while being on treatment. The use of mifepristone in patients with CS has also been associated with reversible decreases in high density lipoprotein- (HDL-) cholesterol and mild increases in serum thyroid stimulating hormone (TSH) levels. Other important considerations include drug-drug interactions (mifepristone is both metabolized by and is an inhibitor of CYP3A).

In summary, this case demonstrates the safe and successful use of mifepristone to rapidly restore the HPA axis in a woman with prolonged secondary adrenal insufficiency (SAI) after adrenalectomy for adrenal Cushing's syndrome (CS). The reader is cautioned that this use of mifepristone is off-label and investigational and requires further study. If these findings are replicated in a structured, IRB-approved protocol, then use of mifepristone to restore HPA function may also be potentially extended to the far more prevalent scenario of HPA axis suppression after exogenous glucocorticoid use.

Acknowledgments

The author thanks Dr. Andreas G. Moraitis and Dr. Precious J. Lim for their guidance and support.

References

[1] C. M. Berr, G. Di Dalmazi, A. Osswald et al., "Time to recovery of adrenal function after curative surgery for Cushing's syndrome depends on etiology," *Journal of Clinical Endocrinology and Metabolism*, vol. 100, no. 4, pp. 1300–1308, 2015.

[2] L. J. Muglia, L. Jacobson, C. Luedke et al., "Corticotropin-releasing hormone links pituitary adrenocorticotropin gene expression and release during adrenal insufficiency," *Journal of Clinical Investigation*, vol. 105, no. 9, pp. 1269–1277, 2000.

[3] H. Oskari, K. Kimmo, C. Horacio, S. Irving, L. Tapani, and L. Pekka, "Plasma concentrations and receptor binding of RU 486 and its metabolites in humans," *Journal of Steroid Biochemistry*, vol. 26, no. 2, pp. 279–284, 1987.

[4] R. C. Gaillard, A. Riondel, A. F. Muller, W. Herrmann, and E. E. Baulieu, "RU 486: a steroid with antiglucocorticosteroid activity that only disinhibits the human pituitary-adrenal system at a specific time of day," *Proceedings of the National Academy of Sciences of the United States of America*, vol. 81, no. 12, pp. 3879–3882, 1984.

[5] X. Bertagna, H. Escourolle, J. L. Pinquier et al., "Administration of RU 486 for 8 days in normal volunteers: antiglucocorticoid effect with no evidence of peripheral cortisol deprivation," *Journal of Clinical Endocrinology and Metabolism*, vol. 78, no. 2, pp. 375–380, 1994.

[6] P. Cohan, "Pasireotide and mifepristone: new options in the medical management of cushing's disease," *Endocrine Practice*, vol. 20, no. 1, pp. 84–93, 2014.

[7] J. Flitsch, D. K. Lüdecke, U. J. Knappe, and W. Saeger, "Correlates of long-term hypocortisolism after transsphenoidal microsurgery for Cushing's disease," *Experimental and Clinical Endocrinology and Diabetes*, vol. 107, no. 3, pp. 183–189, 1999.

[8] T. Maehana, T. Tanaka, N. Itoh, N. Masumori, and T. Tsukamoto, "Clinical outcomes of surgical treatment and longitudinal

non-surgical observation of patients with subclinical Cushing's syndrome and nonfunctioning adrenocortical adenoma," *Indian Journal of Urology*, vol. 28, no. 2, pp. 179–183, 2012.

[9] A. R. Hermus, G. F. Pieters, G. J. Pesman, A. G. H. Smals, T. J. Benraad, and P. W. C. Kloppenborg, "Enhancement of the ACTH response to human CRH by pretreatment with the antiglucocorticoid RU-486," *European Journal of Clinical Pharmacology*, vol. 31, no. 5, pp. 609–611, 1987.

[10] A. C. Wulsin, J. P. Herman, and M. B. Solomon, "Mifepristone decreases depression-like behavior and modulates neuroendocrine and central hypothalamic-pituitary-adrenocortical axis responsiveness to stress," *Psychoneuroendocrinology*, vol. 35, no. 7, pp. 1100–1112, 2010.

[11] M. Fleseriu, B. M. K. Biller, J. W. Findling, M. E. Molitch, D. E. Schteingart, and C. Gross, "Mifepristone, a glucocorticoid receptor antagonist, produces clinical and metabolic benefits in patients with Cushing's syndrome," *The Journal of Clinical Endocrinology & Metabolism*, vol. 97, no. 6, pp. 2039–2049, 2012.

[12] R. Pivonello, M. De Leo, A. Cozzolino, and A. Colao, "The treatment of cushing's disease," *Endocrine Reviews*, vol. 36, no. 4, pp. 385–486, 2015.

8

Type 2 Diabetes Mellitus, a Sequel of Untreated Childhood Onset Growth Hormone Deficiency Developing in a 17-Year-Old Patient

Rohan K. Henry (ID)[1] **and Ram K. Menon**[2]

[1]Division of Endocrinology, Department of Pediatrics, Nationwide Children's Hospital,
 The Ohio State University College of Medicine, Columbus, OH 43205, USA
[2]Division of Endocrinology, Department of Pediatrics, C.S. Mott Children's Hospital, Michigan Medicine,
 University of Michigan Medical School, Ann Arbor, MI 48109, USA

Correspondence should be addressed to Rohan K. Henry; rohan.henry@nationwidechildrens.org

Academic Editor: Lucy Mastrandrea

In a seminal report, a 17-year-old boy with panhypopituitarism had fatty liver (FL) amelioration with growth hormone (GH). By extension, since hepatic insulin resistance (IR) is key to FL and type 2 diabetes mellitus (T2DM), GH then may ameliorate the IR of T2DM. We present a 17-year-old nonobese female with untreated childhood onset growth hormone deficiency (CO-GHD) who developed type 2 diabetes mellitus (T2DM) and steatohepatitis with bridging fibrosis. Based on height z-score of – 3.1 and a history of radiation therapy as treatment for a medulloblastoma at 7 years of age, GHD was quite likely. GH therapy was, however, not initiated at 15 years of age (when growth was concerning) based on full skeletal maturity. After she developed T2DM, GHD was confirmed and GH was initiated. With its initiation, though insulin dose decreased from 2.9 (~155 units) to 1.9 units/kg/day (~ 100 units), her T2DM was, however, not fully reversed. This illustrates the natural history of untreated CO-GHD and shows that though hepatic IR can be ameliorated by GH, full reversal of T2DM may be prevented with irreversible hepatic changes (fibrosis). Clinicians caring for pediatric patients and otherwise should remember that, even in patients beyond the cessation of linear growth, GH can have a crucial role in both glucose and lipid metabolism.

1. Introduction

The role of growth hormone (GH) in growth promotion is well known by clinicians, however, less appreciated is its effect on metabolism in the well state. In 1936, Bernardo Houssay, M.D. in the New England Journal of Medicine, proposed that the anterior pituitary gland after the liver and pancreas plays a key role in glucose metabolism. That key role was later shown to be due in part to GH [1].

The effect of GH on glucose metabolism involves two phases: an initial phase which involves a decrease in glucose (an insulin-like effect) and a second phase which includes its effects on gluconeogenesis and fat mobilization [2]. In both states of growth hormone deficiency and excess, these effects on glucose metabolism will be altered.

Altered glucose and fat metabolism are important components of fatty liver (FL) and type 2 diabetes (T2DM), both states of hepatic insulin resistance (IR). In fact, a seminal case of fatty liver (FL) resolution with GH administration in a 17-year-old patient with panhypopituitarism treated initially with levothyroxine and hydrocortisone alone was reported by *Takano* et al. in 1997 [3]. This suggests that GH treatment of T2DM which may be associated with GHD has the potential to reduce the IR which may be present.

We outline a case of untreated childhood onset growth hormone deficiency (CO-GHD) who presented with type 2 diabetes mellitus (T2DM) and also steatohepatitis. We discuss her management and evidence from the basic sciences and clinical studies which show that her presentation with T2DM and steatohepatitis was likely associated with untreated GHD

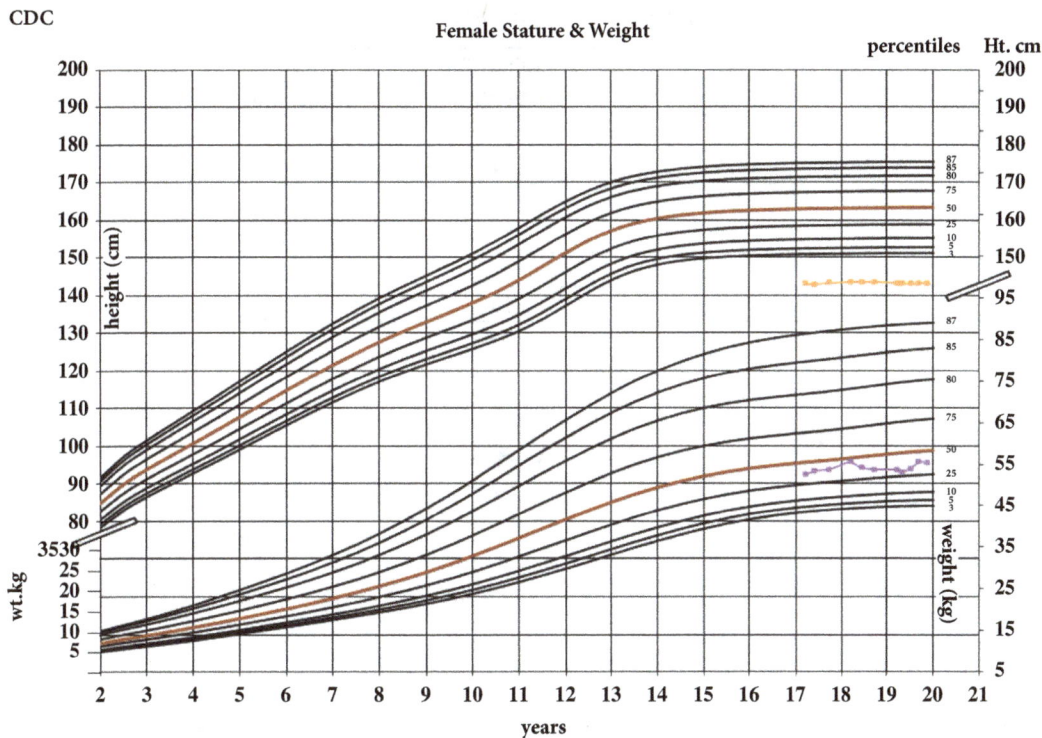

FIGURE 1: Patient's weight for age and height for age on CDC growth charts after being 17 years old.

and that with GH supplementation her condition was ameliorated. Lastly, we discuss the implications of this case.

2. Case Presentation

A 17-year-old nonobese Caucasian female who had a history of a medulloblastoma diagnosed at 7 years of age was treated with radiation therapy. She subsequently developed TSH and GnRH deficiencies. Though GHD was suspected based on height (z-score of – 3.1; see Figure 1), treatment had not been initiated based on the initial management focus being to treat her medulloblastoma. At 15 years of age when her bone age showed full skeletal maturity, her parents were informed that GH therapy could not be pursued because her linear growth was complete.

On presentation, the patient's height was 141.3 cm (z= - 3.1) and weight was 53 kgs (36th percentile for age). Body mass index was 25.8 kg/m^{-2} (86th percentile for age). Surveillance labs done at the oncology clinic showed glucosuria. Further testing showed HbA1c of 9.6% and on another day her fasting glucose was 277 mg/dL. Based on these results, diabetes mellitus was diagnosed.

When glutamic acid decarboxylase (GAD-65; Esoterix), islet-cell (Esoterix), insulin (Esoterix), and zinc transporter 8 (ARUP Laboratories) antibodies as well as DNA panel for maturity onset diabetes of youth (MODY) genes (HNF4α, GCK, IPF1, HNF1α, and HNF1β, [Athena Diagnostics]) returned all negative along with an elevated fasting C-peptide level of 3 ng/mL (normal: 0.4 - 2.1), T2DM was diagnosed. With the initiation of traditional basal/bolus insulin therapy using conventional dosing, a rapid escalation to peak total

daily insulin dose of 2.9 units/kg/day (~ 155 units/day) was required to treat her refractory hyperglycemia. Treatment nonadherence was thought to be the unlikely cause of her increased insulin requirements based on the agreement between her insulin dosing and prescription refill data.

A comprehensive evaluation for conditions associated with IR was negative. However, based on Arginine/Clonidine stimulation testing showing peak GH level of 0.8 (normal: ≥ 10 ng/mL), a diagnosis of GHD was made. GH supplementation was initiated at 0.3 mgs daily and titrated based on IGF-1 levels.

After GH was started, her systolic and diastolic blood pressures (BP) which were mildly elevated between 124-136 and 77-89, respectively, became more normal. Despite this, lisinopril 5 mgs once daily was added for microalbuminuria.

With the diagnosis of T2DM and our patient having a significant family history of adverse cardiovascular risk factors, she was started on atorvastatin 10 mgs once daily. Within 2 months of therapy, her LDL cholesterol (LDL-C) decreased to 74 mg/dL. Table 1 shows serial lipid profiles.

Though her diabetes was not fully reversed with GH, her HbA1c decreased to 5.9% and 5.8% at 6 and 19 months, respectively. Her insulin therapy requirement decreased to 1.9 units/kg/day (~ 100 units) at 12 months after the start of GH.

Magnetic Resonance Imaging (MRI) of the brain and abdomen indicated a small anterior pituitary gland and liver masses, respectively. Liver biopsy showed steatohepatitis with bridging fibrosis (Figure 2). With GH therapy, her liver transaminases trended to normalcy (Table 1). Repeat MRI abdomen at 20 months after the start of GH showed stability of the liver lesions when compared to that done at 14 months.

TABLE 1: Some of the patient's lab tests with reference to growth hormone start.

TEST	RESULT			REFERENCE RANGE
	Baseline	**12 mths**	**22 mths**	
Aspartate aminotransferase	92	36	33	< 40 U/L
Alanine aminotransferase	87	24	56	15- 50 U//L
Total Cholesterol	247	99	132	95- 195 mg/dL
HDL Cholesterol	32	27	43	40- 58 ng/dL
LDL Cholesterol	171	57	65	73- 117 mg/dL
Triglyceride	267	70	120	20-200 mg/dL
IGF-1	74	146	294	121-566 ng/mL

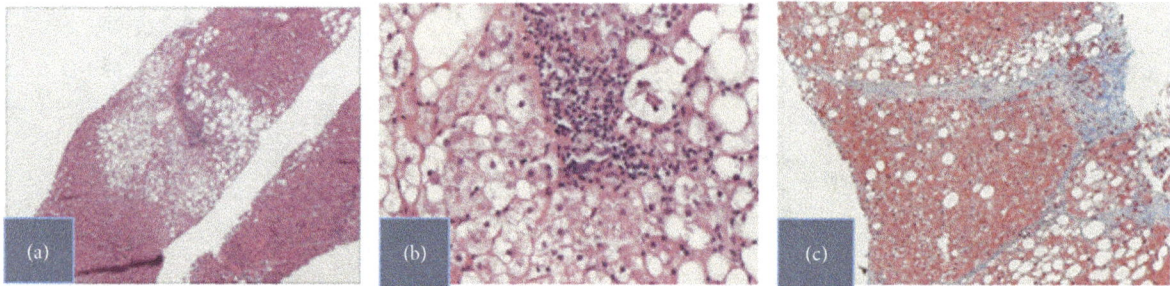

FIGURE 2: Slides from the patient's liver biopsy. (a) Low power liver section, (b) ballooning hepatocyte degeneration, a feature of hepatic cell death, and (c) intervening fibrous tissue seen as a terminal stage of liver injury. These all constitute steatohepatis with moderate steatosis.

These hyperintense lesions like the initial ones were located in the liver's parenchyma and the appearance of the liver was otherwise normal.

With GH therapy, the patient's stamina improved. She was now able to work for 20 hours weekly without becoming fully exhausted and her Quality of Life-Assessment of Growth Hormone Deficiency in Adults (QoL-AGHDA) and Quality of Life Satisfaction (QLS) scores, both questionnaire-based, improved (Figure 3).

3. Discussion

This case demonstrates that GH supplementation in an adolescent with CO-GHD led to improvements in transaminases, insulin requirements, and glucose control.

Several mouse models have corroborated the association of GHD with IR. In mice with liver GH receptor (GH-R) knockout, metabolic syndrome (MetS), steatohepatitis, increased inflammation, liver fibrosis, and hepatic tumor develop [4]. Additionally, a similar mouse model resulted in hyperinsulinemia, hyperglycemia, and IR. With the restoration of the liver's IGF-1 expression, there was an improvement in both insulin sensitivity and serum lipid profile. This, however, did not protect against hepatic inflammation induced by steatosis. This shows that GH and not IGF-1 directly affects lipid uptake and lipogenesis [5]. Also in a prior study again involving a liver specific GH receptor knockout mice, de novo lipogenesis was increased; however, this increase was not associated with the classic insulin mediated pathway [6]. So, our patient's IR and hepatic steatosis can be explained by her GHD based on data from some studies as well as the effect of GH in inhibiting this.

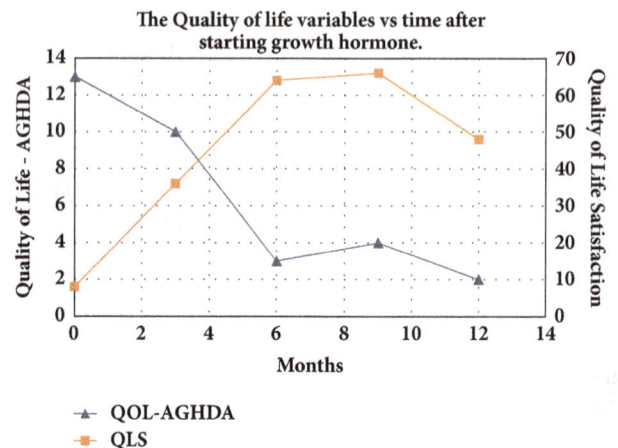

FIGURE 3: The patient's Quality of Life (QoL) scores with time. QoL-AGHDA: Quality of Life-Assessment of Growth Hormone Deficiency in Adults. QLS: Quality of Life Satisfaction. $_1$A decrease in score for QoL-AGHDA indicates an improvement in QoL-AGHDA, whereas an increase in QLS indicates an improvement while taking GH therapy.

Evidence for the association of hepatic steatosis with GHD is also provided by the abnormalities involving the downstream pathway of GH signal transduction. Mice with hepatocyte-specific deletion of Janus kinase 2 (JAK2L), involved in the postreceptor phase of GH signaling, were lean but had FL. They also showed increased levels of GH, triglycerides, and plasma free fatty acids. Since GH in some instances can cause lipolysis, GH-deficient *little* mice which were crossed to JAK2L mice had both a rescuing of the FL and an increased expression of a fatty acid transporter [7]. Though this provides a mechanism for the FL observed with the liver specific disruption of GH signaling, in the same mice, elevated GH levels occurring as a consequence of disrupted signaling can cause an increase in resting energy expenditure [8]. In this situation, steatohepatitis is prevented based on increased fatty acid utilization. So the putative lipolytic action of GH can be offset by hyperinsulinemia; hence, the action of GH is variable and depends on the physiological context.

Additionally, mice with signal transducer and activator of transcription (STAT) 5 mutations, another downstream signal from GH, also develop steatohepatitis [9]. Since pathologies involving the downstream pathways in GH signal transduction are associated with steatohepatitis, this supports the role of GH in lipid metabolism and the notion that the FL changes in our patient may be due to GHD.

Clinical reports about Laron syndrome, primary GH insensitivity involving a molecular defect in human GH-R, have also documented the development of FL, IR, and T2DM [10]. In addition, men with hypopituitarism have a high prevalence of nonalcoholic FL disease (NAFLD) in the absence of GH therapy. When these men were treated with GH, there was histological improvement in the liver. This demonstrates that NAFLD is predominantly attributable to GH [11].

Though a follow-up liver biopsy was not done, the trend to normal in our patient's transaminases (Table 1) supports the effect of GH on the liver and the likelihood that these changes were induced by GHD. Since our patient's steatohepatitis improved with GH treatment, she likely had a reduction in her hepatic IR. The evidence for this was seen in her decreased insulin requirements. This reduction in IR also was associated with her decreased blood pressures and these decreased pressures can be explained since IR negatively impacts endothelial cell function [12].

Moreover, the decrease in our patient's insulin resistance may also be explained by the positive impact of GH on β-cell function which is well described. In adults with lifetime congenital untreated GHD, there is reduced β-cell function [13]. In children with GHD who are supplemented with GH, β-cell secretory capacity is enhanced [14]. Additionally, studies in mice have shown that, with isolated GHD, β-cell function deteriorates. This deterioration is not due to changes in β-cell mass [15]. Studies by *Nielsen* et al. have shown that GH stimulates β-cell proliferation, glucose induced insulin release, and insulin gene expression *in vitro* [16]. These also provide a possible mechanism for the decrease in our patient's IR.

Atorvastatin was added to our patient's treatment because although an amelioration of her LDL-C was expected with GH therapy, this did not happen. Plausible explanations for this include a genetic basis for her hyperlipidemia. This could have been superimposed on an accumulated adverse CV risk profile which developed based on the time period of her untreated CO-GHD [17]. Atorvastatin was also added to her treatment as well since based on her history of T2DM, her LDL-C levels needed improvement.

Based on the points discussed, with evidence from adult studies, clinical reports, and, more recently, mouse models (even with the lack of pediatric studies, especially long-term ones) explaining the important contribution of GH to normal lipid and glucose metabolism, there is enough data to reinforce the benefits of treating GHD even when linear growth is completed.

Pediatric clinicians should highlight and reinforce that GH supplementation has the potential to prevent adverse metabolic consequences in untreated states of severe deficiency. Also important is the fact that, even with growth cessation, supplementation with GH may improve QoL-AGHDA and QLS scores [18]. These questionnaire-based scores address the impact of GHD on issues of relevance to patients with GHD and can be useful for tracking the patient's response to treatment. The QoL-AGHDA tool addresses the general impact of GHD on each patient whereas the QLS score accounts for the level of importance which each individual may place on the issues affecting his/her life and gives a summarized weighted score based on these.

In conclusion, this case illustrates not only that both NAFLD and T2DM are potential associations of untreated GHD but also that they may represent points along the natural history of hepatic IR secondary to untreated GHD. Furthermore, clinicians should ensure that patients with CO-GHD are not only treated in childhood but also appropriately transitioned to adult GH dosing after growth has ceased. This is important as GH can have a crucial role beyond the period of linear growth. With delayed GH initiation, it is possible that, with irreversible hepatic injury (such as bridging fibrosis in this patient), there may not be total amelioration of the metabolic manifestations seen in patients with GHD.

Additional Points

Learning Points. (i) Growth hormone is integral to both glucose and lipid metabolism even after the period of linear growth. (ii) Insulin resistance (IR) can be a feature of untreated growth hormone deficiency (GHD). (iii) Hepatic steatosis and type 2 diabetes mellitus (T2DM) being both hepatic IR states could be a feature of the natural history of untreated GHD. (iv) While growth hormone supplementation may ameliorate IR seen in the setting of T2DM and GHD, it is likely that delayed supplementation may not fully ameliorate IR if simple steatosis progresses to steatohepatitis with fibrosis.

Ethical Approval

No IRB approval was required by our institutions.

Authors' Contributions

Rohan K. Henry and Ram K. Menon contributed to drafting the article. Rohan K. Henry contributed to the critical revision of the article. All authors approved the final version of the article to be published.

Acknowledgments

The authors would like to thank Robert Hoffman, M.D., for his critical review of this manuscript.

References

[1] B. A. Houssay, "Carbohydrate Metabolism," *The New England Journal of Medicine*, vol. 214, no. 20, pp. 971–986, 1936.

[2] S. Melmed, "Medical progress: acromegaly," *The New England Journal of Medicine*, vol. 355, no. 24, pp. 2558–2573, 2006.

[3] S. Takanoj, S. Kanzaki, M. Sato, T. Kubo, and Y. Seino, "Effect of growth hormone on fatty liver in panhypopituitarism," *Archives of Disease in Childhood*, vol. 76, no. 6, pp. 537-538, 1997.

[4] Y. Fan, X. Fang, A. Tajima et al., "Evolution of Hepatic Steatosis to Fibrosis and Adenoma Formation in Liver-Specific Growth Hormone Receptor Knockout Mice," *Frontiers in Endocrinology*, vol. 5, 2014.

[5] Z. Liu, J. Cordoba-Chacon, R. D. Kineman et al., "Growth hormone control of hepatic lipid metabolism," *Diabetes*, vol. 65, no. 12, pp. 3598–3609, 2016.

[6] J. Cordoba-Chacon, N. Majumdar, E. O. List et al., "Growth hormone inhibits hepatic de novo lipogenesis in adult mice," *Diabetes*, vol. 64, no. 9, pp. 3093–3103, 2015.

[7] B. C. Sos, C. Harris, S. M. Nordstrom et al., "Abrogation of growth hormone secretion rescues fatty liver in mice with hepatocyte-specific deletion of JAK2," *The Journal of Clinical Investigation*, vol. 121, no. 4, pp. 1412–1423, 2011.

[8] S. Y. Shi, R. García Martin, R. E. Duncan et al., "Hepatocyte-specific deletion of Janus kinase 2 (JAK2) protects against diet-induced steatohepatitis and glucose intolerance," *The Journal of Biological Chemistry*, vol. 287, no. 13, pp. 10277–10288, 2012.

[9] Y. Cui, A. Hosui, R. Sun et al., "Loss of signal transducer and activator of transcription 5 leads to hepatosteatosis and impaired liver regeneration," *Hepatology*, vol. 46, no. 2, pp. 504–513, 2007.

[10] Z. Laron, "Lessons from 50 years of study of laron syndrome," *Endocrine Practice*, vol. 21, no. 12, pp. 1395–1402, 2015.

[11] H. Nishizawa, G. Iguchi, A. Murawaki et al., "Nonalcoholic fatty liver disease in adult hypopituitary patients with GH deficiency and the impact of GH replacement therapy," *European Journal of Endocrinology*, vol. 167, no. 1, pp. 67–74, 2012.

[12] E. Cersosimo and R. A. DeFronzo, "Insulin resistance and endothelial dysfunction: The road map to cardiovascular diseases," *Diabetes/Metabolism Research and Reviews*, vol. 22, no. 6, pp. 423–436, 2006.

[13] C. R. Oliveira et al., "Insulin sensitivity and beta-cell function in adults with lifetime, untreated isolated growth hormone deficiency," *The Journal of Clinical Endocrinology & Metabolism*, vol. 97, no. 3, pp. 1013–1019, 2012.

[14] F. Baronio, L. Mazzanti, Y. Girtler et al., "The influence of growth hormone treatment on glucose homeostasis in growthhormone-deficient children: A six-year follow-up study,"

Hormone Research in Paediatrics, vol. 86, no. 3, pp. 196–200, 2016.

[15] J. Cordoba-Chacon, M. D. Gahete, N. K. Pokala et al., "Long-But Not Short-Term Adult-Onset, Isolated GH Deficiency in Male Mice Leads to Deterioration of β-Cell Function, Which Cannot Be Accounted for by Changes in β-Cell Mass," *Endocrinology*, vol. 155, no. 3, pp. 726–735, 2014.

[16] J. H. Nielsen, E. D. Galsgaard, A. M ldrup et al., "Regulation of beta-cell mass by hormones and growth factors," *Diabetes*, vol. 50, no. Supplement 1, pp. S25–S29, 2001.

[17] G. Johannsson, K. Albertsson-Wikland, B.-Å. Bengtsson et al., "Discontinuation of growth hormone (GH) treatment: Metabolic effects in GH-deficient and GH-sufficient adolescent patients compared with control subjects," *The Journal of Clinical Endocrinology & Metabolism*, vol. 84, no. 12, pp. 4516–4524, 1999.

[18] S. M. Webb, "Measurements of quality of life in patients with growth hormone deficiency," *Journal of Endocrinological Investigation*, vol. 31, Suppl 9, pp. 52–55, 2008.

9

Severe Short Stature in an Adolescent Male with Prader-Willi Syndrome and Congenital Adrenal Hyperplasia: A Therapeutic Conundrum

Meredith Wasserman,[1] Erin M. Mulvihill,[2] Angela Ganan-Soto,[3] Serife Uysal,[4] and Jose Bernardo Quintos[4]

[1] The Warren Alpert Medical School, Brown University, Providence, RI, USA
[2] College of Human Ecology, Cornell University, Ithaca, NY, USA
[3] Alexian Brothers Women and Children's Hospital and Amita Health Medical Group, Hoffman Estates, IL, USA
[4] Division of Pediatric Endocrinology, Rhode Island Hospital and Hasbro Children's Hospital, The Warren Alpert Medical School, Brown University, Providence, RI, USA

Correspondence should be addressed to Jose Bernardo Quintos; jbquintos@brown.edu

Academic Editor: Wayne V. Moore

Congenital adrenal hyperplasia (CAH) due to 21-hydroxylase deficiency results in excess androgen production which can lead to early epiphyseal fusion and short stature. Prader-Willi syndrome (PWS) is a genetic disorder resulting from a defect on chromosome 15 due to paternal deletion, maternal uniparental disomy, or imprinting defect. Ninety percent of patients with PWS have short stature. In this article we report a patient with simple-virilizing CAH and PWS who was overtreated with glucocorticoids for CAH and not supplemented with growth hormone for PWS, resulting in a significantly short adult height.

1. Introduction

Congenital adrenal hyperplasia (CAH) is a family of autosomal recessive disorders characterized by the inability to synthesize cortisol from cholesterol in the adrenal cortex. 21-hydroxylase deficiency is the most common cause of CAH and results in excess androgen production due to shunting of intermediates in the steroidogenic pathway toward androgen synthesis. Excess androgen production causes the early fusion of epiphyseal plates, which stunts growth. Treatment for patients with CAH involves the delicate balance of suppressing adrenal androgens while maintaining normal growth.

Short adult stature is common in 21-hydroxylase deficiency. Final adult height in patients with CAH is 1.38 SD lower than the population norm and their corrected height (final height minus genetic height potential) is 1.03 SD lower than their genetic height potential [1]. This short stature is seen in CAH patients even in the presence of early glucocorticoid treatment to suppress excess androgen production.

Excess glucocorticoids can inhibit the pituitary production of growth hormone and contribute to short stature [2]. Growth hormone therapy was found to improve final height in patients with CAH by 9.2 cm ± 6.7 cm in males and 10.5 ± 3.7 cm in females [3]. It was also found that treatment with growth hormone can counter the growth-suppressing effects of glucocorticoids [4].

Prader-Willi syndrome (PWS) is a genetic disorder resulting from a defect within the Prader-Willi critical region on chromosome 15 due to paternal deletion, maternal uniparental disomy, or imprinting defect. PWS is characterized by short adult stature, morbid obesity, hypogonadism, and characteristic facial features such as narrow bifrontal diameter, almond-shaped eyes, and small mouth with down-turned corners and thin upper lip [5]. Decreased growth hormone levels and serum levels of insulin-like growth factor 1 (IGF-1) and insulin-like growth factor binding protein 3 (IGFBPG-3) are found in 40–100% of children with PWS [6, 7]. Additionally, 90% of patients with PWS have short stature [7]. In the absence of growth hormone treatment and subsequent pubertal growth spurt, average adult height in male and female patients with PWS is 155 cm and 148 cm, respectively [7]. Patients treated with growth hormone were found to attain a mean adult height SDS of -0.3 ± 1.2 [8]. In addition, growth hormone treatment has been shown to improve body composition by lowering body fat percentage and increasing lean body mass [9].

To our knowledge, no case of simultaneous PWS and CAH has been reported. Here, we report a patient with PWS and CAH who was overtreated with glucocorticoids for CAH and not supplemented with growth hormone for PWS, resulting in a significantly short adult height.

2. Case Report

We report the case of a 20-year-old Puerto Rican male with PWS and CAH who we initially evaluated when he was 17-year-old. He was born full term with birth weight 5 pounds, birth length 21 inches, and physical exam showing bilateral cryptorchidism and hypotonia. Karyotype is 46XY. He experienced feeding difficulties in the first year of life and had delayed milestones. At 3 years of age, he developed pubic hair and his laboratory examination showed 17-hydroxyprogesterone level 8,676 ng/dL and DHEAS 29 ug/dL. He was diagnosed with CAH and prescribed hydrocortisone. He was treated with fludrocortisone for the first 1-2 years after diagnosis. At 9 years of age his dose of hydrocortisone was increased, most likely due to poor compliance to treatment and poor adrenal control. Over the years he struggled with obesity and learning and behavioral problems, including hyperactivity and short attention span. He was diagnosed with PWS at 12 years of age, showing a submicroscopic deletion of chromosome 15 (q11.2q11.2). He was not treated with growth hormone. He also had a bone age of left hand in an outside hospital when he was 12 years old and his bone age was reported as 16 years old.

He came to our clinic for the first time at age 17 years. He was taking hydrocortisone 40 mg in the morning and 20 mg in the evening (equivalent of 37.5 mg/m^2/day). Usual dose of hydrocortisone is 10–20 mg/m^2/day. Physical exam showed a short male with almond-shaped eyes, fair skin, narrow bifrontal diameter, upslanted palpebral fissures (Figure 1), and small hands (Figure 2). His height was 138.6 cm (<5 percentile; −5.3 height SDS), height age 10 years, weight 72.3 kg (72nd percentile; 0.6 SDS), BMI 37.48 kg/m^2 (>99th percentile), and blood pressure 124/56 mmHg. He was Tanner 3 for pubic hair and genitalia and testicular volume was 5-6 cc. His mother measured 159.8 cm and his father's reported height is 167.6 cm. Based on parental heights his midparental target height is 170.2 cm.

Laboratory investigation showed 17-hydroxyprogesterone 16 ng/dL, testosterone 5 ng/dL (normal for 17-year-old male is 348–1197 ng/dL), and renin 10.47 ng/mL/hr. Adrenal hormone assays were done by liquid chromatography tandem mass spectrometry at Esoterix Laboratory Services in Calabasas Hills, California, United States. Bone age of left hand was 17 years of age, consistent with his chronological age.

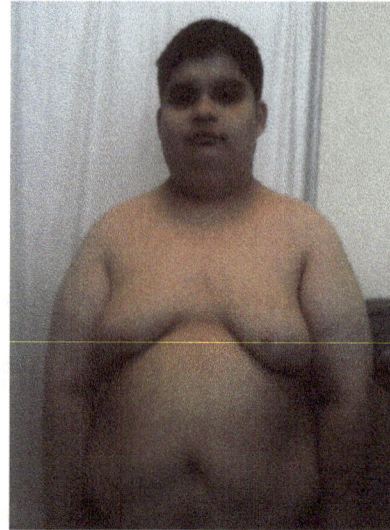

FIGURE 1: Characteristic facial features of Prader-Willi syndrome.

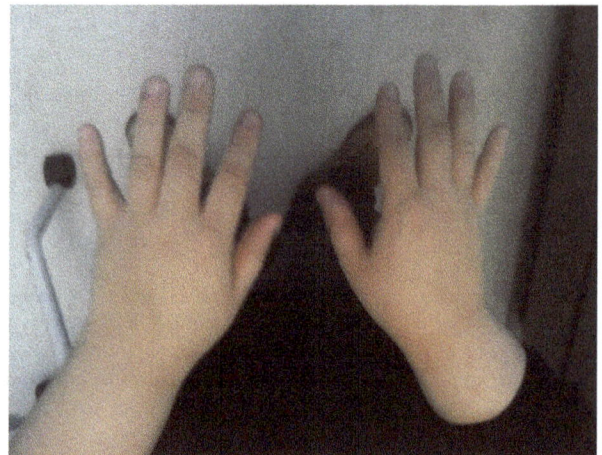

FIGURE 2: Small hands characteristic of Prader-Willi syndrome.

We decreased his hydrocortisone dosage to 20 mg twice a day (equivalent 25 mg/m^2/day) with the goal of 17-hydroxyprogesterone level between 100 and 1000 ng/dL and androstenedione level normal for age and sex. His electrolytes were Na$^+$ 135 mEq/L, Cl$^-$ 100 mEq/L, CO$_2$ 27 mEq/L, and K$^+$ 4.3 mEq/L. Hologic DEXA scan showed bone mass density below expected range for age. Femoral neck Z-score was −3.2, total hip Z-score was −3.3, and total body Z-score was −1.7 (−1.0 to −2.5 SDS).

He returned to our clinic six months later and his laboratory work-up showed 17-hydroxyprogesterone 23 ng/dL, androstenedione < 10 ng/dL (normal 17–72 ng/dL for Tanner 3), renin 3.43 ng/mL/hr, IGFBP-3 2.8 mg/L (normal 2.5–4.8 mg/L), and IGF-1 252 ng/mL (normal 161–467 mg/mL, mean 290 mg/mL). We further decreased hydrocortisone dose to 20 mg in the morning and 10 mg in the evening (equivalent 18 mg/m^2/day), which resulted in normal adrenal control (17-hydroxyprogesterone 426 ng/dL).

TABLE 1: Results of high dose ACTH stimulation test with 250 mcg cosyntropin.

Time (mins)	Cortisol (ug/dl)	17-Hydroxyprogesterone (ng/dl)	Androstenedione (ng/dl)	Testosterone (ng/dl)	DHEA (ng/dl)
0	2.9	9,410	106	31	<20
60	2.7	11,000	77	44	<20

Pituitary gonadal axis evaluation showed LH 9.6 mIU/mL, FSH 21 mIU/mL, testosterone 139 ng/dL, and androstenedione 35 ng/dL, suggesting primary gonadal dysgenesis. Patient has not had testicular ultrasound to evaluate for testicular adrenal rest tumor (TART). An ACTH stimulation test to confirm the CAH diagnosis was done after stopping hydrocortisone for 24 hours. Results were consistent with simple-virilizing CAH due to 21-hydroxylase deficiency (Table 1). Genetic testing for mutations in the 21-hydroxylase gene has not been obtained. Testosterone cypionate 50 mg IM every four weeks was started. This resulted in more aggressive behavior and violent outbursts prompting discontinuation of testosterone treatment.

3. Discussion

We report the case of a 20-year-old male with simple-virilizing CAH and PWS, who probably had both periods of undertreatment and overtreatment of glucocorticoids and lack of growth hormone treatment for PWS, resulting in a significantly short adult height. He also displayed aggressive behavior after being treated with testosterone for hypogonadism associated with PWS. To the best of our knowledge, there has been no other reported case of a patient with both PWS and CAH.

The chance of one patient having both CAH and PWS is extremely rare. The worldwide incidence of severe classic CAH is 1 in 15,000 [10] and the incidence of PWS is estimated to be between 1 in 10,000 and 1 in 30,000 [11].

The late diagnosis of PWS and missed opportunity for growth hormone therapy contributed to his significantly short adult stature. His height is 138.6 cm, or −5.3 height SDS. The average adult height of a male with untreated PWS is 155 cm (−3 height SDS) [7]. In one study, PWS patients treated with growth hormone achieved a mean adult height of −0.3 ± 1.2 SDS, while untreated patients achieved a mean adult height of −3.1 ± 1 SDS [8]. A retrospective study evaluating the effects of hydrocortisone treatment in patients with classical CAH showed that higher doses of glucocorticoids in children with CAH may result in decreased linear growth [12]. Additionally, a study of children with classic CAH found that the average final height for males treated with an average daily hydrocortisone dose of 19.7 ± 2.9 mg/m^2/day was 163.1 ± 6.6 cm [13].

We hypothesize that periods of undertreatment and overtreatment with hydrocortisone contributed to his severe short stature. Factors that cause short adult stature in patients with 21-hydroxylase deficiency are (1) elevated adrenal androgens, which cause advanced epiphyseal maturation and premature epiphyseal fusion, (2) early or precocious puberty, which also leads to premature epiphyseal fusion, and (3) overtreatment with glucocorticoids [14]. Our patient also experienced premature epiphyseal fusion, as his bone age was 16 years at a chronological age 12. This premature epiphyseal fusion could be a result of periods of glucocorticoid undertreatment for CAH. Additionally, overtreatment with glucocorticoids most likely led to growth hormone suppression leading to poor growth velocity. This case reinforces the importance of growth hormone treatment for PWS and reduced glucocorticoid treatment for CAH, especially when both disorders coexist in one patient. Additionally, our patient was born small for gestational age with a birth weight of 5 pounds. It was unclear if he had catch-up growth due to lack of growth charts from the early childhood period. This may also have contributed to his short stature.

Our patient's elevated FSH and LH levels and low testosterone levels indicate that he has primary hypogonadism. Eiholzer et al. found that boys with PWS have a combination of central and primary hypogonadism involving deficiency of LH and testosterone secretion at puberty and damage of the seminiferous tubules and Sertoli cells, resulting in reduced inhibin B levels and elevated FSH levels [15]. Additionally primary hypogonadism may be due to TART. Vanzulli et al. reported a prevalence of 27% of TART in a group of 30 CAH patients with age range 9 to 32 years [16]. It is more commonly seen in patients with salt-wasting CAH; however TART also occurs in patients with simple-virilizing and nonclassical CAH.

He displayed aggressive and violent behavior after testosterone replacement therapy, prompting discontinuation of therapy. It has been suggested that, to avoid aggressive behavior, testosterone should be administered daily as gels or patches instead of monthly depot intramuscular (IM) injections [17, 18]. Depot testosterone preparations cause unpredictable peaks and troughs, which may cause mood instability. Others suggest reducing the testosterone dose for patients with PWS to one-third to one-half of the normally recommended dose [6].

This unique case highlights the importance of careful follow-up and monitoring of adrenal androgens in a patient with CAH. Glucocorticoid dosage should be adjusted to prevent premature epiphyseal fusion and to maximize growth. This case also highlights the importance of early diagnosis of PWS and initiation of growth hormone treatment. When hypotonia, feeding difficulties followed by obesity, characteristic facial features, and characteristics of hypogonadism present in an infant, PWS should be suspected [5]. This case also exemplifies the need for further research on appropriate testosterone therapy for males with PWS.

Authors' Contributions

Meredith Wasserman, M.S., wrote first draft of manuscript and edited. Erin M. Mulvihill edited and revised manuscript drafts. Angela Ganan-Soto, M.D., performed data collection and edited manuscript, with direct care of patient. Serife Uysal, M.D., edited and revised manuscript drafts. Jose Bernardo Quintos, M.D., conceptualized manuscript, edited, and revised, with direct care of patient.

References

[1] K. Muthusamy, M. B. Elamin, G. Smushkin et al., "Adult height in patients with congenital adrenal hyperplasia: a systematic review and metaanalysis," *Journal of Clinical Endocrinology and Metabolism*, vol. 95, no. 9, pp. 4161–4172, 2010.

[2] A. Grigorescu-Sido, M. Bettendorf, E. Schulze, I. Duncea, and U. Heinrich, "Growth analysis in patients with 21-hydroxylase deficiency influence of glucocorticoid dosage, age at diagnosis, phenotype and genotype on growth and height outcome," *Hormone Research*, vol. 60, no. 2, pp. 84–90, 2003.

[3] K. Lin-Su, M. D. Harbison, O. Lekarev, M. G. Vogiatzi, and M. I. New, "Final adult height in children with congenital adrenal hyperplasia treated with growth hormone," *Journal of Clinical Endocrinology and Metabolism*, vol. 96, no. 6, pp. 1710–1717, 2011.

[4] D. B. Allen, J. R. Julius, T. J. Breen, and K. M. Attie, "Treatment of glucocorticoid-induced growth suppression with growth hormone," *Journal of Clinical Endocrinology and Metabolism*, vol. 83, no. 8, pp. 2824–2829, 1998.

[5] V. A. Holm, S. B. Cassidy, M. G. Butler et al., "Prader-Willi syndrome: consensus diagnostic criteria," *Pediatrics*, vol. 91, no. 2, pp. 398–402, 1993.

[6] M. Cataletto, M. Angulo, G. Hertz, and B. Whitman, "Prader-Willi syndrome: a primer for clinicians," *International Journal of Pediatric Endocrinology*, vol. 2011, no. 1, 12 pages, 2011.

[7] P. Burman, E. M. Ritzén, and A. C. Lindgren, "Endocrine dysfunction in Prader-Willi syndrome: a review with special reference to GH," *Endocrine Reviews*, vol. 22, no. 6, pp. 787–799, 2001.

[8] M. A. Angulo, M. Castro-Magana, M. Lamerson, R. Arguello, S. Accacha, and A. Khan, "Final adult height in children with Prader-Willi syndrome with and without human growth hormone treatment," *American Journal of Medical Genetics, Part A*, vol. 143, no. 13, pp. 1456–1461, 2007.

[9] A. L. Carrel, S. E. Myers, B. Y. Whitman, J. Eickhoff, and D. B. Allen, "Long-term growth hormone therapy changes the natural history of body composition and motor function in children with prader-willi syndrome," *Journal of Clinical Endocrinology and Metabolism*, vol. 95, no. 3, pp. 1131–1136, 2010.

[10] D. P. Merke and S. R. Bornstein, "Congenital adrenal hyperplasia," *The Lancet*, vol. 365, no. 9477, pp. 2125–2136, 2005.

[11] B. J. Hurren and N. A. M. S. Flack, "Prader-Willi Syndrome: a spectrum of anatomical and clinical features," *Clinical Anatomy*, vol. 29, no. 5, pp. 590–605, 2016.

[12] W. Bonfig, S. B. Pozza, H. Schmidt, P. Pagel, D. Knorr, and H. P. Schwarz, "Hydrocortisone dosing during puberty in patients with classical congenital adrenal hyperplasia: An evidence-based recommendation," *Journal of Clinical Endocrinology and Metabolism*, vol. 94, no. 10, pp. 3882–3888, 2009.

[13] Z. Aycan, S. Akbuga, E. Cetinkaya, G. Ocal, and M. Berberoglu, "Final height of patients with classical congenital adrenal hyperplasia," *The Turkish Journal of Pediatrics*, vol. 51, no. 6, pp. 539–544, 2009.

[14] J. B. Q. Quintos, M. G. Vogiatzi, M. D. Harbison, and M. I. New, "Growth hormone therapy alone or in combination with gonadotropin-releasing hormone analog therapy to improve the height deficit in children with congenital adrenal hyperplasia," *Journal of Clinical Endocrinology and Metabolism*, vol. 86, no. 4, pp. 1511–1517, 2001.

[15] U. Eiholzer, D. l'Allemand, V. Rousson et al., "Hypothalamic and gonadal components of hypogonadism in boys with Prader-Labhart-Willi syndrome," *Journal of Clinical Endocrinology and Metabolism*, vol. 91, no. 3, pp. 892–898, 2006.

[16] A. Vanzulli, A. DelMaschio, and P. Paesano, "Testicular masses in association with adrenogenital syndrome: US findings," *Radiology*, vol. 183, no. 2, pp. 425–429, 1992.

[17] S. B. Cassidy and D. J. Driscoll, "Prader-Willi syndrome," *European Journal of Human Genetics*, vol. 17, no. 1, pp. 3–13, 2009.

[18] F. Benarroch, H. J. Hirsch, L. Genstil, Y. E. Landau, and V. Gross-Tsur, "Prader-Willi Syndrome: Medical Prevention and Behavioral Challenges," *Child and Adolescent Psychiatric Clinics of North America*, vol. 16, no. 3, pp. 695–708, 2007.

10

Hypogonadotropic Hypogonadism and Kleefstra Syndrome due to a Pathogenic Variant in the *EHMT1* Gene: An Underrecognized Association

Ana Patricia Torga,[1] **Juanita Hodax,**[2] **Mari Mori** ⓘ,[3]
Jennifer Schwab,[3] **and Jose Bernardo Quintos** ⓘ[2]

[1]*Summer Intern, Division of Pediatric Endocrinology and Diabetes, Rhode Island Hospital/Hasbro Children's Hospital,*
111 Plain St, 3rd Floor, Providence, RI 02903, USA
[2]*Division of Pediatric Endocrinology and Diabetes, Rhode Island Hospital/Hasbro Children's Hospital,*
The Warren Alpert Medical School of Brown University, 111 Plain St, 3rd Floor, Providence, RI 02903, USA
[3]*Division of Human Genetics, Hasbro Children's Hospital, The Warren Alpert Medical School of Brown University,*
2 Dudley Street, Suite 460, Providence, RI 02903, USA

Correspondence should be addressed to Jose Bernardo Quintos; jbquintos@brown.edu

Academic Editor: Carlo Capella

Kleefstra syndrome is a genetic condition characterized by intellectual disability, childhood hypotonia, and facial dysmorphisms. Genital anomalies such as micropenis, cryptorchidism, and hypospadias have been reported in 30-40% of males diagnosed with the disease. However, endocrinological investigations have been limited. We describe a case of an adolescent male with Kleefstra syndrome due to a pathogenic variant in the *EHMT1* gene whose workup for isolated micropenis is suggestive of a partial hypogonadotropic hypogonadism. A possible endocrine mechanism of the genital anomaly associated with Kleefstra syndrome is discussed.

1. Introduction

Kleefstra syndrome is characterized by intellectual disability and childhood hypotonia with associated distinctive facial dysmorphisms. A heterozygous microdeletion at chromosome 9q34.3 overlapping the euchromatin histone methyltransferase 1 (*EHMT1*) gene accounts for more than 75% of cases, and the remainder are associated with a heterozygous intragenic pathogenic variant in the *EHMT1 gene* [1, 2]. Prevalence data is limited but it has been estimated at 1 per 200,000 individuals diagnosed with intellectual disability [3]. Typical phenotypes highly associated with the syndrome include heart defects, seizures, obesity, eye abnormalities, behavioral problems, and genital abnormalities. Penetrance is likely 100% with variable expressivity.

Genital anomalies including micropenis, cryptorchidism, and hypospadias have been reported in 30-40% of male patients with Kleefstra syndrome [4]. The mechanisms of genital anomalies among these patients have yet to be established and there are no reports of endocrinological investigations of these patients.

We describe a case of an adolescent male diagnosed with Kleefstra syndrome due to a de novo pathogenic variant c.2712+1G>A in the *EHMT1* gene and isolated micropenis. The boy's clinical presentation, workup, management, and possible endocrine mechanisms underlying his genital anomaly are discussed.

2. Case Presentation

The patient is an 11-year-old boy with Kleefstra syndrome whom we first evaluated in the endocrine clinic at 8 years of age for obesity to rule out Prader-Willi Syndrome. The patient is the male child of nonconsanguineous Guatemalan parents and was born at 41 weeks of gestation by spontaneous vaginal

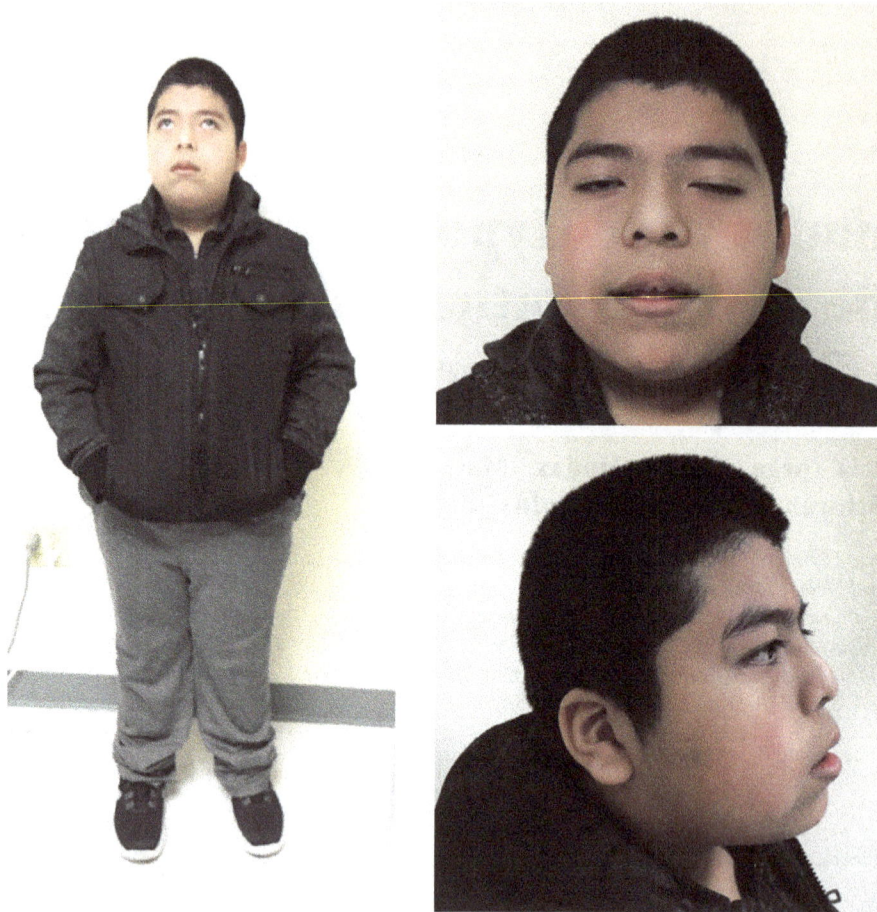

FIGURE 1: Index patient showing facial dysmorphism (prominent eyebrow, low set ears, midfacial retrusion, and mild prognathism).

delivery to a 23-year-old, gravida 2, para 1 mother. The pregnancy was not complicated by any exposure to viral infection or medications. His siblings and both parents are healthy with no family history of miscarriages, stillbirths, congenital abnormalities, or learning difficulties. He was reportedly well until the 19th day of life when he presented with projectile vomiting and was diagnosed with pyloric stenosis. Surgery was uncomplicated; however, he had recurrent surgical site infections which required multiple readmissions.

In the interim, parents reported that he was able to walk at 3 years of age and had his first meaningful word ("Papa") at 16 months. He attended special education classes and received speech, occupational, and physical therapy to address his developmental delays. He had recurrent acute otitis media managed with bilateral myringotomy. Audiologic evaluation also showed conductive hearing loss.

He was evaluated by endocrinology for the first time at age 8 years and 8 months. He was referred by his pediatrician for evaluation of obesity and hyperphagia which raised concern for possible Prader-Willi Syndrome. His height was 134.1 cm (64th percentile), weight 63.5 kg (>99th percentile), and BMI 35.31 kg/m2. Examination was remarkable for facial dysmorphisms (prominent eyebrows, low set ears, midfacial retrusion, and mild prognathism) (see Figure 1) and a genital exam that showed a micropenis. He was prepubertal with

TABLE 1: Summary of initial endocrine hormones done at the age of 9 years and 4 months.

LH (0.02 - 0.3)	<0.005 mIU/mL
FSH (0.26-3)	0.184 mIU/mL
Testosterone (2.5-10)	9 ng/dL
Free T4 (0.8-1.8)	0.81 ng/dL
AM Cortisol (>10)	10.5 mcg/dl

3 cc testicles bilaterally, stretched penile length measured at 3 cm (-2.5 SD for age is 2.8 cm; mean is 6.3 cm), and no hypospadias. Laboratory tests showed LH <0.005 mIU/ml (normal 0.02-0.3), FSH 0.184 mIU/ml (normal 0.26-3), and testosterone 9 ng/dL (normal 2.5-10) (Table 1). Brain MRI was normal.

Due to the low gonadotropins associated with isolated micropenis, treatment was initiated via intramuscular testosterone cypionate injection of 50 mg given once a month for 3 months at the age of 9 years and 9 months. He had a normal response to testosterone injections with an improvement of stretched penile length to 5.5 cm (normal 6.3 ± 1.0 cm) after 4 doses. There were no noted adverse reactions to testosterone injections such as acne, fluid retention, decreased testicular size, or mood swings.

TABLE 2: GnRH agonist stimulation test (leuprolide acetate) done at the age of 10 years and 9 months using 20 mcg/kg/subcutaneous dose.

	Baseline	60 min	120 min	24 hrs
LH (mIU/mL)	1.7	9.2	10	11
FSH (mIU/mL)	2.3	3.4	3.7	4.3
Testosterone (ng/dL)	48	-	-	132

TABLE 3: hCG stimulation test done at the age of 10 years and 10 months with 5000-unit hCG once a day for 3 days.

	Baseline (Day 1)	Day 3	Day 6
Testosterone (ng/dL)	43	300	298
DHT (ng/dL)	4.6	14	15
T:DHT (<35)	9.3	21.4	19.1
Androstenedione (ng/dL)	85	105	66
T:Androstenedione (>0.8)	0.5	2.9	4.5

TABLE 4: Summary of clinical features seen in 21 patients [4] with *EHMT1* mutations and in the index patient.

Clinical Features	% in 21 patients	Index Patient
Short Stature	17	-
Overweight (BMI>25)	42	+
Developmental Delay/Intellectual Disability	100	+
Heart defect	43	-
Genital anomaly (in males)	43	+
Renal anomaly	14	-
Recurrent Infections	64	+
Hearing deficit	24	+
Gastro-esophageal reflux	14	-
Epilepsy	24	-
Behavioral/psychiatric problems	75	-
Anomalies on brain imaging	63	-
Tracheomalacia	5	-
Umbilical/inguinal hernia	10	-
Anal atresia	5	-
Musculoskeletal anomaly	19	-
Respiratory complications	5	-

At 10 years and 9 months, GnRH agonist stimulation testing showed an LH-predominant response with peak LH of 11 mIU/mL and peak FSH of 4.3 mIU/mL at 24 hours. Testosterone rose from 48 ng/dL (normal <7-130 ng/dL) at baseline to 132 ng/dL at 48 hours (Table 2). hCG stimulation testing was done 1 month later for Leydig cell function assessment. Table 3 shows that there was adequate testosterone biosynthesis (testosterone 300 ng/dL at 24 hours after the last dose of hCG) and no evidence of 5-alpha reductase deficiency (T:DHT 21.4; normal T:DHT <35) after the hCG stimulation test.

Genetics referral was initially made at 1 year of age due to global developmental delay, nontypical dysmorphic facial features, and the history of hypertrophic pyloric stenosis. There was no history of hypotonia, feeding difficulties, or seizures. Karyotype showed normal male (46, XY). Fragile X testing was normal. DNA oligonucleotide microarray study revealed a likely benign maternally inherited 563 kb

duplication at 1p22.3. Rett syndrome, although rare in males, was ruled out at the age of 4 by sequencing and deletion/duplication analysis of the MECP2 gene. At 9 years of age, methylation study for Prader-Willi critical region was negative. Whole exome sequencing (WES) revealed a heterozygous de novo pathogenic variant c.2712+1G>A in the *EHMT1* gene, which led to a diagnosis of Kleefstra syndrome. Mitochondrial DNA was sequenced as part of the WES with normal result. Developmental delays, dysmorphic facies, genital abnormalities, obesity, hearing loss, and recurrent infections are consistent with the diagnosis (see Table 4). Screening tests for other associated phenotypic presentations were done. Echocardiogram and renal ultrasound were negative.

Follow-up exam at 11 years of age showed Tanner stage 3 pubic hair, testicular volume of 6 cc bilaterally, and stretched penile length 6 cm (normal 6.4 ± 1.1 cm). Parents deny any new behavioral changes, sleep disturbances, or seizures. He continues to follow up in the endocrine clinic for monitoring of pubertal progression and growth velocity.

3. Discussion

We report the case of an 11-year-old male with Kleefstra syndrome, isolated micropenis, and possible hypogonadotropic hypogonadism. We propose partial hypogonadotropic hypogonadism as an underlying mechanism of micropenis in association with the genetic syndrome. This case report provides an extensive endocrinology workup to further elucidate this mechanism.

Partial hypogonadotropic hypogonadism is known to cause incomplete pubertal development in both boys and girls. Male patients with partial hypogonadotropic hypogonadism can present with micropenis, cryptorchidism, stalled pubertal progression, or hypogonadism with normal testicular volume (Fertile Eunuch Syndrome) [5]. Female patients can present with incomplete breast development and primary amenorrhea [6].

The initial labs of our patient showed undetectable LH and FSH levels suggestive of hypogonadotropic hypogonadism. After testosterone replacement therapy, a normal hypothalamic-pituitary-gonadal axis response on GnRH agonist and hCG stimulation tests was noted. This can be explained by a partial hypogonadotropic hypogonadism. Normalization of gonadotropin levels after treatment has been reported in 10% of males with idiopathic hypogonadotropic hypogonadism in a retrospective study done to reevaluate the need for lifelong hormonal therapy [7]. There are also reports of spontaneous reversal of idiopathic hypogonadotropic hypogonadism associated with the Fertile Eunuch variant [5]. This reflects the plasticity of the reproductive neuroendocrine system. It also highlights the importance of conducting an endocrine evaluation in patients presenting with potentially treatable genital anomalies including those associated with genetic syndromes such as Kleefstra syndrome.

Kleefstra syndrome is a recently identified cause of intellectual disability with associated childhood hypotonia and distinctive facial dysmorphism. More than 75% of the cases reported in the literature have been found to have a subtelomeric deletion at chromosome 9q34.3 while the remaining cases are due to a heterozygous pathogenic variant of the EHMT1 gene [4]. Similar phenotypic presentations such as cardiac defects, obesity, and seizures have been reported for the two genotypes.

Molecular testing confirmed a de novo heterozygous pathogenic variant in the *EHMT1* gene diagnostic of Kleefstra syndrome. The variant destroys a canonical splice donor site and likely leads to a truncated protein [8]. *EHMT1* is expressed in multiple tissues including the brain, eyes, male embryonic germ cells, epididymis, ovary, heart, and aorta [9]. In the brain, it is expressed in the hypothalamus and the pituitary gland showing that it can potentially play a role in gonadotropin secretion.

Only male patients present with genital anomalies such as micropenis, cryptorchidism, and hypospadias but these have been reported in both genotypes (62.5% with microdeletions,

33% with *EHMT1* gene mutation). Case series on Kleefstra syndrome [1, 4, 10] do not report the endocrine evaluation of these patients presenting with associated genital anomalies limiting the available pool of knowledge to identify its underlying mechanism. Micropenis etiology can be classified as primary hypogonadism, insufficient testosterone secretion (hypogonadotropic hypogonadism), testosterone activation defect, developmental, or idiopathic [11]. Chromosome 9q34.3 overlaps the nasal embryonic LH-releasing hormone factor (NELF) gene which is associated with some patients with autosomal dominant idiopathic hypogonadotropic hypogonadism [12]. It can be speculated that loss of function in the gene underlies hypogonadotropic hypogonadism in 9q34.3 deletion-related Kleefstra syndrome. However, in patients with *EHMT1* gene pathogenic variants such as our patient the mechanism remains unclear.

Assessment of the serum gonadotropins, pituitary hormones, testosterone, and its derivatives is a practical starting point to determine the level at which the hypothalamic-pituitary-gonadal axis is affected [13]. Ideally, the GnRH agonist stimulation testing should have been done prior to testosterone therapy. However, both LH and FSH were quite low for age at onset, which makes partial hypogonadotropic hypogonadism a strong differential for micropenis in this patient in the setting of Kleefstra syndrome.

Partial hypogonadotropic hypogonadism could be a potential cause of isolated micropenis in some patients with Kleefstra syndrome. This case is a reminder that genital anomalies associated with Kleefstra syndrome due to an intragenic variant in the *EHMT1* gene warrant investigation of underlying neuroendocrine imbalances that may cause genital anomalies and affect the progression of puberty, especially during adolescence. Continued monitoring of pubertal progression should be done in patients treated with hormone-replacement therapy for micropenis. There is still a possibility of stalled pubertal progression in patients with partial hypogonadotropic hypogonadism. Findings of continuous testicular growth and increase in serum testosterone in the absence of treatment are strong indicators of a normally functioning hypothalamic-pituitary-gonadal axis [7]. Maintenance of a normal hormonal status in patients with partial hypogonadotropic hypogonadism is expected to have positive impacts on other aspects of development (e.g., achievement of genetic potential for height, lean muscle mass, bone mineralization, metabolism, mood, and cognitive function) [14]. Further studies are needed to elucidate the mechanism of the association of hypogonadotropic hypogonadism with pathogenic variants in the *EHMT1* gene.

Authors' Contributions

Ana Patricia Torga, M.D., wrote the first draft of the manuscript and edited it. Juanita Hodax, M.D., performed data collection, edited the manuscript, and was involved with direct care of patient. Mari Mori, M.D., and Jennifer Schwab, M.S., CGC, edited the manuscript, with direct patient care. Jose Bernardo Quintos, M.D., conceptualized, edited, and revised the manuscript, with direct care of patient.

References

[1] D. R. Stewart and T. Kleefstra, "The chromosome 9q subtelomere deletion syndrome," *American Journal of Medical Genetics Part C: Seminars in Medical Genetics*, vol. 145, no. 4, pp. 383–392, 2007.

[2] T. Kleefstra, H. G. Brunner, J. Amiel et al., "Loss-of-function mutations in Euchromatin histone methyl transferase 1 (EHMT1) cause the 9q34 subtelomeric deletion syndrome," *American Journal of Human Genetics*, vol. 79, no. 2, pp. 370–377, 2006.

[3] T. Kleefstra, W. M. Nillesen, and H. G. Yntema, "Kleefstra Syndrome," in *Gene Reviews*, M. P. Adam, H. H. Ardinger, and R. A. Pagon, Eds., pp. 1993–2018, University of Washington, Seattle, WA, USA, 2010, [Updated 2015 May 7].

[4] M. H. Willemsen, A. T. Vulto-Van Silfhout, W. M. Nillesen et al., "Update on Kleefstra syndrome," *Molecular Syndromology*, vol. 2, no. 3–5, pp. 202–212, 2012.

[5] N. Pitteloud, P. A. Boepple, S. Decruz, S. B. Valkenburgh, W. F. Crowley Jr., and F. J. Hayes, "The fertile eunuch variant of idiopathic hypogonadotropic hypogonadism: spontaneous reversal associated with a homozygous mutation in the gonadotropin-releasing hormone receptor," *The Journal of Clinical Endocrinology & Metabolism*, vol. 86, no. 6, pp. 2470–2475, 2001.

[6] M. Beranova, "Prevalence, phenotypic spectrum, and modes of inheritance of gonadotropin-releasing hormone receptor mutations in idiopathic hypogonadotropic hypogonadism," *The Journal of Clinical Endocrinology & Metabolism*, vol. 86, no. 4, pp. 1580–1588, 2001.

[7] V. F. Sidhoum, Y.-M. Chan, and M. F. Lippincott, "Reversal and relapse of hypogonadotropic hypogonadism: resilience and fragility of the reproductive neuroendocrine system," *The Journal of Clinical Endocrinology & Metabolism*, vol. 99, no. 3, pp. 861–870, 2014.

[8] A. Rump, L. Hildebrand, A. Tzschach, R. Ullmann, E. Schrock, and D. Mitter, "A mosaic maternal splice donor mutation in the EHMT1 gene leads to aberrant transcripts and to Kleefstra syndrome in the offspring," *European Journal of Human Genetics*, vol. 21, no. 8, pp. 887–890, 2013.

[9] T. Kleefstra, M. Smidt, M. J. G. Banning et al., "Disruption of the gene euchromatin histone methyl transferase1 (Eu-HMTase1) is associated with the 9q34 subtelomeric deletion syndrome," *Journal of Medical Genetics*, vol. 42, no. 4, pp. 299–306, 2005.

[10] M. Iwakoshi, N. Okamoto, N. Harada et al., "9q34.3 Deletion Syndrome in Three Unrelated Children," *American Journal of Medical Genetics*, vol. 126, no. 3, pp. 278–283, 2004.

[11] N. Hatipoglu and S. Kurtoglu, "Micropenis: etiology, diagnosis and treatment approaches," *Journal of Clinical Research in Pediatric Endocrinology*, vol. 5, no. 4, pp. 217–223, 2013.

[12] N. Xu, H.-G. Kim, B. Bhagavath et al., "Nasal embryonic LHRH factor (NELF) mutations in patients with normosmic hypogonadotropic hypogonadism and Kallmann syndrome," *Fertility and Sterility*, vol. 95, no. 5, pp. 1613.e7–1620.e7, 2011.

[13] R. Fraietta, D. S. Zylberstejn, and S. C. Esteves, "Hypogonadotropic hypogonadism revisited," *Clinics*, vol. 68, no. 1, pp. 81–88, 2013.

[14] V. Mirone, F. Debruyne, G. Dohle et al., "European association of urology position statement on the role of the urologist in the management of male hypogonadism and testosterone therapy," *European Urology*, vol. 72, no. 2, pp. 164–167, 2017.

11

Cerebrovascular Accident due to Thyroid Storm: Should We Anticoagulate?

Alex Gonzalez-Bossolo, Alexis Gonzalez-Rivera, and Santiago Coste-Sibilia

Internal Medicine Training Program, Department of Medicine, University District Hospital, University of Puerto Rico School of Medicine, P.O. Box 365067, San Juan, PR 00936-5067, USA

Correspondence should be addressed to Alex Gonzalez-Bossolo; alex.gonzalez7@upr.edu

Academic Editor: Osamu Isozaki

Thyroid storm is a life-threatening condition that occurs secondary to an uncontrolled hyperthyroid state. Atrial fibrillation is a cardiovascular complication occurring in up to 15% of patients experiencing thyroid storm, and if left untreated this condition could have up to a 25% mortality rate. Thyroid storm with stroke is a rare presentation. This case report details a left middle cerebral artery (MCA) stroke with global aphasia and thyroid storm in a 53-year-old Hispanic male patient. Although uncommon, this combination has been reported in multiple case series. Although it is well documented that dysfunctional thyroid levels promote a hypercoagulable state, available guidelines from multiple entities are unclear on whether anticoagulation therapy is appropriate in this situation.

1. Introduction

Thyroid storm is a life-threatening condition that is associated with an uncontrolled hyperthyroid state caused by a precipitating event, such as recent surgery, trauma, infection, iodine load, or poor adherence to antithyroid medications [1]. Although tachycardia is the most common cardiovascular manifestation of thyroid storm, atrial fibrillation occurs in up to 15% of patients [2, 3]. Thyroid hormone dysregulation affects the coagulation pathway and promotes settings in which a stroke may occur [4]. There is, however, no clear recommendation for anticoagulation therapy in patients experiencing thyroid storm. This case report describes a 53-year-old Hispanic man who experienced a left middle cerebral artery (MCA) stroke and global aphasia with coexisting thyroid storm.

2. Case Presentation

A 53-year-old man with a history of untreated hyperthyroidism (toxic nodule), chronic smoking, and arterial hypertension arrived to the emergency room of our institution complaining of disorientation, restlessness, palpitations, vomiting, abdominal pain, and fever (not quantified) that had begun over 48 hours prior. Worsening symptoms, including right-sided weakness and difficulty understanding verbal language and communication with his spouse in the previous 24 hours, prompted the patient's assistance to our institution. Upon evaluation by the emergency room physician, the patient had a decreased neurological status with poor response to pain and verbal stimuli, for which he was endotracheally intubated to secure his airway. A head computed tomography (CT) scan without intravenous contrast revealed a gross acute left middle cerebral artery (MCA) territory infarction with no associated hemorrhage and minimal compression of the left lateral ventricle (Figures 1 and 2). The patient had a National Institutes of Health stroke scale value of 9/42, so the emergency department consulted the internal medicine department for further management. Thrombolytic therapy was not indicated due to the timing of symptom appearance.

Upon evaluation in our department, we determined that the patient was acutely ill with a Glasgow Coma Scale score 11/15 when assessed while off sedation and on mechanical ventilation support with adequate oxygenation. His vital signs showed that he had a remarkable high fever (39.8°C),

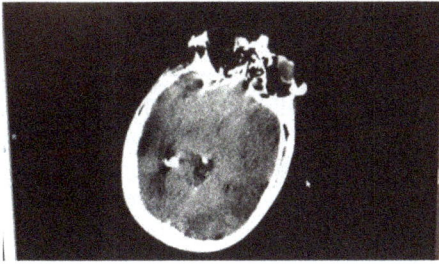

FIGURE 1: Head computed tomography image without contrast, showing left middle cerebral artery territory infarction.

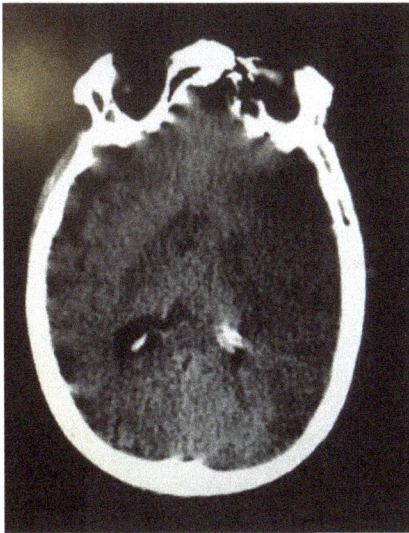

FIGURE 2: High density within left middle cerebral artery territory, corresponding to the site of arterial occlusion.

TABLE 1: Thyroid function tests and serum chemistries.

	Upon hospital arrival	Upon discharge
Thyroid stimulating hormone (μIU/mL)	<0.225	N/A[a]
Total T4 (μg/dL)	16.50	12.2
Free T4 (ng/dL)	5.49	2.3
Sodium (mEq/L)	147	143
Potassium (mEq/L)	3.8	3.5
Blood urea nitrogen (mg/dL)	32	29.5
Creatinine (mg/dL)	0.82	0.50
Calcium (mg/dL)	8.5	8.4
Phosphorus (mg/dL)	3.70	3.5
Magnesium (mg/dL)	2.22	2.0
Albumin (g/dL)	2.7	2.5
Carbon dioxide (mEq/L)	25.2	26.7
Prothrombin time (s)	13	N/A[a]
Partial thromboplastin time (s)	30	N/A[a]
INR (s)	1.0	N/A[a]
White blood cell ($\times 10^3/\mu$L]	8.8	7.5
Hemoglobin (g/dL)	14.7	14.0
Hematocrit (%)	44	42
Platelet count ($\times 10^9$/L)	300	350

[a]Value not available.

tachycardia (heart rate: 107 bpm), and elevated blood pressure 180/90 mmHg. A physical examination revealed right hemiplegia with bibasilar crackles and an irregular rhythm. He also exhibited remarkable pedal edema. An electrocardiogram revealed atrial fibrillation with adequate ventricular response. Due to a patient history of untreated hyperthyroidism secondary to problems with medical insurance as well as clinical signs and symptoms, the patient was diagnosed with thyroid storm. The patient had a Burch and Wartofsky score of 70, which is indicative of thyroid storm [5]. Treatment was initiated immediately, using a beta blocker (60 mg of propranolol) to control adrenergic symptoms, a thionamide (200 mg of propylthiouracil) to block hormone synthesis, and a glucocorticoid (100 mg of hydrocortisone) to reduce T4-T3 conversion. Lugol's iodine solution (10 drops of 8 mg iodine per 0.05 mL drop) used to stop thyroid hormone synthesis was initiated 1 hour after the antithyroid drugs. Additionally, along with statin therapy (atorvastatin 80 mg), clopidogrel 75 mg and enoxaparin 40 mg were administered as secondary stroke prevention. Intravenous diuretics were given to treat fluid overload symptoms.

Laboratory results revealed no leukocytosis or leukopenia, adequate hemoglobin and hematocrit levels, no electrolytes disturbances, and a negative toxicology screen. Thyroid function tests were abnormal (thyroid stimulating hormone: <0.225 μIU/mL, total thyroxine: 16.50 mcg/dL, and free thyroxine: 5.49 ng/dL) (Table 1). A chest radiograph revealed opacity projecting at the right lower lung field with silhouetting of the diaphragm and increased interstitial lung markings, which were consistent with pulmonary edema. A two-dimensional echocardiogram revealed atrial fibrillation at baseline, mild left ventricular systolic dysfunction, no valvulopathies, and mild left atrium and right atrium dilation. Based on the Japanese Thyroid Association criteria for thyroid storm, this case met the criteria for definitive diagnosis of TS1-grade thyroid storm [5].

Our patient was treated aggressively for thyroid storm upon arrival to our institution. Successful extubation was achieve on day 6 following admission. When the patient's mental status recovered, he confirmed that his fever palpitations and nausea preceded the paralysis, confirming that the events of thyrotoxicosis leaded to the stroke. In addition, his sinus rhythm returned to normal after completed hyperthyroidism treatment and his pedal edema improved. The patient was transferred to a rehabilitation center for inpatient physical therapy on the 8th day of admission. Following physical therapy sessions, he was discharged and given thionamide therapy with methimazole for his hyperthyroidism and was followed up by primary endocrinologist for further management. Based on the clinical progression of the patient's illness, we feel that if early anticoagulation had been started, the cerebrovascular accident with associated global aphasia might have been prevented.

3. Discussion

Thyroid storm is a life-threatening condition that occurs due to an accentuated hyperthyroid state. Recent studies report a mortality range from 8 to 25% [6]. Thyroid storm usually presents in patients with a current history of poorly treated thyrotoxicosis. It can also be precipitated by an infection, recent surgery, or recent trauma, among other things. The clinical presentation resembles an accentuated catabolic state. Fever is a very common sign and is often accompanied by sweating. Other manifestations include agitation, diarrhea, nausea, vomiting, abdominal pain, jaundice, seizures, and coma [5, 7]. A link between the cardiovascular system and elevated thyroid function has also been characterized. Sinus tachycardia is the most common electrocardiographic finding, but atrial fibrillation can also occur and is the most common cardiovascular complication, arising in 5–15% of cases [2, 3]. Another important link that was recently discovered is between thyroid hormone and coagulation pathways. Thyrotoxicosis promotes a hypercoagulable state due to a shortened activated partial thromboplastin time, increased fibrinogen levels, and increased factor VIII and factor X activity [4]. These abnormalities predispose a patient to stroke regardless of heart rhythm.

Although these links are known and the mechanisms have been documented, there are no specific or clear-cut recommendations regarding anticoagulation therapy in these patients. Guidelines from multiple entities also do not include hyperthyroidism as a risk factor for stroke. The most recent American Thyroid Association (ATA) guidelines for thyrotoxicosis management do not clearly state that anticoagulation therapy should be included only suggesting its use in the event of heart failure [8]. In 2014, the American Heart Association (AHA), American College Cardiology (ACC), and the Heart Rhythm Society (HRS) published guidelines for atrial fibrillation (AF) management. They stated that the evidence associating thyrotoxicosis with AF was not sufficient enough to recommend anticoagulation therapy administration. Anticoagulation should be guided by the CHA2DS2-VASc risk factors, which do not include hyperthyroidism [9]. Although no large randomized controlled trials have assessed this association, many case reports/series have documented it. Yuen et al. reported a case series of 21 subjects with thyrotoxicosis and atrial fibrillation, in which 23% of the patients had developed systemic emboli [10]. In another study, Bar-Sela and associates describe 30 out of 142 thyrotoxic patients with concomitant atrial fibrillation, 12 (40%) of whom experienced an embolic event [11]. In a recent prospective cohort study from Taiwan, 3176 patients with hyperthyroidism were followed for 5 years and compared with subjects without hyperthyroidism. The risk for developing a stroke was 1.4-fold greater in the hyperthyroidism cohort compared with the control group after adjusting for several confounders [12].

In conclusion, although some clinical evidence exists concerning cardioembolic stroke in thyrotoxic patients, no standard of care exists in this situation, likely because the clinical protocol is based on case reports and methodologically flawed small-scale studies. However, the decision for anticoagulation in thyrotoxicosis should be based on the patient's risk factors, as shown in previous studies, and not solely on the presence of thyroid storm. The case presented here highlights an important unresolved issue regarding the administration of anticoagulation therapy in patients with thyrotoxicosis with atrial fibrillation.

Acknowledgments

The authors wish to thank Editage® for English language editing. The authors are also grateful to Yolianne Lozada Capriles, MD, for invaluable advice and discussion about the paper and Raymond Rivera Vergara for literature review.

References

[1] N. J. Sarlis and L. Gourgiotis, "Thyroid emergencies," *Reviews in Endocrine and Metabolic Disorders*, vol. 4, no. 2, pp. 129–136, 2003.

[2] P. Petersen and J. M. Hansen, "Stroke in thyrotoxicosis with atrial fibrillation," *Stroke*, vol. 19, no. 1, pp. 15–18, 1988.

[3] A. W. Petersen, G. D. Puig-Carrión, and A. López-Candales, "Should we revisit anticoagulation guidelines during thyroid storm?" *Boletín de la Asociación Médica de Puerto Rico*, vol. 107, no. 1, pp. 62–66, 2015.

[4] M. Franchini, M. Montagnana, F. Manzato, and P. P. Vescovi, "Thyroid dysfunction and hemostasis: an issue still unresolved," *Seminars in Thrombosis and Hemostasis*, vol. 35, no. 3, pp. 288–294, 2009.

[5] T. Akamizu, T. Satoh, O. Isozaki et al., "Diagnostic criteria, clinical features, and incidence of thyroid storm based on nationwide surveys," *Thyroid*, vol. 22, no. 7, pp. 661–679, 2012.

[6] T. E. Angell, M. G. Lechner, C. T. Nguyen, V. L. Salvato, J. T. Nicoloff, and J. S. LoPresti, "Clinical features and hospital outcomes in thyroid storm: a retrospective cohort study," *The Journal of Clinical Endocrinology & Metabolism*, vol. 100, no. 2, pp. 451–459, 2015.

[7] R. A. Nordyke, F. I. Gilbert Jr., and A. S. M. Harada, "Graves' disease. Influence of age on clinical findings," *Archives of Internal Medicine*, vol. 148, no. 3, pp. 626–631, 1988.

[8] R. S. Bahn, H. B. Burch, D. S. Cooper et al., "Hyperthyroidism and other causes of thyrotoxicosis: management guidelines of the American Thyroid Association and American Association of Clinical Endocrinologists," *Thyroid*, vol. 21, no. 6, pp. 593–646, 2011.

[9] C. T. January, L. S. Wann, J. S. Alpert et al., "2014 AHA/ACC/HRS guideline for the management of patients with atrial

fibrillation: a report of the American college of Cardiology/American heart association task force on practice guidelines and the heart rhythm society," *Journal of the American College of Cardiology*, vol. 64, no. 21, pp. el–e76, 2014.

[10] R. W. Yuen, D. H. Gutteridge, P. L. Thompson, and J. S. Robinson, "Embolism in thyrotoxic atrial fibrillation," *The Medical Journal of Australia*, vol. 1, no. 13, pp. 630–631, 1979.

[11] S. Bar-Sela, M. Ehrenfeld, and M. Eliakim, "Arterial embolism in thyrotoxicosis with atrial fibrillation," *Archives of Internal Medicine*, vol. 141, no. 9, pp. 1191–1192, 1981.

[12] J.-J. Sheu, J.-H. Kang, H.-C. Lin, and H.-C. Lin, "Hyperthyroidism and risk of ischemic stroke in young adults: a 5-year follow-up study," *Stroke*, vol. 41, no. 5, pp. 961–966, 2010.

12

A Case of Hyperparathyroidism due to a Large Intrathyroid Parathyroid Adenoma with Recurrent Episodes of Acute Pancreatitis

Kazunori Kageyama,[1,2] **Noriko Ishigame,**[1,2] **Aya Sugiyama,**[1,2] **Akiko Igawa,**[3] **Takashi Nishi,**[3] **Satoko Morohashi,**[4] **Hiroshi Kijima,**[4] **and Makoto Daimon**[1]

[1]*Department of Endocrinology and Metabolism, Hirosaki University Graduate School of Medicine, 5 Zaifu-cho, Hirosaki, Aomori 036-8562, Japan*

[2]*Department of Endocrinology and Metabolism, Odate Municipal General Hospital, 3-1 Yutaka-cho, Odate 017-8550, Japan*

[3]*Department of Gastroenterological Surgery, Hirosaki University Graduate School of Medicine, 5 Zaifu-cho, Hirosaki, Aomori 036-8562, Japan*

[4]*Department of Pathology and Bioscience, Hirosaki University Graduate School of Medicine, 5 Zaifu-cho, Hirosaki, Aomori 036-8562, Japan*

Correspondence should be addressed to Kazunori Kageyama; kageyama@hirosaki-u.ac.jp

Academic Editor: Carlo Capella

We report a case of a 66-year-old woman who developed hyperparathyroidism due to a large intrathyroid parathyroid adenoma with episodes of acute pancreatitis. She had previously been treated for acute pancreatitis twice. Serum calcium was 12.4 mg/dL, and intact parathyroid hormone was 253 pg/dL. Ultrasonography and computed tomography of the neck with contrast enhancement revealed a soft tissue mass (28 mm transverse diameter) within the left lobe of the thyroid. ^{99m}Tc-MIBI scintigraphy demonstrated focal accumulation due to increased radiotracer uptake in the left thyroid lobe. Left hemithyroidectomy was performed. Histopathology showed no signs of invasion, and this is consistent with parathyroid adenoma. Immunostaining was positive for expression of chromogranin A and parathyroid hormone. The patient had no episode of pancreatitis after the operation. In a patient with recurrent episodes of pancreatitis, the possibility of complication with hyperparathyroidism should be considered.

1. Introduction

Primary hyperparathyroidism (PHPT) is a common endocrine disorder characterized by hypercalcemia and excessive secretion of parathyroid hormone (PTH) [1]. PHPT is most commonly caused by a single adenoma of the parathyroid gland. Patients with PHPT tend to develop complications such as reduction of bone mineral density, nephrolithiasis, and gastric ulcer, which may impair quality of life [1, 2]. In the management of PHPT, parathyroidectomy of the abnormal gland is the gold standard for effective treatment. Generally, most parathyroid adenomas remain relatively small, measuring under a few centimeters and weighing less than 1 g [3]. Large or giant parathyroid adenomas are seldom seen in patients with PHPT [4], and in such cases differential diagnosis is necessary to rule out malignancy.

Acute pancreatitis may be induced by cholelithiasis and alcohol abuse in adults; however, the incidence of pancreatitis in patients with hyperparathyroidism was reported to be only 1.5% [5]. Here, we report a case of hyperparathyroidism due to a large intrathyroid parathyroid adenoma with episodes of acute pancreatitis. She had been treated for acute pancreatitis twice. However, there was no episode of pancreatitis after the operation.

2. Case Report

A 66-year-old woman was consulted for evaluation of hypercalcemia. She had been treated for acute pancreatitis twice

TABLE 1: General laboratory data.

	Before operation	After operation	(normal values)
Peripheral blood			
White blood cells (/μL)	5690	6210	(3500–8500)
Red blood cells (/μL)	3.50	3.84	(3.80–4.80×10^6)
Hemoglobin (g/dL)	10.7	10.9	(11.5–15.0)
Hematocrit (%)	31.5	32.7	(34.0–45.0)
Platelets (/μL)	18.1	20.5	(13.0–35.0×10^4)
Blood biochemistry			
Total protein (g/dL)	6.9	7.0	(6.7–8.3)
Albumin (g/dL)	4.0	4.0	(3.9–4.9)
Total bilirubin (mg/dL)	0.8	0.6	(0.2–1.1)
Aspartate aminotransferase (U/L)	28	25	(10–35)
Alanine aminotransferase (U/L)	20	16	(7–38)
γ-Glutamyltranspeptidase (U/L)	28	35	(0–65)
Alkaline phosphatase (IU/L)	263	213	(104–340)
Urea nitrogen (mg/dL)	17	14	(8–25)
Creatinine (mg/dL)	0.81	0.89	(0.40–1.10)
Sodium (mmol/L)	145	143	(137–146)
Chloride (mmol/L)	112	107	(99–110)
Potassium (mmol/L)	4.4	4.0	(3.5–4.9)
Calcium (mg/dL)	12.4	9.6	(8.3–10.3)
Phosphorus (mg/dl)	2.4	3.3	(2.4–4.7)
Total cholesterol (mg/dl)	215	182	(115–220)
Triglyceride (mg/dL)	185	215	(20–150)
Plasma glucose (mg/dL)	98	132	(70–110)
Hemoglobin A1c (%)	5.1	5.8	(4.6–6.2)
Intact PTH	253.0	59.3	(8.7–79.5)

(3 years and 6 months earlier) and had a long history of hypercalcemia (calcium 12.3 mg/dL (albumin 3.5 g/dL) and calcium 12.7 mg/dL (albumin 4.7 g/dL), resp.). Abdominal computed tomography (CT) had shown the presence of multiple renal stones, but not gall stones or pancreatic calcifications (not shown). She usually consumed 350 mL of beer 4 times/week. She had no palpable mass in her neck. Endocrine evaluation was performed according to relevant clinical guidelines, and the patient gave written informed consent for all tests performed. Renal function was within normal. As shown in Table 1, serum calcium was 12.4 mg/dL (reference range: 8.3–10.3), albumin 4.0 g/dL, and intact PTH (iPTH) level 253 pg/dL (reference range: 8.7–79.5). Urinary calcium/creatinine ratio was 0.39. Serum phosphorus was 2.4 mg/dL (reference range: 2.4–4.7).

Contrast-enhanced CT of the neck revealed a heterogeneous soft tissue mass (28 mm transverse diameter), clearly defined, within the left thyroid (Figure 1(a)). T-scores of femoral and lumbar bone mineral density were −1.3 and −2.7, respectively. Technetium-99m-methoxyisobutylisonitrile (^{99m}Tc-MIBI) scintigraphy demonstrated focal accumulation of increased radiotracer uptake in the left lobe of the thyroid on both early and delayed images (Figure 1(b)).

Left hemithyroidectomy was performed due to the clearly defined soft tissue mass within the left thyroid. Histopathology showed no signs of invasion, and this is consistent with parathyroid adenoma. The adenoma was composed mainly of chief cells and oxyphil cells, covered with a fibrous capsule (Figure 2(a)). Evaluation of chromogranin A expression showed positive chromogranin A immunostaining (Figure 2(b)). Evaluation for PTH expression showed positive PTH immunostaining (Figure 2(c)). Soon after surgery, the elevated calcium and iPTH were normalized. The patient has had no episodes of pancreatitis for one year after the operation.

3. Discussion

This is an unusual case of hyperparathyroidism due to a large parathyroid adenoma. This present patient had been treated for acute pancreatitis twice. Pooled clinical data suggest an association between PHPT and pancreatitis [6, 7]. Serum calcium levels in PHPT with pancreatitis were found to be higher than those in PHPT without pancreatitis [6, 8]. Acute pancreatitis may be caused by calcium-induced activation of intrapancreatic trypsinogen to trypsin. However, only a

(a)

Early

Delay

Tc MIBI Early

Tc MIBI Delay

(b)

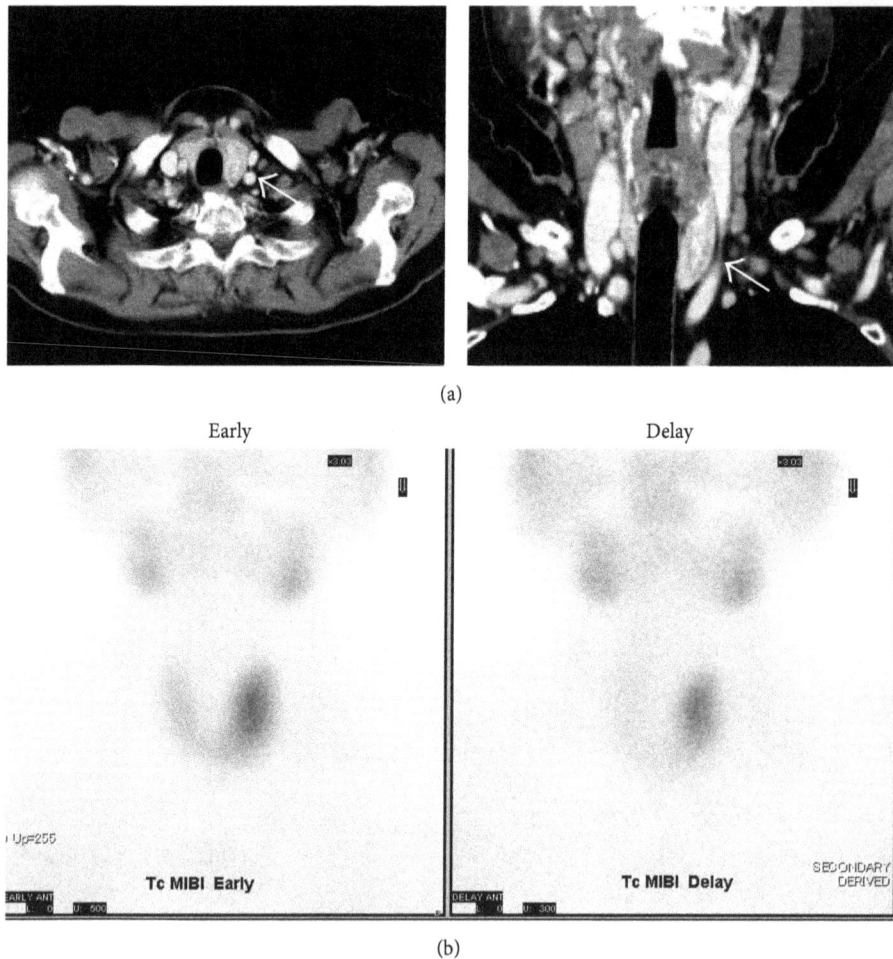

FIGURE 1: (a) Computed tomography of the neck. The scan with contrast enhancement shows a large heterogeneous soft tissue mass (28 mm transverse diameter), clearly defined, within the left thyroid lobe (white arrow). (b) ^{99m}Tc-MIBI scintigraphy. Early and delayed scintigrams reveal focal accumulation of increased radiotracer uptake in the left lobe of the thyroid.

minority of patients with PHPT would develop pancreatitis. Felderbauer et al. found that mutations in the serine protease inhibitor Kazal type I (SPINK1) and cystic fibrosis transmembrane conductance regulator (CFTR) genes increase the risk for pancreatitis, and mutations in the Chymotrypsin C gene (CTRC) modulate susceptibility for pancreatitis [9, 10]. Therefore, markedly elevated serum calcium may contribute to pancreatitis, together with additional genetic or environmental insults [6].

Parathyroid adenomas usually measure less than 2 cm and weigh less than 1 g. In parathyroid lesions larger than 2 cm, the differential diagnosis between giant parathyroid adenomas and parathyroid carcinomas would be considered [11]. Parathyroid cysts or cystic adenomas often show large parathyroid ones [12]. No signs of malignancy, such as presence of capsular invasion, angioinvasion, and invasion of the surrounding structures, were observed by morphological analysis in our case. The weight or size of the adenoma may have been correlated with the functional status of the gland and the severity of biochemical abnormalities. For example, larger adenomas may be associated with a more severe form

of primary hyperparathyroidism [13]. Conversely, in some cases of giant adenoma, there was no correlation with clinical symptoms or functional status [14].

The incidence of intrathyroid parathyroid adenoma is rare: true one is 0.7%, and partial one is 1.9% [15]. Imaging may miss the pathologic gland [16]. Generally, different imaging techniques, such as high resolution ultrasonography, CT, arteriography, venous sampling, and magnetic resonance imaging, have been used for detection of the abnormal parathyroid glands [17, 18]. Radionuclide imaging has also been used in the detection and localization of parathyroid adenomas. ^{99m}Tc-MIBI has been used for preoperative evaluation of PHPT [19], as demonstrated in our case.

Hypercalcemia may mediate the development of pancreatitis and our patient had earlier been treated for acute pancreatitis twice. However, during short-term follow-up, she had not experienced any episodes of pancreatitis after surgery. In a patient with recurrent episodes of pancreatitis, the possibility of complication with hyperparathyroidism should be considered.

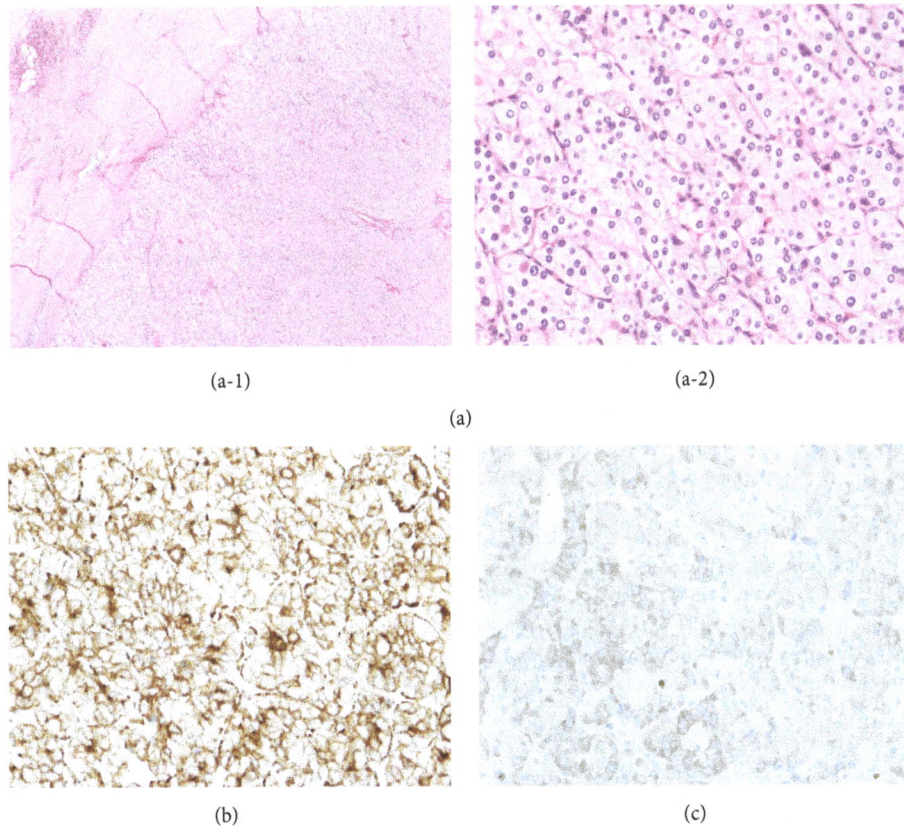

FIGURE 2: (a) Hematoxylin-eosin stained sections of the adenoma (original magnification ×4 (a-1) and ×40 (a-2)). The adenoma was composed mainly of chief cells and oxyphil cells, covered with a fibrous capsule. No signs of malignancy, such as presence of capsular invasion, angioinvasion, and invasion of the surrounding structures, were observed. (b) Immunostaining for chromogranin A (brown precipitates). Section shows expression of chromogranin A. (c) Immunostaining for PTH (brown precipitates). Section shows expression of PTH.

In summary, we report an unusual case of hyperparathyroidism due to a large intrathyroid parathyroid adenoma with episodes of acute pancreatitis.

Authors' Contributions

All authors contributed to the management of the patient and drafting of the manuscript, and all have approved the final submission.

References

[1] J. P. Bilezikian, J. T. Potts Jr., G. El-Hajj Fuleihan et al., "Summary statement from a workshop on asymptomatic primary hyperparathyroidism: a perspective for the 21st century," *The Journal of Clinical Endocrinology and Metabolism*, vol. 87, no. 12, pp. 5353–5361, 2002.

[2] F. R. Bringhurst, M. B. Demay, and H. M. Kronenberg, "Hormones and disorders of mineral metabolism," in *Williams Textbook of Endocrinology*, J. D. Wilsonn, D. W. Foster, H. M. Kronenberg, and P. R. Larsen, Eds., pp. 1155–1209, W.B. Saunders Company, Philadelphia, USA, 9th edition, 1998.

[3] R. M. Neagoe, D. T. Sala, A. Borda, C. A. Mogoanta, and G. Muhlfay, "Clinicopathologic and therapeutic aspects of giant parathyroid adenomas - three case reports and short review of the literature," *Romanian Journal of Morphology and Embryology*, vol. 55, pp. 669–674, 2014.

[4] A. Krishnamurthy, G. Raghunandan, and V. Ramshankar, "A rare case of giant parathyroid adenoma presenting with recurrent episodes of pancreatitis," *Indian Journal of Nuclear Medicine*, vol. 31, no. 1, pp. 36–38, 2016.

[5] M. A. Bess, A. J. Edis, and J. A. van Heerden, "Hyperparathyroidism and pancreatitis. Chance or a causal association?" *The Journal of the American Medical Association*, vol. 243, no. 3, pp. 246-247, 1980.

[6] H. X. Bai, M. Giefer, M. Patel, A. I. Orabi, and S. Z. Husain, "The association of primary hyperparathyroidism with pancreatitis," *Journal of Clinical Gastroenterology*, vol. 46, no. 8, pp. 656–661, 2012.

[7] S. K. Bhadada, H. P. Udawat, A. Bhansali, S. S. Rana, S. K. Sinha, and D. K. Bhasin, "Chronic pancreatitis in primary hyperparathyroidism: comparison with alcoholic and idiopathic chronic pancreatitis," *Journal of Gastroenterology and Hepatology*, vol. 23, no. 6, pp. 959–964, 2008.

[8] V. N. Shah, S. K. Bhadada, A. Bhansali et al., "Effect of gender, biochemical parameters and parathyroid surgery on gastrointestinal manifestations of symptomatic primary hyperparathyroidism," *Indian Journal of Medical Research*, vol. 139, pp. 279–284, 2014.

[9] P. Felderbauer, E. Karakas, V. Fendrich et al., "Pancreatitis risk in primary hyperparathyroidism: relation to mutations in the *SPINK1* trypsin inhibitor (N34S) and the cystic fibrosis gene," *The American Journal of Gastroenterology*, vol. 103, no. 2, pp. 368–374, 2008.

[10] P. Felderbauer, E. Karakas, V. Fendrich, R. Lebert, D. K. Bartsch, and K. Bulut, "Multifactorial genesis of pancreatitis in primary hyperparathyroidism: Evidence for protective (PRSS2) and destructive (CTRC) genetic factors," *Experimental and Clinical Endocrinology and Diabetes*, vol. 119, no. 1, pp. 26–29, 2011.

[11] M. Araujo Castro, A. A. López, L. M. Fragueiro, and N. P. García, "Giant parathyroid adenoma: differential aspects compared to parathyroid carcinoma," *Endocrinology, Diabetes & Metabolism Case Reports*, 2017.

[12] M. Ahmad, M. Almohaya, N. Al Johani, and M. Almalki, "Intrathyroidal Parathyroid Cyst: An Unusual Neck Mass," *Clinical Medicine Insights: Endocrinology and Diabetes*, vol. 10, no. 0, 2017.

[13] W. A. Zamboni and R. Folse, "Adenoma weight: A predictor of transient hypocalcemia after parathyroidectomy," *The American Journal of Surgery*, vol. 152, no. 6, pp. 611–615, 1986.

[14] C. Power, D. Kavanagh, A. D. K. Hill, N. O'Higgins, and E. McDermott, "Unusual presentation of a giant parathyroid adenoma: Report of a case," *Surgery Today*, vol. 35, no. 3, pp. 235–237, 2005.

[15] A. Goodman, D. Politz, J. Lopez, and J. Norman, "Intrathyroid parathyroid adenoma: Incidence and location - The case against thyroid lobectomy," *Otolaryngology - Head and Neck Surgery*, vol. 144, no. 6, pp. 867–871, 2011.

[16] G. Bahar, R. Feinmesser, B.-Z. Joshua et al., "Hyperfunctioning intrathyroid parathyroid gland: A potential cause of failure in parathyroidectomy," *Surgery*, vol. 139, no. 6, pp. 821–826, 2006.

[17] A. J. Krubsack, S. D. Wilson, T. L. Lawson et al., "Prospective comparison of radionuclide, computed tomographic, sonographic, and magnetic resonance localization of parathyroid tumors," *Surgery*, vol. 106, no. 4, pp. 639–644, 1989.

[18] A. Bhansali, S. R. Masoodi, S. Bhadada, B. R. Mittal, A. Behra, and P. Singh, "Ultrasonography in detection of single and multiple abnormal parathyroid glands in primary hyperparathyroidism: Comparison with radionuclide scintigraphy and surgery," *Clinical Endocrinology*, vol. 65, no. 3, pp. 340–345, 2006.

[19] M. J. O'Doherty, A. G. Kettle, P. Wells, R. E. C. Collins, and A. J. Coakley, "Parathyroid imaging with technetium-99m-sestamibi: Preoperative localization and tissue uptake studies," *Journal of Nuclear Medicine*, vol. 33, no. 3, pp. 313–318, 1992.

13

Myxedema Crisis Presenting with Seizures: A Rare Life-Threatening Presentation—A Case Report and Review of the Literature

Sonali Sihindi Chapa Gunatilake and Uditha Bulugahapitiya

Endocrinology, Colombo South Teaching Hospital, Kalubowila, Sri Lanka

Correspondence should be addressed to Sonali Sihindi Chapa Gunatilake; sonaligunatilake@gmail.com

Academic Editor: Osamu Isozaki

Myxedema crisis is a life-threatening extreme form of hypothyroidism with a high mortality rate if left untreated. Myxedema crisis is commonly seen in older patients, especially in women, and is associated with signs of hypothyroidism, hypothermia, hyponatraemia, hypercarbia, and hypoxemia. Patients might present with different organ specific symptoms. Seizures are a recognized but rare manifestation of myxedema with a very high mortality rate. Prompt diagnosis and appropriate management may improve the prognosis. Many contributory factors may involve development of seizures in a patient with myxedema. Hyponatraemia is one such cause, which is seen in moderate-severe form in the background of myxedema. We report an elderly male who presented with generalized tonic clonic seizure preceded by memory impairment and drowsiness. He had moderate hyponatraemia and very high thyroid stimulatory hormone levels in association with low free thyroxin levels. Diagnosis of myxedema crisis was made and patient was successfully treated with sodium correction and thyroid hormone replacement.

1. Case Presentation

A 68-year-old male patient was brought to the Emergency Treatment Unit with first episode of generalized tonic clonic seizure, which lasted for 15 minutes.

Detailed history revealed that he was having mild memory impairment and drowsiness for the past 1 month prior to the index admission. There was no associated fever, diarrheal illness, respiratory symptoms, morning headache with vomiting, or focal neurological deficit prior to the development of fits. There was no history of trauma to head. He did not have any chronic illness or fits in the past, did not undergo any surgeries, and was not on any medications. There was no family history of cardiovascular events or epilepsy. He is a nonsmoker and has not consumed alcohol. He was not an illicit drug abuser.

Following admission, patient remained drowsy with only a mild improvement of conscious level following the seizure.

On examination, his body mass index was 27 kg/m^2 (height, 1.65 cm; weight, 73.5 kg). He had a puffy face with significant periorbital swelling and bilateral nonpitting ankle edema. His skin was dry and coarse. Neck examination revealed no lymphadenopathy or goiter. His body temperature was $36°C$. Vital parameters revealed a heart rate of 45 beats/min, blood pressure of 140/100 mmHg, and a respiratory rate of 12 cycles/min with an oxygen saturation of 94% on air. Glasgow coma scale (GCS) was 10/15 on admission which had improved to 12/15 with persisting drowsiness. He did not have any evidence of external injuries. There was no neck stiffness or detectable focal limb weakness. His ankle jerk was slow relaxing, planta response was flexor, and his fundi were normal. Examination of the respiratory system and abdomen was normal.

Following the clinical evaluation, meningoencephalitis, intracranial space occupying lesion, myxedema, metabolic encephalopathy, and toxin induced disease were taken as differential diagnoses. Preceding memory disturbances, facial puffiness, dry skin, hypothermia, bradycardia, low respiratory rate, and slow relaxing reflexes were supportive of the diagnosis of myxedema.

Basic investigations revealed, haemoglobin, 10.5 g/dL, with macrocytosis, normal white cell count, and normal inflammatory markers. His random blood sugar was 85 mg/dL, liver profile revealed AST of 50 U/L (<20), ALT of 65 U/L (<17), and serum creatinine of 1.3 mg/dL (0.8–1.2). Noncontrast computed tomography of the brain was normal excluding the possibility of intracranial lesion. Electroencephalogram revealed diffuse slow waves and was suggestive of metabolic encephalopathy. Electrocardiogram showed sinus bradycardia with small QRS complexes. ST segments were depressed and T waves showed inverted pattern in all the leads. Echocardiogram showed a mild-to-moderate amount of pericardial effusion with good left ventricular functions but had no evidence of cardiac tamponade. In addition, his creatinine kinase (CK) value was 455 U/L (24–195). Septic screening was negative.

His serum sodium level (Na^+) was 125 mmol/L and potassium was 4.0 mmol/L. Further evaluation revealed a low serum osmolality (260 mOsm/L) with a urinary osmolality of 426 mOsm/L and urinary sodium excretion of 54 mmol/L. His random cortisol level prior to initiating treatment was 560 nmol/L and thyroid stimulating hormone (TSH) and free thyroxin level (fT4) were >100 mU/L (0.4–4) and 0.32 ng/dL (0.9–1.7), respectively. Lumbar puncture and cerebrospinal fluid analysis was performed to exclude the possibility of meningoencephalitis and CSF results were normal.

Diagnosis of myxedema was made on clinical as well as biochemical evidence. In addition to the very high TSH and low fT4 levels, patient had macrocytic anaemia, mild pericardial effusion on echocardiography, hyponatraemia in the background of normal hydration status, elevated liver enzymes, and high CK value in support of the above diagnosis. It was further supported by the high total cholesterol level of 310 mg/dL (<200 mg/dL) found on subsequent evaluation. A definitive precipitation factor was not identified in our patient.

As the possible causes for the presentation with fits and persistent drowsiness, hyponatraemia and/or myxedema were considered. Our patient had moderate degree of hyponatraemia (125–129 mmol/L). Although overt neurological symptoms are seen in severe hyponatraemia (<125 mmol/L), especially when the Na^+ < 115 mmol/L [1], as the patient was having persistent drowsiness, he was initially managed with Na^+ correction. He was given one bolus of 3% NaCl 100 ml over 20 min on admission following which his GCS had improved to 13/15. Thereafter, hyponatraemia was managed with fluid restriction. After 4 hours, serum Na^+ was 128 mmol/L. In addition, general supportive measures including gradual rewarming were initiated.

Patient was commenced on intravenous (IV) glucocorticoids (hydrocortisone 50 mg 6 hourly) after taking a blood sample for random cortisol and treatment was continued until glucocorticoid deficiency was ruled out. After initiating glucocorticoids, he was treated with oral levothyroxine 400 µg initial dose via nasogastric tube followed by oral levothyroxine 100 µg daily. Oral form was used instead of recommended IV form due to the unavailability of intravenous levothyroxine. Recommended dose is IV levothyroxine 200–400 µg followed by 1.6 µg/kg replacement dose,

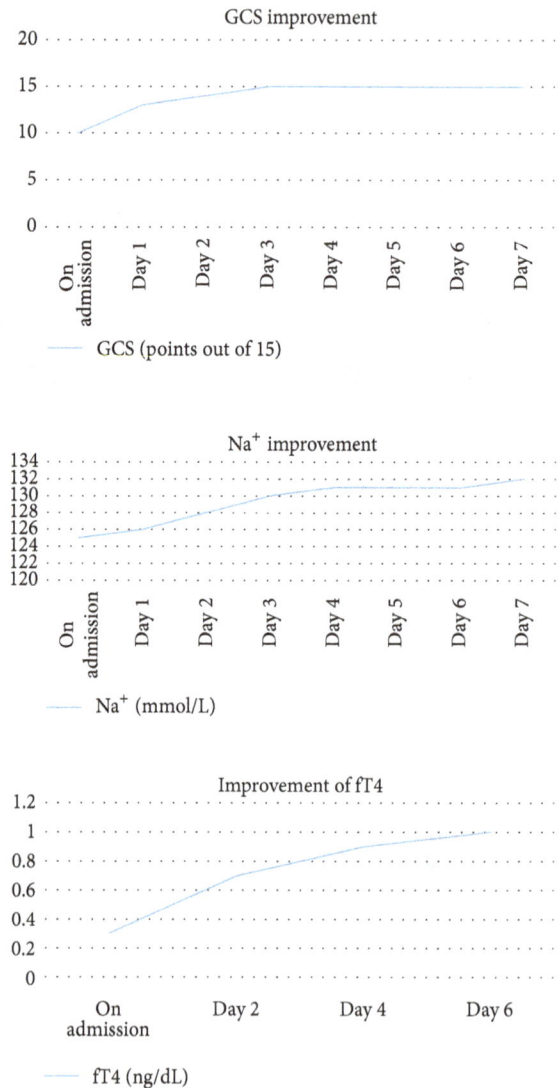

FIGURE 1: Improvement of parameters following treatment.

where 75% of it is given if the daily replacement is done with IV levothyroxine [2]. A lower dose was used in our patient after the initial dose (calculated dose is 1.6 µg/Kg × 80 Kg = 128 µg/day) as he was elderly and to prevent any cardiovascular morbidity.

Careful monitoring was done with regard to clinical improvement, serum Na^+ level daily, and fT4 every 2 days as in Figure 1.

Following good clinical recovery, he was discharged and reviewed in six weeks. His fT4 was 1.12 ng/dL and TSH was 10.4 mU/L. Slow titration was done in order to achieve normal TSH range. His memory and cognition had markedly improved with resolution of facial puffiness. Biochemical parameters including Na^+, liver enzymes, serum creatinine, CK, red cell indices, and echocardiogram had also normalized at 3 months of follow-up.

2. Discussion

Myxedema crisis/coma is a rare life-threatening clinical condition that represents severe hypothyroidism with physiological decompensation [3]. The term myxedema coma is a misnomer, and myxedema crisis may be an appropriate term as quite a few patients are obtunded, rather than frankly comatose [4]. It is rare and unrecognized. Exact prevalence of myxedema coma is unknown. Even with early detection and appropriate treatment, mortality ranges from 30 to 60% where most die due to respiratory failure, sepsis, and gastrointestinal bleeding [5, 6]. Myxedema crises occur mostly in persons 60 years or older and nearly 80% of cases occur in females [7]. However, myxedema coma occurs in younger patients as well, with more than 30 documented cases of pregnant women [8].

Low intracellular triiodothyronine (T3) secondary to hypothyroidism is the basic underlying pathology in myxedema crisis which leads to hypothermia and suppression of cardiac activity. The body tries to compensate by neurovascular adaptations including chronic peripheral vasoconstriction, mild diastolic hypertension, and diminished blood volume. Decreased central nervous system sensitivity to hypoxia and hypercapnia leads to respiratory failure. Altered vascular permeability leads to effusions and anasarca. Water retention and hyponatraemia occurs secondary to reduced glomerular filtration rate, decreased delivery to the distal nephron, and excess vasopressin [9]. Decreased gluconeogenesis, precipitating factors like sepsis and concomitant adrenal insufficiency, may contribute to hypoglycemia. In addition to the generalized depression of cerebral function, hyponatraemia, hypoglycemia, hypoxemia, and reduced cerebral blood flow can precipitate focal or generalized seizures and worsen the level of consciousness as in the index case.

Most of the patients with myxedema crisis have primary hypothyroidism and secondary hypothyroidism account to 5% of the cases [10]. Dutta et al. reported that 39% of patients present with myxedema crisis had hypothyroidism detected only at the time of crisis [11] as in our patient.

Clinical presentation may vary but almost all patients have altered mentation and 80% have hypothermia. In addition to the characteristic features of hypothyroidism, patients may present with some atypical features as heart blocks, prolonged QT interval and arrhythmias, myocardial infarction, pericardial/pleural effusions, respiratory depression, hypercapnia, bleeding manifestations with prolonged APTT, and acquired von Willebrand factor defects and psychosis [12, 13]. Neurological manifestations in myxedema may range from alteration of mental status with slowness, decreased concentration and lethargy, headache, cranial nerve palsies, hoarseness, myopathy, neuropathy, reflex changes, ataxia, psychotic episodes, and fits. Ultimate result would be a coma state and role of hypothermia, CO_2 narcosis, cerebral edema, and other metabolic disturbances in the genesis of coma should be looked into.

Occurrence of seizures in myxedema can have several mechanisms but myxedema itself can precipitate seizure activity. The cause of epileptic seizure activity in hypothyroidism is unknown. It may be due to cerebral oedema secondary to expansion of the extracellular fluid volume [14]. This may be related to inappropriate antidiuretic hormone (ADH) secretion and hyponatraemia or hypoventilation with postanoxic encephalopathy, which can further precipitate seizure activity.

Hyponatraemia is reported in up to 10% of hypothyroid patients, although it is usually mild and rarely causes symptoms [15]. In water-loading studies, patients with hypothyroidism have a diminished ability to excrete free water and fail to achieve maximum urine dilution. Although some studies have reported elevated ADH levels in patients with hypothyroidism the literature is inconsistent [15]. The reduction in cardiac output and glomerular filtration rate observed in severe hypothyroidism may be a nonosmotic stimuli to ADH release. However, recent data suggests that the hypothyroidism induced hyponatraemia is rather rare and probably occurs only in severe hypothyroidism and myxedema [16]. Patients with a low plasma sodium had a lower mean Free T4 concentration and higher mean TSH concentration than Free T4 concentration and mean TSH concentration of the patients with a normal plasma sodium concentration. Treatment of hypothyroidism and fluid restriction are usually adequate for the management of mild hyponatraemia in hypothyroidism. Patients with possible hyponatraemic encephalopathy should be urgently treated according to the protocols of management of severe hyponatraemia but caution must be taken to avoid rapid correction of chronic hyponatraemia, which might put patients at risk for central pontine myelinolysis.

Patient in the index case presented with a generalized tonic clonic seizure in the background of newly diagnosed severe hypothyroidism and moderate hyponatraemia, which is relatively rarely reported in the literature in association with myxedema and fits. Both factors could have contributed for the development of seizures although classically Na^+ level of <120 mmol/L is known to cause seizures. He was initially managed with 3% NaCl as he was having a lower level of GCS on admission in the background of fits followed by persistent drowsiness.

Management of myxedema crisis involves replacement of thyroxin hormones with additional supportive care. Prior to thyroxin replacement, glucocorticoid replacement should be considered as the clinical features of myxedema crisis and cortisol deficiency may overlap; hence thyroid hormone replacement may increase cortisol clearance and may aggravate cortisol deficiency. In addition, precipitant cause should be sought and treated.

Thyroxin replacement is recommended in the form of intravenous (IV) tetraiodothyronine (T4), mainly to avoid poor gastrointestinal absorption. T4 therapy provides a smooth, steady, and slow onset of action with relatively lesser number of adverse events [4]. T4 therapy avoids major peaks and troughs in body. Values of serum T4 may be easy to interpret. However, triiodothyronine (T3) is the active hormone in the body, and in a setting of severe illness there may be a decreased conversion of T4 to T3. Advantages of using T3 include a rapid onset of action, an earlier beneficial effect on neuropsychiatric symptoms, and significant clinical improvement within 24 hours. Several options are available for the treatment of myxedema [2]:

(1) IV T4 loading dose of 200–400 μg bolus (to replenish body stores) followed by 75% of the calculated dose of [1.6 μg/Kg × 75%] IV T4 per day till patient is alert to take oral thyroxin

(2) IV T3 10–20 μg followed by 2.5–10 μg every 8 hours during first 2 days till patient is alert to take oral thyroxin

(3) Combination of IV T4 4 μg/Kg (or 200–300 μg) + IV T3 10 μg bolus followed by T4 100 μg in 24 hours and 50 μg/day thereafter with T3 2.5–10 μg every 8 hours till patient recovers

Although there are beneficial effects, poor availability, fluctuations in serum levels of T3, adverse cardiac effects, and limited availability may limit the use of IV T3. There is a controversy on the ideal modality of treatment and American Thyroid Association recommends combination of IV T4 and T3 [2]. Measurement of thyroid hormones every 1-2 days is suggested. Yamamoto et al. reported that doses of LT4 more than 500 μg per day and LT3 more than 75 μg/day were associated with increased mortality [17].

Oral administration of T4 through nasogastric tube has proved to be equally effective with a drawback that gastric atony may prevent absorption and put the patient at risk for aspiration. Dutta and colleagues compared 500 μg of oral loading dose of T4 with 150 μg of maintenance dose orally and 200 μg of T4 intravenously followed by 100 μg T4 intravenously until they regained their vital functions and were able to take oral medications in patients with myxedema crisis and did not find any difference in outcome among the patients [11]. Arlot et al. reported that oral absorption of T4 is variable, but clinical response occurs quickly even in myxoedema ileus after comparing oral T4 500 μg stat dose followed by 100 μg/day with IV T4 in patients with myxedema [6]. But all above studies had used higher doses of oral T4 compared to the IV T4 dose. A lower initial dose of T4 should be administered to patients who are frail or have other comorbidities, particularly cardiovascular disease. Thyroid hormones may be measured every 1 to 2 days to identify the response. We used oral T4 for our patient who had shown marked improvement clinically as well as biochemically over 1 week.

Abbreviations

ADH: Antidiuretic hormone
ALT: Alanine transaminase
APTT: Activated partial thrombin time
AST: Aspartate transaminase
CK: Creatinine kinase
CSF: Cerebrospinal fluid
CT: Computed tomogram
GCS: Glasgow coma scale
IV: Intravenous
NaCl: Sodium chloride
TSH: Thyroid stimulating hormone
fT4: Free tetraiodothyronine
fT3: Free triiodothyronine.

Disclosure

Details of the patient are available in the hospital notes.

Authors' Contributions

Uditha Bulugahapitiya made the clinical diagnosis. Sonali Sihindi Chapa Gunatilake drafted the manuscript, reviewed the literature, and was involved in direct management of the patient. All authors read and approved the final manuscript.

References

[1] E. E. Simon and V. Batuman, "Medscape," Hyponatremia. Medscape 2016, http://emedicine.medscape.com/article/242166-overview.

[2] J. Jonklaas, A. C. Bianco, A. J. Bauer et al., "Guidelines for the treatment of hypothyroidism: prepared by the American thyroid association task force on thyroid hormone replacement," Thyroid, vol. 24, no. 12, pp. 1670–1751, 2014.

[3] J. Klubo-Gwiezdzinska and L. Wartofsky, "Thyroid emergencies," Medical Clinics of North America, vol. 96, no. 2, pp. 385–403, 2012.

[4] V. Mathew, R. A. Misgar, S. Ghosh et al., "Myxedema coma: a new look into an old crisis," Journal of Thyroid Research, vol. 2011, Article ID 493462, 7 pages, 2011.

[5] S. C. Werner, S. H. Ingbar, L. E. Braverman, and R. D. Utiger, Werner and Ingbar's The thyroid: a fundamental and clinical text, Lipincott Williams and Wilkins, Philadelphia, Pa, USA, 8th edition, 2000.

[6] S. Arlot, X. Debussche, J.-D. Lalau et al., "Myxoedema coma: response of thyroid hormones with oral and intravenous high-dose L-thyroxine treatment," Intensive Care Medicine, vol. 17, no. 1, pp. 16–18, 1991.

[7] B. K. Bailes, "Hypothyroidism in elderly patients," AORN Journal, vol. 69, no. 5, pp. 1026–1030, 1999.

[8] S. Patel, S. Robinson, R. Bidgood, and C. Edmonds, "A pre-eclamptic-like syndrome associated with hypothyroidism during pregnancy," QJM, vol. 79, no. 2, pp. 435–441, 1991.

[9] Y.-C. Chen, M. A. Cadnapaphornchai, J. Yang et al., "Nonosmotic release of vasopressin and renal aquaporins in impaired urinary dilution in hypothyroidism," American Journal of Physiology—Renal Physiology, vol. 289, no. 4, pp. F672–F678, 2005.

[10] L. Wartofsky, "Myxedema coma," Endocrinology and Metabolism Clinics of North America, vol. 35, no. 4, pp. 687–698, 2006.

[11] P. Dutta, A. Bhansali, S. Masoodi, S. Bhadada, N. Sharma, and R. Rajput, "Predictors of outcome in myxoedema coma: a study from a tertiary care centre," *Critical Care*, vol. 12, no. 1, article R1, 2008.

[12] J. B. Schenck, A. A. Rizvi, and T. Lin, "Severe primary hypothyroidism manifesting with torsades de pointes," *American Journal of the Medical Sciences*, vol. 331, no. 3, pp. 154–156, 2006.

[13] H. C. Ford and J. M. Carter, "Haemostasis in hypothyroidism," *Postgraduate Medical Journal*, vol. 66, no. 774, pp. 280–284, 1990.

[14] E. C. Evans, "Neurological complications of myxedema: convulsions," *Annals of Internal Medicine*, vol. 52, pp. 434–444, 1960.

[15] J. Montenegro, O. Gonzalez, R. Saracho, R. Aguirre, O. Gonzalez, and I. Martinez, "Changes in renal function in primary hypothyroidism," *American Journal of Kidney Diseases*, vol. 27, no. 2, pp. 195–198, 1996.

[16] G. Liamis, T. D. Filippatos, A. Liontos, and M. S. Elisaf, "Management of endocrine disease: hypothyroidism-associated hyponatremia: mechanisms, implications and treatment," *European Journal of Endocrinology*, vol. 176, no. 1, pp. R15–R20, 2016.

[17] T. Yamamoto, J. Fukuyama, and A. Fujiyoshi, "Factors associated with mortality of myxedema coma: report of eight cases and literature survey," *Thyroid*, vol. 9, no. 12, pp. 1167–1174, 1999.

14

Surgical Management of Life-Threatening Thyroid Haematoma following Occult Blunt Neck Trauma

Ronak Ved, Neil Patel, and Michael Stechman

University Hospital of Wales, Cardiff CF14 4XW, UK

Correspondence should be addressed to Ronak Ved; vedr@cf.ac.uk

Academic Editor: Osamu Isozaki

A 42-year-old man arrived at the emergency department in severe respiratory distress, requiring immediate intubation and ventilation. An emergency computed tomography (CT) neck scan identified a substantial haematoma within a multinodular goitre, necessitating an emergency total thyroidectomy. It was later discovered that the patient had been the victim of an assault involving blunt trauma to the anterior neck. Five days postoperatively the patient was extubated and was well enough to self-discharge the following day. Pathology revealed the lesion to be a ruptured follicular adenoma within his multinodular goitre. Signs of this rare but life-threatening condition may be subtle on initial presentation, particularly if the patient is obtunded. Patients with suspected blunt neck trauma should be observed for signs of respiratory distress. If this develops, the patient should be intubated to facilitate CT scan, and if thyroid haematoma is confirmed, emergency thyroidectomy is the definitive treatment.

1. Introduction

In cases of blunt trauma involving the neck, a high index of suspicion is warranted for thyroid haematoma, as signs may not be present on initial examination. We report a case of occult blunt injury to the neck of a 42-year-old homeless male patient with a preexisting multinodular goitre (MNG). Invasive airway management, cross-sectional imaging, and emergency thyroidectomy were necessary.

2. Case Presentation

The patient was admitted by ambulance after workers in a hostel observed him develop gradual onset difficulty of breathing and swelling of the throat. There was no other history available at this time. He arrived at the emergency department in severe respiratory distress and with fluctuating consciousness. His vital signs at presentation were respiratory rate of 28 breaths per minute, heart rate of 110 beats per minute, 100% saturation on 100% O_2, BP 170/109, and temperature 37.4°. His neck was markedly swollen and tender, necessitating immediate nasotracheal intubation and ventilation. He was then taken for emergency computed tomography (CT) of the neck and thorax to determine the cause. The patient had an established multinodular goitre, took 200 mcg levothyroxine daily, had no known allergies, and was an alcoholic. Admission biochemistry demonstrated no evidence of hyperthyroidism with TSH 5.52 mU/L (0.30–4.40) and fT4 12.3 pmol/L (9.0–19.1). Neither anti-TPO nor TSH-R antibody titres were elevated.

Whilst being transferred to the CT scanner he was commenced on empirical intravenous antibiotics and steroids. A substantial neck collection and multinodular goitre were identified on the arterial phase neck CT. The $3.5 \times 10 \times 10$ cm (anterior-posterior × lateral × superior-inferior) mass was anterior to the thyroid and displaced the trachea to the left. The great vessels were displaced laterally by the collection but remained undamaged (Figures 1–3).

The thyroid gland was noted to contain multiple cystic structures, and one of these in the right lobe was of increased density (Figure 3) suggesting haemorrhage within that nodule. A direct connection was strongly suspected between this haemorrhagic lesion and the anterior neck collection.

This necessitated an emergency total thyroidectomy. The cause was identified as an arterial vessel within the wall of a ruptured right-sided thyroid nodule (Video 1 in Supplementary Material available online at

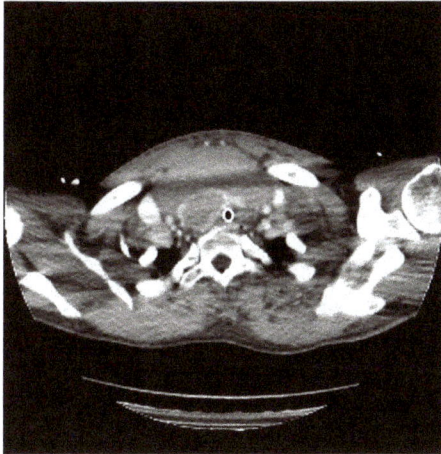

FIGURE 1: Arterial phase CT neck: axial view of neck haematoma demonstrating compression of the intubated trachea.

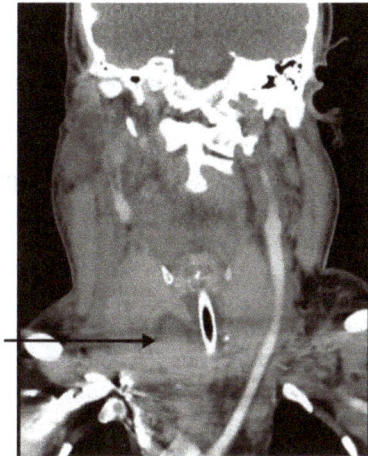

FIGURE 2: Arterial phase CT neck: coronal view of neck haematoma demonstrating lateral displacement of the great vessels and trachea and hyperdense haemorrhage within right-sided thyroid nodule (arrow).

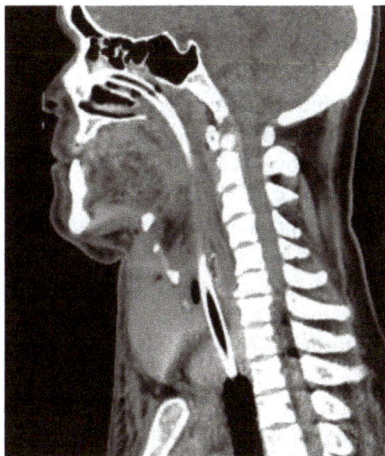

FIGURE 3: Arterial phase CT neck: parasagittal view of neck haematoma.

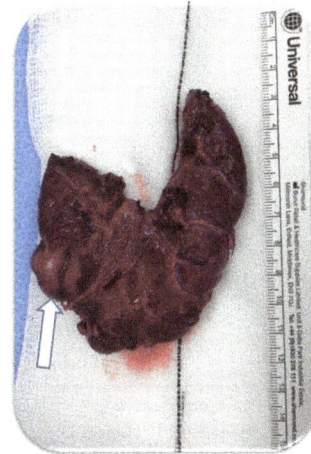

FIGURE 4: Postoperative specimen of the goitrous right lobe of the thyroid gland, with the right-sided nodule clearly visible adjacent to the isthmus (white arrow), from which the pulsatile arterial haemorrhage was identified intraoperatively.

http://dx.doi.org/10.1155/2016/4307695). A right thyroid lobectomy was performed after evacuation of the haematoma. A left lobectomy was also carried out as persistent bleeding originating from the enlarged left lobe, which may have been related to venous bleeding within the lobe caused by the blunt neck injury. The nodule is visible in Figure 4.

During the patient's convalescence on the intensive care unit postoperatively, it was discovered that he had been the victim of an assault, involving blunt trauma to the anterior neck a few hours before his arrival in the emergency department. Pathology results revealed the lesion to be a ruptured 35 mm follicular adenoma within a multinodular goitre, without any features of papillary nuclear features nor any evidence of capsular or vascular invasion. The nodule was expanding from the lower right pole into the isthmus (Figure 4). A number of small follicular adenomas were identified in the left lobe of the thyroid gland. However, none of these were as enlarged as the right-sided nodule responsible for the arterial bleeding.

Flexible nasendoscopy on the 3rd postoperative day revealed moderate supraglottic oedema. Intravenous dexamethasone and antibiotics were therefore continued until 5 days postoperatively, when repeat visualisation of the laryngopharynx revealed resolution of the oedema. The patient was successfully extubated and converted to oral antibiotics and steroids. His recovery thereafter was rapid, and on the 6th postoperative day he was well enough to self-discharge from hospital. He did not attend arranged follow-up with endocrine surgery but has since been reviewed by local internal medicine and substance misuse teams, and there have been no further concerns regarding his neck.

3. Discussion

Neck trauma is common. However secondary haemorrhage of the thyroid gland as a result of trauma is rare [2].

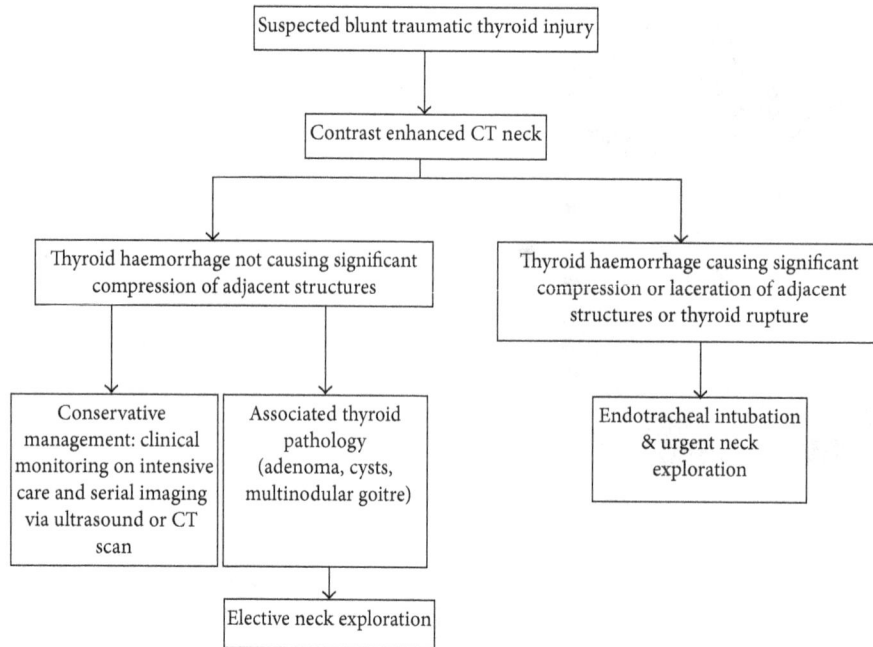

FIGURE 5: Adapted algorithm for the assessment and management of suspected thyroid haematoma from Heizmann et al. [1].

Goitrous glands, with their increased size and vascularity, carry an increased risk for posttraumatic haemorrhage [3]. Haemorrhage into a normal gland has also been reported [4].

Symptoms of traumatic thyroid haematoma may not be apparent immediately after a neck injury. The trauma may be direct impact, but cervical hyperflexion/extension, deceleration injuries, and even Valsalva manoeuvres can all cause thyroid haemorrhage [3]. The onset of airway compromise is also variable: it may develop within minutes [4], days [5], or not at all [6]. Other than frank airway compromise and respiratory distress, symptoms of thyroid haematoma include a painful neck mass, dysphagia, and hoarseness [5]. Clinical assessment can be difficult, particularly if there is incomplete history or low GCS, as in this case. Therefore, a high index of suspicion is required if there is any indication of neck trauma, with or without a palpable neck mass.

Radiological investigations can establish the diagnosis of thyroid gland injury. Emergency arterial phase CT scanning was the investigation of choice in our case as the patient presented with rapid onset respiratory distress out of hours; a CT scan permitted assessment for both thyroid haemorrhage and great vessel injury within the neck. Ultrasound has been utilised as a diagnostic tool in cases without rapid onset of airway compromise [5]. Fiberoptic laryngoscopy can also prove helpful in these stable cases to rule out laryngeal injury, as this may not be demonstrated on imaging [4].

Thyrotoxicosis has been reported after thyroid trauma [3], although it is not universal, as illustrated by the absence of hyperthyroidism in our case. Thyroid function should therefore be checked if there is suspicion of thyroid injury, even in the absence of a palpable neck mass. Given the increased risk of thyroid haemorrhage for patients with goitres, which may potentially be undiagnosed until the event, appropriate investigations to determine causes of hyper/hypothyroidism should be undertaken if a traumatic thyroid haematoma is identified.

Traumatic thyroid haematomas may be successfully managed both surgically and conservatively [3]. Increasing size and/or suspicion of airway compromise are indications for immediate intubation, imaging, and neck exploration. Signs of respiratory distress were readily apparent in our case, which necessitated emergency surgical intervention. Heizmann et al. proposed a simple algorithm to aid in the investigation and treatment after blunt neck trauma [1]. This algorithm advocates CT neck for all patients with suspected blunt neck injury, after which the severity of any thyroid injury then dictates the requirement for urgent neck exploration (Figure 5). The pathway also suggests elective thyroidectomy for patients with minor haemorrhage in the presence of structural thyroid abnormalities, owing to the established association between significant bleeding and thyroid disease. This is a useful paradigm for management of suspected thyroid trauma; however it is dependent upon an index of suspicion for thyroid injury in the first instance, which may not be obvious in the absence of a clear history of trauma, as in our case. It is also imperative that airway stability is obtained prior to CT neck scanning if necessary and that there should be a low threshold for patients following the conservative or elective surgical management pathway to be reviewed for urgent surgical intervention, as life-threatening features of an expanding neck haematoma can evolve rapidly.

This algorithm does not specify which procedures should be performed if thyroid haemorrhage is identified at neck exploration. In the presented case a pulsatile arterial haemorrhage was identified from an individual right-sided thyroid nodule, and therefore a hemithyroidectomy could have been performed in the first instance. However, we elected to perform a total thyroidectomy to (a) obviate the risk of continued, delayed bleeding from the enlarged left lobe, which was noted intraoperatively, and (b) avoid the potential need for reoperative left hemithyroidectomy in the future in an already goitrous patient, who was known to regularly fail to attend medical follow-up appointments. The decision between hemi- and total thyroidectomy in these cases may often need to be made intraoperatively, after evacuation of the haematoma when macroscopic assessment of likely bleeding sources from the thyroid gland can be carried out.

The presentation of thyroid haematoma may be subtle or delayed, and in these cases substantial thyroid haematomas may be missed [3–5]. Such cases could rapidly evolve into life-threatening scenarios. Regular and comprehensive monitoring of airway and breathing is paramount if conservative management is contemplated.

4. Clinical Significance

Cases of blunt neck trauma should be observed meticulously for signs of respiratory distress in the first instance. If this develops, the patient should be intubated to facilitate CT scan. If thyroid haematoma is confirmed, emergency thyroidectomy is the definitive treatment. There must be a low threshold for these interventions if a conservative approach is adopted.

Authors' Contributions

All authors contributed to the data collection, analysis, and manuscript preparation and review.

Acknowledgments

The authors would like to thank Ms. Ann Dilger for her assistance with the administrative tasks required to develop this manuscript.

References

[1] O. Heizmann, R. Schmid, and D. Oertli, "Blunt injury to the thyroid gland: proposed classification and treatment algorithm," *The Journal of Trauma*, vol. 61, no. 4, pp. 1012–1015, 2006.

[2] M. Blaivas, D. B. Hom, and J. G. Younger, "Thyroid gland hematoma after blunt cervical trauma," *The American Journal of Emergency Medicine*, vol. 17, no. 4, pp. 348–350, 1999.

[3] R. L. Behrends and R. B. Low, "Acute goiter hematoma following blunt neck trauma," *Annals of Emergency Medicine*, vol. 16, no. 11, pp. 1300–1301, 1987.

[4] C. Weeks, F. D. Moore Jr., S. J. Ferzoco, and J. Gates, "Blunt trauma to the thyroid: a case report," *The American Surgeon*, vol. 71, no. 6, pp. 518–521, 2005.

[5] B. Saylam, B. Çomçali, M. V. Ozer, and F. Coskun, "Thyroid gland hematoma after blunt neck trauma," *The Western Journal of Emergency Medicine*, vol. 10, no. 4, pp. 247–249, 2009.

[6] W. B. Armstrong, G. F. Funk, and D. H. Rice, "Acute airway compromise secondary to traumatic thyroid hemorrhage," *Archives of Otolaryngology—Head and Neck Surgery*, vol. 120, no. 4, pp. 427–430, 1994.

15

Posttransplant Tacrolimus-Induced Diabetic Ketoacidosis: Review of the Literature

Zaid Ammari,[1] Stella C. Pak,[1] Mohammed Ruzieh [ID],[1] Osama Dasa [ID],[1] Abhinav Tiwari [ID],[1] Juan C. Jaume,[1,2,3] and Maria A. Alfonso-Jaume [ID][1,3,4]

[1]Department of Medicine, College of Medicine and Life Sciences, University of Toledo, Toledo, OH, USA
[2]Division of Endocrinology, Diabetes and Metabolism, College of Medicine and Life Sciences, University of Toledo, Toledo, OH, USA
[3]Center for Diabetes and Endocrine Research (CeDER), College of Medicine and Life Sciences, University of Toledo, Toledo, OH, USA
[4]Division of Nephrology, College of Medicine and Life Sciences, University of Toledo, Toledo, OH, USA

Correspondence should be addressed to Maria A. Alfonso-Jaume; Maria.Alfonso-Jaume@utoledo.edu

Academic Editor: John Broom

Diabetic ketoacidosis (DKA) in patients receiving tacrolimus as part of their immunosuppressive regimen is a rarely reported adverse event. We report a patient with autosomal dominant polycystic kidney disease (ADPKD) and no known history of diabetes mellitus who presented with DKA, 3 months after kidney transplantation.

1. Introduction

For 2 decades now, kidney allograft survival has been shortening despite an obvious decrease in acute allograft rejection. The possibility of a single agent capable of both outcomes is being considered. Tacrolimus, the most potent calcineurin inhibitor, may be the reason for both. Its popularity is clearly a consequence of the excellent short term outcome. However, as second kidney transplant becomes the norm because of the reduced allograft survival, alternative immunosuppressive regimens ought to be considered.

New-onset diabetes mellitus after transplantation (NODAT) is now a well-established adverse effect of calcineurin inhibitors, mostly tacrolimus. NODAT has been reported to occur in 32% of patients after solid organ transplantation and may be the most important contributing factor for decreased long-term allograft survival [1]. Immunosuppressant accounts for 74% of the occurrence of NODAT [2], with a higher incidence in patients receiving tacrolimus than cyclosporine (16.6–33.6% versus 9.8–26%) [3, 4]. Failure to identify and manage glucose homeostasis in a timely manner in these patients lead to a life-threatening complication, DKA.

The case presented here describes an accelerated development of tacrolimus-induced DKA 3 months after kidney transplantation. To our knowledge, only 14 cases of tacrolimus-induced DKA have been reported.

2. Case Description

A 44-year-old Caucasian male, with no past medical history of diabetes mellitus, was admitted to the hospital with DKA, three months after receiving a deceased-donor kidney transplant for end stage renal disease (ESRD) secondary to ADPKD. The posttransplant course was unremarkable. Patient's immunosuppressive regimen included tacrolimus 1.5 mg BID, mycophenolate sodium 720 mg BID, and low dose prednisone of 5 mg daily. Patient presented to the emergency department with nausea, polyuria, and abdominal pain. He did not have family history of diabetes mellitus. Physical exam was unremarkable except for mild overweight, body mass index of 27 kg/m^2. Laboratory work-up revealed hyperglycemia, high anion gap metabolic acidosis, significant ketosis with a beta-hydroxybutyrate level of 4.45 mmol/l (reference range 0.02–0.27 mmol/l), ketonuria, and normal lactate levels. Glycated hemoglobin (A1C) was 9.8% compared to 4.8%, 30 days after transplant. Tacrolimus trough level was 13.9 ng/ml. Glutamic acid decarboxylase (GAD-65) autoantibodies were negative. Infectious etiology for hyperglycemia was ruled out.

The patient received intravenous fluids and a bolus of intravenous insulin followed by continuous insulin infusion which was gradually switched to subcutaneous insulin. Daily insulin requirements were approximately 40 units. He was educated about his new diagnosis and discharged on diabetic diet and subcutaneous insulin therapy. Upon follow-up, tacrolimus dose was adjusted to a lower therapeutic index. Insulin requirements markedly decreased and patient was able to be taken off insulin 9 months after. Glycated hemoglobin (A1C) checked at 9 months was 5.2%.

3. Discussion

Many of the risk factors that predispose nontransplant patients to diabetes mellitus have been identified as risk factors for NODAT. Some risk factors are unique to the transplant population. Immunosuppressive agents that contribute to NODAT include glucocorticoids, calcineurin inhibitors, and mTOR inhibitors. Both cyclosporine and tacrolimus increase the risk of NODAT. Tacrolimus is more diabetogenic than cyclosporine [3, 4]. Other risk factors are hepatitis C virus and cytomegalovirus infections, impaired glucose tolerance, perioperative hyperglycemia, HLA matching and donor characteristics, and hypomagnesemia [1, 2, 5]. Interestingly, ADPKD, the cause of ESRD in the present case may confer an increased risk of NODAT [6].

In a study using data from the United States Renal Data System (USRDS), 21,489 patients were enrolled, of whom 4,105 developed NODAT by 3 years after transplant. Diabetes complications developed in 58.3% of patients. DKA developed in 8.1% of patients with NODAT [7]. In most of these cases exposure to high dose steroids (steroid-induced diabetes) appears to be a determining factor. Different from many other protocols, our transplant protocol includes a very short (3 days) exposure to high dose steroids.

Including our case, there are 15 cases of tacrolimus associated DKA presentation in organ transplant patients reported in the literature [8–18]. Summary of these cases focused on clinical presentation and management is described in Table 1. Out of the 15 cases, 6 had kidney transplant [8, 10, 13, 16, 17], 6 had liver transplant [9, 12, 13, 18], 2 had heart transplant [11, 14], and 1 had bone marrow transplant [15]. The mean age of patients was 29.9±15.2 years with no gender predominance (8 females and 7 males). None of the patients had history of diabetes mellitus prior to the transplant. 40% of patients, including our patient presented with DKA within the first 3 months after transplant, with median of 7 months.

Higher body mass index (BMI) has been associated with increased risk for NODAT [2]. However, lower BMI has been reported with tacrolimus-associated DKA in organ transplant patients, with mean of $22.1 \pm 4.7 \, kg/m^2$ as in our case.

Female gender, African American ethnicity, recipients of deceased donor kidney transplant, younger age (33–44 versus >55 years), and recent transplant patients had significantly higher risk of DKA after kidney transplantation [19].

Maintenance immunosuppressive therapy is essential to prevent rejection in renal transplant recipients. Calcineurin inhibitors play an integral role in immunosuppressive regimens, with tacrolimus being the preferred agent over cyclosporine, as several studies showed lower incidence of acute rejections with its use [4, 20]. In addition to lower rates of acute rejections, tacrolimus is better tolerated and preferred by patients compared with cyclosporine. Moreover, tacrolimus does not lower mycophenolate levels unlike cyclosporine and, therefore, relatively lower doses of mycophenolate are needed when tacrolimus is used.

Transplant patients on tacrolimus as part of their immunosuppressive regimen had increased risk of DKA compared to cyclosporine based immunosuppressive regimens [7, 19]. Both calcineurin inhibitors cause toxicity to pancreatic islet beta cells and may directly affect transcriptional regulation of insulin expression [21, 22]. Some evidence suggests however that tacrolimus causes more severe swelling-vacuolization, endoplasmic reticulum stress, and apoptosis of pancreatic islet beta cells [23]. Toxic levels of tacrolimus and higher steroid doses potentiate each other's diabetogenic effects [24]. Tacrolimus's diabetogenic effects therefore threaten the health and longevity of the allograft by predisposing the recipients to microvascular and macrovascular diabetes complications which consequently reduce allograft survival.

Decreased insulin requirement after DKA is suggestive of transient pancreatic damage by toxic levels of tacrolimus which is usually dose dependent and appears reversible [24]. Both tapering tacrolimus regimens and cyclosporine substitution for tacrolimus have been associated with decreased insulin requirements. There is one case report in which everolimus substitution for tacrolimus provided sufficient decline in insulin requirements [17].

Importantly, DKA in renal transplant patients has been associated with increased mortality [19].

4. Conclusion

Tacrolimus remains the preferred immunosuppressive agent after kidney transplantation given lower incidence of acute rejections and better patients' tolerance. However, tacrolimus's contribution to new-onset diabetes ketoacidosis, as a consequence of pancreatic islet beta cell toxicity, adds to the accumulating evidence of reduced allograft survival observed since its introduction as the immunosuppressant of choice. Despite rarity of reported cases of posttransplant tacrolimus-induced DKA, it seems possible that the decrease in allograft survival observed in the last two decades is just the consequence of tacrolimus-induced diabetes and its complications. The successful decrease in acute allograft rejection provided by tacrolimus has likely confounded this observation. The development of diabetes mellitus with ketoacidosis in patients on therapeutic tacrolimus levels, with no risk factors for diabetes, highlights the need for alternative immunosuppressive agents that will not compromise patients' allografts long-term survival at the expense of inducing a devastating chronic disease. This case

TABLE 1: Comparison of different characteristics of transplant recipients with tacrolimus-induced diabetes ketoacidosis [8–18] and our case.

	Age (years), Gender	Organ transplant	BMI (kg/m2)	Duration since transplantation (month)	Maintenance immunosuppressant regimen	Presentation	Glucose (mg/dl)/pH/HCO_3^- (mmol/l)	HbA$_1$C (%)	Glucosuria, ketonuria, proteinuria	IA-2 Ab/GAD-65 Ab	Tacrolimus level (ng/ml)	Management	Discharge regimen/outcome
Our case	44 M	Kidney	27.0	3	TAC + PDN + MPS	*Nausea, polyuria, abdominal pain*	493/7.32/15	9.8	+/+/−	NA/−	13.9	*IV saline and insulin Tapering TAC regimen*	*SC insulin Off insulin in 9 months*
Cho et al.	35 F	Kidney	21.8	6	TAC + PDL + MMF	Polydipsia, dry mouth, weight loss, anorexia, fatigue, confusion	712/6.80/1.4	14.7	NA/+/NA	NA/−	11.1	IV saline and insulin CYC substituted for TAC	Diabetic diet
Dehghani et al.	13 F	Liver	NA	7	TAC + MMF	Anorexia, fatigue, dizziness, ascites	742/7.22/10	NA	+/+/NA	NA/NA	16.2	IV saline and insulin	Inpatient death secondary to bacterial sepsis
Dehghani et al.	14 M	Liver	NA	3	TAC + PDL	Nausea, vomiting, fever	390/7.26/10	NA	+/+/NA	NA/NA	14.8	IV saline and insulin	SC insulin
Dehghani et al.	14 M	Liver	NA	4	TAC + MMF	Abdominal pain, fever	432/7.21/12.2	NA	NA/+/NA	NA/NA	16.5	IV saline and insulin	SC insulin
Ersoy et al.	42 F	Kidney	29.8	36	TAC + PDL + AZT	Polyuria, polydipsia, confusion, fatigue	520/7.16/7.9	11.6	+/+/+	NA/NA	30	IV saline and insulin CYC substituted for TAC MMF substituted for AZT	SC insulin Switched to OHA in 6 months
Im et al.	22 F	Heart	22.4	7	TAC	Polydipsia, anorexia, abdominal pain	702/6.9/4	12.1	+/+/NA	NA/NA	>30	IV saline and insulin Tapering TAC regimen	SC insulin Switched to OHA in 3 months
Keshavarz et al.	14 F	Liver	NA	12	TAC + PDN	Chest pain, dyspnea	980/7.08/11	10.5	+/+/+	NA/NA	24	IV saline and insulin CYC substituted for TAC	SC insulin
Masood et al.	17 M	Kidney	NA	12	TAC + PDL + MMF	Polyuria, nocturia, dry mouth, anorexia, vomiting, confusion	702/7.10/6	NA	NA/+/NA	−/−	NA	IV saline and insulin CYC substituted for TAC	SC insulin

Table 1: Continued.

	Age (years), Gender	Organ transplant	BMI (kg/m2)	Duration since transplantation (month)	Maintenance immunosuppressant regimen	Presentation	Glucose (mg/dl)/pH/HCO$_3^-$ (mmol/l)	HbA$_1$C (%)	Glucosuria, ketonuria, proteinuria	IA-2 Ab/GAD-65 Ab	Tacrolimus level (ng/ml)	Management	Discharge regimen/outcome
Masood et al.	55 F	Liver	NA	24	TAC + PDL + MMF	Polyuria, dizziness	474/NA/16.4	8.9	NA/+/NA	NA/NA	NA	IV saline and insulin	SC insulin
Öztürk et al.	17 M	Heart	15.4	3	TAC + PDL + MMF	Dyspnea, fatigue	574/7.22/13.3	9.7	NA/+/NA	−/−	45.4	IV saline and insulin Tapering TAC regimen	SC insulin
Solmaz et al.	24 F	Bone marrow	20.8	2	TAC	Loss of consciousness	890/6.9/4	9.1	+/+/NA	NA/NA	NR	IV saline and insulin CYC substituted for TAC	NA
Toyonaga et al.	43 M	Kidney	18.2	12	TAC + MPL	Polyuria, polydipsia, fatigue, weight loss	925/7.34/23.8	11.8	+/+/+	−/−	9.4	IV saline and insulin Tapering TAC regimen	Diabetic diet
Tuğcu et al.	44 M	Kidney	NA	1	TAC + PDL + MMF	Polyuria, polydipsia, weakness	862/7.27/15	10.7	+/+/NA	−/−	9.4	IV saline and insulin Everolimus substituted TAC	SC insulin
Yoshida et al.	50 F	Liver	NA	9	TAC + PDN + AZT	Polyuria, polydipsia, visual blurring	1227/6.93/3	NA	NA/+/NA	NA/NA	21.2	IV saline and insulin	SC insulin

Abbreviations. BMI, body mass index; HgbA1C, hemoglobin A1C; IA-2 Ab; IA-2-2 Ab, islet antigen 2 antibody; GAD-65 Ab, glutamic acid decarboxylase antibody; M, male; F, female; NA, not available; TAC, tacrolimus; PDN, prednisone; MPS, mycophenolate sodium; PDL, prednisolone; CYC, cyclosporine; NR, normal range; IV, intravenous; SC, subcutaneous; MPL, methylprednisolone; MMF, mycophenolate mofetil; AZT, azathioprine; OHA, oral hypoglycemic agents.

study highlights the importance of regular monitoring of fasting blood glucose in transplant patients on tacrolimus based regimen for early detection of NODAT in order to prevent life-threatening complications. It is also another call for attention on the toxic effects of this potent calcineurin inhibitor.

Abbreviations

DKA: Diabetic ketoacidosis
ADPKD: Autosomal dominant polycystic kidney disease
NODAT: New-onset diabetes mellitus after transplantation
ESRD: End stage renal disease.

Authors' Contributions

Zaid Ammari was responsible for conception and design of the article, data collection, data analysis and interpretation, drafting of the article, and final approval of the version to be published. Stella C. Pak, Mohammed Ruzieh, Osama Dasa, and Abhinav Tiwari were responsible for data collection, data analysis and interpretation, drafting of the article, and final approval of the version to be published. Juan C. Jaume and Maria A. Alfonso-Jaume were responsible for critical revision of the article and final approval of the version to be published.

References

[1] E. L. Porrini, J. M. Díaz, F. Moreso et al., "Clinical evolution of post-transplant diabetes mellitus," *Nephrology Dialysis Transplantation* , vol. 31, no. 3, pp. 495–505, 2016.

[2] Z. Kaposztas, E. Gyurus, and B. D. Kahan, "New-onset diabetes after renal transplantation: Diagnosis, incidence, risk factors, impact on outcomes, and novel implications," *Transplantation Proceedings*, vol. 43, no. 5, pp. 1375–1394, 2011.

[3] O. Heisel, R. Heisel, R. Balshaw, and P. Keown, "New Onset Diabetes Mellitus in Patients Receiving Calcineurin Inhibitors: A Systematic Review and Meta-Analysis," *American Journal of Transplantation*, vol. 4, no. 4, pp. 583–595, 2004.

[4] F. Vincenti, S. Friman, E. Scheuermann et al., "Results of an international, randomized trial comparing glucose metabolism disorders and outcome with cyclosporine versus tacrolimus," *Am J Transplant*, vol. 7, no. 6, pp. 1506–1514, 2007.

[5] J. W. Huang, O. Famure, Y. Li, and S. J. Kim, "Hypomagnesemia and the Risk of New-Onset Diabetes Mellitus after Kidney Transplantation," *J Am Soc Nephrol*, vol. 27, no. 6, pp. 1793–1800, 2016.

[6] R. A. Hamer, C. L. Chow, A. C. M. Ong, and W. S. McKane, "Polycystic kidney disease is a risk factor for new-onset diabetes after transplantation," *Transplantation*, vol. 83, no. 1, pp. 36–40, 2007.

[7] T. E. Burroughs, J. Swindle, S. Takemoto et al., "Diabetic complications associated with new-onset diabetes mellitus in renal transplant recipients," *Transplantation*, vol. 83, no. 8, pp. 1027–1034, 2007.

[8] Y. M. Cho, K. S. Park, H. S. Jung, Y. S. Kim, S. Y. Kim, and H. K. Lee, "A case showing complete insulin independence after severe diabetic ketoacidosis associated with tacrolimus treatment.," *Diabetes Care*, vol. 25, no. 9, p. 1664, 2002.

[9] S. M. Dehghani, S. Nikeghbalian, A. Eshraghian et al., "New-onset diabetes mellitus presenting with diabetic ketoacidosis after pediatric liver transplantation," *Pediatric Transplantation*, vol. 13, no. 5, pp. 536–539, 2009.

[10] A. Ersoy, C. Ersoy, H. Tekce, I. Yavascaoglu, and K. Dilek, "Diabetic ketoacidosis following development of de novo diabetes in renal transplant recipient associated with tacrolimus," *Transplantation Proceedings*, vol. 36, no. 5, pp. 1407–1410, 2004.

[11] M.-S. Im, H.-S. Ahn, H.-J. Cho, K.-B. Kim, and H.-Y. Lee, "Diabetic ketoacidosis associated with acute pancreatitis in a heart transplant recipient treated with tacrolimus," *Experimental and Clinical Transplantation*, vol. 11, no. 1, pp. 72–74, 2013.

[12] R. Keshavarz, M.-A. Mousavi, and C. Hassani, "Diabetic ketoacidosis in a child on FK506 immunosuppression after a liver transplant," *Pediatric Emergency Care*, vol. 18, no. 1, pp. 22–24, 2002.

[13] M. Q. Masood, M. Rabbani, W. Jafri, M. Habib, and T. Saleem, "Diabetic ketoacidosis associated with tacrolimus in solid organ transplant recipients," *Journal of the Pakistan Medical Association*, vol. 61, no. 3, pp. 288–290, 2011.

[14] Z. Öztürk, E. Nazlı Gönç, L. Akcan, S. Kesici, İ. Ertuğrul, and B. Bayrakçı, "A rare but important adverse effect of tacrolimus in a heart transplant recipient: Diabetic ketoacidosis," *The Turkish Journal of Pediatrics*, vol. 57, no. 5, pp. 533–535, 2015.

[15] S. Solmaz, Z. Gokgoz, and C. Gereklioglu, "Tacrolimus-Induced Diabetic Ketoacidosis After Allogeneic Bone Marrow Transplant," *Exp Clin Transplant*, 2015.

[16] T. Toyonaga, T. Kondo, N. Miyamura et al., "Sudden onset of diabetes with ketoacidosis in a patient treated with FK506/tacrolimus," *Diabetes Research and Clinical Practice*, vol. 56, no. 1, pp. 13–18, 2002.

[17] M. Tuğcu, U. Kasapoglu, B. Boynuegri et al., "Tacrolimus-induced diabetic ketoacidosis and effect of switching to everolimus: a case report," *Transplantation Proceedings*, vol. 47, no. 5, pp. 1528–1530, 2015.

[18] E. M. Yoshida, A. K. Buczkowski, S. M. Sirrs et al., "Post-transplant diabetic ketoacidosis - A possible consequence of immunosuppression with calcineurin inhibiting agents: A case series," *Transplant International*, vol. 13, no. 1, pp. 69–72, 2000.

[19] K. C. Abbott, V. J. Bernet, L. Y. Agodoa, and C. M. Yuan, "Diabetic ketoacidosis and hyperglycemic hyperosmolar syndrome after renal tranplantation in the United States," *BMC Endocrine Disorders*, vol. 3, article no. 1, 2003.

[20] M. Kamel, M. Kadian, T. Srinivas, D. Taber, and M. A. Salas, "Tacrolimus confers lower acute rejection rates and better renal allograft survival compared to cyclosporine," *World Journal of Transplantation*, vol. 6, no. 4, p. 697, 2016.

[21] L. A. Øzbay, K. Smidt, D. M. Mortensen, J. Carstens, K. A. Jørgensen, and J. Rungby, "Cyclosporin and tacrolimus impair insulin secretion and transcriptional regulation in INS-1E beta-cells," *British Journal of Pharmacology*, vol. 162, no. 1, pp. 136–146, 2011.

[22] I. Hernández-Fisac, J. Pizarro-Delgado, C. Calle et al., "Tacrolimus-induced diabetes in rats courses with suppressed insulin gene expression in pancreatic islets," *American Journal of Transplantation*, vol. 7, no. 11, pp. 2455–2462, 2007.

16

Thyrotoxicosis Associated with a Hypopharyngeal Toxic Nodular Thyroid

S. Ali Imran,[1] Adam Hinchey,[2] Rob Hart,[3] Martin Bullock,[4] Andrew Ross,[5] and Steven Burrell[5]

[1]Division of Endocrinology and Metabolism, Department of Medicine, Dalhousie University, Halifax, NS, Canada
[2]Dalhousie Medical School, Halifax, NS, Canada
[3]Division of Otolaryngology, Department of Surgery, Dalhousie University, Halifax, NS, Canada
[4]Department of Pathology, Dalhousie University, Halifax, NS, Canada
[5]Division of Nuclear Medicine, Department of Diagnostic Radiology, Dalhousie University, Halifax, NS, Canada

Correspondence should be addressed to S. Ali Imran; ali.imran@nshealth.ca

Academic Editor: Toshihiro Kita

Ectopic thyroid is a rare developmental anomaly which may be either asymptomatic or present with thyroid dysfunction as well as pressure symptoms. Here we present a novel case of thyrotoxicosis associated with a hypopharyngeal multinodular thyroid in a female. Removal of the ectopic thyroid led to normalization of the thyroid status.

1. Case Description

A 32-year-old female was referred to the endocrine clinic for assessment of hyperthyroidism. She was previously known to have mild depression that was controlled on Cipralex 10 mg daily. She had originally gone to her family physician for frequent palpitations and excessive sweating for the past 3 months. Preliminary work-up showed thyroid stimulating hormone (TSH) of <0.01 mIU/L (normal: 0.35–5.50) and serum free thyroxine (fT4) of 20 pmol/L (9.5–19.0). The family physician prescribed methimazole, 5 mg twice a day, and 8 weeks later her TSH became 6.01 mIU/L and serum fT4 dropped to 9.0 pmol/L. Methimazole was discontinued and she remained biochemically euthyroid until a follow-up blood test around 9 months later showed TSH of <0.01 mIU/L, fT4 of 17.4, and free triiodothyronine (fT3) of 7.2 pmol/L (normal: 3.5–6.5) at which point she was referred to endocrinology.

She denied any family history of thyroid disorders and, on initial assessment, her pulse was 82/minute (regular), blood pressure was 110/84, she had mild tremor and moist skin, and her reflexes were brisk (grade 3). There was no evidence of thyroid associated ophthalmopathy. Methimazole 5 mg twice a day was again initiated and the preliminary investigations revealed that thyroid receptor antibody was <1 IU/L (normal < 1) and antithyroid peroxidase antibody was < 10 IU/mL (normal ≤ 40). A ^{99m}Tc-pertechnetate thyroid scan was performed (Figure 1(a)) after discontinuing methimazole for 4 days, which revealed heterogeneous uptake in a large lobulated mass superior to the right lobe of the thyroid. Uptake throughout the thyroid itself was relatively homogenous. The 6-hour radioiodine (^{131}Iodine) uptake was measured at 27.1% (normal < 20%) but may have been underestimated as counts from the mass above the thyroid may not have been fully detected by the probe. Her thyroid indices normalized with methimazole 5 mg daily, which was continued for one year and then stopped. However, within few weeks of stopping methimazole she experienced recurrence of thyrotoxic symptoms including palpitations, excessive sweating, and anxiety and repeat testing showed suppression of serum TSH to <0.01 mIU/L with fT4 being 16.1 pmol/. ^{99m}Tc-pertechnetate was repeated which was similar in appearance (not shown). This time SPECT-CT (Single Photon Emission Computed Tomography-Computed Tomography) imaging was also performed to better localize the mass, revealing it to be in the

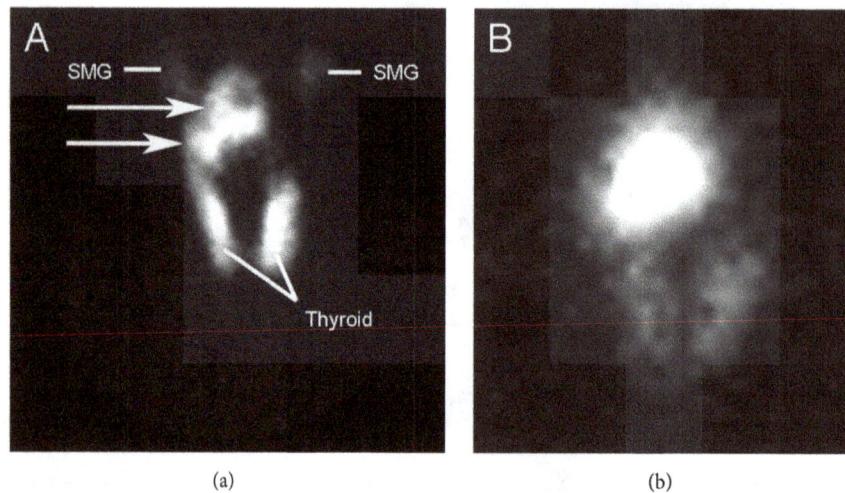

(a)   (b)

FIGURE 1: (a) Anterior view from initial ^{99m}Tc-pertechnetate thyroid scan. There is heterogeneous uptake in a lobulated mass (arrows) superior to the right lobe of the thyroid. Uptake in the thyroid gland is relatively homogeneous. There is normal physiologic uptake in the submandibular glands (SMG). ^{131}Iodine scan (b) demonstrates intense radioiodine uptake in the mass.

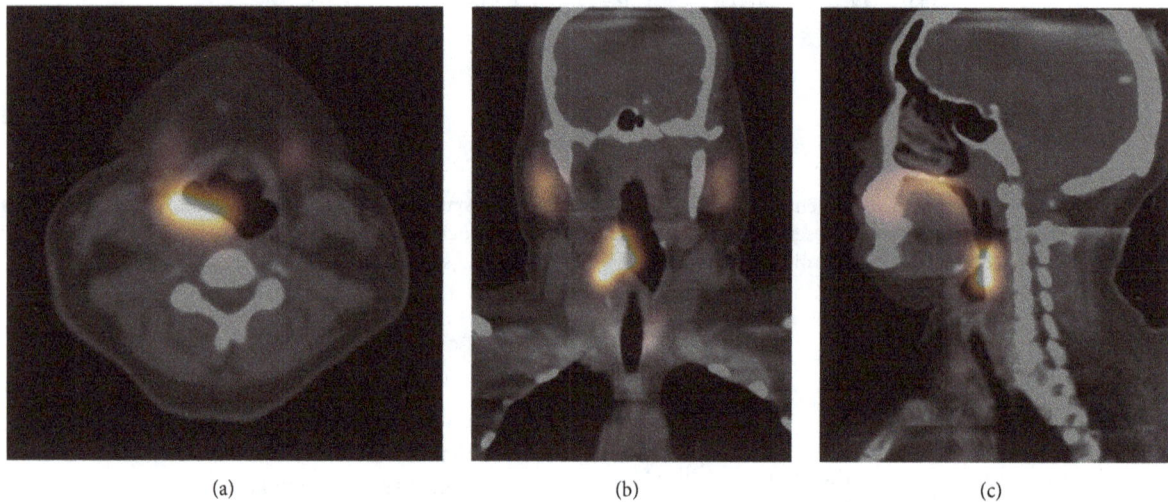

(a)   (b)   (c)

FIGURE 2: SPECT-CT images from the second ^{99m}Tc-pertechnetate thyroid scan ((a) axial, (b) coronal, and (c) sagittal) localize the mass to the posterior right hypopharynx.

right posterior hypopharynx, measuring up to 4 cm cranial-caudal (Figure 2). A thyroid ultrasound was performed which showed a 9.0 × 9.5 CM slightly heterogeneous mass with internal vascularity just above the superior aspect of the right thyroid with no other focal lesion in the right lobe and a small 5 mm mixed echogenicity nodule in the lower left lobe. An ^{131}Iodine scan was then performed (Figure 1(b)) that revealed intense radioiodine uptake in the mass, confirming that it was indeed thyroidal in origin. The uptake in the mass was more intense than the uptake in the thyroid gland, in keeping with a hyperfunctioning ("hot") nodule.

The patient did not complain of any symptoms due to mass effect of the lesion. The finding and management options including continuing medical therapy with methimazole, radioiodine therapy, and surgical excision were discussed with the patient, who opted for surgical excision of

the mass. She was maintained in a euthyroid state on methimazole and surgical excision of the lateral hypopharyngeal mass was conducted. Given the uncommon location, care was taken to avoid injury to the superior laryngeal nerve, which was proven normal on postoperative endoscopy. The surgical specimen consisted of a 16 g, 5.3 cm mass of thyroid tissue. Some normal thyroid parenchyma was present that contained several small hyperplastic nodules, but the specimen was dominated by an attached 3.5 cm circumscribed nodule of hyperplastic thyroid tissue. This consisted of a mixed population of microfollicles, macrofollicles, and small cysts containing pale colloid. Focal papillary infoldings of hyperplastic follicular cells extended into the dilated follicles (Figure 3). The nodule was partially fibrotic and focally calcified. There was no significant inflammation in the nodule or the adjacent normal thyroid parenchyma. There was no

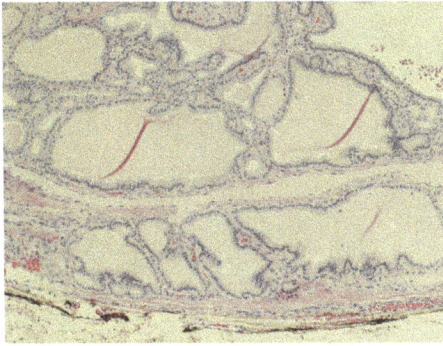

FIGURE 3: Photomicrograph of the edge of the dominant nodule, showing irregularly dilated follicles with pale colloid and subtle infoldings of the follicular epithelium. The follicular cells are uniform and evenly spaced, without features of papillary thyroid carcinoma (H&E, 100x).

evidence of malignancy. Methimazole was discontinued after surgery and the patient remains biochemically euthyroid.

2. Discussion

Ectopic thyroid tissue is a rare developmental abnormality involving defects in the embryogenesis of the thyroid gland during its embryological descent. Its prevalence is reported to be approximately 1 per 100,000–300,000 people but it is likely much commoner as the autopsy studies have suggested the prevalence being as high as 7–10% [1]. In the reported larger series, ectopia of the thyroid is commoner in females [2, 3]. The thyroid gland is derived from the endoderm and an understanding of the development of the gland can aid in identifying typical locations where ectopic thyroid tissue can develop. The thyroid is one of the earliest glands to develop with the formation of the medial anlage on gestation days 16 and 17. The expanding thyroid remains attached to the pharyngeal floor by the stalk called the thyroglossal duct. The medial portion of the thyroid is associated with the developing heart and with the descent of the heart the thyroid is pulled caudally into its position at the base of the neck with the consequent elongation of the thyroglossal duct which generally degenerates. Although the ectopic thyroid tissue can develop anywhere along the developmental pathway, the base of the tongue remains the most common site accounting for up to 90% of the cases of ectopic thyroid [4]. However, ectopic thyroid tissue has been reported around the hyoid bone, infrahyoid and lateral portions of the neck, and rarely in peripheral sites such as the mediastinum, adrenal glands, and the duodenum.

Symptoms of the ectopic thyroid can vary depending upon its location. The commonest location is the base of the tongue where it can present with dysphonia, dysphagia, cough, sleep apnea, and rarely with obstruction [5, 6]. Other sites include submandibular thyroid which can present as a localized swelling in the carotid triangle, whereas intratracheal thyroid has also been described which can present with cough, dyspnea, hemoptysis, and stridor. Rarely reported intrathoracic and intracardiac thyroid can present

with signs of obstruction, chest pain, and palpitations [7, 8]. Neoplasia of the ectopic thyroid tissue has also previously been described. Typically, neoplasms of the thyroglossal duct tend to be papillary carcinoma; however, follicular thyroid cancer has also been described [9]. Thyrotoxicosis associated with ectopic thyroid tissue has also been described as a result of retrotracheal and intrathoracic toxic nodules and lingual thyroid as well as submandibular thyroid [10–13]. To our knowledge no case of an ectopic pharyngeal multinodular thyroid has been described previously, particularly in the setting of an otherwise normally positioned thyroid gland.

Although the most appropriate therapeutic option for an ectopic thyroid remains unclear, most reported cases underwent surgery. Surgical excision would obviously be required in case of obstructive symptoms; yet in asymptomatic cases nonsurgical follow-up may be sufficient. Others have reported I-131 ablation therapy for ectopic thyroid [14]; however, it is suggested that a significantly higher dose of I-131 [15] may be needed for ablation in such cases. Therefore, ablation therapy should be carefully assessed in younger individuals.

In summary, this case highlights an unusual case of thyrotoxicosis due to an ectopic hyperfunctioning thyroid mass in the lateral hypopharynx, localized preoperatively with SPECT-CT imaging. The pathology showed a multinodular thyroid.

References

[1] G. Guerra, M. Cinelli, M. Mesolella et al., "Morphological, diagnostic and surgical features of ectopic thyroid gland: a review of literature," *International Journal of Surgery*, vol. 12, supplement 1, pp. S3–S11, 2014.

[2] J. S. Yoon, K. C. Won, I. H. Cho, J. T. Lee, and H. W. Lee, "Clinical characteristics of ectopic thyroid in Korea," *Thyroid*, vol. 17, no. 11, pp. 1117–1121, 2007.

[3] R. A. Gopal, S. V. Acharya, T. Bandgar, P. S. Menon, H. Marfatia, and N. S. Shah, "Clinical profile of ectopic thyroid in asian indians: a single-center experience," *Endocrine Practice*, vol. 15, no. 4, pp. 322–325, 2009.

[4] G. Noussios, P. Anagnostis, D. G. Goulis, D. Lappas, and K. Natsis, "Ectopic thyroid tissue: anatomical, clinical, and surgical implications of a rare entity," *European Journal of Endocrinology*, vol. 165, no. 3, pp. 375–382, 2011.

[5] A. Toso, F. Colombani, G. Averono, P. Aluffi, and F. Pia, "Lingual thyroid causing dysphagia and dyspnoea. Case reports and review of the literature," *Acta Otorinorhinolaryngologica Italica*, vol. 29, no. 4, pp. 213–217, 2009.

[6] F. Muysoms, M. Boedts, and D. Claeys, "Intratracheal ectopic thyroid tissue mass," *CHEST*, vol. 112, no. 6, pp. 1684-1685, 1997.

[7] I. Richmond, J. S. Whittaker, A. K. Deiraniya, and R. Hassan, "Intracardiac ectopic thyroid: A case report and review of published cases," *Thorax*, vol. 45, no. 4, pp. 293-294, 1990.

[8] B. Özpolat, O. V. Doğan, G. Gökaslan, S. Erekul, and E. Yücel, "Ectopic thyroid gland on the ascending aorta with a partial

pericardial defect: Report of a case," *Surgery Today*, vol. 37, no. 6, pp. 486–488, 2007.

[9] J. Klubo-Gwiezdzinska, R. P. Manes, S. H. Chia et al., "Ectopic cervical thyroid carcinoma—Review of the literature with illustrative case series," *The Journal of Clinical Endocrinology & Metabolism*, vol. 96, no. 9, pp. 2684–2691, 2011.

[10] M. Salvatori, V. Rufini, S. M. Corsello et al., "Thyrotoxicosis due to ectopic retrotracheal adenoma treated with radioiodine," *The Journal of Nuclear Biology and Medicine*, vol. 37, no. 2, pp. 69–72, 1993.

[11] B. D. Serim, U. Korkmaz, U. Can, and G. Altun, "Intrathoracic toxic thyroid nodule causing hyperthyroidism with a multin-odular normal functional cervical thyroid gland," *Indian Journal of Nuclear Medicine*, vol. 31, no. 3, pp. 229–231, 2016.

[12] M. P. Abdallah-Matta, P. H. Dubarry, J. J. Pessey, and P. Caron, "Lingual thyroid and hyperthyroidism: a new case and review of the literature," *Journal of Endocrinological Investigation*, vol. 25, no. 3, pp. 264–267, 2002.

[13] R. Kumar, R. Gupta, C. S. Bal, S. Khullar, and A. Malhotra, "Thyrotoxicosis in a patient with submandibular thyroid," *Thyroid*, vol. 10, no. 4, pp. 363–365, 2000.

[14] P. Iglesias, R. Olmos-García, B. Riva, and J. J. Díez, "Iodine 131 and lingual thyroid," *The Journal of Clinical Endocrinology & Metabolism*, vol. 93, no. 11, pp. 4198-4199, 2008.

[15] F. W. Neinas, C. A. Gorman, K. D. Devine, and L. B. Woolner, "Lingual thyroid: Clinical characteristics of 15 cases," *Annals of Internal Medicine*, vol. 79, no. 2, pp. 205–210, 1973.

17

Patients with Acromegaly Presenting with Colon Cancer: A Case Series

Murray B. Gordon,[1] Samer Nakhle,[2] and William H. Ludlam[3]

[1]Allegheny Neuroendocrinology Center, Departments of Medicine and Neurosurgery, Allegheny General Hospital, 320 East North Avenue, Pittsburgh, PA 15212, USA
[2]Palm Research Center, 9280 West Sunset Road, Suite 306, Las Vegas, NV 89148, USA
[3]Novartis Pharmaceuticals, 1 Health Plaza, East Hanover, NJ 07936, USA

Correspondence should be addressed to Murray B. Gordon; mgordon740@msn.com

Academic Editor: Wayne V. Moore

Introduction. Frequent colonoscopy screenings are critical for early diagnosis of colon cancer in patients with acromegaly. *Case Presentations*. We performed a retrospective analysis of the incidental diagnoses of colon cancer from the ACCESS trial (ClinicalTrials.gov identifier: NCT01995734). Colon cancer was identified in 2 patients (4.5%). Case 1 patient was a 36-year-old male with acromegaly who underwent transsphenoidal surgery to remove the pituitary adenoma. After surgery, the patient underwent routine colonoscopy screening, which revealed a 40 mm tubular adenoma in the descending colon. A T1N1a carcinoma was surgically removed, and 1 of 22 lymph nodes was positive for metastatic disease, leading to a diagnosis of stage 3 colon cancer. Case 2 patient was a 50-year-old male with acromegaly who underwent transsphenoidal surgery to remove a 2 cm pituitary adenoma. The patient reported severe cramping and lower abdominal pain, and an invasive 8.1 cm^3 grade 2 adenocarcinoma with signet rings was identified in the ascending colon and removed. Of the 37 lymph nodes, 34 were positive for the presence of tumor cells, and stage 3c colon cancer was confirmed. *Conclusion*. Current guidelines for colonoscopy screening at the time of diagnosis of acromegaly and at appropriate follow-up intervals should be followed.

1. Introduction

Acromegaly is a disease most often caused by benign somatotrophic pituitary adenomas that lead to elevated secretion of growth hormone (GH), which stimulates increased expression of insulin-like growth factor 1 (IGF-1) [1]. A persistent increase in GH and IGF-1 leads to known acromegaly-associated comorbidities, including congestive heart failure, arthritis, and impaired glucose tolerance [1]. In some studies, colon polyps or cancer have also been reported to occur more frequently in patients with acromegaly than in the general population [2]. However, data from other studies have not supported the association between acromegaly and colon cancer [2, 3]. Here, we present case studies of 2 patients who were diagnosed with colon cancer from a small cohort of patients with acromegaly.

2. Case Presentations

We performed a retrospective analysis of the incidental diagnoses of colon cancer in the ACCESS trial (ClinicalTrials.gov identifier: NCT01995734), an open-label, multicenter study that allowed for expanded access to pasireotide long-acting while regulatory approval was being pursued. To be included in the cohort, patients with acromegaly must have undergone surgery to remove the pituitary tumor (unless they were not eligible for surgery or refused surgery) and had uncontrolled acromegaly, as defined by IGF-1 levels greater than the upper limit of normal and random GH greater than 1 ng/mL. Patients were excluded if they had been diagnosed with active malignant disease within the last 5 years (with the possible exception of basal cell carcinoma or carcinoma in situ of the cervix). Colon cancer was diagnosed using colonoscopy, and

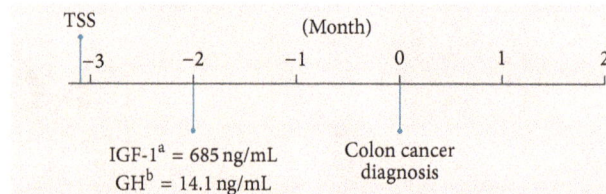

FIGURE 1: Patient timeline from removal of pituitary adenoma to colon cancer diagnosis. GH, growth hormone; IGF-1, insulin-like growth factor 1; TSS, transsphenoidal surgery. [a]Reference range, 109–329 ng/mL. [b]Reference range, ≤3 ng/mL.

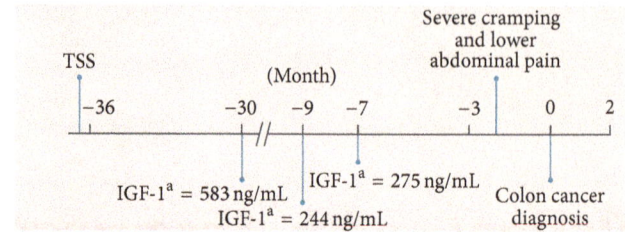

FIGURE 2: Patient timeline from removal of pituitary adenoma to colon cancer diagnosis. IGF-1, insulin-like growth factor 1; TSS, transsphenoidal surgery. [a]Reference range, 70–205 ng/mL.

histological examination of tumor resections was used for cancer staging.

The cohort was composed of 44 patients (female, 56.8%). The mean age was 45.5 years, and the mean body mass index was 32.9 kg/m^2. Impaired fasting glucose and type 2 diabetes mellitus were observed in 1 (2.3%) and 9 (20.5%) patients, respectively. Two men (4.5%) were incidentally diagnosed with stage 3 colon cancer soon after they entered the study (after 1 week for 1 patient and after 5 months for the other patient); however, the cancer-related events were considered to be unrelated to treatment with the study drug.

Case 1 patient was a 36-year-old white male with a reported family history of colon cancer (grandmother) who presented with acromegaly, weight loss, and skin tags. The patient had not been screened by colonoscopy before diagnosis of acromegaly. Three months before case presentation, transsphenoidal surgery was performed with resection of a pituitary adenoma (Figure 1). Approximately 6 weeks after surgery, the patient's IGF-1 level was 685 ng/mL, more than twice the upper limit of normal (reference range, 109–329 ng/mL), and his GH level was 14.1 ng/mL (reference range, ≤3 ng/mL). Magnetic resonance imaging revealed no evidence of pituitary adenoma 3 months after surgery.

The patient enrolled in the study 1 week before case presentation. One week after study enrollment, the patient underwent routine colonoscopy screening, which revealed a 40 mm tubular adenoma in the descending colon. A T1N1a carcinoma was surgically removed 2 weeks later; 1 of 22 lymph nodes was positive for metastatic disease. The patient was diagnosed with stage 3 colon cancer and started oxaliplatin every 3 weeks (targeting 10 treatments) and capecitabine 4 g once daily. The patient reported cold sensitivity, some nausea, soft stools (resolved), weight loss, metallic mouth, depression, and anxiety associated with chemotherapy treatment. The colon tumor was subsequently resected, and the patient is now in remission without evidence of tumor recurrence.

Case 2 patient was a 50-year-old male who originally presented with headache, hypogonadism, and fatigue. Initial colonoscopy (performed 3 years before the diagnosis of acromegaly) was negative. Magnetic resonance imaging showed a 2 cm pituitary adenoma that was removed with transsphenoidal surgery. The patient's IGF-1 levels were uncontrolled after surgery and ranged from 244 to 583 ng/mL (reference range, 70–205 ng/mL) during 16 months of lanreotide Autogel treatment (Figure 2). The patient switched

to pasireotide long-acting at the beginning of the trial and continued to receive pasireotide.

Six months later, the patient reported severe cramping and lower abdominal pain, and a colonoscopy was performed. Two polyps were revealed, and an invasive 8.1 cm^3 grade 2 adenocarcinoma with signet rings was removed from the ascending colon. Of the 37 lymph nodes, 34 were positive for the presence of tumor cells. Histology confirmed stage 3c colon cancer, and the patient started treatment with capecitabine and oxaliplatin. The patient subsequently died in hospice care because of metastatic colon cancer. The death was not considered related to pasireotide treatment.

3. Discussion

These case studies detail the identification of advanced-stage colon cancer in 2 patients (4.5%) from a cohort of patients who were being treated for uncontrolled acromegaly. The incidence of colon cancer in this cohort is comparable to and within the range of other reported epidemiological findings of colon cancer in acromegaly (1.1%–20.0%) [4]. It should be noted that the identification of colon cancer was not considered to be related to the study drug, which is not surprising given that the 2 patients had only been in the study for 1 week in case 1 and 5 months in case 2, and colon cancer is associated with various stages that occur over many years. Because many patients with uncontrolled acromegaly are undiagnosed for years, it is possible that persistently elevated GH and IGF-1 levels could be a factor in the relatively high incidence of colon cancer in this cohort compared with the general population [5]. Therefore, biochemical control of GH and IGF-1 levels may reduce the risk of colon cancer in patients with acromegaly. There are currently no prospective interventional studies demonstrating to what extent therapies that reduce GH and IGF-1 levels affect the incidence and prognosis of colon cancer in acromegaly.

The extent of the association between colon cancer risk and acromegaly has been unclear. In a preclinical model, local increases in colon GH generated a tumor microenvironment that was permissive for neoplastic colon growth in mice [6]. In addition, in a meta-analysis that included 9 controlled studies of 701 patients with acromegaly and 1573 controls, there was a higher risk of colon cancer in patients with acromegaly (14/304 [4.6%]) than in control patients (8/627 [1.2%]) [2]. In contrast, a study by Renehan et al. found no difference in the prevalence of colon cancer or colonic polyps between patients with acromegaly using colonoscopy and control patients without acromegaly using autopsy examinations [7]. However, autopsy examinations may have detected a higher rate of adenomas/carcinomas in the general population because the examinations could be more extensive.

Other factors may contribute to the increased risk of colon cancer in patients with acromegaly. Hyperplastic polyps and carcinoma have been associated with higher levels of serum GH [8], although higher IGF-1 levels are also associated with increased risks [9, 10]. In addition, the risk of colonic lesions is 2.4- to 5.8-fold higher in patients with impaired glucose regulation (impaired fasting glucose, impaired glucose tolerance, or diabetes) than in those with normal glucose tolerance [11]. This effect may be mediated by hyperinsulinemia, because the risk of developing adenomatous polyps was 14.8 times higher in patients with fasting insulin levels in the highest tertile than in those with levels in the lowest tertile [11]. Additionally, genetic factors have also been associated with more frequent incidences of colorectal cancer and may increase the risk of colorectal cancer in patients with acromegaly [12].

Acromegaly treatment guidelines from the American Association of Clinical Endocrinologists (AACE) and the Endocrine Society suggest screening for colon neoplasia with colonoscopy at the time of diagnosis of acromegaly [13, 14]. Furthermore, AACE guidelines suggest that follow-up colonoscopy be performed at time intervals "appropriate for patients at higher-than-average risk for colon cancer" [13], whereas the Endocrine Society guidelines suggest screening every 5 years for patients with elevated IGF-1 levels or polyps and every 10 years for patients with normalized IGF-1 levels and no polyps [14]. In contrast, guidelines from the British Society of Gastroenterology recommend screening every 3 years for patients with adenoma(s) at initial colonoscopy and/or elevated IGF-1, while those from the Acromegaly Consensus Group recommend screening every 3 to 5 years depending on the number and size of the adenomas [4]. These guidelines provide 3 points of consideration. First, colonoscopy was shown to be superior to fecal occult blood testing in identifying adenomas and cancer and is the suggested method of screening for colon neoplasms [15]. Second, colonoscopies should be performed at diagnosis, as evidenced in a study that showed that up to 19.3% of patients with acromegaly who were aged <40 years compared with 4.4% of controls had colonic neoplasia at diagnosis [10]. Third, follow-up colonoscopies should occur, although the frequency has not been firmly established. In this study, there was no evidence of colon cancer in 1 patient at his previous colonoscopy (3 years before the diagnosis of acromegaly and 5 years before the diagnosis of colon cancer). In a retrospective study of patients with acromegaly who were screened by colonoscopy at a mean interval of approximately every 4 years, new polyps were identified in roughly one-third of patients at each screening [16]. Additionally, in this study, a patient with a family history of colon cancer was reported. A cohort analysis previously showed a potential association between increased risk of colon cancer and acromegaly in

male patients with a family history of colon cancer [17]. A joint guideline from the American Cancer Society, US Multi-Society Task Force on Colorectal Cancer, and American College of Radiology recommends that patients with a family history of colon cancer should have a colonoscopy at an earlier age (i.e., before the generally recommended age of 50 years) and more frequently than individuals at average risk [18]. Therefore, based on this case series and in conjunction with a literature review, we suggest an evidence-based guideline of follow-up screening with colonoscopy at relatively shorter intervals (e.g., every 3 years) in patients with acromegaly who are ≤50 years of age, particularly in cases with a positive family history of colon cancer.

4. Conclusion

The diagnoses of colon cancer in this cohort of patients with acromegaly suggests that physicians should perform a routine colonoscopy screening at the time of diagnosis of acromegaly and at appropriate follow-up intervals after the diagnosis. Furthermore, control of GH and IGF-1 levels should be paramount to mitigate comorbidities such as colon cancer.

Disclosure

Dr. Ludlam is now with Chiasma, Inc, 60 Wells Avenue, Newton, MA 02459.

Acknowledgments

Support for this study was provided by Novartis Pharmaceuticals Corporation. Medical editorial assistance was provided by Andrea Eckhart and Meredith MacPherson of MedThink SciCom (Raleigh, NC) and was sponsored by Novartis Pharmaceuticals Corporation.

References

[1] G. Lugo, L. Pena, and F. Cordido, "Clinical manifestations and diagnosis of acromegaly," *International Journal of Endocrinology*, vol. 2012, Article ID 540398, 10 pages, 2012.

[2] T. Rokkas, D. Pistiolas, P. Sechopoulos, G. Margantinis, and G. Koukoulis, "Risk of colorectal neoplasm in patients with acromegaly: a meta-analysis," *World Journal of Gastroenterology*, vol. 14, no. 22, pp. 3484–3489, 2008.

[3] P. J. Jenkins, A. Mukherjee, and S. M. Shalet, "Does growth hormone cause cancer?" *Clinical Endocrinology*, vol. 64, no. 2, pp. 115–121, 2006.

[4] L. Vilar, L. A. Naves, C. Caldato et al., "Acromegaly and colorectal cancer," *Translational Gastrointestinal Cancer*, vol. 4, no. 1, pp. 28–38, 2015.

[5] K. Lois, J. Bukowczan, P. Perros, S. Jones, M. Gunn, and R. A. James, "The role of colonoscopic screening in acromegaly revisited: review of current literature and practice guidelines," *Pituitary*, vol. 18, no. 4, pp. 568–574, 2015.

[6] V. Chesnokova, S. Zonis, C. Zhou et al., "Growth hormone is permissive for neoplastic colon growth," *Proceedings of the National Academy of Sciences*, vol. 113, no. 23, pp. E3250–E3259, 2016.

[7] A. G. Renehan, P. Bhaskar, J. E. Painter et al., "The prevalence and characteristics of colorectal neoplasia in acromegaly," *The Journal of Clinical Endocrinology and Metabolism*, vol. 85, no. 9, pp. 3417–3424, 2000.

[8] Y. Matano, T. Okada, A. Suzuki, T. Yoneda, Y. Takeda, and H. Mabuchi, "Risk of colorectal neoplasm in patients with acromegaly and its relationship with serum growth hormone levels," *The American Journal of Gastroenterology*, vol. 100, no. 5, pp. 1154–1160, 2005.

[9] P. J. Jenkins, V. Frajese, A.-M. Jones et al., "Insulin-like growth factor I and the development of colorectal neoplasia in acromegaly," *The Journal of Clinical Endocrinology and Metabolism*, vol. 85, no. 9, pp. 3218–3221, 2000.

[10] M. Terzolo, G. Reimondo, M. Gasperi et al., "Colonoscopic screening and follow-up in patients with acromegaly: a multi-center study in Italy," *The Journal of Clinical Endocrinology and Metabolism*, vol. 90, no. 1, pp. 84–90, 2005.

[11] A. Colao, R. Pivonello, R. S. Auriemma et al., "The association of fasting insulin concentrations and colonic neoplasms in acromegaly: a colonoscopy-based study in 210 patients," *The Journal of Clinical Endocrinology & Metabolism*, vol. 92, no. 10, pp. 3854–3860, 2007.

[12] M. L. Torre, G. T. Russo, M. Ragonese et al., "MTHFR C677T polymorphism, folate status and colon cancer risk in acrome-galic patients," *Pituitary*, vol. 17, no. 3, pp. 257–266, 2014.

[13] L. Katznelson, J. L. D. Atkinson, D. M. Cook et al., "Amer-ican Association of Clinical Endocrinologists medical guide-lines for clinical practice for the diagnosis and treatment of acromegaly—2011 update: executive summary," *Endocrine Practice*, vol. 17, no. 4, pp. 636–646, 2011.

[14] L. Katznelson, E. R. Laws Jr., S. Melmed et al., "Acromegaly: an endocrine society clinical practice guideline," *The Journal of Clinical Endocrinology and Metabolism*, vol. 99, no. 11, pp. 3933–3951, 2014.

[15] F. Bogazzi, M. Lombardi, I. Scattina et al., "Comparison of colonoscopy and fecal occult blood testing as a first-line screening of colonic lesions in patients with newly diagnosed acromegaly," *Journal of Endocrinological Investigation*, vol. 33, no. 8, pp. 530–533, 2010.

[16] D. Dworakowska, M. Gueorguiev, P. Kelly et al., "Repeated colonoscopic screening of patients with acromegaly: 15-year experience identifies those at risk of new colonic neoplasia and allows for effective screening guidelines," *European Journal of Endocrinology*, vol. 163, no. 1, pp. 21–28, 2010.

[17] J. E. Brunner, C. C. Johnson, S. Zafar, E. L. Peterson, J. F. Brunner, and R. C. Mellinger, "Colon cancer and polyps in acromegaly: increased risk associated with family history of colon cancer," *Clinical Endocrinology*, vol. 32, no. 1, pp. 65–71, 1990.

[18] E. C. Cabebe, Colorectal Cancer Guidelines, Medscape, http://emedicine.medscape.com/article/2500006-overview.

Primary Hyperparathyroidism in Pregnancy: Successful Parathyroidectomy during First Trimester

Niranjan Tachamo (ID),[1] **Bidhya Timilsina,**[1] **Rashmi Dhital** (ID),[1] **Theresa Lynn** (ID),[1] **Vasudev Magaji,**[2] **and Ilan Gabriely**[2]

[1]*Department of Internal Medicine, Reading Hospital, Reading, PA, 19611, USA*
[2]*Section of Endocrinology, Reading Hospital, Reading, PA, 19611, USA*

Correspondence should be addressed to Niranjan Tachamo; niranjan.tachamo@towerhealth.org

Academic Editor: Wayne V. Moore

Primary hyperparathyroidism in pregnancy can result in significant maternal and fetal complications. When indicated, prompt parathyroidectomy in the early second trimester is considered the treatment of choice. Pregnant patients with primary hyperparathyroidism who have an indication for parathyroidectomy during the first trimester represent a therapeutic challenge. We present the case of a 32-year-old primigravida who presented with symptomatic hypercalcemia from her primary hyperparathyroidism. She remained symptomatic despite aggressive conservative management and underwent parathyroidectomy in her first trimester with excellent outcomes.

1. Introduction

Primary hyperparathyroidism (PHP) is rarely diagnosed during pregnancy. It is associated with serious maternal and fetal complications including maternal pancreatitis, nephrolithiasis, hyperemesis, miscarriage, fetal demise, low birth weight, neonatal hypocalcaemia, and tetany. Most cases of PHP during pregnancy are mild, are asymptomatic, and often go undiagnosed [1]. When diagnosed, PHP associated with hypercalcemia should be managed promptly. Surgery (removal of the parathyroid adenoma) in the early second trimester is considered the treatment of choice in selected women [2–4]. We present a case of a primigravida with significant symptomatic hypercalcemia who was diagnosed with PHP and underwent successful parathyroidectomy during her first trimester of pregnancy.

2. Case Presentation

A 32-year-old primigravida presented to the Emergency Department (ED) during her 7th week of gestation with complaints of two weeks of progressively worsening intermittent lower abdominal pain. She denied any visual disturbances, headache, nausea, vomiting, constipation or diarrhea, vaginal bleeding, or uterine contractions. Her medical history was significant for a pituitary microadenoma (6.5 × 6 × 5 mm) diagnosed 12 months prior. At that time her serum prolactin was slightly elevated at 35 ng/mL (Ref: 3.34 - 26.72 ng/mL); however, other pituitary hormones were within the normal limits. There was no family history of parathyroid disease, hypercalcemia, nephrolithiasis, or other endocrinopathies except for hypothyroidism affecting her mother. Admission medications included daily prenatal vitamins.

On presentation to the ED, her review of systems was otherwise negative with no genitourinary or gastrointestinal or neurological symptoms. Her vital signs were within normal limits. Her physical examination was unremarkable.

Her blood tests demonstrated hypercalcemia (serum calcium 12.2 mg/dL [Ref: 8.6-10.3 mg/dL], ionized calcium 1.67 mmol/L [Ref: 1.15 - 1.33 mmol/L]), and hyperparathyroidism (PTH 135 pg/mL [Ref: 12-88 pg/mL]). Her serum albumin was 3.2 g/dL (3.5-5.7 g/dL), phosphorus 2.2 mg/dL (Ref: 2.5-5 mg/dL), and magnesium 1.5 mg/dL (Ref: 1.9-2.7 mg/dL). Other relevant labs included a 24-hour urinary calcium of 712

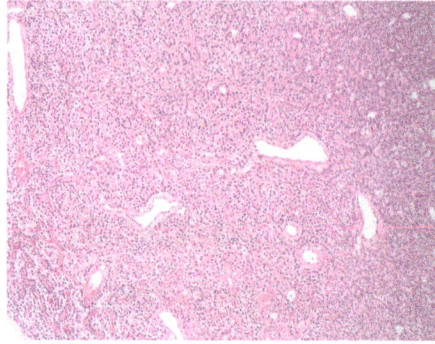

FIGURE 1: Section of the lesion, showing a diffuse proliferation of cells with loss of the acinar architecture. The lesion show patchy foci of glandular luminal formation (H&E stain, 100x original magnification).

mg/24 hour (Ref: 100-300 mg/24 hr), 25-hydroxyvitamin D 18.5 ng/mL (Deficient if <20 ng/mL), 1,25-dihydroxyvitamin D 94.9 pg/mL (Ref: 19.9-79.3 pg/mL), and thyroid stimulating hormone (TSH) 0.43 uIU/mL (Ref: 0.45-5.33 uIU/mL). Renal ultrasound was unremarkable with no nephrolithiasis or hydronephrosis. Thyroid ultrasound revealed a 28 × 11 × 11 mm hypervascular, heterogeneous mass along the posterior margin of the left thyroid gland. A fine needle aspiration from the mass demonstrated scant cells and was reported as benign cytology. The FNA needle washout resulted in high levels of parathyroid hormone.

She was diagnosed with primary hyperparathyroidism and started conservative treatment with IV fluid and magnesium supplements with improvement in her serum calcium levels (11.4 mg/dL). Unfortunately the patient subsequently became symptomatic with nausea, vomiting, and maintaining serum calcium levels of 12 mg/dL despite sufficient hydration. She was started on aggressive hydration (lactated ringers at 125 ml/hr followed by normal saline at 125 ml/hr) continuously until the day of surgery. She received a total of 23 L of intravenous fluids over 10 days; however the serum calcium ranged between 10.6 and 11.6 mg/dL with most values at >11 mg/dL. Just prior to surgery, her serum calcium level was 10.7 mg/dL and her ionized calcium level was 1.38 mmol/L. She underwent left superior parathyroidectomy and the pathology was consistent with a 3.0 × 1.8 × 1.2 cm parathyroid adenoma (Figures 1 and 2). Intraoperative PTH measurement was not performed to reduce the time of anesthesia. Following surgery, her serum calcium and PTH levels normalized. She did not develop hypocalcaemia after surgery. In subsequent follow-up weekly visits after discharge, her serum calcium and PTH levels have been within the normal limits.

With her history of pituitary adenoma and a large parathyroid adenoma, multiple endocrine neoplasia type 1 (MEN1) was considered. However, direct DNA testing for MEN1, RET, AIP, and CDKN1B gene mutations were negative.

3. Discussion

Primary hyperparathyroidism is a common endocrine disorder and has a prevalence estimate of about one to seven

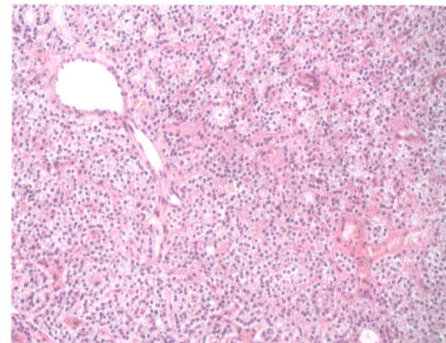

FIGURE 2: High power view of a representative area, showing that the lesion is composed of uniform-appearing cells, indicating a single cell type proliferation, consistent with adenoma (H&E stain, 400x original magnification).

cases per 1000 adults. The true incidence of PHP is difficult to estimate; however it is considered to vary between 0.4 and 21.6 cases per 100000 person-years [5]. The incidence increases with age, and it is two to three times more common in women [5], with peak incidence in women aged 50-60. The exact incidence of PHP in pregnancy is unknown, and most data derives from case reports.

The exact cause of PHP is not known. It was demonstrated that irradiation to the neck (for benign conditions or in survivors of an atomic bomb) was associated with a significantly increasing incidence of PHP [6]. MEN 1 and MEN 2 are examples of genetic mutations associated with PHP [4].

PHP is rarely diagnosed in pregnancy as many cases are mild and asymptomatic. Moreover, many of the nonspecific symptoms of pregnancy, such as nausea, vomiting, fatigue, and constipation, are similar to those associated with hyperparathyroidism, which leads to missed or delayed diagnosis [2]. It is considered that as many as 80% of cases of PHP during pregnancy may be asymptomatic. However, untreated PHP can be associated with significant and serious maternal (e.g., hypercalcemic crisis, pancreatitis, nephrolithiasis, and preeclampsia) and fetal (e.g., neonatal tetany, hypoparathyroidism, stillbirth, and miscarriage) complications which may be as high as 67% and 80% respectively [1, 4]. This may be an overestimate, taking into account that most cases are mild, asymptomatic and undiagnosed, and only clinically evident cases are likely to be reported [4].

Moreover, a large retrospective study by Abood et al. did not find any significant difference in pregnancy outcomes between patients with PHP during pregnancy and age-matched controls [7]. Norman et al., however, showed that hyperparathyroidism in pregnancy had a 3.5 times higher rate of abortion when compared to the general population. As expected, the rate of complications increased with the escalating levels of maternal serum calcium [3].

The diagnosis of PHP during pregnancy is similar to nonpregnant patients with the exception that physiological changes in pregnancy (plasma volume expansion) result in low total serum calcium level; the upper limit of normal total calcium in pregnancy is considered 9.5 mg/dL [1]. Alternatively, ionized calcium does not change significantly with pregnancy and may represent a better assay to assess serum calcium levels during pregnancy [2, 4].

Neck ultrasound is used to identify the parathyroid adenoma (sensitivity 69%, specificity 94%) as nuclear scans are contraindicated in pregnancy due to concern for fetal risk from ionizing radiation [2]. Fine needle aspiration and needle washout for PTH are not routinely recommended (it carries a particular risk in patients with parathyroid cancer). However, since surgery in the first trimester carries a substantial risk, we wanted to ensure that the nodule identified in the thyroid ultrasound was indeed a parathyroid adenoma prior to subjecting the patient to surgery. In the overall risk calculation, we took into account the facts that the prevalence of parathyroid carcinoma in the general population is very low and it usually occurs in the higher age group. Furthermore, parathyroid carcinoma is associated with significantly higher serum calcium and PTH levels. Thus, taking into account the patient's demographic data, the clinical presentation and serum calcium, and PTH level, we considered that her risk of having parathyroid carcinoma was very low.

In the differential diagnosis, familial hypocalciuric hypercalcemia and hereditary syndromes such as MEN-1 and MEN-2 should always be considered [2], both of which were ruled out in our patient.

There are no clear guidelines for management of PHP during pregnancy. Treatment should be tailored based on symptoms, severity of hypercalcemia, gestational age, and the risk-benefit assessment [8].

Mild cases of asymptomatic PHP in pregnancy may be managed conservatively with a low calcium diet, adequate hydration, and close monitoring of serum calcium. A small dose of vitamin D may be supplemented cautiously in deficient patients to decrease PTH levels, as well as lower the risk of hungry bone syndrome postoperatively if parathyroidectomy is planned. However, excess and rapid supplementation can lead to aggravation of the hypercalcemia and hypercalcemic crisis [4]. In more severe cases, cinacalcet and calcitonin may be used with temporary results. Bisphosphonates are not indicated in pregnancy because of the risk of fetal bone toxicity and modeling abnormality [2].

Parathyroidectomy remains the only curative treatment. In multiple reports, conservative management was shown to have higher fetal complications when compared to parathyroidectomy in pregnancy [9, 10]. The current recommendation is to perform parathyroidectomy during the second trimester of pregnancy due to incomplete organogenesis in first trimester, and risk of preterm labor in the third trimester [4]. While there are multiple reports of successful second and third trimester parathyroidectomy, there are only limited data on parathyroidectomy during the first trimester. In a review by Carella et al. [11], parathyroidectomies were reported for all trimesters with 34/38 live births (7/7 in first trimester, 17/18 in second trimester, 9/12 in third trimester, and 1/1 unspecified). When feasible, a minimally invasive approach rather than open procedures and intraoperative PTH monitoring is recommended [2]. Our patient underwent minimally invasive parathyroidectomy; however, intraoperative PTH monitoring was not performed in order to reduce time under anesthesia.

In a retrospective study, Norman et al. [3] reported that 71% of the study participants had prior history of miscarriage and were able to achieve 100% successful pregnancy outcome after parathyroidectomy with no subsequent maternal or fetal complications, demonstrating the efficacy of parathyroidectomy in PHP during pregnancy. Furthermore, the study emphasized the detrimental effects of increasing maternal serum calcium levels on pregnancy outcome, with 73% pregnancy loss when maternal serum calcium levels were 11.4 mg/dL or higher. While pregnancy loss occurred even with mild elevations in serum calcium at 10.7 mg/dL, fetal death was more likely to occur when the serum calcium level was 11.4 mg/dL or higher. The study also showed that the majority of pregnancy loss occurred in the late first or early second trimester with the majority of pregnancy losses at 10-15 weeks gestation. Hence, the authors proposed surgical intervention in the late first or early second trimester rather than waiting until mid-second trimester, especially with elevated maternal serum calcium levels of >11.4 mg/dL and prior history of miscarriage [3]. Our patient underwent parathyroidectomy in the first trimester, having both symptomatic hypercalcemia and a serum calcium level >11.4 mg/dL (uncontrollable with conservative treatment).

Acknowledgments

The authors would like to thank Dr. Brian Le, MD (Department of Pathology, Reading Hospital, West Reading, PA), for providing them with the pathology slides of the parathyroid adenoma.

References

[1] S. Malekar-Raikar and B. P. Sinnott, "Primary hyperparathyroidism in pregnancy – A rare cause of life-threatening hypercalcemia: Case report and literature review," *Case Reports in Endocrinology*, vol. 2011, Article ID 520516, 6 pages, 2011.

[2] V. Dochez and G. Ducarme, "Primary hyperparathyroidism during pregnancy," *Archives of Gynecology and Obstetrics*, vol. 291, no. 2, pp. 259–263, 2015.

[3] J. Norman, D. Politz, and L. Politz, "Hyperparathyroidism during pregnancy and the effect of rising calcium on pregnancy loss: a call for earlier intervention," *Clinical Endocrinology*, vol. 71, no. 1, pp. 104–109, 2009.

[4] G. Diaz-Soto, A. Linglart, M.-V. Sénat, P. Kamenicky, and P. Chanson, "Primary hyperparathyroidism in pregnancy," *Endocrine Journal*, vol. 44, no. 3, pp. 591–597, 2013.

[5] M. W. Yeh, P. H. G. Ituarte, H. C. Zhou et al., "Incidence and prevalence of primary hyperparathyroidism in a racially mixed population," *The Journal of Clinical Endocrinology & Metabolism*, vol. 98, no. 3, pp. 1122–1129, 2013.

[6] T. Tsunoda, N. Mochinaga, T. Eto, and H. Maeda, "Hyperparathyroidism following the atomic bombing in Nagasaki," *The Japanese Journal of Surgery*, vol. 21, no. 5, pp. 508–511, 1991.

[7] A. Abood and P. Vestergaard, "Pregnancy outcomes in women with primary hyperparathyroidism," *European Journal of Endocrinology*, vol. 171, no. 1, pp. 69–76, 2014.

[8] M. T. Truong, M. L. Lalakea, P. Robbins, and M. Friduss, "Primary hyperparathyroidism in pregnancy: a case series and review," *The Laryngoscope*, vol. 118, no. 11, pp. 1966–1969, 2008.

[9] T. R. Kelly, "Primary hyperparathyroidism during pregnancy," *Surgery*, vol. 110, no. 6, pp. 1028–1033, 1991.

[10] A. Kristoffersson, S. Dahlgren, F. Lithner, and J. Jarhult, "Primary hyperparathyroidism in pregnancy," *Surgery*, vol. 97, no. 3, pp. 326–330, 1985.

[11] M. J. Carella and V. V. Gossain, "Hyperparathyroidism and pregnancy - Case report and review," *Journal of General Internal Medicine*, vol. 7, no. 4, pp. 448–453, 1992.

19

Nonislet Cell Tumor Hypoglycemia in a Patient with Adrenal Cortical Carcinoma

Se Won Kim,[1] **Seung-Eun Lee,**[2] **Young Lyun Oh,**[3] **Seokhwi Kim,**[4]
Sun Hee Park,[1] **and Jae Hyeon Kim**[2]

[1]*Division of Endocrinology, Department of Internal Medicine, Sahmyook Medical Center, Seoul, Republic of Korea*
[2]*Department of Medicine, Samsung Medical Center, Sungkyunkwan University School of Medicine, Seoul, Republic of Korea*
[3]*Department of Pathology, Samsung Medical Center, Sungkyunkwan University School of Medicine, Seoul, Republic of Korea*
[4]*Graduate School of Medical Science and Engineering, Korea Advanced Institute of Science and Technology, Daejeon, Republic of Korea*

Correspondence should be addressed to Jae Hyeon Kim; jaehyeonkim26@gmail.com

Academic Editor: Michael P. Kane

Nonislet cell tumor hypoglycemia (NICTH) is a rare but serious paraneoplastic syndrome in which a tumor secretes incompletely processed precursors of insulin-like growth factor-II (IGF-II), causing hypoglycemia. Here, we report an exceptional case of NICTH caused by nonfunctioning adrenocortical carcinoma in a 39-year-old male with recurrent hypoglycemia. The patient's serum IGF-II/IGF-I ratio had increased to 27.8. The serum level of the IGF-II/IGF-I ratio was normalized after removal of the tumor, and the hypoglycemic attacks no longer occurred after the operation.

1. Introduction

Hypoglycemia is a common medical emergency that can sometimes be the first manifestation of tumor disease [1]. Hypoglycemia can be caused by several tumors, including islet and nonislet tumors. Nonislet cell tumor hypoglycemia (NICTH) is a rare but serious complication of malignancy [2, 3]. It has been estimated that NICTH is four times less common than insulinoma [4]. It is believed that insulin-like growth factor-II (IGF-II, 7.5 kDa) or its high-weight precursor ("Big"-IGF-II, 10–20 kDa) produced by tumors is the primary hormonal mediator of NICTH. In 1988, Daughaday et al. reported the first description of NICTH due to aberrant expression of an immature form of IGF-II in a patient with leiomyosarcoma [5]. In a previous extensive review of this topic in 2007, De Groot et al. reported that, of the IGF-II-producing tumors causing hypoglycemia, 41% had a mesenchymal origin, 43% had an epithelial origin, 1% had a neuroendocrine and hematopoietic origin, and 14% had an unknown origin [6]. The tumors are typically large and slow growing.

NICTH has been rarely reported in cases of adrenocortical carcinoma. In this report, we describe a case of adrenocortical carcinoma with recurrent hypoglycemia that was diagnosed as NICTH associated with the production of IGF-II.

2. Case Presentation

A 39-year-old male patient initially presented to his general practitioner in May 2015 with nonsensical ramblings, sweating, and light-headedness. His past medical history consisted of hypertension a year earlier, but there was no other relevant history. His plasma glucose level was 40 mg/dL. The patient was referred to our hospital for further evaluation. His height was 177.1 cm and body weight was 64.0 kg. On physical examination, the patient appeared to be well developed and well nourished, and there were no signs of an excessive production of adrenocortical steroids. He had blood pressure of 130/86 mmHg, pulse of 73/min, and respiratory rate of 18/min. When the patient developed hypoglycemia, his serum insulin concentration was 1.7 μIU/mL, C-peptide was 0.04 ng/mL, and blood glucose was 40 mg/dL. The patient's insulin antibodies were not detected. We confirmed significant hypoglycemia with suppression of endogenous insulin secretion.

TABLE 1: Endocrinological data from a patient with hypoglycemia.

	Levels	Normal range	Units
Blood glucose	40	70–109	mg/dL
Hemoglobin A1c	4.8	4–6	%
Insulin	1.7	1.1–11.2	μIU/mL
C-peptide	0.04	0.69–3.59	ng/mL
Anti-insulin antibody	3.8	0–7	%
GAD II antibody	0.27	0–1	U/mL
IGF-I	20	49–642	ng/mL
IGF-II	555	288–736	ng/mL
ACTH	63.9	0–60	pg/mL
Cortisol	10	1.8–26.0	μg/dL
DHEAS	359.2	34.9–479.4	μg/dL

ACTH, adrenocorticotropic hormone; DHEAS, dehydroepiandrosterone sulfate; IGF, insulin-like growth factor.

TABLE 2: 24-hour urinary catecholamines and plasma metanephrines before surgery.

	Levels	Normal range	Units
Plasma metanephrines			
Metanephrine	0.12	<0.35	nmol/L
Normetanephrine	0.34	<0.64	nmol/L
24-hour urinary catecholamines			
Metanephrine	95.7	<229.5	μg/day
Normetanephrine	168.2	<502	μg/day
Norepinephrine	184.8	15–80	μg/day
Epinephrine	32.0	0–20	μg/day
VMA	5.4	<6.8	mg/day
Cortisol	180	14–97	μg/day

VMA, vanillylmandelic acid.

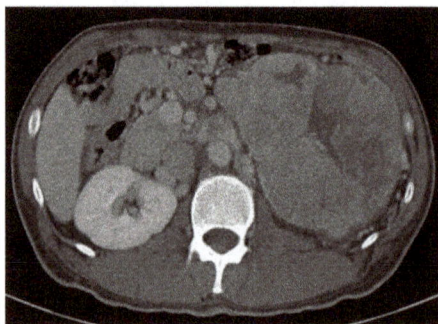

FIGURE 1: Abdominal computed tomography demonstrating a heterogeneously enhanced mass, 14 × 12 cm in diameter, with internal necrotic changes in the left adrenal region.

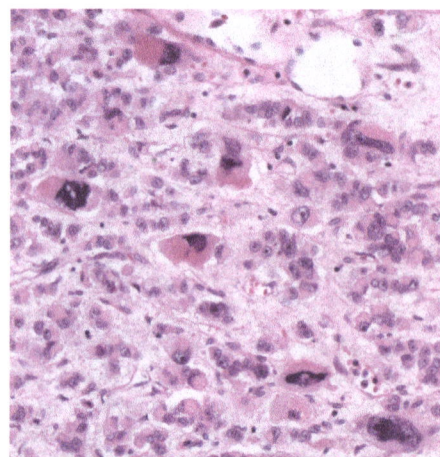

FIGURE 2: Histopathology showing malignant cells in the adrenocortical site (HE stain, ×400), with abundant eosinophilic cytoplasm, enlarged hyperchromatic nuclei, and prominent nucleoli. Several anaplastic cells were also shown in the field.

A 14-centimeter left adrenal mass was found on abdominal computed tomography (CT), obtained as part of the evaluation for recurrent hypoglycemia (Figure 1). The mass was solid, but partly cystic, and the findings of these examinations suggested that the mass may have had a necrotic lesion in the center. CT of the chest revealed no evidence of metastasis. On further questioning, he did not experience traditional attacks of pheochromocytoma, such as headaches, flushing, or palpitations. Urea and electrolytes, aldosterone, plasma renin activity, and testosterone were normal. A complete blood count with platelet count and measurement of serum calcium, creatinine, alanine aminotransferase, and aspartate aminotransferase levels were normal. Glycosylated hemoglobin (HbA1c) was 4.8%. The patient's 24-hour urine vanillylmandelic acid (VMA), metanephrine, and normetanephrine levels were normal. However, urinary epinephrine, norepinephrine, and cortisol levels were elevated. These results likely indicate compensation for hypoglycemia. The serum level of IGF-II was within normal range (555 ng/mL; normal, 288–736 ng/mL), but serum IGF-I level was decreased to 20 ng/mL (normal, 49–642 ng/mL). The serum IGF-II/IGF-I ratio had increased to 27.8 (normal, <10), suggesting a diagnosis of NICTH. The laboratory data on admission are shown in Tables 1 and 2.

During hospitalization, symptoms associated with hypoglycemia occurred frequently, mostly in the morning, and required continuous hypertonic glucose infusion (220 g per day by intravenous administration). A left adrenalectomy, left nephrectomy, and left renal vein thrombectomy were performed, with the histopathology confirming an adrenocortical carcinoma measuring 18 × 16 × 9 cm. Macroscopically, the mass was closely attached to renal capsule but direct invasion into renal parenchyme was not identified. The cut section showed round and lobulated soft pinkish mass with multifocal hemorrhage and necrosis. Microscopic examination of the adrenal tumor revealed high nuclear grade (Fuhrman grade IV), 13 mitoses per HPF, vascular invasion, and necrosis. The clear cells accounted for less than 25% in the tumor (Figure 2). Based on the above findings, the pathological diagnosis of the adrenocortical carcinoma was made according to the diagnostic criteria of malignancy of adrenocortical tumors defined by Lau and Weiss [7]. Immunohistochemistry showed the tumor cells to be positive for inhibin-α, calretinin, and negative for chromogranin A.

He received adjuvant treatment with mitotane and replacement therapy with hydrocortisone postoperatively. After tumor excision, serum levels of glucose, insulin, and C-peptide normalized. The patient's postoperative IGF-I and IGF-II/IGF-I ratio levels returned to the normal range (188 ng/mL and 3.2, resp.), and he experienced no further hypoglycemic episodes. The follow-up abdominal CT was done 6 months after the operation, which revealed multiple hepatic metastases. We considered additional combined chemotherapy, but he was lost to follow-up.

3. Discussion

NICTH is a rare paraneoplastic syndrome and is the second most common cause of tumor-related hypoglycemia following insulinoma. In the review by Bodnar et al. [3], there were nearly 290 cases of NICTH reported in the English language medical literature in the past 25 years. This condition is usually associated with slow-growing and mesenchymal tumors such as sarcomas, fibromas, and mesotheliomas. Among primary epithelial tumors, episodes of hypoglycemia were described in patients with hepatocellular carcinoma, gastric cancer, renal cell carcinoma, phyllodes tumor of breast, and ovarian adenocarcinoma [3].

Adrenocortical carcinoma (ACC) is a rare malignancy with an annual incidence of 1-2 per million population [8]. The natural clinical course of ACC is not well known because of its poor prognosis. Only four cases of NICTH accompanied by ACC were recognized in a PubMed search from 1984 onward [9–12]. When we consider that many ACCs are associated with IGF-II overexpression, ACC might be a potential candidate causing NICTH through incomplete processing of pro-IGF-II [8].

No single pathogenetic mechanism can explain all cases of NICTH. However, the major cause of NICTH could be as follows: increased glucose utilization by large tumors, inhibition of glycogenolysis and gluconeogenesis from the liver, and suppression of counterregulatory hormones for insulin or insulin-like factors secreted by the tumor. NICTH is mediated via IGF-II, which exhibits a high degree of structural homology to proinsulin. In NICTH, 70% of the patients have high molecular weight IGF-II, so-called "big" IGF-II (10–20 kDa), although the total IGF-II values are within normal range [13]. "Big"-IGF-II forms binary complexes with IGF-binding protein (IGFBP), instead of the normal ternary complex, and these small binary complexes have greater capillary permeability and therefore increase IGF bioavailability to the tissues [14].

In the clinical setting, diagnosing NICTH is difficult because serum IGF-II levels are not always elevated in these patients. Hizuka et al. suggested that the IGF-II/IGF-I ratio in serum is useful for detecting IGF-II-producing NICTH [13]. They reported that the IGF-II/IGF-I ratio in serum exceeded 20 in patients with NICTH. In these patients, IGF-I production could be suppressed by an insulin-like factor, big IGF-II. Their data indicated that serum big IGF-II and IGF-II/IGF-I ratio are useful for screening patients with IGF-II-producing NICTH. However, assays for big IGF-II are not commercially available. Thus, the IGF-II/IGF-I ratio is used

as a surrogate marker for big IGF-II concentration. A ratio of IGF-II/IGF-I > 10 indicates NICTH [15].

In NICTH, the best treatment for hypoglycemia is surgical resection of the tumor. The metabolic alterations caused by NICTH are fully reversible after successful surgical removal of a big IGF-II-producing tumor. In our case, we only measured total IGF-II including normal and big IGF-II and did not distinguish big IGF-II. Unfortunately, we could not investigate IGF-II expression in cancer tissues. The serum IGF-II level was not elevated, but the IGF-II/IGF-I ratio was increased to 27.8. The serum IGF-II/IGF-I ratio before surgery decreased and normalized after the removal of the tumor, and hypoglycemic attacks no longer occurred after the operation.

In conclusion, we have reported a very rare case of adrenocortical carcinoma associated with NICTH. We have found five cases, including our own case, of adrenocortical carcinoma causing NICTH during 30 years. The possibility of NICTH is suggested by low serum insulin and C-peptide during a hypoglycemic episode, with low IGF-I level. However, the circulating level of total IGF-II may be increased, decreased, or normalized, with an IGF-II/IGF-I ratio of 10 or more. In subjects with recurrent hypoglycemia and no history of diabetes, NICTH should be included in the differential diagnosis.

References

[1] M. L. Virally and P. J. Guillausseau, "Hypoglycemia in adults," *Diabetes and Metabolism*, vol. 25, no. 6, pp. 477–490, 1999.

[2] K. Scott, "Non-islet cell tumor hypoglycemia," *Journal of Pain and Symptom Management*, vol. 37, no. 4, pp. e1–e3, 2009.

[3] T. W. Bodnar, M. J. Acevedo, and M. Pietropaolo, "Management of non-islet-cell tumor hypoglycemia: a clinical review," *Journal of Clinical Endocrinology and Metabolism*, vol. 99, no. 3, pp. 713–722, 2014.

[4] V. Marks and J. D. Teale, "Tumours producing hypoglycaemia," *Endocrine-Related Cancer*, vol. 5, no. 2, pp. 111–129, 1998.

[5] W. H. Daughaday, M. A. Emanuelle, M. H. Brooks, A. L. Barbato, M. Kapadia, and P. Rotwein, "Synthesis and secretion of insulin-like growth factor II by a leiomyosarcoma with associated hypoglycemia," *The New England Journal of Medicine*, vol. 319, no. 22, pp. 1434–1440, 1988.

[6] J. W. B. De Groot, B. Rikhof, J. Van Doorn et al., "Non-islet cell tumour-induced hypoglycaemia: a review of the literature including two new cases," *Endocrine-Related Cancer*, vol. 14, no. 4, pp. 979–993, 2007.

[7] S. K. Lau and L. M. Weiss, "The Weiss system for evaluating adrenocortical neoplasms: 25 years later," *Human Pathology*, vol. 40, no. 6, pp. 757–768, 2009.

[8] M. Fassnacht, M. Kroiss, and B. Allolio, "Update in adrenocortical carcinoma," *The Journal of Clinical Endocrinology & Metabolism*, vol. 98, no. 12, pp. 4551–4564, 2013.

[9] T. I. M. Korevaar, F. Ragazzoni, A. Weaver, N. Karavitaki, and A. B. Grossman, "IGF2-induced hypoglycemia unresponsive to

everolimus," *Quarterly Journal of Medicine*, vol. 107, no. 4, pp. 297–300, 2014.

[10] J. Soutelo, M. Saban, F. Borghi Torzillo, R. Lutfi, and M. Leal Reyna, "Adrenal carcinoma induced hypoglycemia," *Medicina*, vol. 73, no. 4, pp. 339–342, 2013.

[11] K. Ishikura, T. Takamura, Y. Takeshita et al., "Cushing's syndrome and big IGF-II associated hypoglycaemia in a patient with adrenocortical carcinoma," *BMJ Case Reports*, vol. 2010, 2010.

[12] T. Eguchi, A. Tokuyama, Y. Tanaka et al., "Hypoglycemia associated with the production of insulin-like growth factor II in adrenocortical carcinoma," *Internal Medicine*, vol. 40, no. 8, pp. 759–763, 2001.

[13] N. Hizuka, I. Fukuda, K. Takano, Y. Okubo, K. Asakawa-Yasumoto, and H. Demura, "Serum insulin-like growth factor II in 44 patients with non-islet cell tumor hypoglycemia," *Endocrine Journal*, vol. 45, supplement, pp. S61–S65, 1998.

[14] C. L. Alvino, S. C. Ong, K. A. McNeil et al., "Understanding the mechanism of insulin and insulin-like growth factor (IGF) receptor activation by IGF-II," *PLoS ONE*, vol. 6, no. 11, Article ID e27488, 2011.

[15] J. D. Teale and V. Marks, "Inappropriately elevated plasma insulin-like growth factor II in relation to suppressed insulin-like growth factor I in the diagnosis of non-islet cell tumour hypoglycaemia," *Clinical Endocrinology*, vol. 33, no. 1, pp. 87–98, 1990.

20

Treatment of Concurrent Thrombotic Thrombocytopenic Purpura and Graves' Disease: A Report on Two Cases

Karl Lhotta ⓘ,[1] Emanuel Zitt,[1] Hannelore Sprenger-Mähr,[1] Lorin Loacker,[2] and Alexander Becherer[3]

[1]*Department of Internal Medicine 3, Academic Teaching Hospital Feldkirch, Feldkirch, Austria*
[2]*Central Institute for Medical and Chemical Laboratory Diagnostics, Medical University Innsbruck, Innsbruck, Austria*
[3]*Department of Nuclear Medicine, Academic Teaching Hospital Feldkirch, Feldkirch, Austria*

Correspondence should be addressed to Karl Lhotta; karl.lhotta@lkhf.at

Academic Editor: Thomas Grüning

Graves' disease (GD) and thrombotic thrombocytopenic purpura (TTP) are autoimmune diseases caused by autoantibodies against the TSH receptor (TRAb) and the enzyme ADAMTS13. We here report on two patients with concurrent GD and TTP, who achieved sustained remission of both conditions with the TTP treatment regimen and thiamazole. Both patients suffered from relapsing TTP and were diagnosed with GD concomitantly at the time of relapse. They were treated with steroids, plasma exchange, rituximab, and thiamazole. This therapy induced complete remission of TTP. TRAb levels also decreased rapidly and both patients developed subclinical hypothyroidism three and five weeks later. Our observations suggest that TTP and GD may be concomitant and that GD possibly triggers a relapse of TTP. The combination of thyrostatic treatment and immunosuppression with PE, rituximab, and steroids is able to induce rapid and prolonged remission of GD.

1. Introduction

Graves' disease (GD) is the most common cause of hyperthyroidism with a lifetime risk of 3% for women and 0.5% for men [1]. The disease is caused by activating autoantibodies directed against the alpha subunit of the TSH receptor (TRAb) on thyroid follicular cells [2]. Graves' disease is currently treated with either thyrostatic drugs such as thiamazole or propylthiouracil, which block thyroid hormone synthesis, radioactive iodine, or surgical thyroidectomy [3]. Remission after medical thyrostatic therapy is achieved in about 50% of patients. Although a theoretical option, targeting autoimmunity with immunosuppression is currently not pursued in patients with the disorder. We here report on two patients with concurrent thrombotic thrombocytopenic purpura (TTP), an autoimmune disease caused by autoantibodies against the von Willebrand factor-cleaving protease ADAMTS13, and GD. Treatment consisting of steroids, plasma exchange, and rituximab induced rapid and sustained remission of both conditions.

2. Patient 1

A 40-year-old woman sought medical treatment because of petechia, hematuria, and headache. Laboratory analysis revealed severe hemolytic anemia with schistocytosis and thrombopenia. ADAMTS13 activity was absent (<24 ng/mL, reference range 530-800 ng/mL), but no inhibitor could be detected. A diagnosis of thrombotic thrombocytopenic purpura was made despite a negative test for anti-ADAMTS13 antibodies [4]. She made a quick recovery with steroids and daily plasma exchange (PE) using fresh frozen plasma as a substitution fluid. After one week she experienced a severe relapse with microangiopathic involvement of the brain, heart, lung, kidneys, liver, spleen, stomach, and gut. PE was performed twice daily. Altogether, the patient had 41 exchanges over a six-week period. In addition, she received two 1g infusions of rituximab. Thyroid function was normal. The patient made a complete recovery and ADAMTS13 activity remained in the normal range.

TABLE 1: Laboratory results of Patients 1 and 2 at time of TTP diagnosis and over the course after TTP therapy.

Patient 1		Patient 2	
TSH (0.34.4.94 mIU/L)			
basal	<0.1	basal	<0.1
3 weeks	0.53	5 weeks	4.36
24 months	2.78	6 months	1.66
31 months	2.48	15 months	0.99
FT3 (1.71-3.71 pg/ml)			
basal	7.00	basal	12.7
3 weeks	1.01	5 weeks	3.40
24 months	3.16	6 months	3,17
31 months	3.24	15 months	3.64
FT4 (9.3-17.0 pg/ml)			
basal	19.7	basal	30.7
3 weeks	5.4	5 weeks	6.9
24 months	11.5	6 months	12.4
31 months	11.8	15 months	15.7
TRAb (<1.75 U/L)			
basal	28.3	basal	10.1
after 1. PE	5.4		
10 days	1.8	2 weeks	2.7
24 months	0.3	8 months	1.5
31 months	1.8	15 months	<0.8

Six years later the patient experienced a relapse of her TTP, again with absent ADAMTS13 activity but undetectable inhibitor. She had mild involvement of the brain (headache), kidneys (microhematuria and albuminuria), and gut (abdominal pain). She received oral steroids (starting dose methylprednisolone: 1 mg/kg bodyweight), eleven PEs and two 1g rituximab infusions two weeks apart, and completely recovered. The patient also reported weight loss, nervousness, and increased sweating before clinical relapse. TSH was suppressed, and FT3 and FT4 were mildly elevated (Table 1). Ultrasound of the thyroid showed increased perfusion. TSH receptor antibodies (TRAb) were also elevated. A diagnosis of GD was made and thiamazole 20 mg and propranolol 20 mg twice a day were started. TRAb levels decreased by 50% after the first PE and further 50% after ten days (Table 1). Thyroid function also normalized rapidly and the patient developed peripheral hypothyroidism three weeks later. Thiamazole and propranolol were discontinued. The patient subsequently had normal thyroid function and a negative test for TRAb. Two and a half years later TRAbs were of borderline value and TSH, FT3, and FT4 remained normal. ADAMTS13 activity was in the normal range. Thyroid function is being closely monitored in order to avoid hyperthyroidism and relapse of TTP.

3. Patient 2

A 25-year-old female was admitted because of petechiae, hematuria, and menorrhagia. Blood tests showed hemolytic anemia and thrombopenia. ADAMTS13 activity was reduced

(59 ng/mL) and an inhibitor was detectable (0.75 BU/mL, reference: <0.2 BU/mL). The patient made a quick and complete recovery with steroids, three PEs and a single 1g dose of rituximab. At that time her TSH was normal (0.98 mIU/L).

Two years later, after an uneventful pregnancy and a cesarean section, she relapsed with ADAMTS13 of 38 ng/mL and a positive inhibitor test (2.6 BU/mL). She was treated with steroids, ten PEs, and 1g rituximab followed by 0.5g after the first PE and 1g after the plasma exchange series. At that time, her thyroid function was not assessed, but TSH had been normal (0.93 mIU/L) three months earlier.

Another two years later the patient had a second relapse with severe headache and petechiae. Again, ADAMTS13 activity was reduced (128 ng/mL) and anti-ADAMTS13 antibodies were present (1.89 BU/mL). Besides, she had tachycardia of 120 beats per minute and thyroid function tests confirmed a thyrotoxicosis (Table 1). A retrospective analysis of a stored blood sample taken before the first plasma exchange showed elevated TRAbs. Sonography revealed thyroidal hyperperfusion, and pertechnetate uptake was increased upon scintigraphy. TTP was treated with methylprednisolone 1mg/kg body weight as starting dose, thirteen PEs, and 1g rituximab followed by two doses of 0.5 g. Two weeks later the TRAb titer had fallen by three-quarters. GD was treated with thiamazole 20 mg and propranolol 20 mg, each twice a day. Five weeks later the patient had developed subclinical hypothyroidism with low FT4 (Table 1). Thiamazole was reduced to 5 mg daily. Three months later the patient had reached a stable euthyroid state and thiamazole was further reduced to 5 mg on alternate days. Eight and twelve months after diagnosis of GD, TRAb levels were in the normal range below 1.75 U/L.

4. Discussion

We here report on two patients with concomitant TTP and GD. This combination has been described before in four case reports [5–8]. An association between both TTP [9] and GD [10] and other autoimmune diseases is well described, but concurrence of TTP and GD is not mentioned in those publications, probably because of the rarity of TTP. TTP has a low incidence of 3 cases per million persons per year [11], whereas GD is rather common with 20 to 50 cases per 100.000 [1]. In our patients TTP presented before GD and GD was associated with a relapse of TTP. Whether this is a coincidence or whether GD is indeed the cause of the TTP relapse remains unknown, but we assume a causal relationship is very likely. The nature of this causal link remains to be determined, but could be by augmented stimulation of synthesis of (possibly preformed) ADAMTS13 autoantibodies or some endothelial activation, thus triggering a TTP relapse. A causal link is also supported by one of the case reports describing remission of TTP without PE after successful treatment of GD with radioactive iodine [5].

The four previous case reports all describe good response of TTP to PE and of GD to PE and either antithyroid drugs [6, 8], radioiodine [7], or radioiodine and surgery [5]. The current therapy for relapsing TTP is a combination of steroids, PE with FFP as substitution fluid and rituximab [12, 13]. In our two patients, this therapy caused complete remission of TTP, but also rapid recovery from hyperthyroidism. One reason for that may be that PE is able to remove TRABs, as shown in our patients, in whom TRAb levels fell rapidly (Table 1) compared to the expected normal half-life of 21 days of IgG TRAbs [14]. Number and frequency of PE sessions (11 in Patient 1 and 13 in Patient 2) were determined by TTP response to treatment. PE is also considered to be a therapeutic option in thyroid storm, not only because it removes TRABs, but also because it lowers the pool of T3 and T4 bound to plasma proteins [15]. Rituximab is an anti-CD20 monoclonal antibody that eliminates B lymphocytes. It is used in B-cell lymphomas and autoimmune diseases such as rheumatoid arthritis or anti-neutrophil cytoplasmic antibody-associated vasculitis. In TTP, rituximab and steroids are applied to block ADAMTS13 autoantibody synthesis. It can be expected that this therapy also affects TRAb formation. Indeed, our patients quickly became TRAb-negative and remained in remission thereafter. In Patient 1, a borderline TRAb level was detected two and a half years after the attack, when recovery from rituximab-induced B-cell depletion is likely.

In addition to removal and suppression of TRAb synthesis, our patients also received standard therapy with thiamazole to block thyroid hormone synthesis. This combination therapy actually led to subclinical hypothyroidism with low FT4 levels after three and five weeks, respectively, and to normalization of TSH levels after four and six weeks, when thiamazole was able to be discontinued or the dose dramatically reduced.

Rituximab has been used in the treatment of GD and especially Graves' orbitopathy (GO) with mixed results. One small study described sustained remission in four out of ten GD patients after rituximab compared to none of the ten patients not on rituximab. Rituximab seemed to be effective in patients with low TRAb levels but had no effect on TRAb titers in addition to thiamazole [16]. Another study in relapsing patients found a persistent remission in nine out of 13 patients [17]. In addition, rituximab led to a decrease in TRAb levels. Two studies in GO compared rituximab and iv methylprednisolone. In the first study including 32 patients, rituximab was superior to iv methylprednisolone [18], whereas in the second study comprising 21 patients, it was not [19]. In both studies TRAb titers fell with rituximab. The decrease in TRAb levels induced by rituximab occurs slowly over several months [17, 20], which is comparable to the effect of antithyroid drugs on TRAb levels [21]. Rituximab, however, has been shown to specifically reduce the production of thyroid-stimulating autoantibodies, whereas methimazole has no such effect [22]. In conclusion, we report on two patients, in whom GD possibly caused a relapse of preexisting TTP. GD should be considered as a risk factor for TTP recurrence and we suggest routine assessment of thyroid function in such patients. Initiation of TTP treatment with steroids, PE, and rituximab with the addition of thiamazole caused rapid and prolonged remission of GD. This treatment regimen could also be considered, for example, in GD patients with thyroid storm. Further studies are required to prove its effectiveness and to determine the optimal dose of steroids, PE, and rituximab.

References

[1] M. B. Zimmermann and K. Boelaert, "Iodine deficiency and thyroid disorders," *The Lancet Diabetes & Endocrinology*, vol. 3, no. 4, pp. 286–295, 2015.

[2] T. J. Smith and L. Hegedüs, "Graves' disease," *The New England Journal of Medicine*, vol. 375, no. 16, pp. 1552–1565, 2016.

[3] H. B. Burch and D. S. Cooper, "Management of Graves Disease: A Review," *Journal of the American Medical Association*, vol. 314, no. 23, pp. 2544–2554, 2015.

[4] H. M. Tsai, "Measurement of ADAMTS13," *Int Rev Thromb*, vol. 1, pp. 272–280, 2006.

[5] F. Bellante, P. Redondo Saez, C. Springael, and S. Dethy, "Stroke in thrombotic thrombocytopenic purpura induced by thyrotoxicosis: A case report," *Journal of Stroke and Cerebrovascular Diseases*, vol. 23, no. 6, pp. 1744–1746, 2014.

[6] B. T. Chaar, G. C. Kudva, T. J. Olsen, A. B. Silverberg, and B. J. Grossman, "Thrombotic thrombocytopenic purpura and graves disease," *The American Journal of the Medical Sciences*, vol. 334, no. 2, pp. 133–135, 2007.

[7] S. Chhabra and G. Tenorio, "Thrombotic thrombocytopenic purpura precipitated by thyrotoxicosis," *Journal of Clinical Apheresis*, vol. 27, no. 5, pp. 265–266, 2012.

[8] W.-L. Zheng, G.-S. Zhang, and M.-Y. Deng, "Thrombotic thrombocytopenic purpura complicating Graves disease: Dramatic response to plasma exchange and infusion," *Transfusion Medicine*, vol. 21, no. 5, pp. 354-355, 2011.

[9] P. Coppo, D. Bengoufa, A. Veyradier et al., "Severe ADAMTS13 deficiency in adult idiopathic thrombotic microangiopathies defines a subset of patients characterized by various autoimmune manifestations, lower platelet count, and mild renal involvement," *Medicine*, vol. 83, no. 4, pp. 233–244, 2004.

[10] K. Boelaert, P. R. Newby, M. J. Simmonds et al., "Prevalence and relative risk of other autoimmune diseases in subjects with autoimmune thyroid disease," *American Journal of Medicine*, vol. 123, no. 2, pp. 183.e1–183.e9, 2010.

[11] J. A. Reese, D. S. Muthurajah, J. A. K. Hovinga, S. K. Vesely, D. R. Terrell, and J. N. George, "Children and adults with thrombotic thrombocytopenic purpura associated with severe, acquired Adamts13 deficiency: comparison of incidence, demographic and clinical features," *Pediatric Blood & Cancer*, vol. 60, no. 10, pp. 1676–1682, 2013.

[12] Y. Benhamou, G. Paintaud, E. Azoulay et al., "Efficacy of a rituximab regimen based on B cell depletion in thrombotic thrombocytopenic purpura with suboptimal response to standard treatment: Results of a phase II, multicenter noncomparative study," *American Journal of Hematology*, vol. 91, no. 12, pp. 1246–1251, 2016.

[13] W. F. Clark, G. Rock, D. Barth et al., "A phase-II sequential case-series study of all patients presenting to four plasma exchange centres with presumed relapsed/refractory thrombotic thrombocytopenic purpura treated with rituximab," *British Journal of Haematology*, vol. 170, no. 2, pp. 208–217, 2015.

[14] L. S. Zuckier, L. D. Rodriguez, and M. D. Scharff, "Immunologic and pharmacologic concepts of monoclonal antibodies," *Seminars in Nuclear Medicine*, vol. 19, no. 3, pp. 166–186, 1989.

[15] J. Schwartz, A. Padmanabhan, N. Aqui et al., "Guidelines on the Use of Therapeutic Apheresis in Clinical Practice-Evidence-Based Approach from the Writing Committee of the American Society for Apheresis: The Seventh Special Issue," *Journal of Clinical Apheresis*, vol. 31, no. 3, pp. 149–162, 2016.

[16] D. El Fassi, C. H. Nielsen, S. J. Bonnema, H. C. Hasselbalch, and L. Hegedüs, "B lymphocyte depletion with the monoclonal antibody rituximab in graves' disease: A controlled pilot study," *The Journal of Clinical Endocrinology & Metabolism*, vol. 92, no. 5, pp. 1769–1772, 2007.

[17] K. A. Heemstra, R. E. Toes, J. Sepers et al., "Rituximab in relapsing Graves' disease, a phase II study," *European Journal of Endocrinology*, vol. 159, no. 5, pp. 609–615, 2008.

[18] M. Salvi, G. Vannucchi, N. Currò et al., "Efficacy of B-cell targeted therapy with rituximab in patients with active moderate to severe graves' orbitopathy: a randomized controlled study," *The Journal of Clinical Endocrinology & Metabolism*, vol. 100, no. 2, pp. 422–431, 2015.

[19] M. N. Stan, J. A. Garrity, B. G. C. Leon, T. Prabin, E. A. Bradley, and R. S. Bahn, "Randomized controlled trial of rituximab in patients with graves' orbitopathy," *The Journal of Clinical Endocrinology & Metabolism*, vol. 100, no. 2, pp. 432–441, 2015.

[20] A. L. Mitchell, E. H. Gan, M. Morris et al., "The effect of B cell depletion therapy on anti-TSH receptor antibodies and clinical outcome in glucocorticoid-refractory Graves' orbitopathy," *Clinical Endocrinology*, vol. 79, no. 3, pp. 437–442, 2013.

[21] P. Laurberg, G. Wallin, L. Tallstedt, M. Abraham-Nordling, G. Lundell, and O. Törring, "TSH-receptor autoimmunity in Graves' disease after therapy with anti-thyroid drugs, surgery, or radioiodine: A 5-year prospective randomized study," *European Journal of Endocrinology*, vol. 158, no. 1, pp. 69–75, 2008.

[22] D. El Fassi, J. P. Banga, J. A. Gilbert, C. Padoa, L. Hegedüs, and C. H. Nielsen, "Treatment of Graves' disease with rituximab specifically reduces the production of thyroid stimulating autoantibodies," *Clinical Immunology*, vol. 130, no. 3, pp. 252–258, 2009.

21

Atypical Complications of Graves' Disease: A Case Report and Literature Review

Khaled Ahmed Baagar,[1] **Mashhood Ahmed Siddique,**[1] **Shaimaa Ahmed Arroub,**[1] **Ahmed Hamdi Ebrahim,**[2] **and Amin Ahmed Jayyousi**[1]

[1]*Endocrine Department, Hamad Medical Corporation, Doha, P.O. Box 3050, Qatar*
[2]*Emergency Department, Hamad Medical Corporation, Doha, P.O. Box 3050, Qatar*

Correspondence should be addressed to Khaled Ahmed Baagar; kbaagar@hamad.qa

Academic Editor: Toshihiro Kita

Graves' disease (GD) may display uncommon manifestations. We report a patient with rare complications of GD and present a comprehensive literature review. A 35-year-old woman presented with a two-week history of dyspnea, palpitations, and edema. She had a raised jugular venous pressure, goiter, and exophthalmos. Laboratory tests showed pancytopenia, a raised alkaline phosphatase level, hyperbilirubinemia (mainly direct bilirubin), and hyperthyroidism [TSH: <0.01 mIU/L (reference values: 0.45–4.5), fT4: 54.69 pmol/L (reference values: 9.0–20.0), and fT3: >46.08 pmol/L (reference values: 2.6–5.7)]. Her thyroid uptake scan indicated GD. Echocardiography showed a high right ventricular systolic pressure: 60.16 mmHg. Lugol's iodine, propranolol, cholestyramine, and dexamethasone were initiated. Hematologic investigations uncovered no reason for the pancytopenia; therefore, carbimazole was started. Workup for hepatic impairment and pulmonary hypertension (PH) was negative. The patient became euthyroid after 3 months. Leukocyte and platelet counts and bilirubin levels normalized, and her hemoglobin and alkaline phosphatase levels and right ventricular systolic pressure (52.64 mmHg) improved. This is the first reported single case of GD with the following three rare manifestations: pancytopenia, cholestatic liver injury, and PH with right-sided heart failure. With antithyroid drugs treatment, pancytopenia should resolve with euthyroidism, but PH and liver injury may take several months to resolve.

1. Introduction

Graves' disease (GD) is an autoimmune thyroid disease first described by Robert Graves in 1835 [1]. Patients with GD usually present with common manifestations such as palpitations, tremors, heat intolerance, and weight loss. However, some patients may present with unusual gastrointestinal, hematologic, neurologic, and cardiopulmonary complications [2]. We report a patient who presented to our institution with pancytopenia and pulmonary hypertension (PH) with right-sided heart failure and raised liver enzymes. She was found to have GD. Further, there was no other explanation for her manifestations as the workup failed to reveal any other pathologic conditions. The pathogenesis of these complications in patients with GD is not completely understood. However, the prognosis is good if the underlying hyperthyroidism is treated with antithyroid drugs (ATDs). In this review, we discuss the prevalence of each complication,

possible mechanisms of their development in the context of GD, and the clinical course during treatment of the underlying hyperthyroidism.

2. Case Presentation

A 35-year-old woman presented to our emergency department with a two-week history of breathlessness, palpitations, and generalized edema. She had a history of having lost approximately 10 kg of weight over a 3-month period but had regained weight in the month before presentation. She had no chronic illness and was not on any medication(s). On examination, she looked tired, was afebrile, and had a blood pressure of 103/58 mmHg, pulse rate of 92/min, and a respiratory rate of 20/min. She had exophthalmos, a raised jugular venous pressure, a diffuse goiter with a positive bruit, and bilateral pedal edema extending to the thighs. She had a third heart sound and bilateral fine basal lung

TABLE 1: Laboratory investigations at presentation and in the 3 months following carbimazole treatment.

	Presentation	Next day	2 weeks	3 months
TSH (mIU/L)	<0.01		<0.01	<0.01
FT4 (pmol/L)	54.69		23.99	6.6
FT3 (pmol/L)	>46.08		12.98	3.97
WBC ($\times10^9$/L)	2.9	3.6	3.9	6.8
Neutrophils ($\times10^9$/L)	1.1	2.2	2.1	3.8
Hemoglobin (g/L)	84	96	87	111
Hematocrit (%)	26.6	33.7	30.4	36.7
MCV (femtoliter)	83.1	91.9	92.3	89.1
Platelets ($\times10^9$/L)	113	143	211	285
T. bilirubin (μmol/L)	35.3	31.1	21.9	11.7
D. bilirubin (μmol/L)	27.4	23.2	17.6	7.3
I. bilirubin (μmol/L)	6.9			
ALP (U/L)	304	262	303	311
GGT (U/L)			128	98
ALT (U/L)	14	13	12	18
AST (U/L)	24	25	16	26
Albumin (g/L)	29	25	25	34
Weight (kg)	96			91

TSH: thyroid-stimulating hormone (0.45–4.5 mIU/L), FT4: free T4 (9–20 pmol/L), FT3: free T3 (2.6–5.7 pmol/L), WBC: white blood cells (4–10 $\times 10^9$/L), neutrophils (2–7 $\times 10^9$/L), hemoglobin (120–150 g/L), hematocrit (36–46%), MCV: mean corpuscular volume (83–101 femtoliter), platelets (150–400 $\times 10^9$/L), T. bilirubin: total bilirubin (3.4–20.5 μmol/L), D. bilirubin: direct bilirubin (0–8.6 μmol/L), I. bilirubin: indirect bilirubin (0–3 μmol/L), ALP: alkaline phosphatase (40–150 U/L), GGT: gamma-glutamyl transferase (9–36 U/L), ALT: alanine aminotransferase (0–55 U/L), AST: aspartate aminotransferase (5–34 U/L), albumin (35–50 g/L).

crepitations. Her abdominal examination was unremarkable with no tenderness or organomegaly. An electrocardiogram showed a sinus rhythm with right bundle branch block and right ventricular strain.

Laboratory investigations (detailed in Table 1) showed pancytopenia; raised bilirubin (mainly direct bilirubin) and alkaline phosphatase (ALP); and normal creatinine, alanine aminotransferase (ALT), and aspartate aminotransferase (AST) levels. Her thyroid functions were as follows: thyroid-stimulating hormone (TSH), <0.01 mIU/L (reference values: 0.45–4.5); FT4, 54.69 pmol/L (reference values: 9–20); FT3, >46.08 pmol/L (reference values: 2.6–5.7); and antithyroid peroxidase, >1000 U.

Echocardiography showed an ejection fraction of 50–55%, a right ventricular systolic pressure (RVSP) of 60.16 mmHg measured by Doppler, and severe tricuspid regurgitation. Therefore, a computed tomography pulmonary angiogram was performed; it was negative for pulmonary embolism. A thyroid uptake scan showed diffusely increased uptake, indicating GD, and ultrasound examination showed a diffuse goiter with no nodules. She was initially started on Lugol's iodine, 7 drops (8 mg/drop) every 8 hours, propranolol, 40 mg every 8 hours, dexamethasone, 1 mg every 8 hours, and cholestyramine, 4 grams every 6 hours, to control thyrotoxicosis and to prevent further worsening of the patient's complications which were suspected to be related to GD. Also, 2 doses of intravenous furosemide 40 mg were given on the first hospital day then it was discontinued and the basal lungs crepitations disappeared on the following day.

Workup did not reveal any specific reason other than GD for her pancytopenia, PH, and raised alkaline phosphatase (ALP) and bilirubin. Regarding the pancytopenia, a peripheral blood smear showed a moderate normocytic anemia with mild hypochromia; a few ovalocytes, burr cells, and schistocytes; and increased rouleaux formation. There was leukopenia with neutropenia, some toxic features, a few reactive lymphocytes, and minor platelet clumps. The reticulocyte count was 3.2% (reference values: 0.5–2.5%), erythrocyte sedimentation rate was 3 mm/h (reference values: 2–37), C-reactive protein was 9 mg/L (reference values: 0–5), and hemoglobin electrophoresis was normal. The levels of all the following parameters were normal: lactate dehydrogenase, 184 U/L (reference values: 135–214); haptoglobin, 95 mg/dL (reference values: 35–250); folate, 34.5 nmol/L (reference values: 4.0–45.3); and vitamin B12, 617 pmol/L (reference values: 133–675). Iron studies showed the following: iron, 5 μmol/L (reference values: 5.83–34.5); total iron binding capacity, 32 μmol/L (reference values: 45–80); iron saturation, 15% (reference values: 15–45); transferrin, 1.29 g/L (reference values: 2–3.6); and ferritin, 38 μg/L (reference values: 11–304). Coombs test and HIV serology were negative. Additional workup for cholestatic liver impairment, viral hepatitis serology, and antimitochondrial antibodies (AMA) was negative. The patient's abdominal ultrasound was unremarkable, with no hepatic or splenic enlargement. Further investigations for PH, rheumatoid factor, and antinuclear (ANA), anti-neutrophil cytoplasmic, anti-RO, anti-LA, anti-JO, anti-scleroderma 70, anti-RNP, and anti-smith antibodies were negative. Complements 3 (C3) and 4 (C4) were 110 mg/dL (reference values: 90–180) and 18.4 mg/dL (reference values: 10–40), respectively.

Bone marrow examination was not performed as the reticulocyte count was high and in the following two days of the initial treatment patient's white blood cells and platelets improved; at that point carbimazole 60 mg/day was started. After six days, she was ready for discharge from hospital on the same dose of carbimazole and propranolol, and furosemide was added for the lower limbs edema.

Follow-up investigations nine days later showed improvement in white blood cell and platelet counts. In addition, the gamma-glutamyl transferase (GGT) level was high (128 U/L [normal: 9–36]).

Two months after her initial presentation, the lower limb edema had improved but had not resolved completely. A month later (3 months after presentation), the lower limb edema disappeared. Moreover, the clinical and laboratory features of hyperthyroidism resolved with carbimazole therapy, and her bilirubin level and white blood cell and platelet counts normalized; and her hemoglobin, ALP, and GGT levels improved. ALP isoenzymes were checked; the raised ALP level was mainly of hepatic origin. Repeat echocardiography showed improvement of RVSP (52.64 mmHg) measured by Doppler, with moderate tricuspid regurgitation.

3. Discussion

GD is caused by autoantibodies that stimulate TSH receptors in the thyroid gland; it is the most common cause of hyperthyroidism [3]. Our patient is the first reported case to have these three rare complications of GD: pancytopenia, cholestatic hepatic injury, and PH with right-sided heart failure.

3.1. Pancytopenia. It is rare for patients with GD to have pancytopenia; there are only a few documented reports in the literature [1, 4–9]. However, single lineage abnormalities (anemia, leukopenia, or thrombocytopenia) are more common in patients with hyperthyroidism (34%, 5.8%, and 3.3%, resp.) [5, 10]. Leukopenia with a relative lymphocytosis is not an uncommon blood abnormality in GD, named "Kocher's blood picture." [11]. There was no identifiable cause for this patient's anemia and it was similar to an anemia of chronic disease, commonly called "GD anemia," that affects 22% of patients with GD [12]. Bone marrow examination in patients with GD, although was not performed in our case, could show hypercellular [8], normocellular [1, 5, 6], or, very rarely, hypoplastic [4] changes.

Initially, thionamides were not used. We chose a more conservative approach to treatment in this patient with multiple complications, using alternatives such as Lugol's solution and cholestyramine, as we did not want to aggravate her pancytopenia. The use of radioactive iodine at the time of presentation might have precipitated a thyroid storm [13]; thus, it was not considered. However, once the workup for pancytopenia showed no other causes and the neutrophil and platelet counts were improving, we initiated treatment with carbimazole. Generally, the use of thionamides is contraindi-

cated in patients with a baseline neutrophil count $<0.5 \times 10^9$/L [13] and should be stopped if the neutrophil count drops after their initiation below 1.0×10^9/L [14]. Thus, although ATDs can be used in patients with hyperthyroidism-associated pancytopenia, their use is recommended only after a full hematologic assessment has been performed, as ATDs carry a minimal risk of pancytopenia [15]. Dexamethasone was added to the initial management because of the severe thyrotoxic state of the patient with pancytopenia. However, the evidence for its use in this situation was weak, being derived from a previous case report [5].

The duration of hyperthyroidism related pancytopenia is variable, from 2 weeks [1] to several months [4]; it resolves only when the patient is euthyroid. Pancytopenia should resolve by the time euthyroidism is reestablished; if it does not, hematologic evaluation should be revisited. It was reported that a patient with GD-related pancytopenia started on methimazole showed no improvement despite becoming euthyroid; investigations revealed methimazole-associated aplastic anemia [8].

The pathogenesis of GD-related pancytopenia is not fully understood and different theories exist [1, 4, 5, 10], including the following: (i) high level of circulating thyroid hormones, resulting in ineffective hematopoiesis; (ii) shortened blood cell lifespan, either by immune destruction or by sequestration; (iii) autoimmune mechanisms, given the presence of antineutrophil and antiplatelet antibodies; and (iv) direct bone marrow toxicity, as excessive thyroid hormones may adversely affect the pluripotent stem cells.

The mechanism of pancytopenia is most likely multifactorial as no single theory could explain it completely. The association between GD and other autoimmune hematologic disorders that respond to ATDs (e.g., autoimmune hemolytic anemia, immune thrombocytopenic purpura, and Evan's syndrome [6]) supports the autoimmune theory. However, pancytopenia has also been reported with other forms of hyperthyroidism that are not immunologically mediated, such as toxic multinodular goiter [10], toxic adenoma [16], and even levothyroxine overtreatment in a patient previously treated for GD [17].

3.2. Cholestatic Hepatic Injury. The hepatic derangement in patients with GD ranges from mild laboratory abnormalities without clinical features to overt hepatitis [18], with either hepatitic or cholestatic injury [19]. Our patient had a cholestatic pattern of liver impairment with raised bilirubin (predominantly direct bilirubin), ALP, and GGT. After 3 months of carbimazole treatment with resolution of hyperthyroidism, ALP and GGT levels were better, and bilirubin normalized. Moreover, ANA and AMA were negative, thereby excluding concomitant autoimmune liver disease such as primary biliary cirrhosis. The patient had no clinical or ultrasonographic manifestations of hepatic congestion (i.e., hepatic tenderness and hepatomegaly); thus, this was excluded as a reason for cholestatic hepatic injury.

ALP is the commonest liver enzyme to be increased in hyperthyroid patients at diagnosis (25–64%) [20, 21]. In a study of 30 patients with GD [22], the reported increase in different liver enzymes was as follows: ALP (33%), ALT

(26%), GGT (24%), AST (17%), and total bilirubin (8%). The initial increase in ALP may originate from the liver, bone, or both, so it is important to check for GGT and bilirubin levels to diagnose cholestasis [21]. With treatment of hyperthyroidism, improvement of GGT has been reported while the ALP level was increasing, mainly from the bone [20]. The ALP level can take several months to normalize after euthyroidism is reestablished; this is because of increased osteoblast activity [20]. However, our patient's ALP after three months of treatment was mainly of liver origin.

The possible mechanisms of liver injury in hyperthyroidism are as follows [22, 23]: (i) relative hypoxia due to increased oxygen demand while the splanchnic blood supply is unchanged, leading to liver impairment and cholestasis in the centrilobular hepatocytes; (ii) congestive heart failure; (iii) direct toxicity by high thyroid hormones, although this has not been confirmed; and (iv) associated autoimmune liver disease.

Treatment of hyperthyroidism in patients with raised liver enzymes is challenging, as ATDs are hepatotoxic (0.5%) [24]. Carbimazole and methimazole usually cause cholestasis while propylthiouracil usually causes hepatocyte damage by an idiosyncratic mechanism unrelated to the dose [19, 24]. Thus, it is advised to investigate for a concomitant liver disease; if the workup is negative, thionamides can be used with careful monitoring; otherwise it is better to use an alternative, such as radioactive iodine ablation or thyroidectomy [2].

3.3. Pulmonary Hypertension. The association between hyperthyroidism and PH was first described in 1950 [25]. PH can be found in patients with GD or nodular goiter with hyperthyroidism [26]. In one study, PH was the most common cardiac complication detected by echocardiography in hyperthyroid patients [27], with a reported prevalence of 36–65% [28, 29]. However, most cases are mild and asymptomatic and are not identified in daily practice [27].

At presentation, the patient had bilateral basal lung crepitations indicative of left ventricular compromise; this can occur with hyperthyroidism. However, the left ventricular dysfunction was mild; the crepitations disappeared on the second day of hospitalization and the ejection fraction was 50–55% on initial echocardiographic examination. On the other hand, the lower limb edema secondary to right-sided heart failure took 3 months to resolve, indicating that this was the main impairment of cardiac function.

Our patient demonstrated an improvement of her RVSP, from 60.16 mmHg at presentation to 52.64 mmHg after 3 months of carbimazole with the resolution of hyperthyroid state. The weight changes that the patient experienced were interesting, as she initially lost weight secondary to hyperthyroidism but then regained some weight because of the right-sided heart failure with resultant edema. Subsequently, once treatment for GD had been initiated, unlike other patients who often gain weight, our patient lost weight as her right heart failure and edema improved. Most cases of PH recover by the time euthyroidism is reestablished. In one report, 79.2% of patients had normal pulmonary artery pressures after 11–21 weeks of ATD treatment [27]. However, in other reports, 3–14 months were needed until normalization of PH occurred [30, 31].

Theories to explain the relationship between hyperthyroidism and PH [32, 33] include the following: (i) autoimmune-mediated endothelial remodeling; (ii) mechanical endothelial damage caused by the high cardiac output; (iii) accelerated metabolism of pulmonary vasodilators (nitric oxide and prostacyclin); (iv) inhibited metabolism of pulmonary vasoconstrictors (endothelin-1, serotonin, and thromboxane); and (v) enhanced pulmonary vascular response to catecholamines. It has been found that pulmonary artery systolic pressure has a significant linear correlation with thyroid-stimulating hormone receptor antibody, pulmonary vascular resistance, and cardiac output [28].

In a study by Marvisi et al. [26] the group of patients who received methimazole showed a more rapid improvement in PH than those who received partial thyroidectomy without pretreatment with methimazole or β-blockers; the difference in the pulmonary pressure drop was significant after 15 days, but not after 90 days, of treatment. The methimazole effect may be due to its ability to suppress Ng-nitro-l-arginine methyl ester production, which acutely inhibits nitric oxide synthesis, resulting in increased levels of nitric oxide [34]. In addition, methimazole might cause direct vasodilatation of the pulmonary vasculature [26]. The possibility of thyroid dysfunction should be considered in patients with unexplained PH, as long-standing untreated hyperthyroidism may lead to refractory PH [32, 35].

4. Conclusion

Patients with GD may present with rare manifestations that have partially understood mechanisms. With ATDs treatment, pancytopenia should resolve as euthyroidism is reestablished. Liver enzyme levels and PH may normalize, or at least show some improvement, once normal thyroid function is established, with full recovery several months later.

When treating patients with GD, it is generally recommended that liver function tests and a complete blood count be performed before initiating ATDs [13]. Having this baseline information gives insight about the abnormal laboratory findings primarily related to the hyperthyroid state, which is reversible with ATD treatment, and eliminates doubt around whether subsequent abnormal test results are secondary to the use of ATDs.

It is crucial to test the thyroid function of a patient presenting with any of the complications described in our patient where no clear explanation is found. Lack of awareness of such associations with GD may lead to misdiagnosis or delayed diagnosis, with a redundant workup being performed [2].

References

[1] A. N. Rafhati, C. K. See, F. K. Hoo, and L. B. Badrulnizam, "A report of three cases of untreated Graves' disease associated with

pancytopenia in Malaysia," *Electronic Physician*, vol. 6, no. 3, pp. 877–882, 2014.

[2] M. O. Hegazi and S. Ahmed, "Atypical clinical manifestations of Graves' disease: an analysis in depth," *Journal of Thyroid Research*, vol. 2012, Article ID 768019, 8 pages, 2012.

[3] J. A. Franklyn and K. Boelaert, "Thyrotoxicosis," *The Lancet*, vol. 379, no. 9821, pp. 1155–1166, 2012.

[4] J. Garcia, L. D. França, V. Ellinger, and M. Wolff, "Marrow hypoplasia: a rare complication of untreated grave's disease," *Arquivos Brasileiros de Endocrinologia e Metabologia*, vol. 58, no. 9, pp. 953–957, 2014.

[5] T. H. Kim, J. S. Yoon, B. S. Park et al., "A Case of pancytopenia with hyperthyroidism," *Yeungnam University Journal of Medicine*, vol. 30, no. 1, pp. 47–50, 2013.

[6] P. Naji, G. Kumar, S. Dewani, W. A. Diedrich, and A. Gupta, "Graves' disease causing pancytopenia and autoimmune hemolytic anemia at different time intervals: a case report and a review of the literature," *Case Reports in Medicine*, vol. 2013, Article ID 194542, 4 pages, 2013.

[7] S. Raina, R. Kaul, and M. Mruthyunjaya, "Pancytopenia with cellular bone marrow related to Graves' hyperthyroidism," *Indian Journal of Endocrinology and Metabolism*, vol. 16, no. 3, pp. 478–479, 2012.

[8] C. S. P. Lima, D. E. Zantut Wittmann, V. Castro et al., "Pancytopenia in untreated patients with Graves' disease," *Thyroid*, vol. 16, no. 4, pp. 403–409, 2006.

[9] L. Kebapçilar, S. Yeşil, F. Bayraktar et al., "Recovery from pancytopaenia and liver dysfunction after administration of propylthiouracil for Graves' disease," *New Zealand Medical Journal*, vol. 118, no. 1220, 2005.

[10] P. Jha, Y. P. R. Singh, B. Ghimire, and B. K. U. Jha, "Pancytopenia in a surgical patient, a rare presentation of hyperthyroidism," *BMC surgery*, vol. 14, article 108, 2014.

[11] W. J. Irvine, F. C. W. Wu, S. J. Urbaniak, and F. Toolis, "Peripheral blood leucocytes in thyrotoxicosis (Graves' disease) as studied by conventional light microscopy," *Clinical & Experimental Immunology*, vol. 27, no. 2, pp. 216–221, 1977.

[12] A. G. Gianoukakis, M. J. Leigh, P. Richards et al., "Characterization of the anaemia associated with Graves' disease," *Clinical Endocrinology*, vol. 70, no. 5, pp. 781–787, 2009.

[13] R. S. Bahn, H. B. Burch, D. S. Cooper et al., "Hyperthyroidism and other causes of thyrotoxicosis: management guidelines of the american thyroid association and American association of clinical endocrinoloigists," *Endocrine Practice*, vol. 17, no. 3, pp. 456–520, 2011.

[14] D. S. Cooper, "Antithyroid drugs," *The New England Journal of Medicine*, vol. 352, no. 9, pp. 905–917, 2005.

[15] N. Watanabe, H. Narimatsu, J. Y. Noh et al., "Antithyroid drug-induced hematopoietic damage: a retrospective cohort study of agranulocytosis and pancytopenia involving 50,385 patients with Graves' disease," *Journal of Clinical Endocrinology and Metabolism*, vol. 97, no. 1, pp. E49–E53, 2012.

[16] M. Duquenne, D. Lakomsky, J. C. Humbert, S. Hadjadj, G. Weryha, and J. Leclere, "Resolutive pancytopenia with effective treatment of hyperthyroidism," *Presse Medicale*, vol. 24, no. 17, pp. 807–810, 1995.

[17] A. L. Talansky, P. Schulman, V. P. Vinciguerra, D. Margouleff, D. R. Budman, and T. J. Degnan, "Pancytopenia complicating Graves' disease and drug-induced hypothyroidism," *Archives of Internal Medicine*, vol. 141, no. 4, pp. 544–545, 1981.

[18] M. O. Hegazi and M. R. El-Sonbaty, "Unusual presentations of hyperthyroidism," in *Handbook of Hyperthyroidism: Etiology, Diagnosis and Treatment*, L. Mertens and J. Bogaert, Eds., pp. 265–270, Nova Science Publishers, 2010.

[19] R. Malik and H. Hodgson, "The relationship between the thyroid gland and the liver," *The Quarterly Journal of Medicine*, vol. 95, pp. 559–569, 2002.

[20] V. Sarinnapakorn, P. Noppavetchwich, T. Sunthorntepwarakul, C. Deerochanawong, and S. Ngongamrut, "Abnormal liver function test in Graves' disease: a prospective study of comparison between the hyperthyroid state and the euthyroid state," *Journal of the Medical Association of Thailand*, vol. 94, supplement 2, pp. S11–S16, 2011.

[21] G. R. Doran, "Serum enzyme disturbances in thyrotoxicosis and myxoedema," *Journal of the Royal Society of Medicine*, vol. 71, no. 3, pp. 189–194, 1978.

[22] M. Biscoveanu and S. Hasinski, "Abnormal results of liver function tests in patients with Graves' disease," *Endocrine Practice*, vol. 6, no. 5, pp. 367–369, 2000.

[23] S. Khemichian and T.-L. Fong, "Hepatic dysfunction in hyperthyroidism," *Gastroenterology & Hepatology*, vol. 7, no. 5, pp. 337–339, 2011.

[24] D. S. Cooper, "Hyperthyroidism," *The Lancet*, vol. 362, no. 9382, pp. 459–468, 2003.

[25] J. D. Myers, E. S. Brannon, and B. C. Holland, "A correlative study of the cardiac output and the hepatic circulation in hyperthyroidism," *The Journal of Clinical Investigation*, vol. 29, no. 8, pp. 1069–1077, 1950.

[26] M. Marvisi, P. Zambrelli, M. Brianti, G. Civardi, R. Lampugnani, and R. Delsignore, "Pulmonary hypertension is frequent in hyperthyroidism and normalizes after therapy," *European Journal of Internal Medicine*, vol. 17, no. 4, pp. 267–271, 2006.

[27] S. Muthukumar, D. Sadacharan, K. Ravikumar, G. Mohanapriya, Z. Hussain, and R. V. Suresh, "A prospective study on cardiovascular dysfunction in patients with hyperthyroidism and its reversal after surgical cure," *World Journal of Surgery*, vol. 40, no. 3, pp. 622–628, 2016.

[28] T. Sugiura, S. Yamanaka, H. Takeuchi, N. Morimoto, M. Kamioka, and Y. Matsumura, "Autoimmunity and pulmonary hypertension in patients with Graves' disease," *Heart and Vessels*, vol. 30, no. 5, pp. 642–646, 2015.

[29] M. Armigliato, R. Paolini, S. Aggio et al., "Hyperthyroidism as a cause of pulmonary arterial hypertension: a prospective study," *Angiology*, vol. 57, no. 5, pp. 600–606, 2006.

[30] I. A. Nakchbandi, J. A. Wirth, and S. E. Inzucchi, "Pulmonary hypertension caused by Graves' thyrotoxicosis: normal pulmonary hemodynamics restored by ^{131}I treatment," *Chest*, vol. 116, no. 5, pp. 1483–1485, 1999.

[31] M. O. Hegazi, A. El Sayed, and H. El Ghoussein, "Pulmonary hypertension responding to hyperthyroidism treatment," *Respirology*, vol. 13, no. 6, pp. 923–925, 2008.

[32] A. Frogoudaki, A. S. Triantafyllis, E. Vassilatou, C. Tsamakis, A. Zacharoulis, and J. Lekakis, "Shortness of breath and lower limb edema in a 54-year-old woman, is there any cure?" *Research in Cardiovascular Medicine*, vol. 5, no. 1, Article ID e30549, 2015.

[33] B. Biondi and G. J. Kahaly, "Cardiovascular involvement in patients with different causes of hyperthyroidism," *Nature Reviews Endocrinology*, vol. 6, no. 8, pp. 431–443, 2010.

22

Severe Thyrotoxicosis Secondary to Povidone-Iodine from Peritoneal Dialysis

Kirstie Lithgow and Christopher Symonds

Department of Medicine, Cumming School of Medicine, University of Calgary, Calgary, AB, Canada

Correspondence should be addressed to Kirstie Lithgow; kirstie.lithgow@ahs.ca

Academic Editor: Osamu Isozaki

A 73-year-old male on home peritoneal dialysis (PD) with recent diagnosis of atrial fibrillation presented with fatigue and dyspnea. Hyperthyroidism was diagnosed with TSH < 0.01 mIU/L and FT4 > 100 pmol/L. He had no personal or family history of thyroid disease. There had been no exposures to CT contrast, amiodarone, or iodine. Technetium thyroid scan showed diffusely decreased uptake. He was discharged with a presumptive diagnosis of thyroiditis. Three weeks later, he had deteriorated clinically. Possible iodine sources were again reviewed, and it was determined that povidone-iodine solution was used with each PD cycle. Methimazole 25 mg daily was initiated; however, he had difficulty tolerating the medication and continued to clinically deteriorate. He was readmitted to hospital where methimazole was restarted at 20 mg bid with high dose prednisone 25 mg and daily plasma exchange (PLEX) therapy. Biochemical improvement was observed with FT4 dropping to 48.5 pmol/L by day 10, but FT4 rebounded to 67.8 pmol/L after PLEX was discontinued. PLEX was restarted and thyroidectomy was performed. Pathology revealed nodular hyperplasia with no evidence of thyroiditis. Preoperative plasma iodine levels were greater than 5 times the upper limit of normal range. We hypothesize that the patient had underlying autonomous thyroid hormone production exacerbated by exogenous iodine exposure from a previously unreported PD-related source.

1. Case

A 73-year-old male with end-stage renal failure on home peritoneal dialysis (PD) and a recent diagnosis of atrial fibrillation presented to hospital with fatigue and dyspnea. At presentation, he had a heart rate of 100 beats per minute. On examination, profound muscle weakness was observed but there were no other findings of thyrotoxicosis. He was found to be thyrotoxic with TSH < 0.01 mIU/L (reference range 0.20–4.0 mIU/L) and free T4 (FT4) >100 pmol/L (reference range 10.0–25.0 pmol/L). The patient had no personal or family history of thyroid disease. There had been no exposures to CT contrast, amiodarone, or iodine. Thyroid peroxidase antibodies were within normal limits at presentation (17.4 kIU/L, reference range 0.0–34.0 kIU/L). C-reactive protein was elevated at 30.6 mg/L (0.0–8.0 mg/L), and white blood cell count was within normal limits. Thyroid ultrasound revealed a mildly bulky thyroid gland with the right lobe measuring 6.6×2.9×2.8 cm and the left lobe measuring 5.7×1.7×1.4 cm,

with no evidence of increased thyroid vascularity or nodules. A thyroid radionuclide scan showed diffusely decreased uptake in the thyroid gland. A presumptive diagnosis of thyroiditis was made. The patient was discharged once his atrial fibrillation was under good control and his dyspnea had resolved. He did not receive anticoagulation as his bleeding risk was felt to be elevated. He did not have any neck pain and was already treated with metoprolol 62.5 mg bid for his atrial fibrillation, so no additional medical therapy for hyperthyroidism was initiated.

At follow-up, three weeks later, he had deteriorated clinically with ongoing weight loss and generalized fatigue. His thyroid biochemistry was persistently above the upper limit of the reference range with FT4 > 100 pmol/L. Possible iodine sources were again reviewed. After further discussion with the patient and consultation with a dialysis nurse, it was determined that a plastic cap containing a small sponge soaked in povidone-iodine solution was used between the PD catheter and draining bag following each daily cycle, revealing a potential source of exogenous iodine exposure. Methimazole was initiated at a dose of 25 mg daily. However, the patient had difficulty tolerating the medication due to gastrointestinal upset. He continued to clinically deteriorate with weight loss and debilitating fatigue, leading him to discontinue the drug. He was readmitted to hospital where methimazole was restarted at 20 mg bid along with prednisone 25 mg and daily plasma exchange (PLEX) therapy, a therapeutic procedure where patient plasma is extracted from the blood and a colloid replacement is infused, decreasing both free and protein bound T3 and T4 [1]. Biochemical improvement was observed with FT4 decreasing to 48.5 pmol/L by the tenth day of hospital admission. PLEX was subsequently stopped, and the FT4 rebounded to 67.8 pmol/L. PLEX was restarted and a thyroid surgeon was consulted. A thyroidectomy was performed successfully, 64 days after the initial presentation. On the day of surgery, the patient was biochemically hyperthyroid with FT4 of 60.2 pmol/L.

Pathology revealed nodular hyperplasia with no evidence of thyroiditis. TSH-receptor antibody levels were undetectable at <0.3 IU/L (reference range < 1.75 IU/L). Preoperative plasma iodine levels were markedly elevated at 3.55 Umol/L (reference range 0.24–0.63 Umol/L). Urine iodine measurement was not possible given the patient's anuria. We hypothesize that the patient's hyperthyroidism was secondary to either an underlying autonomously functioning multinodular goiter or antibody-negative Graves' disease, exacerbated by significant exogenous iodine exposure from a previously unreported PD-related source.

2. Discussion

Iodine is a requirement for thyroid hormone synthesis [2]. Iodine is actively transported into thyroid follicular cells by the sodium-iodide symporter (NIS) at the basolateral membrane. Within the follicular lumen, thyroid peroxidase (TPO) oxidizes iodine and then catalyzes the organification of tyrosine residues in thyroglobulin. This result is mono- and dihydrotyrosines (MIT AND DIT), which are then coupled by TPO to form T3 and T4 [3]. Exposure to excessive amounts of exogenous iodine is a recognized cause of thyroid dysfunction. Under normal physiology, regulatory mechanisms can maintain euthyroidism in the presence of iodine excess. Initially, increased intrathyroidal iodine concentration decreases thyroid hormone synthesis by inhibiting TPO, thus preventing organification; this is known as the Wolff-Chaikoff effect [2–4]. In most individuals, this effect is transient as escape from the Wolff-Chaikoff effect occurs via downregulation of NIS mRNA and protein expression. This decreases intrathyroidal iodine so that thyroid hormone synthesis can resume [3, 4].

In individuals that are predisposed to thyroid disease, exogenous iodine can serve as a substrate for increased thyroid hormone synthesis, causing autonomous thyroid function and subsequent hyperthyroidism. This is most frequently observed in individuals with nontoxic multinodular goiter, iodine deficiency, and latent Graves' disease [2, 4]. Common sources of excess iodine include supplements containing

seaweed or kelp, radiocontrast media, and amiodarone [4]. Elevations of serum iodine levels in peritoneal dialysis patients have been observed previously with povidone-iodine antiseptic use and were shown to significantly decrease once the antiseptics were withdrawn [5]. A similar case report described surreptitious thyrotoxicosis in a patient with a spinal cord injury who used povidone-iodine swabs for chronic self-catheterization, which resolved after swab discontinuation [6]. Despite the widespread use of the povidone-iodine PD cap, there are no previous reports linking its use to hyperthyroidism. It is possible that other cases exist but perhaps are less severe and therefore misdiagnosed or under-recognized.

The diagnosis of iodine-induced thyrotoxicosis required careful exclusion of other causes. The findings from the thyroid ultrasound and radionuclide scan argued against auto-immune thyroid disease or toxic adenoma. Negative thyroid autoantibodies further supported a nonimmune mediated disease process. The remaining diagnostic possibilities were between thyroiditis and hyperthyroidism due to exogenous iodine. Thyroiditis has a self-limited course, with FT4 levels declining over weeks to months [7]. Thus, iodine-induced thyrotoxicosis was the leading diagnosis; the markedly elevated serum iodine levels were supportive of this. From the thyroid pathology, we are still unable to definitively determine the exact etiology of the underlying disease process. In a small case series, previous authors showed that antibody-negative Graves' disease may share features with antibody-positive disease including nodular hyperplasia and colloid enlargement; however, patients with antibody-negative disease also showed significant lymphocytic infiltration, which was not seen in the antibody-positive patients [8]. Our own case's histopathology was significant for nodular hyperplasia but did not reveal any lymphocytic infiltration, nor did it demonstrate any other infiltrative or inflammatory changes that would support a diagnosis of thyroiditis. We therefore presume that the patient's hyperthyroidism was secondary to either underlying toxic multinodular goiter or antibody-negative Grave's disease exacerbated by exogenous iodine from a previously unreported peritoneal dialysis source. We ensured that other potential sources of exogenous iodine were excluded. A detailed history and thorough review of the patient's medical records revealed no previous administration of radiocontrast media, exposure to amiodarone, ingestion of iodine containing supplements, or consumption of drinking water with high iodine content. To our knowledge, our report is the first case of thyrotoxicosis secondary to povidone-iodine from peritoneal dialysis.

Patients with chronic kidney disease have been shown to have a higher prevalence of thyroid disease compared to the general population [9]. A recent observational study evaluated the prevalence of thyroid dysfunction in 1484 patients on peritoneal dialysis and found that 7% and 18%, respectively, had hyperthyroidism and hypothyroidism and that both lower and higher TSH values were associated with increased mortality [10]. The mechanisms leading to thyroid dysfunction in this population have not yet been fully elucidated. Loss of thyroid binding proteins in the peritoneal dialysis effluent, inflammation, malnutrition, nonthyroidal illness, mineral deficiencies, and metabolic acidosis have all been suggested as potential causes [11]. Erythropoietin and zinc supplementation are medical therapies used in the chronic kidney disease population and have been shown to increase TSH-responsiveness to TRH [12]. Exogenous iodine exposure from povidone-iodine used in peritoneal dialysis has previously been proposed as a possible mechanism of thyroid dysfunction in this patient population. In a previous case series, 2 infants acquired hypothyroidism following initiation of PD, leading the authors to hypothesize that this was a consequence of povidone-iodine exposure due to the Wolff-Chaikoff effect, especially given lack of renal clearance of iodine in this circumstance [13]. However, povidone-iodine from PD causing severe thyrotoxicosis has not been previously reported. Though further investigation is needed to delineate the mechanisms underlying thyroid dysfunction in peritoneal dialysis, our case suggests that povidone-iodine exposure may be an important and underrecognized contributor.

3. Conclusion

This case highlights the importance of a careful review of possible sources of exogenous iodine when the etiology of thyrotoxicosis is unclear. Furthermore, low uptake on thyroid radionuclide scan should raise high suspicion of exogenous iodine if thyroiditis is not in keeping with the clinical picture [14]. Patients on peritoneal dialysis are at risk of thyroid dysfunction, and symptoms may overlap with those of uremia and other existing comorbidities. Health care providers should therefore have a low threshold to screen these patients for thyroid disease. This case was exceptionally challenging in that it proved refractory to medical therapies. Thionamides can be used as first-line therapy for iodine-induced thyrotoxicosis, but it may take months to achieve a euthyroid state [15]. This represents a critical situation for the patient, given the high mortality rate that has been associated with this condition [16]. As shown by previous authors, PLEX was an effective strategy for acute treatment of severe thyrotoxicosis and bridge to surgery [1, 14]. In the setting of iodine-induced hyperthyroidism with low radionuclide uptake, thyroid gland ablation with radioactive iodine is not a viable option as the gland is already saturated with iodine [17]. This clinical scenario was highly reminiscent of severe amiodarone-induced thyrotoxicosis due to its severity and therapeutic challenges [14, 17]. While thyroidectomy represents a rapid and effective cure in such cases, there are concerns about precipitating thyroid storm or exacerbating underlying cardiac disease [17]. However, a previous case series demonstrated that thyroidectomy could be performed safely with good outcomes even in high risk cardiac patients [15]. Thus, when iodine-induced thyrotoxicosis is severe and medical management fails, thyroidectomy is the definitive treatment. This approach requires close coordination in a tertiary care setting with a multidisciplinary team including surgery, anesthesia, endocrinology, and critical care.

References

[1] A. Ezer, K. Caliskan, A. Parlakgumus, S. Belli, I. Kozanoglu, and S. Yildirim, "Preoperative therapeutic plasma exchange in patients with thyrotoxicosis," *Journal of Clinical Apheresis*, vol. 24, no. 3, pp. 111–114, 2009.

[2] E. Roti and E. D. Uberti, "Iodine excess and hyperthyroidism," *Thyroid*, vol. 11, no. 5, pp. 493–500, 2001.

[3] L. E. Braverman, R. D. Utiger, and A. P. Farwell, "The thyroid," in *A Fundamental and Clinical Text*, Lippincott Williams & Wilkins, Philadelphia, Pa, USA, 9th edition, 2005, Utiger RD Farwell AP. The Thyroid. A Fundamental and Clinical Text. Ninth edition. Lippincott Williams Wilkins.

[4] A. M. Leung and L. E. Braverman, "Consequences of excess iodine," *Nature Reviews Endocrinology*, vol. 10, no. 3, pp. 136–142, 2014.

[5] D. F. Gardner, D. R. Mars, R. G. Thomas, C. Bumrungsup, and R. I. Misbin, "Iodine retention and thyroid dysfunction in patients on hemodialysis and continuous ambulatory peritoneal dialysis," *American Journal of Kidney Diseases*, vol. 7, no. 6, pp. 471–476, 1986.

[6] P. Pramyothin, A. M. Leung, E. N. Pearce, A. O. Malabanan, and L. E. Braverman, "Clinical problem-solving: a hidden solution," *The New England Journal of Medicine*, vol. 365, no. 22, pp. 2123–2127, 2011.

[7] E. N. Pearce, A. P. Farwell, and L. E. Braverman, "Thyroiditis," *The New England Journal of Medicine*, vol. 348, no. 26, pp. 2646–2655, 2003.

[8] K. Kawai, H. Tamai, T. Mori et al., "Thyroid histology of hyperthyroid Graves' disease with undetectable thyrotropin receptor antibodies," *Journal of Clinical Endocrinology and Metabolism*, vol. 77, no. 3, pp. 716–719, 1993.

[9] J. C. Lo, G. M. Chertow, A. S. Go, and C.-Y. Hsu, "Increased prevalence of subclinical and clinical hypothyroidism in persons with chronic kidney disease," *Kidney International*, vol. 67, no. 3, pp. 1047–1052, 2005.

[10] C. M. Rhee, V. A. Ravel, E. Streja et al., "Thyroid functional disease and mortality in a national peritoneal dialysis cohort," *Journal of Clinical Endocrinology and Metabolism*, vol. 101, no. 11, pp. 4054–4061, 2016.

[11] C. M. Rhee, G. A. Brent, C. P. Kovesdy et al., "Thyroid functional disease: an under-recognized cardiovascular risk factor in kidney disease patients," *Nephrology Dialysis Transplantation*, vol. 30, no. 5, pp. 724–737, 2015.

[12] E. M. Kaptein, "Thyroid hormone metabolism and thyroid diseases in chronic renal failure," *Endocrine Reviews*, vol. 17, no. 1, pp. 45–63, 1996.

[13] R. Brough and C. Jones, "Iatrogenic iodine as a cause of hypothyroidism in infants with end-stage renal failure," *Pediatric Nephrology*, vol. 21, no. 3, pp. 400–402, 2006.

[14] M. Piga, A. Serra, F. Boi, M. L. Tanda, E. Martino, and S. Mariotti, "Amiodarone-induced thyrotoxicosis: a review," *Minerva Endocrinologica*, vol. 33, no. 3, pp. 213–228, 2008.

[15] J. Gough and I. R. Gough, "Total thyroidectomy for amiodarone-associated thyrotoxicosis in patients with severe cardiac disease," *World Journal of Surgery*, vol. 30, no. 11, pp. 1957–1961, 2006.

[16] A. J. O'Sullivan, M. Lewis, and T. Diamond, "Amiodarone-induced thyrotoxicosis: left ventricular dysfunction is associated with increased mortality," *European Journal of Endocrinology*, vol. 154, no. 4, pp. 533–536, 2006.

23

Unusual Cushing's Syndrome and Hypercalcitoninaemia due to a Small Cell Prostate Carcinoma

Antonio Balestrieri,[1] Elena Magnani,[2] and Fiorella Nuzzo[3]

[1]*Endocrinology and Diabetology Unit, "M. Bufalini" Hospital, ASL of Romagna, Cesena, Italy*
[2]*Internal Medicine Unit, "M. Bufalini" Hospital, ASL of Romagna, Cesena, Italy*
[3]*Pathology Unit, "M. Bufalini" Hospital, ASL of Romagna, Cesena, Italy*

Correspondence should be addressed to Antonio Balestrieri; antonio.balestrieri@auslromagna.it

Academic Editor: Michael P. Kane

A 75-year-old man was hospitalized because of severe hypokalaemia due to ACTH dependent Cushing's syndrome. Total body computed tomography (TBCT) and 68 Gallium DOTATATE PET/CT localized a voluminous prostate tumour. A subsequent transurethral prostate biopsy documented a small cell carcinoma positive for ACTH and calcitonin and negative for prostatic specific antigen (PSA) at immunocytochemical study; serum prostatic specific antigen (PSA) was normal. Despite medical treatments, Cushing's syndrome was not controlled and the patient's clinical condition progressively worsened. Surgical resection was excluded; the patient underwent a cycle of chemotherapy followed by febrile neutropenia and fatal intestinal perforation. This case report describes a rare case of Cushing's syndrome and hypercalcitoninaemia due to a small cell carcinoma of the prostate, a rare tumour with very few therapeutic options and negative prognosis.

1. Introduction

Ectopic Cushing's syndrome (CS) due to adrenocorticotropic hormone (ACTH) secretion accounts for about 10–15% of all ACTH dependent CS. Ectopic ACTH syndrome is frequently related to small cell carcinomas of the lung or neuroendocrine tumours such as bronchial carcinoids, thymic carcinoids, and pancreatic NETs; more rarely, other neuroendocrine tumours involving gastrointestinal and genitourinary tracts, pheochromocytomas, or medullary thyroid carcinomas may be involved [1, 2]. Plasma calcitonin is a marker of medullary thyroid carcinoma, generally useless in other clinical settings even if sometimes hypercalcitoninaemia can be associated with nonthyroid pathologies or other neuroendocrine tumours [3, 4].

We describe a rare case of Cushing syndrome due to an aggressive small cell prostate carcinoma associated with high levels of plasma calcitonin, an aggressive tumour with very few therapeutic options and a negative prognosis.

2. Case Presentation

A 75-year-old man was hospitalized for mental confusion, muscular weakness, and severe hypokalaemia (2.5 mEq/L). The patient's medical history included hypertension and benign prostatic hyperplasia; he took ramipril 5 mg and dutasteride 0.5 mg daily. Few months before he had felt an increasing asthenia, he noted weight gain and the worsening of hypertension control and he experienced some episodes of low urinary tract infections. The laboratory tests evidenced the onset of diabetes (fasting glycaemia 160 mg/dL and HBA1C 50 mmol/L); prostate-specific antigen (PSA) was normal (2.39 μg/L). His wife reported that lastly he was physically exhausted and mentally confused. At physical examination the patient was 165 cm in height and he weighed 70 kgs (BMI 25.7); he showed slight round face and thin arms and legs; his arterial pressure was 160/105 mmHg. Digital evaluation revealed that the prostate was enlarged and firm in consistency. Laboratory tests (Table 1) confirmed severe

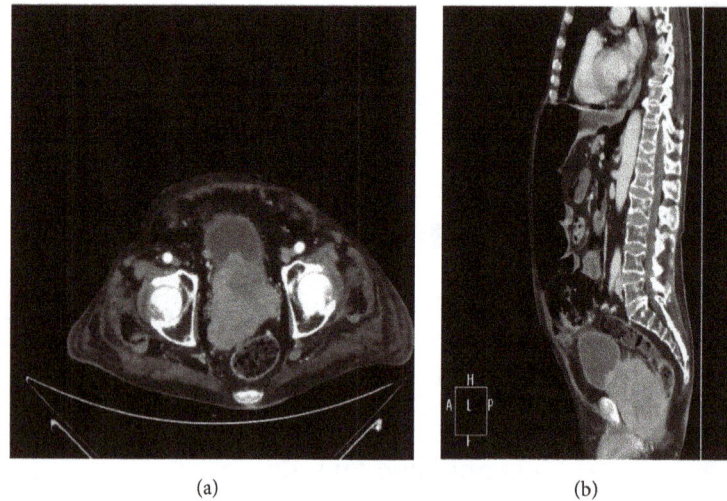

(a)　　　　　　　　　　　　　　(b)

FIGURE 1: Computed tomography (CT) images, axial (a) and coronal (b), of the pelvis showing a huge mass involving bladder and rectum.

TABLE 1: Blood test results.

Investigations	Results	Reference range
White blood cell count	12.210	4.00–10.00 10^9/L
Hemoglobin	15.5	13.5–17.0 g/dL
Creatinine	0.60	0.70–1.2 mg/dL
Potassium	2.5	3.5–5.1 mMol/L
Fasting glucose	160	60–100 mg/dL
Total bilirubin	0.73	<1.2 mg/dL
Alanine aminotransferase	29	<41 U/L
Albumin	31	35–50 g/L
Prostate specific antigen (PSA)	1.7	<4.1 μg/L
Chromogranin A (CGA)	215	<120 μg/L
Plasma ACTH	155.4	7.2–63.3 ng/L
Plasma cortisol	398	62–180 μg/L
Salivary cortisol	50.6	<2.1 μg/L
Testosterone	2.57	4.6–31 nmoli/L
Phosphate	2.6	2.7–4.5 mg/dL
Calcium	8.8	8.6–10.2 mg/dL
Calcitonin	272	<20 ng/L

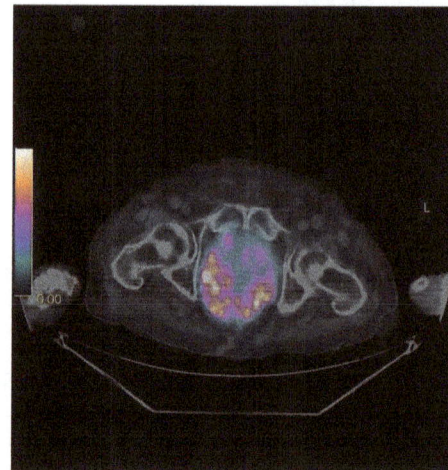

FIGURE 2: 68 Gallium DOTATATE PET/CT image showing a high and diffuse uptake of the prostate.

hypokalaemia (2.3 mmol/L) and documented high levels of midnight salivary cortisol (50.6 μg/L), elevated levels of plasma ACTH (155.4 ng/L), and plasma cortisol (398 μg/L). The overnight 8 mg dexamethasone suppression test did not properly suppress plasma cortisol (198 μg/L); high levels of plasma chromogranin A and calcitonin (272 ng/L) were also documented; PSA was confirmed to be normal (1.7 μg/L) (Table 1).

Magnetic Resonance Imaging (RMI) of the pituitary gland was normal; no nodules were found by thyroid ultrasonography. Total body computed tomography (TBCT) (Figures 1(a)-1(b)) revealed a voluminous prostate gland (maximum diameter of 10 cm) heterogeneously enhancing the contrast medium. The tumour of the prostate had invaded the bladder; the rectum and multiple pathological retroperitoneal lymph nodes as well as bilateral enlarged adrenal glands were evident. A subsequent 68 Gallium DOTATATE PET/CT found a high uptake of the whole prostate (SUV max 12.7) and of the adjacent lymph nodes, confirming the presence of a neuroendocrine tumour in that site and excluding other distant metastases (Figure 2). The patient underwent a transurethral prostate biopsy that showed a small cell prostate cancer focally positive for ACTH and calcitonin and negative for chromogranin A and PSA at immunocytochemistry (Figures 3(a) and 3(b)). Continuous intravenous potassium infusion, potassium sparing drugs (Aldactone), and antihypertensive drugs were administered to the patient. Ketoconazole was also administered with an uptitrating dose of 400 mg/twice daily for 5 weeks and because of the poor control of cortisol secretion, octreotide 0.1 mg every 8 hours subcutaneously was added for further 13 days. Despite a reduction of plasma cortisol (195 mcg/L) after 6 weeks of treatment, no significant clinical benefit was achieved; in fact the patient continued rapidly to worsen

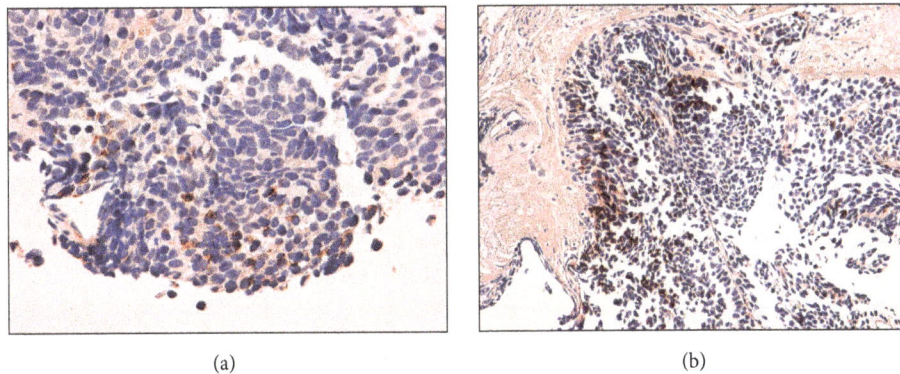

(a)   (b)

FIGURE 3: (a) Immunohistochemical stain showing tumour cell positive for ACTH (×40). (b) Immunohistochemical stain showing tumour cell positive for calcitonin (×20).

becoming more asthenic and confused since he developed a glucocorticoid induced psychosis. The surgeon urologist excluded prostate resection and bilateral surrenectomy because they were considered too dangerous for the patient. The patient started a cycle of chemotherapy with epirubicin and carboplatin, but few weeks after the first cycle, febrile neutropenia, sepsis, and intestinal perforation occurred and the patient died.

3. Discussion

Extrapulmonary small cell carcinomas are rare cancers that may involve many tissues. Genital urinary tract (bladder and prostate) and gastroenteric tract are the mostly affected extrapulmonary sites [5]. The prostate is affected in about 10% of all extrapulmonary small cell carcinomas and accounts for 0.2% of all prostate carcinomas [6, 7]. The pathogenesis of the tumour is still poorly understood; it may arise de novo or represent an aggressive terminal phase of a preexisting prostate adenocarcinoma; generally the tumour is not responsive to androgen ablation therapy [6, 8, 9]. In the case described, we suppose a primary form of a neuroendocrine cancer; of note is the fact that the patient was taking dutasteride, an antiandrogen drug known to reduce the risk of prostate cancer [10].

Cushing's syndrome (CS) due to ACTH secreting small cell prostate carcinoma was first described many decades ago [11]; sporadic cases have been reported subsequently, but it remains a very rare and not easily recognized pathology. CS is the consequence of an ectopic secretion of ACTH; hardly and only in this case is it associated with pituitary hyperplasia [12]. To our knowledge, CS of small cell prostate carcinoma has rarely been described in association with high levels of plasma calcitonin [9]; recently CS and hypercalcitoninaemia have been reported in a small cell lung cancer [13]. Small cell carcinoma of the prostate is characterized by poor prognosis because it is quite often metastatic at the diagnosis [7, 14]. Generally PSA is not elevated, in particular in primary type [6], as probably occurring in the patient described. The normality of PSA, which is routinely used in the follow-up of prostatic diseases, may contribute to delay

of the diagnosis. It is very aggressive and a rapidly evolving cancer, more resistant to chemotherapy and radiotherapy with respect to the typical adenocarcinoma, showing a high propensity to metastasize. It has been postulated that the poor prognosis is related to the stage of the disease, but the options of cure are limited even in the early stages and, at the moment, there are no defined care plans for this tumour [7]. It has been suggested that TBCT is the most useful first radiological choice in the evaluation of ectopic CS and that a subsequent nuclear medicine modality is requested to confirm or detect a neuroendocrine tumour. Many nuclear medicine imaging modalities like F-FDGPET, octreoscan, or MIBG scintigraphy can be used in order to detect a neuroendocrine tumour, but it has been proven that 68 Gallium-SSTR-PET/CT, when available, can show the highest sensitivity in localizing ectopic ACTH secreting tumours, specially in occult diseases [15]. In particular 68 Gallium DOTATATE, which has a predominant affinity for somatostatin receptors type 2 (SSTR2), can dramatically improve the spatial resolution and lesion detectability compared to octreoscan, MIBG scintigraphy, and F-FDGPET/CT in neuroendocrine tumours and non-GEP-NETs tumours, being mostly accurate in staging patients in whom metastatic cancers spread, particularly to the bone is suspected [16, 17]. 68 Gallium DOTATATE is particularly useful in the early stages when neuroendocrine tumours are generally well differentiated and express significant SSTR2, while F-FDGPET/CT scan may be more appropriate in the late stages when neuroendocrine tumours become poorly differentiated [16].

Radiolabelled somatostatin analogue imaging is a primary indication for neuroendocrine tumours; of note is the fact that prostate cancer expresses all of the five subtypes of somatostatin receptors (SSTR), so gallium labelled somatostatin analogues may be also indicated in the evaluation and staging of this disease [17]. 68 Gallium DOTATATE is considered one of the best modalities to detect neuroendocrine tumours and relative distant metastases useful to guide the choice of the following treatments, directing patients to curative surgery when only a primary site is identified or to systemic therapy when metastases are documented [16]. Beyond the presence of distant metastasis, it has to be considered that, similarly to small cell lung cancer [18], CS is a further marker of poor prognosis because cortisol overproduction induces a rapid worsening of general health. In fact, intense weakness, severe hypokalaemia, metabolic alkalosis, hypertension, hyperglycaemia, and immunodepression are characteristic features at the time of the diagnosis [19] even when the classic signs of CS may be absent, as in the patient described. An early diagnosis and treatment of CS may give a better chance of recovery for the subsequent treatments. To this view, bilateral surrenectomy has been recently reconsidered as a valid treatment in Cushing's disease [20] and it has been proposed as the first therapeutic treatment [19]. Moreover, we must consider that, given the rarity of the disease, no definitive data can be collected and, at the moment, successful therapeutic choices are lacking [5, 19]. Calcitonin is the typical clinical marker of medullary thyroid cancer (MTC) generally useless in other clinical settings even if, rarely, it can be related to other neuroendocrine tumours [3]. Really, it has been proven for decades that calcitonin, as well as other neuroendocrine markers (serotonin, chromogranin A, and enolase neurone specific antigen NSE), is highly expressed in prostate tissue and that the neuroendocrine differentiation of prostate cancer is generally associated with tumours progression and poor prognosis [9, 21]. Recently calcitonin and calcitonin receptor (CTR) have been demonstrated to be highly expressed in advanced grades of prostate carcinoma; calcitonin and CTR are supposed to be involved in a favourable paracrine axis able to induce the progression from a localized to a metastatic cancer [22]. In the case reported here, we can suppose that the presence of high calcitonin serum levels and the positive immunocytochemical stain for calcitonin in the carcinoma can probably be considered a further marker of poor prognosis. Therefore the dosage of plasma calcitonin can be useful not only in the diagnosis of MTC, but even in the evaluation of ectopic ACTH secretion, because high levels of plasma calcitonin can be, although rarely, related to other neuroendocrine tumours.

4. Conclusions

ACTH secreting Cushing's syndrome due to small cell prostate cancer is a very rare disease with very few options of cure. Prostate-specific antigen (PSA) is generally not elevated, so finding a normal PSA can be misleading. Gallium labelled somatostatin analogues and in particular 68 Gallium DOTATATE are useful imaging modalities to localize and stage a neuroendocrine tumour of the prostate. In the presence of CS the rapid control of glucocorticoid overproduction must precede the cure of the cancer in order to give a better chance of recovery and a longer survival time for the patient. Bilateral surrenectomy, whenever possible, may be considered a valid therapeutic option.

High levels of plasma calcitonin in the presence of CS may be useful in the differential diagnosis of ACTH dependent CS. Even if it is not possible to drag any conclusion about the role of calcitonin in prostate cancer, on the basis of the case described here, we can suppose that high levels of calcitonin, due to a small cell carcinoma of the prostate, as well as CS, can be related to an unfavourable prognosis.

References

[1] I. Ilias, D. J. Torpy, K. Pacak, N. Mullen, R. A. Wesley, and L. K. Nieman, "Cushing's syndrome due to ectopic corticotropin secretion: twenty years' experience at the National Institutes of Health," *Journal of Clinical Endocrinology and Metabolism*, vol. 90, no. 8, pp. 4955–4962, 2005.

[2] A. M. Isidori, G. A. Kaltsas, C. Pozza et al., "The ectopic adrenocorticotropin syndrome: clinical features, diagnosis, management, and long-term follow-up," *The Journal of Clinical Endocrinology & Metabolism*, vol. 91, no. 2, pp. 371–377, 2006.

[3] S. P. A. Toledo, D. M. Lourenço Jr., M. A. Santos, M. R. Tavares, R. A. Toledo, and J. E. D. M. Correia-Deur, "Hypercalcitoninemia is not pathognomonic of medullary thyroid carcinoma," *Clinics*, vol. 64, no. 7, pp. 699–706, 2009.

[4] M. Kováčová, M. Filková, M. Potočárová, S. Kiňová, and U. Pajvani, "Calcitonin-secreting pancreatic neuroendocrine tumors: a case report and review of the literature," *Endocrine Practice*, vol. 20, no. 8, pp. e140–e144, 2014.

[5] C. S. R. Dakhil, J. A. Wick, A. K. L. Kumar, M. T. Satyan, and P. Neupane, "Extrapulmonary small cell carcinoma: the University of Kansas experience and review of literature," *Medical Oncology*, vol. 31, no. 10, article 187, 2014.

[6] P. Furtado, M. V. A. Lima, C. Nogueira, M. Franco, and F. Tavora, "Review of small cell carcinomas of the prostate," *Prostate Cancer*, vol. 2011, Article ID 543272, 5 pages, 2011.

[7] S. Ahmed, S. Neufeld, T. J. Kroczak et al., "Small cell cancer of the bladder and prostate: a retrospective review from a tertiary cancer center," *Cureus*, vol. 7, no. 8, article e296, 2015.

[8] D. S. Schron, T. Gipson, and G. Mendelsohn, "The histogenesis of small cell carcinoma of the prostate: an immunohistochemical study," *Cancer*, vol. 53, no. 11, pp. 2478–2480, 1984.

[9] P. A. Di Sant'Agnese, "Neuroendocrine differentiation in carcinoma of the prostate. Diagnostic, prognostic, and therapeutic implications," *Cancer*, vol. 70, supplement 1, pp. 254–268, 1992.

[10] G. L. Andriole, D. G. Bostwick, O. W. Brawley et al., "Effect of dutasteride on the risk of prostate cancer," *New England Journal of Medicine*, vol. 362, no. 13, pp. 1192–1202, 2010.

[11] R. E. Wenk, B. S. Bhagavan, R. Levy, D. Miller, and W. Weisburger, "Ectopic ACTH, prostatic oat cell carcinoma, and marked hypernatremia," *Cancer*, vol. 40, no. 2, pp. 773–778, 1977.

[12] R. M. Carey, S. K. Varma, C. R. Drake Jr. et al., "Ectopic secretion of corticotropin-releasing factor as a cause of Cushing's syndrome. A clinical, morphologic, and biochemical study," *New England Journal of Medicine*, vol. 311, no. 1, pp. 13–20, 1984.

[13] K. Coners, S. E. Woods, and M. Webb, "Dual paraneoplastic syndromes in a patient with small cell lung cancer: a case report," *Journal of Medical Case Reports*, vol. 5, article no. 318, 2011.

[14] K. Chang, B. Dai, Y.-Y. Kong et al., "Genitourinary small-cell carcinoma: 11-year treatment experience," *Asian Journal of Andrology*, vol. 16, no. 5, pp. 705–709, 2014.

[15] A. M. Isidori, E. Sbardella, M. C. Zatelli et al., "Conventional and nuclear medicine imaging in ectopic Cushing's syndrome: a systematic review," *The Journal of Clinical Endocrinology & Metabolism*, vol. 100, no. 9, pp. 3231–3244, 2015.

[16] A. Mojtahedi, S. Thamake, I. Tworowska, D. Ranganathan, and E. S. Delpassand, "The value of Ga-DOTATATE PET /CT in the diagnosis and management of neuroendocrine tumors compared to current FDA approved imaging modalities: a review of literature," *American Journal of Nuclear Medicine and Molecular Imaging*, vol. 4, no. 5, pp. 426–434, 2014.

[17] M. Sollini, P. A. Erba, A. Fraternali et al., "PET and PET/CT with [68]Gallium-Labeled somatostatin analogues in non GEP-NETs tumors," *The Scientific World Journal*, vol. 2014, Article ID 194123, 19 pages, 2014.

[18] H. Nagy-Mignotte, O. Shestaeva, L. Vignoud et al., "Prognostic impact of paraneoplastic Cushing's syndrome in small-cell lung cancer," *Journal of Thoracic Oncology*, vol. 9, no. 4, pp. 497–505, 2014.

[19] S. Nimalasena, A. Freeman, and S. Harland, "Paraneoplastic Cushing's syndrome in prostate cancer: a difficult management problem," *British Journal of Urology International*, vol. 101, no. 4, pp. 424–427, 2008.

[20] M. Reincke, K. Ritzel, A. Obwald et al., "A critical reappraisal of bilateral adrenalectomy for ACTH-dependent Cushing's syndrome," *European Journal of Endocrinology*, vol. 173, no. 4, pp. M23–M32, 2015.

[21] P. A. Di Sant'Agnese, "Neuroendocrine differentiation in prostatic carcinoma. Recent findings and new concepts," *Cancer*, vol. 75, supplement 7, pp. 1850–1859, 1995.

[22] S. Thomas, A. Muralidharan, and G. V. Shah, "Knock-down of calcitonin receptor expression induces apoptosis and growth arrest of prostate cancer cells," *International Journal of Oncology*, vol. 31, no. 6, pp. 1425–1437, 2007.

24

A Case of Male Osteoporosis: A 37-Year-Old Man with Multiple Vertebral Compression Fractures

Suhaib Radi and Andrew C. Karaplis

Division of Endocrinology, Department of Medicine, Jewish General Hospital, McGill University, Montreal, QC, Canada H3T 1E2

Correspondence should be addressed to Andrew C. Karaplis; andrew.karaplis@mcgill.ca

Academic Editor: Michael P. Kane

While the contributing role of testosterone to bone health is rather modest compared to other factors such as estradiol levels, male hypogonadism is associated with low bone mass and fragility fractures. Along with stimulating physical puberty by achieving virilization and a normal muscle mass and improving psychosocial wellbeing, the goals of testosterone replacement therapy in male hypogonadism also include attainment of age-specific bone mineral density. We report on a 37-year-old man who presented with multiple vertebral compression fractures several years following termination of testosterone replacement therapy for presumed constitutional delay in growth and puberty. Here, we discuss the management of congenital hypogonadotropic hypogonadism with hyposmia (Kallmann syndrome), with which the patient was ultimately diagnosed, the role of androgens in the acquisition of bone mass during puberty and its maintenance thereafter, and outline specific management strategies for patients with hypogonadism and high risk for fragility fractures.

1. Introduction

Osteoporosis in men is a serious disease that is under-diagnosed, undertreated, and often complicated by fragility fractures and their associated morbidity and mortality [1, 2]. Worldwide, nearly forty percent of all osteoporotic fractures in individuals over the age of 50 occur in men [3]. The mortality rate following a hip fracture in men is 37% in the first year, higher than that observed in women [4]. Male osteoporosis is often secondary, with the most common causes being corticosteroid use, excessive alcohol intake, and hypogonadism, including androgen deprivation therapy for prostate cancer [4]. To increase awareness of this disorder and the characteristics of its presentation, we report the case of a 37-year-old man presenting with multiple vertebral compression fractures.

2. Case Report

A 37-year-old man presented to the emergency department at our hospital on October 2012 with a 4-month history of worsening lower back pain. There was no history of trauma or falls. He was unemployed and lived with his mother. He took no medications or supplements, did not smoke, consume excessive alcohol, or use illegal drugs, and had never been treated with corticosteroids. He had no history of prior fractures. Family history was negative for gonadal, endocrine, or bone diseases. Review of systems was remarkable for markedly delayed puberty for which he had received testosterone injections starting at 16 years of age. Three years later, testosterone replacement therapy was terminated by the treating physician, after he responded well in terms of growth and development of secondary male sexual characteristics. He remarked decreased libido for several years and absence of morning erections.

On examination, he was a well-nourished gentleman in obvious distress due to pain at the level of the lower thoracic/lumbar spine. He had an eunuchoidal body habitus with the arm span (181 cm) exceeding the height (174 cm). The pupils were round, equal, and reactive to light. Visual fields were normal to confrontation. The skin turgor was normal, the mucous membranes were moist and the teeth were in good condition with no decay. Examination of the head and neck was remarkable for hyposmia to a number

TABLE 1: Serum biochemistry.

Test	Result	Normal range
Creatinine	54	55–110 μmol/L
Calcium	2.27	2.12–2.62 mmol/L
Phosphorus	1.31	0.70–1.45 mmol/L
Magnesium	0.76	0.70–1.23 mmol/L
Parathyroid hormone (PTH)	29	10–70 ng/L
Alkaline phosphatase	96	40–125 U/L
Osteocalcin	52.3	5–35 mg/L
25(OH) vitamin D	73	>75 nmol/L
Thyroid stimulating hormone (TSH)	0.89	0.4–4.50 mU/L
Free T4	16.1	9.0–26 pmol/L
Prolactin	4.9	2.7–16.9 mg/L
Cortisol (random)	397	nmol/L
Testosterone	<0.7	6.8–20 nmol/L
Estradiol	<18	55–165 pmol/L
Follicle stimulating hormone (FSH)	0.5	1.6–11 U/L
Luteinizing hormone (LH)	<0.1	0.8–6.1 U/L
Hemoglobin	117	140–175 g/L

of odorants. The cardiovascular, respiratory, and abdominal exams were within normal limits. There was no edema in the extremities and neurological assessment was normal. Examination of the integument was remarkable for sparsity of pubic hair. The penile length was normal but testicular volume was decreased (approximately 5 cm^3 as determined using the Prader orchidometer).

On biochemistry, serum levels for luteinizing hormone (LH), follicle-stimulating hormone (FSH), testosterone, and estradiol were extremely low while baseline values for serum creatinine, electrolytes, thyroid function tests [thyroid-stimulating hormone (TSH) and free T4], prolactin, cortisol, parathyroid hormone (PTH), and alkaline phosphatase activity were all within normal limits. Osteocalcin levels were increased while serum 25(OH) vitamin D levels were insufficient (Table 1). Complete blood count showed a normochromic normocytic anemia. Serum protein electrophoresis was unremarkable.

Radiographic examination of the spine disclosed diffuse osteopenia with moderate wedging of several mid-thoracic vertebrae along with severe compression fractures of T11, T12, and L1 (80%–90% vertebral height loss). There was a 10% superior endplate collapse at L5. Dual-energy X-ray absorptiometry (DXA) scan of the skeleton reported a Z-score of −6.9 at the lumbar vertebrae (L2–L4), −3.3 at the femoral neck, and −4.1 at the total hip (Figure 1(a)).

Magnetic resonance imaging (MRI) of the brain with particular attention to the hypophysis was carried out. The pituitary gland was normal except for a 2.4 × 2.6 mm left anterior pituitary cyst with no evidence of a mass effect.

Based on the aforementioned history, physical examination, radiographic evaluation, and biochemical data indicative of hypogonadotropic hypogonadism with hyposmia, the patient was diagnosed with Kallmann syndrome with severe osteoporosis due to hypogonadism. He was given analgesia and was started on calcium (500 mg/day),

vitamin D (2000 IU/day), and testosterone replacement therapy (Androgel™ 1% 2.5 g daily) while awaiting for government approval for teriparatide (Forteo™) use.

Three weeks later, he presented again to the emergency department with a 4-day history of being unable to ambulate due to severe low back pain following a fall from standing height. A CT scan of the spine disclosed a new L3 compression fracture, with 75% loss of height, along with an interval progression of the L5 superior endplate collapse (from 10% to 40% loss of height). The T11-L1 fractures remained unchanged (Figure 1(b), left panel). Given that the area of maximal pain was at the L5 level, the patient underwent L5 vertebroplasty with good analgesic response and near complete ambulatory recovery (Figure 1(b), right panel).

While convalescing, his application for teriparatide use was approved and treatment was initiated. Skeletal response to the drug was monitored using osteocalcin and procollagen type 1 N-terminal propeptide (P1NP) serum levels as surrogate markers of bone formation (Figure 1(c)). Concurrently, the dose of Androgel was gradually increased to 10 g daily. While on this dose, serum testosterone levels normalized and the anemia resolved. On December 2014, after completing 24 months of teriparatide treatment, he was switched over to sequential treatment with denosumab (Prolia™) 60 mg s/c q6 months. A repeat DXA scan performed on May 2015 (following two doses of denosumab) showed improvement of the bone mineral density at the lumbosacral spine, femoral neck, and total hip [Z score of −5 (from −6.9), −3.3 (from −3.3), and −3.9 (from −4.1)] (Figure 1(d)). He has been doing well since then, and while continuing with calcium, vitamin D, testosterone, and denosumab therapy, he has remained pain-free and has not sustained further fractures.

3. Discussion

Hypogonadism is a common cause of osteoporosis in men (rates ranging from 16 to 30% as the attributable cause) [reviewed in [5]]. It is classified either as hypergonadotropic (primary gonadal failure) or hypogonadotropic (secondary to a defect in the hypothalamic-pituitary axis) hypogonadism [6, 7], with the latter being due to congenital (defects in gonadotropin releasing hormone (GnRH) neurons, GnRH regulating neurons, and LH and FSH secreting cells) or acquired etiologies (structural defects or reversible causes). Congenital hypogonadotropic hypogonadism is subclassified into normosmic, where the sense of smell is intact (40%), or anosmic/hyposmic (absent/decreased sense of smell), the latter also being referred to as Kallmann syndrome (60%).

Kallmann syndrome is a rare developmental disorder, more prevalent in men (1 : 10,000 compared to 1 : 50,000 in women) [7]. It arises as a consequence of failed migration of gonadotropin-releasing hormone (GnRH) and olfactory neurons to the forebrain during intrauterine development. Clinically characterized by failure to initiate puberty due to insufficient gonadotropin release, it results in failure to develop secondary sexual characteristics and a mature reproductive system. Although the disease is often named after the German-American psychiatrist Dr. Kallmann who described its genetic aspects in 1944 [8], it was first described

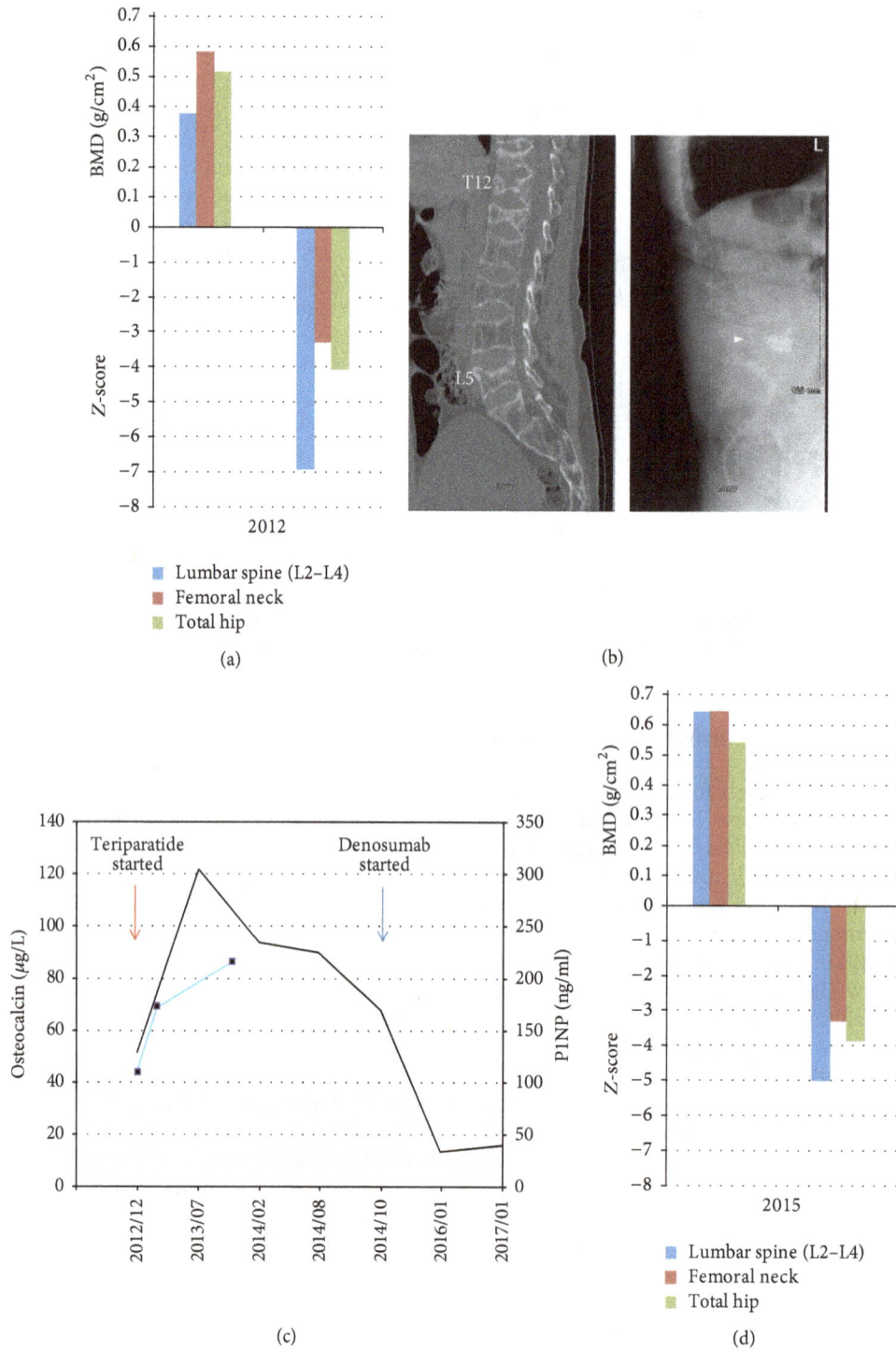

FIGURE 1: (a) BMD measurements and Z-scores at lumbar spine, femoral neck, and total hip at initial presentation. (b) Left: sagittal view of spine CT scan showing compression fractures of T12, L1, L3, and L5, with diffuse osteopenia. Right: lateral spine X-ray showing cement in the body of L5 following vertebroplasty (arrowhead) and severe wedging of L1 and L3. (c) Changes in serum levels of osteocalcin (—) and P1NP (■—■) during the course of treatment. Shaded area represents normal reference values. (d) BMD measurements and Z-scores after completing two years of treatment with teriparatide followed by one year of denosumab.

in 1856 by Maestre de San Juan in a man with absent pubic hair, shrunken testes, decreased sense of smell, and aplasia of the olfactory bulbs at autopsy. Kallmann syndrome is mainly sporadic but can be familial. Multiple genetic mutations have been reported to underlie its pathogenesis, the most common one being *KAL1*, encoding the extracellular glycoprotein anosmin-1, that is responsible for the X chromosome-linked recessive form of the disease. Mutations in a number of other genes have also been reported although all together they may account for less than 30% of these cases. Kallmann syndrome is usually a clinical diagnosis defined by the presence of idiopathic hypogonadotropic hypogonadism and anosmia or hyposmia. Additional abnormalities that may aid in the early diagnosis of the disease including synkinesia *(KAL1)*, dental agenesis and bony anomalies *(FGF8/FGFR1* or *KAL2)*, hearing loss *(CHD7, SOX10)*, renal agenesis, and cleft lip and palate [reviewed in [9]]. A number MRI findings have been reported in patients with Kallmann syndrome, including absent or hypoplastic olfactory bulb and sulci in addition to hypoplastic anterior pituitary [10]. Although these findings may be useful if the clinical picture is not clear, they are not necessary for the diagnosis.

Androgens along with estrogens support the acquisition of bone mass during puberty and its maintenance thereafter [extensively reviewed in [11]]. In men, 15% of estrogen is secreted directly from the testes, and the remaining 85% is derived from peripheral conversion of testosterone by the aromatase (CYP19A1) enzyme [12]. Testosterone on the other hand is made by the Leydig cells of the testicles and acts unmodified or following conversion to the more potent dihydrotestosterone (DHT). The circulating estrogen and androgen levels are controlled by the gonadotropins FSH and LH via the hypothalamic-pituitary-gonadal axis. However, only 1–5% of circulating sex hormones is biologically active, comprising the free fraction not bound to sex hormone-binding globulin (SHBG), albumin, and other proteins.

The effects of androgens on bone are exerted upon binding with high affinity to the androgen receptor (AR; NR3C4) [13]. The androgen receptor has been identified in osteoblasts (bone cells responsible for the deposition of new bone matrix and its mineralization), osteocytes (osteoblasts entombed within the mineralized matrix and interconnected by processes via a canalicular system that extends all the way to the surface of bone used to sense and respond to changes in mechanical forces) and their progenitors, the pluripotent mesenchymal bone stromal cells, and osteoclasts (bone cells that resorb the mineralized matrix arising from hematopoietic precursors).

In both sexes, prepubertal growth velocity is greater in the appendicular skeleton (comprising long bones like the femur and radius) than in the axial (skull, spine, sternum, and the ribs) skeleton. Therefore, patients like ours with disorders of puberty exhibit so-called eunuchoid proportions, characterized by long limbs (arm span) relative to the spine (height).

The role of androgens on male bone metabolism is twofold. First, androgens stimulate bone formation during puberty. Second, androgens prevent bone resorption during and after puberty [14]. During growth, bone is shaped by modeling, a process that ensures the acquisition of the appropriate bone morphology and shapes skeletal elements and mass. Periosteal bone apposition is, for the most part, responsible for the enlargement of bones during growth. The periosteum is a thin layer of connective tissue that covers the external surfaces of most bones and is rich in osteogenic cells. Greater periosteal expansion during puberty accounts for larger bones and hence increased strength and reduced fracture risk. Interestingly, mouse models with targeted AR deletion at different stages of the differentiation program of the osteoblast lineage demonstrate no effect on cortical bone mass while those with global deletion of AR do show a delay in cortical bone mass accrual during puberty. Therefore, androgens do not exert their effects on cortical bone directly through actions on osteoblasts and their progenitors but rather indirectly via actions on some other cell type(s) or tissue(s), yet to be identified [15]. In contrast, the effects of androgens on cancellous bone are direct actions in cells of the osteoblast lineage. AR signaling in osteoblasts leads to a decrease in osteoclast numbers and bone resorption and is responsible for the protective effects of androgens on cancellous bone mass [16]. Finally, genetic evidence from mice with osteoclast-specific AR deletion indicates that androgen signaling in osteoclasts plays no role in the antiresorptive effect of androgens on the cancellous or cortical bone compartments [17].

In addition to bone development and growth, androgens are known to affect the maintenance of bone in men [11, 14]. The maintenance of skeletal mass in adulthood depends on the balance between bone resorption and formation during the continuous regeneration of the skeleton by the process of remodeling. Here, mature bone tissue is removed from the skeleton by resorption and new bone tissue is formed by ossification. Under physiological conditions, bone resorption and formation during remodeling are linked in time and space, being referred to as coupling. Androgens help to maintain bone mass during adult life by slowing the rate of bone remodeling and preserving the balance between resorption and formation, thus explaining the reduction in bone mass at all sites in our patient. In elderly and young hypogonadal men, loss of androgens contributes to the development of low BMD and bone fragility (osteoporosis), a prevalent and impactive metabolic disease.

It is also important to point out that, in men, in addition to androgens, a threshold level of bioavailable estradiol is needed to prevent bone loss, as it has a more dominant role than testosterone [12, 18]. Support for the concept of estrogen being more of a determinant on bone health than testosterone comes from "experiments of nature," that is, from male patients with either estrogen resistance caused by mutations in the estrogen receptor gene [19] or aromatase deficiency, the enzyme responsible for aromatization of androgens into estrogen in extragonadal sites, including fat, brain, skin, endothelium, and bone [20]. The latter group of patients exhibited reduced bone mass at all sites and unfused epiphyses, with normal to high testosterone levels. Interestingly, restoration of bone mass and epiphyseal closure were reported following estrogen replacement, underlining the importance of estrogens in these processes [21]. Finally, selective estrogen receptor modulators (SERMs) which stimulate estrogenic action in bone can block bone loss in orchiectomy-induced, testosterone-depleted male mice [22].

Male patients treated for androgen deficiency can initiate replacement doses of testosterone if fertility is not desired and when there are contraindications [reviewed in [23]]. Testosterone therapy in Kallmann syndrome will achieve full virilization but will not achieve normal testicular volume nor fertility. If fertility is desired, it will need to be replaced with either combined FSH and human chorionic gonadotropin (hCG) or GnRH pump therapy [24]. Testosterone therapy of young, hypogonadal men such as our patient is associated with improvements in overall sexual activity scores, hair growth in several androgen-sensitive areas, fat-free mass, and muscle strength [23]. Although testosterone therapy in healthy, hypogonadal men increases bone mineral density [25, 26], the effects of testosterone on fracture risk are unknown. Different forms of testosterone application are available, such as intramuscular injections, oral, patch/gel/liquid for topical application, or intranasal application. These modalities are all equally effective in normalizing serum testosterone levels and the choice is usually based on patient's preference and cost [23]. However, appropriate dosing should be instituted. Based on the Endocrine Society Clinical Practice Guidelines, the starting dose for Androgel is 5–10 grams daily. In our patient, we opted to initiate treatment with a lower initial dose (2.5 g/day) and increase it progressively, given the long-term absence to testosterone exposure.

In our patient, testosterone replacement therapy had been terminated at the age of 19, after he responded well in terms of growth and development of secondary male sexual characteristics. Conflicting data has been reported about reversibility of hypogonadism in Kallmann syndrome. Some have reported reversibility, even after prolonged discontinuation of therapy [27], while others showed recurrence of the disease [28]. In the report by Raivio et al., sustained reversal of idiopathic hypogonadotropic hypogonadism was achieved in 10% after a mean treatment duration of 6 weeks [29]. The authors concluded that it is reasonable to do a treatment holiday for those patients. However, if a trial of therapy is to be instituted, continuous surveillance should be performed so as to detect and treat any recurrence [28, 30].

Approved treatments for men with low bone mass and high risk for fractures, including those due to hypogonadism, are bisphosphonates (alendronate, risedronate, and zoledronic acid), teriparatide, a recombinant form of human parathyroid hormone amino acids 1–34 [4], and denosumab [31], based on the findings of the ADAMO trial [32]. In addition, optimal calcium and vitamin D intake should be encouraged and specific life style changes be instituted, as needed. For those with hypogonadism and high risk of fractures, treatment should be added to testosterone therapy, whereas, in patients at medium risk of fracture, testosterone alone is usually sufficient. Our patient was treated with teriparatide for 24 months followed by denosumab, in addition to being on testosterone. Patients treated with teriparatide, when switched to denosumab, continue to show increase in bone mineral density, as reported in the DATA-Switch study [33]. Conversely, in the absence of consolidation therapy with

denosumab, the large teriparatide-induced gains in BMD are abruptly lost [34]. Novel bone anabolic agents such as romosozumab or abaloparatide could be considered as alternatives to teriparatide in the near future. Osteocalcin and P1NP are bone turnover markers that can assist in monitoring the response to therapy. With bone anabolic agents like teriparatide, a rise in serum osteocalcin and P1NP levels is expected during the first 6 months of treatment, while serum levels decrease with antiresorptive agents, such as bisphosphonates and denosumab, suggestive of a satisfactory response to treatment [33, 35]. The anticipated bone turnover marker response was observed in our patient, as shown in Figure 1(c). Indeed, there was a concomitant improvement in bone mineral density measurements and he has not sustained additional fractures while continuing therapy.

Finally, it is well recognized that low testosterone causes anemia through decreased erythropoiesis, even in the absence of chronic disease, that is corrected following testosterone replacement therapy [36, 37]. A recent randomised trial in older men with low testosterone and anemia showed that testosterone treatment significantly increased hemoglobin levels in men with unexplained anemia and in those with anemia from known causes [38]. This was also demonstrated here, as the patient's normochromic normocytic anemia corrected completely after serum-free testosterone levels normalized. In addition to the known effect of testosterone in increasing erythropoietin concentrations which stimulate erythropoiesis, testosterone treatment is associated with the suppression of hepcidin and an increase in the expression of ferroportin and transferrin receptor [39]. These changes would potentially facilitate a greater bioavailability of iron from the storage/absorption sites, an increase in iron transport in the circulation, and the uptake at iron utilization sites, thereby further facilitating erythropoiesis. The effect of testosterone on erythropoiesis is dose-dependent and polycythaemia in response to overreplacement with testosterone is well-known [40].

In conclusion, Kallmann syndrome is an uncommon condition that should be suspected in patients with hypogonadotropic hypogonadism irrespective of age, and special attention should be paid to the clinical history for the presence of anosmia/hyposmia. It is a disease that is easily missed but at the same time readily treated with testosterone replacement therapy. Associated osteoporosis is quite common, and when associated with fragility fractures, it is best treated with bone anabolic agents followed by antiresorptive agents, specifically denosumab, in addition to testosterone. It is also important not to stop testosterone therapy without close surveillance as the rate of recurrence is high. Primary care physicians and specialists alike need to maintain awareness of male osteoporosis so that patients who are at risk for fractures are assessed and treated appropriately and in timely fashion.

Acknowledgments

The authors thank Anthony Karaplis for assisting with the preparation of the manuscript and figure.

References

[1] E. Gielen, D. Vanderschueren, F. Callewaert, and S. Boonen, "Osteoporosis in men," *Best Practice & Research Clinical Endocrinology & Metabolism*, vol. 25, no. 2, pp. 321–335, 2011.

[2] P. R. Ebeling, "Clinical practice: osteoporosis in men," *The New England Journal of Medicine*, vol. 358, no. 14, pp. 1474–1482, 2008.

[3] O. Johnell and J. A. Kanis, "An estimate of the worldwide prevalence and disability associated with osteoporotic fractures," *Osteoporosis International*, vol. 17, no. 12, pp. 1726–1733, 2006.

[4] N. B. Watts, R. A. Adler, and J. P. Bilezikian, "Osteoporosis in men: an endocrine society clinical practice guideline," *The Journal of Clinical Endocrinology & Metabolism*, vol. 97, no. 6, pp. 1802–1822, 2012.

[5] G. Golds, D. Houdek, and T. Arnason, "Male hypogonadism and osteoporosis: the effects, clinical consequences, and treatment of testosterone deficiency in bone health," *International Journal of Endocrinology*, Article ID 4602129, 2017.

[6] L. G. L. Amato, A. C. Latronico, and L. F. G. Silveira, "Molecular and genetic aspects of congenital isolated hypogonadotropic hypogonadism," *Endocrinology Metabolism Clinics of North America*, vol. 46, no. 2, pp. 283–303, 2017.

[7] R. Balasubramanian and W. F. Crowley Jr., "Isolated Gonadotropin-Releasing Hormone (GnRH) Deficiency," in *GeneReviews(R)*, R. A. Pagon, M. P. Adam, and H. H. Ardinger, Eds., Seattle, WA, USA, 1993.

[8] FJ. Kallmann, WA. Schoenfeld, and SE. Barrera, "The genetic aspects of primary eunuchoidism," *American Journal of Mental Deficiency*, vol. 48, no. 3, pp. 203–236, 1944.

[9] A. K. Topaloglu and L. D. Kotan, "Genetics of hypogonadotropic hypogonadism," *Endocrine Development*, vol. 29, pp. 36–49, 2016.

[10] Z. Zhang, X. Sun, C. Wang, G. Wang, and B. Zhao, "Magnetic resonance imaging findings in kallmann syndrome: 14 cases and review of the literature," *Journal of Computer Assisted Tomography*, vol. 40, no. 1, pp. 39–42, 2016.

[11] M. Almeida, M. R. Laurent, V. Dubois et al., "Estrogens and androgens in skeletal physiology and pathophysiology," *Physiological Reviews*, vol. 97, no. 1, pp. 135–187, 2016.

[12] L. Gennari, R. Nuti, and J. P. Bilezikian, "Aromatase activity and bone homeostasis in men," *The Journal of Clinical Endocrinology & Metabolism*, vol. 89, no. 12, pp. 5898–5907, 2004.

[13] P. Pihlajamaa, B. Sahu, and O. A. Janne, "Determinants of receptor- and tissue-specific actions in androgen signaling," *Endocrine Reviews*, vol. 36, no. 4, pp. 357–384, 2015.

[14] D. Vanderschueren, J. Gaytant, S. Boonen, and K. Venken, "Androgens and bone," *Current Opinion in Endocrinology, Diabetes and Obesity*, vol. 15, no. 3, pp. 250–254, 2008.

[15] S. Ucer, S. Iyer, S. M. Bartell et al., "The effects of androgens on murine cortical bone do not require AR or ERα signaling in osteoblasts and osteoclasts," *Journal of Bone and Mineral Research*, vol. 30, no. 7, pp. 1138–1149, 2015.

[16] A. J. Notini, J. F. McManus, A. Moore et al., "Osteoblast deletion of exon 3 of the androgen receptor gene results in trabecular bone loss in adult male mice," *Journal of Bone and Mineral Research*, vol. 22, no. 3, pp. 347–356, 2007.

[17] M. Sinnesael, F. Jardi, L. Deboel et al., "The androgen receptor has no direct antiresorptive actions in mouse osteoclasts," *Molecular and Cellular Endocrinology*, vol. 411, pp. 198–206, 2015.

[18] S. Khosla, L. J. Melton, and B. L. Riggs, "Clinical review 144: Estrogen and the male skeleton," *The Journal of Clinical Endocrinology & Metabolism*, vol. 87, no. 4, pp. 1443–1450, 2002.

[19] E. P. Smith, J. Boyd, G. R. Frank et al., "Estrogen resistance caused by a mutation in the estrogen-receptor gene in a man," *The New England Journal of Medicine*, vol. 331, no. 16, pp. 1056–1061, 1994.

[20] E. R. Simpson, "Role of aromatase in sex steroid action," *Journal of Molecular Endocrinology*, vol. 25, no. 2, pp. 149–156, 2000.

[21] J. P. Bilezikian, A. Morishima, J. Bell, and M. M. Grumbach, "Increased bone mass as a result of estrogen therapy in a man with aromatase deficiency," *The New England Journal of Medicine*, vol. 339, no. 9, pp. 599–603, 1998.

[22] Y. Sato, T. Tando, M. Morita et al., "Selective estrogen receptor modulators and the vitamin D analogue eldecalcitol block bone loss in male osteoporosis," *Biochemical and Biophysical Research Communications*, vol. 482, no. 4, pp. 1430–1436, 2017.

[23] S. Bhasin, G. R. Cunningham, F. J. Hayes et al., "Testosterone therapy in men with androgen deficiency syndromes: an endocrine society clinical practice guideline," *The Journal of Clinical Endocrinology & Metabolism*, vol. 95, no. 6, pp. 2536–2559, 2010.

[24] P. Surampudi, R. S. Swerdloff, and C. Wang, "An update on male hypogonadism therapy," *Expert Opinion on Pharmacotherapy*, vol. 15, no. 9, pp. 1247–1264, 2014.

[25] H. M. Behre, S. Kliesch, E. Leifke, T. M. Link, and E. Nieschlag, "Long-term effect of testosterone therapy on bone mineral density in hypogonadal men," *The Journal of Clinical Endocrinology & Metabolism*, vol. 82, no. 8, pp. 2386–2390, 1997.

[26] C. Wang, G. Cunningham, A. Dobs et al., "Long-term testosterone gel (AndroGel) treatment maintains beneficial effects on sexual function and mood, lean and fat mass, and bone mineral density in hypogonadal men," *Journal of Clinical Endocrinology and Metabolism*, vol. 89, no. 5, pp. 2085–2098, 2004.

[27] L. Maione, S. Brailly-Tabard, J. Nevoux, J. Bouligand, and J. Young, "Reversal of congenital hypogonadotropic hypogonadism in a man with Kallmann syndrome due to SOX10 mutation," *Clinical Endocrinology*, vol. 85, no. 6, pp. 988-989, 2016.

[28] A. A. Dwyer, T. Raivio, and N. Pitteloud, "Management of endocrine disease: reversible hypogonadotropic hypogonadism," *European Journal of Endocrinology*, vol. 174, no. 6, pp. R267–274, 2016.

[29] T. Raivio, J. Falardeau, A. Dwyer et al., "Reversal of idiopathic hypogonadotropic hypogonadism," *The New England Journal of Medicine*, vol. 357, no. 9, pp. 863–873, 2007.

[30] V. F. Sidhoum, Y.-M. Chan, M. F. Lippincott et al., "Reversal and relapse of hypogonadotropic hypogonadism: resilience and fragility of the reproductive neuroendocrine system," *Journal of Clinical Endocrinology and Metabolism*, vol. 99, no. 3, pp. 861–870, 2014.

[31] K. M. Sidlauskas, E. E. Sutton, and M. A. Biddle, "Osteoporosis in men: epidemiology and treatment with denosumab," *Clinical Interventions in Aging*, vol. 9, pp. 593–601, 2014.

[32] B. L. Langdahl, C. S. Teglbjaerg, and P. R. Ho, "A 24-month study evaluating the efficacy and safety of denosumab for the treatment of men with low bone mineral density: results from

the ADAMO trial," *The Journal of Clinical Endocrinology & Metabolism*, vol. 100, no. 4, pp. 1335–1342, 2015.

[33] B. Z. Leder, J. N. Tsai, A. V. Uihlein et al., "Denosumab and teriparatide transitions in postmenopausal osteoporosis (the DATA-Switch study): extension of a randomised controlled trial," *The Lancet*, vol. 386, no. 9999, pp. 1147–1155, 2015.

[34] B. Z. Leder, J. N. Tsai, L. A. Jiang, and H. Lee, "Importance of prompt antiresorptive therapy in postmenopausal women discontinuing teriparatide or denosumab: the denosumab and teriparatide follow-up study (DATA-follow-up)," *Bone*, pp. 98-54, 2017.

[35] T. Sugimoto, T. Nakamura, Y. Nakamura, Y. Isogai, and M. Shiraki, "Profile of changes in bone turnover markers during once-weekly teriparatide administration for 24 weeks in post-menopausal women with osteoporosis," *Osteoporosis International*, vol. 25, no. 3, pp. 1173–1180, 2014.

[36] Y. S. Shin, J. H. You, J. S. Cha, and J. K. Park, "The relationship between serum total testosterone and free testosterone levels with serum hemoglobin and hematocrit levels: a study in 1221 men," *Aging Male*, vol. 19, no. 4, pp. 209–214, 2016.

[37] Zhang L. T., Y. S. Shin, J. Y. Kim, and J. K. Park, "Could testos-terone replacement therapy in hypogonadal men ameliorate anemia, a cardiovascular risk factor? an observational, 54-week cumulative registry study," *Journal of Urology*, vol. 195, Part 1, no. 4, pp. 1057–1064, 2016.

[38] E. Orwoll, "Further elucidation of the potential benefits of testosterone therapy in older men," *JAMA Internal Medicine*, vol. 177, no. 4, pp. 480–490, 2017.

[39] S. Dhindsa, H. Ghanim, M. Batra et al., "Effect of testosterone on hepcidin, ferroportin, ferritin and iron binding capacity in patients with hypogonadotropic hypogonadism and type 2 diabetes," *Clinical Endocrinology*, vol. 85, no. 5, pp. 772–780, 2016.

[40] A. D. Coviello, B. Kaplan, K. M. Lakshman, T. Chen, A. B. Singh, and S. Bhasin, "Effects of graded doses of testosterone on erythropoiesis in healthy young and older men," *Journal of Clinical Endocrinology and Metabolism*, vol. 93, no. 3, pp. 914–919, 2008.

25

Dapagliflozin-Associated Euglycemic Diabetic Ketoacidosis in a Patient Presenting with Acute Pancreatitis

Karun Badwal ⓘ, Tooba Tariq, and Diane Peirce

Western Michigan University Homer Stryker M.D. School of Medicine, USA

Correspondence should be addressed to Karun Badwal; karun.badwal@med.wmich.edu

Academic Editor: Osamu Isozaki

Sodium-glucose cotransporter 2 (SGLT-2) inhibitors are a class of medications used for glycemic control in type II diabetes mellitus. Their mechanism of action involves preventing resorption of glucose at the proximal kidney, thereby promoting glucosuria and weight loss. However, they have also been found to be associated with euglycemic diabetic ketoacidosis (euDKA). This case describes a 25-year-old male with a history of type II diabetes on metformin, sitagliptin, and dapagliflozin who was admitted with his third episode of pancreatitis secondary to hypertriglyceridemia. His home oral glycemic agents were continued as inpatient. Despite tight euglycemic control, the patient developed profound metabolic acidosis and was found to have an elevated beta-hydroxybutyrate level and normal lactic acid level. He was admitted into the intensive care unit and started on an insulin drip, and after resolution of his acidosis he was transitioned to basal insulin successfully. He was discharged with an insulin regimen while his oral glycemic agents were discontinued indefinitely. SGLT-2 inhibitors are associated with euDKA, most likely as a result of their non-insulin-dependent glucose clearance, hyperglucagonemia, and decreased ketone clearance. The aim of this case report is to inform the physician about the possibility of euDKA in a patient with type II diabetes on a SGLT-2 inhibitor presenting with an acute illness.

1. Introduction

Sodium-glucose cotransporter 2 inhibitors are a novel class of medications used for glycemic control in type II diabetes mellitus. They exert their effect by inhibiting SGLT-2 receptors in the kidney which are responsible for the resorption of glucose. This promotes glucosuria and in turn also decreases blood glucose levels [1].

This mechanism leads to the added benefit of weight loss by caloric loss in the urine, removing the energy source that drives excess adipose tissue formation resulting in improved insulin sensitivity [2, 3]. As dietary modifications and exercise are the mainstay of treatment in type II diabetes, SGLT-2 inhibitors can be used as monotherapy or as an adjunctive to other classes of oral glycemic agents. Common adverse effects reported in the literature are an increased incidence of genitourinary tract infections and orthostatic hypotension as a result of increased urinary frequency and volume. Recently, postmarketing surveillance has revealed an increased incidence of diabetic ketoacidosis in patients taking SGLT-2 inhibitor medications [4].

This case will illustrate a unique example of euglycemic diabetic ketoacidosis in a type II diabetic patient on a SGLT-2 inhibitor presenting with acute pancreatitis secondary to hypertriglyceridemia.

2. Case Presentation

The patient is a 25-year-old gentleman who presented with a one-day history of abdominal pain, nausea, and emesis. He has had two episodes of pancreatitis in the past secondary to hypertriglyceridemia, with the last episode occurring three years ago. He also has type II diabetes controlled with dapagliflozin (SGLT-2 inhibitor), sitagliptin, and metformin. In the emergency department, the patient's initial labs showed a WBC of 23,000 cells/μL, lipase of 2,530U/L, triglyceride level above 5,000mg/dL, bicarbonate 23mEq/L, and glucose 285mg/dL. His initial urinalysis and chest X-ray were unremarkable. A CT scan of his abdomen and pelvis with contrast was performed showing a large amount of peripancreatic inflammatory change consistent with acute pancreatitis (Figure 1). There was no evidence

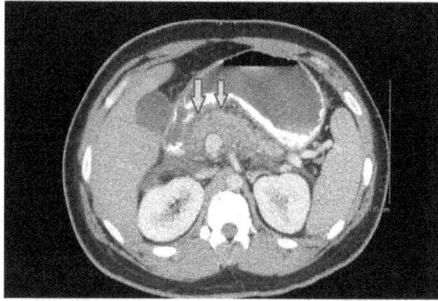

FIGURE 1: Peripancreatic inflammatory changes consistent with acute pancreatitis (arrows).

of cholelithiasis or cholecystitis, and the bile duct diameter was within normal limits. Based on these laboratory findings and imaging results, it was concluded that the patient had acute pancreatitis secondary to elevated triglycerides. He was admitted to the inpatient service and dapagliflozin, sitagliptin, and metformin were continued.

The patient was transitioned from nothing by mouth status on admission to a full-liquid diet on day 3 of hospital stay. By day 5, the lipase level trended down to 158U/L. His blood sugar remained consistently between 120mg/dl and 220mg/dl since admission. Despite maintaining tight euglycemic control, the patient developed profound metabolic acidosis with a gradual downward trend of his bicarbonate level from 23mEq/L to 5mEq/L and a high anion gap of 32 by day 5. This was accompanied by the acute development of tachypnea and tachycardia with a heart rate up to 130bpm. He was immediately started on an IV infusion drip of sodium bicarbonate. The beta-hydroxybutyrate level was 6.06mmol/L with a blood sugar of 161mg/dL and a lactic acid level of 1.5mmol/L. An arterial blood gas revealed a pH of 7.14 and pCO2 of 13mmHg. Although metformin was also continued, the normal lactic acid and elevated beta-hydroxybutyrate supported the diagnosis of DKA. It was concluded that the acidosis was secondary to diabetic ketosis induced by dapagliflozin. All oral glycemic agents were immediately discontinued, and he was transferred to the intensive care unit where he was started on an insulin drip. The nephrology service was consulted and by their recommendations the patient also underwent plasma exchange therapy for hypertriglyceridemia.

After being stabilized in the intensive care unit over the course of 24 hours, he was transferred to the general medical floor on an insulin drip and was transitioned to basal insulin. His diet was cautiously advanced in the setting of acute pancreatitis. Mealtime insulin coverage was added as the patient increased his oral intake. His blood sugars continued to remain well controlled between 120mg/dl and 200mg/dl while his insulin regimen was optimized according to his oral intake. He was discharged on an insulin regimen with insulin detemir and insulin lispro with the recommendation to stop all oral glycemic agents.

3. Discussion

SGLT receptors are a family of sodium glucose cotransporters that are primarily located at the brush border of the proximal convoluted tubules in the kidney [5]. SGLT-2 receptors are a high capacity, low affinity transporter that utilizes the sodium gradient to drive the reabsorption of approximately 90% of the filtered glucose in the S1 segment of the proximal renal tubule. The remaining glucose is reabsorbed by SGLT-1 receptors, which are placed more distally in the S3 segment of the proximal tubule and have a higher affinity but lower capacity for glucose [6]. The SGLT-2 inhibitor class of medications specifically inhibit the SGLT-2 transporters and therefore prevent the reabsorption of the majority of filtered glucose [4, 7, 8]. An added benefit of SGLT-2 inhibitors is the induction of modest weight loss by caloric loss of glucose in the urine leading to decreased visceral and subcutaneous adipose tissue and thereby further improving insulin sensitivity [2]. Finally, some of these agents have also been shown to have cardiovascular mortality benefits [9].

Canagliflozin, dapagliflozin, and empagliflozin are the three SGLT-2 inhibitors currently approved by the FDA for treatment of type II diabetes. However, since the approval of canagliflozin in March 2013, more than 70 cases of DKA have been reported. In May 2015, the FDA issued a warning about the risk of ketoacidosis with the use of SGLT-2 inhibitors [10–12]. Since then, further studies have investigated the incidence of SGLT-2 inhibitor-associated DKA. One study looking at the FDA Adverse Effect Reporting System database identified 7836 patients taking a SGLT-2 inhibitor, out of which 51 patients developed DKA with metabolic data. Of those 51 patients, 20 patients were type I diabetics, 25 patients were type II diabetics, and 6 patients were an unspecified type of diabetes. The study estimated a 7-fold increase in the incidence of DKA with patients on a SGLT-2 inhibitor when compared to patients on DPP-4 inhibitors with type II diabetes [13].

Diabetic ketoacidosis is a serious and potentially life-threatening complication of diabetes mellitus which occurs as a result of profound insulin deficiency. It is more commonly associated with poorly controlled type I diabetes as opposed to type II diabetes, in which case an added stress is required to trigger DKA such as infection or surgery [9]. Euglycemic DKA is an uncommon form of ketoacidosis which is characterized by metabolic acidosis with a pH <7.3 and a serum bicarbonate of <18mEq/L, ketosis, and a blood glucose level of <200 mg/dL [14].

The pathogenesis of DKA is well-known and involves low insulin levels triggering lipolysis and subsequent increased levels of free fatty acids in the blood which stimulates glucagon production. Glucagon promotes the oxidation of fatty acids and results in the production of ketone bodies, which are water-soluble acidic molecules directly responsible for ketoacidosis. Interestingly, the euDKA caused by SGLT-2 inhibitors follows a different mechanism of action. SGLT-2 inhibitors deplete the circulating glucose in the serum by promoting glucosuria, removing the stimulus for beta cells to secrete insulin. This in turn causes enhanced glucagon production by alpha cells in the pancreas. Furthermore,

Bonner et al. demonstrated that both SGLT-1 and SGLT-2 cotransporters are also present on the alpha cells in the pancreas by confocal imaging analysis. Additionally, they found that the inhibition of SGLT-2 cotransporters by dapagliflozin in human islets was correlated with increased glucagon secretion by alpha cells [15]. Finally, there are studies suggesting that SGLT-2 inhibitors may decrease renal excretion of ketone bodies, therefore raising the level of ketone bodies in the blood. The end result of these combined mechanisms is hyperketonemia in the setting of euglycemia [9, 16]. Additionally, euDKA associated with SGLT-inhibitors causes twice the amount of renal glucose clearance compared to DKA [17].

At this time, SGLT-2 inhibitors are not approved by regulatory authorities for the treatment of type I diabetes. However, they are currently being used off-label due to their beneficial effects of weight reduction and maintenance of lower blood glucose levels in conjunction with insulin therapy [18, 19].

It is important to note that it is not common for individuals on a SGLT-2 inhibitor to develop euDKA. In a meta-analysis published by Burke et al. in 2017, the leading risk factors that predispose an individual on a SGLT-2 inhibitor to DKA include medication noncompliance, infection, major surgeries, and underlying autoimmune diabetes in patients previously diagnosed with T2DM [20]. In our patient, acute pancreatitis secondary to hypertriglyceridemia was thought to be the main driving force that led to the development of ketoacidosis. The patient was also not eating for the initial 48 hours of admission, possibly leading to a catabolic state with subsequent ketone body formation in the setting of a SGLT-2 inhibitor. This is supported by a randomized control trial study by Yabe et al. which randomized individuals on the SGLT-2 inhibitor luseogliflozin to diets of differing carbohydrate intake and found a higher incidence of ketoacidosis among individuals in the lower carbohydrate group [21].

SGLT-2 inhibitor-induced DKA is treated in a similar fashion as conventional DKA with the goal of driving the acidemia down with aggressive fluid resuscitation, insulin infusion, and close electrolyte monitoring. SGLT-2 inhibitors should be reinitiated only after consultation with an endocrinologist.

4. Conclusion

Historically, the majority of the cases of euDKA were missed due to presence of euglycemia on presentation [22]. Similarly, in our patient the diagnosis was delayed since his anion gap acidosis was initially attributed to starvation ketosis due to his nothing by mouth status in the setting of pancreatitis. However, after careful consideration a diagnosis of dapagliflozin-induced euDKA precipitated by acute pancreatitis was made. This case elaborates the fact that SGLT-2 inhibitors should be initiated by a clinician cautiously and only after adequately weighing the risks and benefits of treatment, particularly in those with type I diabetes. Patients should be instructed to check their serum and urine ketones in case they feel unwell even if they have a normal blood glucose level. Hospitalized patients (particularly those undergoing surgery or suffering from infectious/inflammatory process) who are on SGLT-2 inhibitors at home should be evaluated and closely monitored for the development of ketonemia or ketonuria during the hospital course.

Acknowledgments

This case report was presented as a poster presentation at the American Thoracic Society conference in San Diego, California, USA, May 2018. This case report was presented as a poster presentation at the American College of Physicians Michigan Chapter Scientific Meeting in Sterling Heights, Michigan, USA, May 2017.

References

[1] J. Girard, "Role of the kidneys in glucose homeostasis. Implication of sodium-glucose cotransporter 2 (SGLT2) in diabetes mellitus treatment," *Néphrologie & Thérapeutique*, vol. 13, no. 1, pp. S35–S41, 2017.

[2] J. Bolinder, Ö. Ljunggren, J. Kullberg et al., "Effects of dapagliflozin on body weight, total fat mass, and regional adipose tissue distribution in patients with type 2 diabetes mellitus with inadequate glycemic control on metformin," *The Journal of Clinical Endocrinology & Metabolism*, vol. 97, no. 3, pp. 1020–1031, 2012.

[3] P. Fioretto, A. Giaccari, and G. Sesti, "Efficacy and safety of dapagliflozin, a sodium glucose cotransporter 2 (SGLT2) inhibitor, in diabetes mellitus," *Cardiovascular Diabetology*, vol. 14, no. 1, 2015.

[4] S. S. Schwartz and I. Ahmed, "Sodium-glucose cotransporter 2 inhibitors: An evidence-based practice approach to their use in the natural history of type 2 diabetes," *Current Medical Research and Opinion*, vol. 32, no. 5, pp. 907–919, 2016.

[5] H. Bays, "Sodium glucose co-transporter type 2 (SGLT2) inhibitors: Targeting the kidney to improve glycemic control in diabetes mellitus," *Diabetes Therapy*, vol. 4, no. 2, pp. 195–220, 2013.

[6] E. M. Wright, B. A. Hirayama, and D. F. Loo, "Active sugar transport in health and disease," *Journal of Internal Medicine*, vol. 261, no. 1, pp. 32–43, 2007.

[7] R. A. DeFronzo, J. A. Davidson, and S. del Prato, "The role of the kidneys in glucose homeostasis: a new path towards normalizing glycaemia," *Diabetes, Obesity and Metabolism*, vol. 14, no. 1, pp. 5–14, 2012.

[8] M. A. Abdul-Ghani and R. A. Defronzo, "Inhibition of renal glucose reabsorption: A novel strategy for achieving glucose control in type 2 diabetes mellitus," *Endocrine Practice*, vol. 14, no. 6, pp. 782–790, 2008.

[9] W. Ogawa and K. Sakaguchi, "Euglycemic diabetic ketoacidosis induced by SGLT2 inhibitors: Possible mechanism and contributing factors," *Journal of Diabetes Investigation*, vol. 7, no. 2, pp. 135–138, 2016.

[10] N. Candelario and J. Wykretowicz, "The DKA that wasn't: A case of euglycemic diabetic ketoacidosis due to empagliflozin," *Oxford Medical Case Reports*, vol. 2016, no. 7, pp. 144–146, 2016.

[11] F. Zaccardi, D. R. Webb, Z. Z. Htike, D. Youssef, K. Khunti, and M. J. Davies, "Efficacy and safety of sodium-glucose cotransporter-2 inhibitors in type 2 diabetes mellitus: systematic review and network meta-analysis," *Diabetes, Obesity and Metabolism*, vol. 18, no. 8, pp. 783–794, 2016.

[12] FDA, "FDA Drug Safety Communication: FDA revises labels of SGLT2 inhibitors for diabetes to include warnings about too much acid in the blood and serious urinary tract infections," 2015.

[13] J. E. Blau, S. H. Tella, S. I. Taylor, and K. I. Rother, "Ketoacidosis associated with SGLT2 inhibitor treatment: Analysis of FAERS data," *Diabetes/Metabolism Research and Reviews*, vol. 33, no. 8, Article ID e2924, 2017.

[14] A. Modi, A. Agrawal, and F. Morgan, "Euglycemic diabetic ketoacidosis: A review," *Current Diabetes Reviews*, vol. 13, no. 3, pp. 315–321, 2017.

[15] C. Bonner, J. Kerr-Conte, V. Gmyr et al., "Inhibition of the glucose transporter SGLT2 with dapagliflozin in pancreatic alpha cells triggers glucagon secretion," *Nature Medicine*, vol. 21, no. 5, pp. 512–517, 2015.

[16] S. I. Taylor, J. E. Blau, and K. I. Rother, "SGLT2 inhibitors may predispose to ketoacidosis," *The Journal of Clinical Endocrinology & Metabolism*, vol. 100, no. 8, pp. 2849–2852, 2015.

[17] J. A. Benmoussa, M. Clarke, A. Penmetsa et al., "Euglycemic diabetic ketoacidosis: The clinical concern of SGLT2 inhibitors," *Journal of Clinical and Translational Endocrinology: Case Reports*, vol. 2, pp. 17–19, 2016.

[18] H. Ahmadieh, N. Ghazal, and S. T. Azar, "Role of sodium glucose cotransporter-2 inhibitors in type I diabetes mellitus," *Diabetes, Metabolic Syndrome and Obesity: Targets and Therapy*, vol. 10, pp. 161–167, 2017.

[19] J. Chen, F. Fan, J. Y. Wang et al., "The efficacy and safety of SGLT2 inhibitors for adjunctive treatment of type 1 diabetes: a systematic review and meta-analysis," *Scientific Reports*, vol. 7, no. 1, Article ID 44128, 2017.

[20] K. R. Burke, C. A. Schumacher, and S. E. Harpe, "SGLT2 Inhibitors: A Systematic Review of Diabetic Ketoacidosis and Related Risk Factors in the Primary Literature," *Pharmacotherapy*, vol. 37, no. 2, pp. 187–194, 2017.

[21] D. Yabe, M. Iwasaki, H. Kuwata et al., "Sodium-glucose cotransporter-2 inhibitor use and dietary carbohydrate intake in Japanese individuals with type 2 diabetes: A randomized, open-label, 3-arm parallel comparative, exploratory study," *Diabetes, Obesity and Metabolism*, vol. 19, no. 5, pp. 739–743, 2017.

[22] A. L. Peters, E. O. Buschur, J. B. Buse, P. Cohan, J. C. Diner, and I. B. Hirsch, "Euglycemic diabetic ketoacidosis: a potential complication of treatment with sodium-glucose cotransporter 2 inhibition," *Diabetes Care*, vol. 38, no. 9, pp. 1687–1693, 2015.

26

Adrenal Oncocytic Neoplasm with Paradoxical Loss of Important Mitochondrial Steroidogenic Protein: The 18 kDA Translocator Protein

Roberto Ruiz-Cordero,[1] **Alia Gupta,**[2] **Arumugam R. Jayakumar,**[3] **Gaetano Ciancio,**[4] **Gunnlaugur Petur Nielsen,**[5] **and Merce Jorda**[2,6]

[1]*Department of Hematopathology, University of Texas MD Anderson Cancer Center, Houston, TX 77030, USA*
[2]*Department of Pathology, Jackson Memorial Hospital/University of Miami Miller School of Medicine, Miami, FL 33136, USA*
[3]*South Florida Foundation for Research and Education Inc., Veterans Affairs Medical Center, Miami, FL 33125, USA*
[4]*Department of Surgery, Jackson Memorial Hospital/University of Miami Miller School of Medicine, Miami, FL 33136, USA*
[5]*Department of Pathology and Center for Cancer Research, Massachusetts General Hospital, Charlestown, MA 02129, USA*
[6]*Department of Urology, Jackson Memorial Hospital/University of Miami Miller School of Medicine, Miami, FL 33136, USA*

Correspondence should be addressed to Roberto Ruiz-Cordero; robertoruizcordero@gmail.com and
Arumugam R. Jayakumar; avrj_2000@yahoo.com

Academic Editor: Osamu Isozaki

The adrenal glands produce a variety of hormones that play a key role in the regulation of blood pressure, electrolyte homeostasis, metabolism, immune system suppression, and the body's physiologic response to stress. Adrenal neoplasms can be asymptomatic or can overproduce certain hormones that lead to different clinical manifestations. Oncocytic adrenal neoplasms are infrequent tumors that arise from cells in the adrenal cortex and display a characteristic increase in the number of cytoplasmic mitochondria. Since the rate-limiting step in steroidogenesis includes the transport of cholesterol across the mitochondrial membranes, in part carried out by the 18-kDa translocator protein (TSPO), we assessed the expression of TSPO in a case of adrenal oncocytic neoplasm using residual adrenal gland of the patient as internal control. We observed a significant loss of TSPO immunofluorescence expression in the adrenal oncocytic tumor cells when compared to adjacent normal adrenal tissue. We further confirmed this finding by employing Western blot analysis to semiquantify TSPO expression in tumor and normal adrenal cells. Our findings could suggest a potential role of TSPO in the tumorigenesis of this case of adrenocortical oncocytic neoplasm.

1. Introduction

Adrenal oncocytic neoplasms (AON) are infrequent, usually benign, nonfunctional tumors arising in the adrenal cortex that occasionally display borderline or malignant clinical courses. Histologic classification systems (i.e., Weiss system) can usually predict aggressive behavior in regular (nononco-cytic) adrenocortical neoplasms; however, histomorphologic features in AON do not always correlate with clinical outcome [1–3].

AON are composed of oncocytes, defined as large eosinophilic cells approximately twice the size of a normal adrenocortical cell with a large central nucleus, a prominent nucleolus, and a characteristic abundant and granular eosinophilic cytoplasm secondary to markedly increased mitochondria [4]. Ultrastructurally, oncocytes are packed with swollen mitochondria. Recent reports strongly support an important role of abnormal steroidogenic events in the pathogenesis of AON [5].

The 18-kDa translocator protein (TSPO) is a ubiquitous mitochondrial nuclear-encoded protein that is upregulated in steroidogenic organs like the adrenal glands and the gonads [6, 7]. Its main function consists in facilitating the migration of cholesterol from the outer to the inner mitochondrial

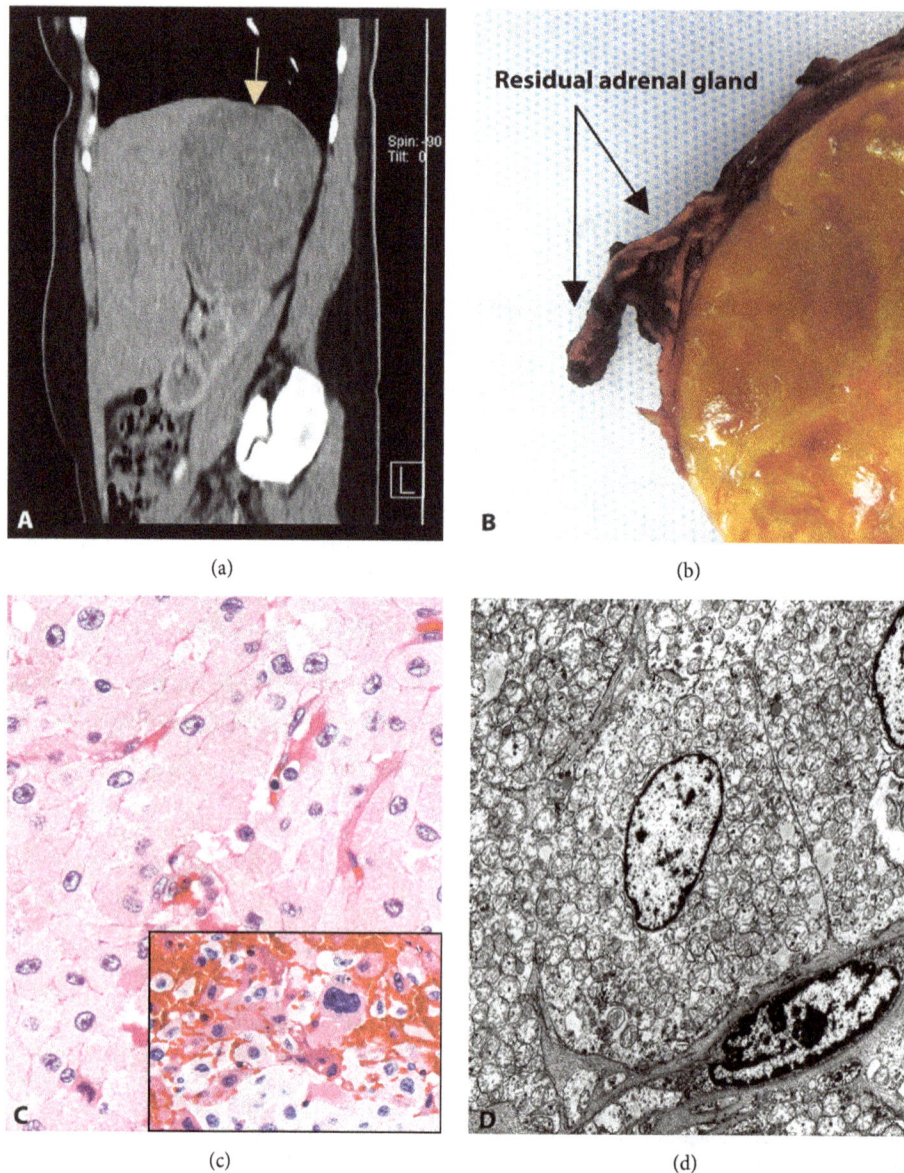

FIGURE 1: Composite figure illustrating imaging, surgical, histologic, and ultrastructural findings. (a) Sagittal CT scan shows a large ovoid mass (arrow) abutting the liver and the superior pole of the right kidney. (b) Surgical resection specimen highlights the bright yellow tumor parenchyma as well as a portion of the patient's residual adrenal gland (arrows). (c) Microscopic examination of adrenal oncocytic neoplasm composed of large cells with abundant pink granular cytoplasm and irregular nuclei with prominent nucleoli (H&E, 20x). The insert highlights the presence of areas displaying marked nuclear pleomorphism and atypia (H&E, 40x). (d) Transmission electron microscopy illustrating a tumor cell at the center of the image with a large centrally located oval nucleus and abundant mitochondria occupying most of the cytoplasm. H&E: hematoxylin and eosin.

membrane for its conversion into pregnenolone by the cholesterol side-chain cleavage enzyme (CYP11A1) [8, 9]. Thus, transport of cholesterol through the mitochondrial membranes is considered the rate-limiting step in steroidogenesis [8]. Since conspicuous increase in intracytoplasmic mitochondria is sine qua non of AON, we decided to study TSPO expression in one case of AON by means of immunofluorescence. Interestingly, we found a paradoxical loss of TSPO expression in AON cells and confirmed the loss of TPSO expression by Western blot semiquantification.

2. Case Presentation

A 49-year-old woman with no significant past medical or surgical history other than sporadic migraines presented to the emergency room at Jackson Memorial Hospital complaining of a 2-week episode of abdominal distention and flank pain. Initial examination revealed an otherwise normal female with vital signs within normal limits and discomfort in the right flank, suspicious for a kidney stone. As part of her initial workup, the patient had an abdominal CT scan that revealed a 15 cm right adrenal mass (Figure 1(a)). No stones or signs of hydronephrosis or pyelonephritis were identified. Laboratory workup, including serum determination of cortisol (5.7 mcg/dL, normal range: 4.3–22.4 mcg/dL at 8 am), aldosterone (<4.0 ng/dL, reference: ≤21 ng/dL), and adrenocorticotropic hormone (12 pg/mL, reference: <47 pg/mL), was unremarkable. The patient underwent surgical excision of the mass. The resected specimen consisted of a well-encapsulated oval mass with a bright golden-yellow parenchyma. The right adrenal gland was found adjacent to the mass (Figure 1(b)). Microscopic examination of the tumor after formalin fixation demonstrated a neoplasm composed of large oncocytic cells (Figure 1(c)) with focal areas of nuclear pleomorphism (Figure 1(c), insert). The presence of increased intracytoplasmic mitochondria was confirmed by electron microscopy (Figure 1(d)). Mitotic figures were not observed. According to the proposed classification by Bisceglia et al. [1], the tumor size and the absence of mitoses, necrosis, capsular, and sinusoidal invasion indicate that this AON could harbor borderline malignant potential. The patient's postsurgical course was unremarkable and no further treatment was required. Currently, four years after surgery, the patient is alive, tumor-free, and in her normal state of health.

2.1. TSPO Expression Assessed by Immunofluorescence Is Markedly Decreased in Tumor Cells. In order to assess the expression of TSPO we obtained additional unstained slides from formalin-fixed paraffin-embedded (FFPE) tissue including a representative section of the tumor with adjacent normal adrenal gland (internal control) of the patient. Two slides were deparaffinized after incubation at room temperature (RT, 24°C) in xylene (twice for 10 minutes). The deparaffinized tissue sections were then rehydrated with a graded series of ethanol (100%, 100%, 70%, 70%, and 50%) and incubated in phosphate buffered saline (PBS) for 15 minutes at RT. After incubation, slides were stained for TSPO by immunofluorescence as previously described [10]. Primary antibody to detect TSPO (FL-169, Santa Cruz Biotechnology, Inc., Dallas, Texas, cat# 20120) was used at 1 : 75 dilution, according to the manufacturer instructions. Fluorescent HRP-conjugated secondary antibody (Alexa Flour-488 goat anti-rabbit IgG (H+L)) was used at 1 : 200 dilutions. The slides were reviewed with a Zeiss LSM510/UV Axiovert 200 M confocal microscope (Carl Zeiss, Peabody, MA, USA). Multiple images captured from tumor cells and normal adrenal gland showed strong immunofluorescence positivity in the normal adjacent adrenal gland (Figure 2(a)) and significant loss of TSPO expression in the tumor cells (Figure 2(b)).

2.2. TSPO Semiquantification by Western Blot Confirms Partial Loss of Expression in Tumor Cells. To more precisely evaluate the loss of nuclear and cytoplasmic TSPO expression in tumor cells and confirm the immunofluorescence findings, we dissected mapped tumor and normal adrenal tissue from FFPE unstained slides and performed immunoblots. Briefly, FFPE tissue sections were deparaffinized by incubation at RT in xylene (twice for 10 minutes). The deparaffinized tissue sections were then rehydrated with a graded series of ethanol (100%, 100%, 70%, 70%, and 50%) and incubated at RT in PBS for 15 minutes. After incubation, tumor and normal adrenal

tissue were dissected off the slides and placed in two separate plastic tubes. The tubes were pelleted at 16,000 ×g for 5 minutes, and the incubation/centrifugation steps were repeated twice. Tissue samples were briefly air-dried in a fume hood. The cell pellet was resuspended in 200 μl cold buffer A, consisting of 10 mM HEPES (pH 7.9), 10 mM KCl, 0.1 mM EDTA, 0.1 mM EGTA, 1 μM dithiothreitol (DTT), and a complete protease inhibitor cocktail (Roche, Mannheim, Germany). The pellet was then incubated on ice for 15 minutes to allow cells to swell, after which 15 μl of 10% NP-40 was added, and the sample was vortexed thoroughly for 40 seconds and centrifuged at 3,000 rpm for 3 minutes at 4°C. The resulting supernatant was used for cytosolic TSPO measurement (equal amount of protein, 12.4 μg was loaded on an SDS-polyacrylamide gel and Western blot analysis with TSPO antibody was performed as described previously [11]) and the pellet (nuclear fraction) was resuspended in 30 μl cold buffer B consisting of 20 mM HEPES (pH 7.9), 0.4 M NaCl, 1 mM EDTA, 1 mM EGTA, 1 μM DTT, and protease inhibitors. The pellet was then incubated on ice and vortexed for 15 seconds every 2 min for up to 15 min. The nuclear extract was then centrifuged at 13,000 rpm for 5 minutes at 4°C. Equal amounts of protein (21.6 μg) from the supernatant (containing the nuclear extract) were loaded and Western blot analysis with TSPO antibody was performed as described above. The quality of the nuclear extract was analyzed by propidium iodide staining, which indicated a purity of 92–96%. Primary TSPO antibody (Santa Cruz Biotechnology, Inc., Dallas, Texas, cat# 20120) was used at 1 : 1000 dilution. Beta actin (ACTBD11B7, sc-81178, Santa Cruz Biotechnology, Dallas, TX, USA) and lamin a/c (Cell Signaling Technology, Beverly, MA, USA) antibodies were used at 1 : 5000 and 1 : 750, respectively. Anti-rabbit and anti-mouse secondary antibodies (Vector Laboratories, Burlingame, CA, USA) were used at 1 : 3000 dilution. Optical density of the bands was determined with the Chemi-Imager (Alpha Innotech, San Leandro, CA, USA) digital imaging system and the results were quantified with the Sigma Scan Pro (Jandell Scientific, San Jose, CA, USA) program as a proportion of the signal of housekeeping protein bands (lamin a/c and β-actin, nuclear and cytosolic markers, resp.). The experiment was performed using 4 different tissue sections from the same sample and the mean intensity of Western blot bands was subjected to Tukey's multiple comparison test. Statistical significance was set at p value = 0.05. As illustrated in Figures 2(a) and 2(b) (cytosolic fraction) and Figures 2(c) and 2(d) (nuclear fraction), the representative semiquantitative immunoblots from two different tumor sections show a significant decrease in TSPO expression in the tumor sample of 72.4 and 72.8% decrease in the cytosol and 77.1 and 76.8% decrease in the nuclear fraction as compared to respective controls (p = 0.03).

3. Discussion

The Weiss classification system for adrenocortical neoplasms has been widely adopted and used to distinguish benign from malignant tumors based on major (high mitotic rate, atypical mitoses, and lymphovascular invasion) and minor criteria

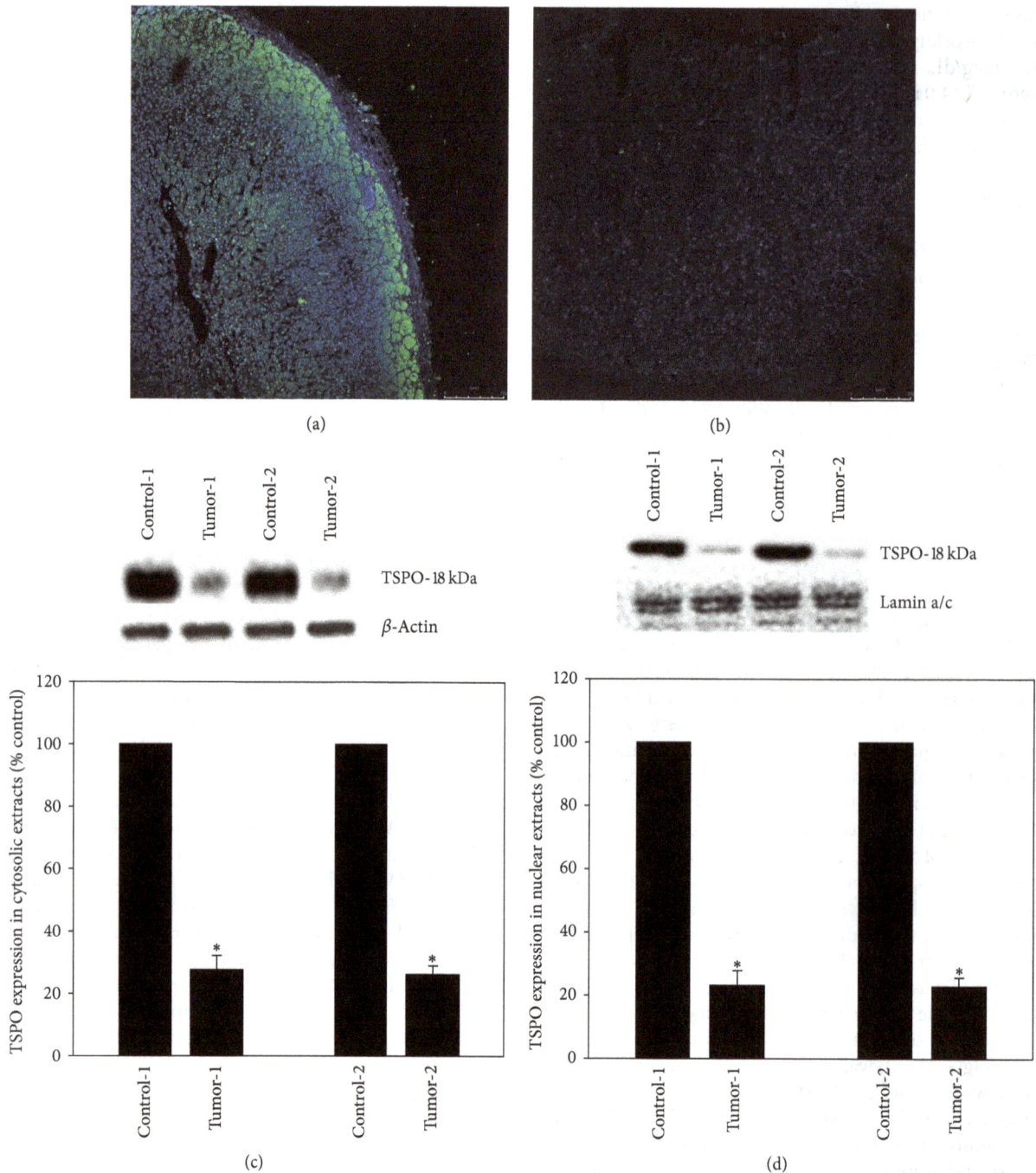

FIGURE 2: Composite figure illustrating TSPO protein expression findings. (a) Expression of TSPO by immunofluorescence in normal adrenal gland demonstrates diffuse immunofluorescence for TSPO protein, particularly in the zona glomerulosa (IF, 10x). (b) Diffuse loss of TSPO expression assessed by immunofluorescence in adrenal oncocytic tumor cells (IF, 10x). Polyacrylamide gels of the experiments performed in duplicate including normal adrenal cortex from the patient as internal control and tumor, normalized to β-actin for cytosolic extracts (c) and lamin a/c for nuclear extracts (d) as housekeeping genes, show a noticeable decrease in the concentration of TSPO in tumor compared to the patient's normal adrenal gland. Western blot semiquantification bar graphs demonstrate 72.4 and 72.8% decrease in cytosolic and 77.1 and 76.8% decrease in nuclear TSPO expression as compared to respective controls. IF: immunofluorescence.

(large-size and increased weight, necrosis, capsular invasion, and sinusoidal invasion) [3]. The presence of one major criterion indicates malignancy, 1 to 4 minor criteria indicate uncertain malignant potential (borderline), and the absence of all major and minor criteria suggests a benign clinical behavior [3]. While this classification system has been useful in accurately predicting the biologic behavior of conventional (nononcocytic) adrenocortical tumors, its use in the setting of AON is questionable. In a series of 10 cases of AON, the Weiss system criteria were reviewed and modified to assess its possible application to the oncocytic tumor variant. Using this new grading system, 1 of the 10 cases had to be revised to a final interpretation of malignant after tumor recurrence [1]. In terms of imaging studies, a cutoff below 4-5 cm in tumor size is used to suggest a benign behavior [12]. In cases of oncocytic neoplasms, however, the size of the mass has not demonstrated to reliably predict tumor behavior. Some nonspecific findings such as fat concentration (almost all malignant lesions are lipid poor) and lower attenuation (10 Hounsfield units or less) on CT scan have proven to be helpful in making this differentiation [12, 13].

It has been extensively documented that these oncocytic tumors display characteristic eosinophilic staining secondary to the accumulation of mitochondria, which may occupy up to 60% of the cytoplasm [4]. The increased concentration of mitochondria is accompanied by a gradual compression and sometimes disappearance of other cytoplasmic organelles [14]. Because of the rarity of this type of adrenocortical tumors and because immunohistochemical studies were not consistently performed in most of the reported cases, their immunophenotypic profile has not been completely characterized [4, 15]. Nevertheless, studied cases demonstrate diffuse positivity for vimentin, melan-A, synaptophysin, and inhibin, while S-100 and chromogranin have been consistently negative [15]. In some cases, immunopositivity with an anti-mitochondrial antibody has been used to corroborate that the tumors are truly oncocytic [16].

TSPO is found in the outer mitochondrial membrane of almost every tissue in the body [17]. It is part of a complex of proteins (i.e., StAR, PKA, ACBD3, and VDAC1) that function together by forming a tansduceosome that facilitates cholesterol transport from the outer to the inner mitochondrial membrane for its conversion into pregnenolone by cholesterol side-chain cleavage cytochrome P450 enzyme CYP11A1 [8, 9]. Recently, there has been controversy regarding the critical role that TSPO plays in cellular homeostasis and steroidogenesis. While some authors initially suggested a crucial role based on experiments with TSPO knockout mice whose embryos did not survive, others have replicated similar experiments with different results [18–23]. Nevertheless, in the realm of cancer, several studies have found an increased TSPO protein expression in cancer cell lines and in tumor biopsies of colon, breast, and prostate [19–21]. Moreover, in the particular case of prostatic adenocarcinoma, TSPO protein expression was the highest in metastatic prostate cancer samples where increased expression also correlated with disease progression [19]. More recently, TSPO has been shown to be part of the mitochondria-to-nucleus signaling pathway that modulates nuclear gene expression and TSPO levels have been directly correlated with increased tumorigenicity and/or malignancy, probably as a mechanism to promote apoptosis and reduce tumorigenicity, thereby suggesting that benign tumors do not have increased TSPO levels [6, 24–26]. However, we have observed conventional adrenocortical carcinomas with a wide range of TSPO expression, ranging from no expression to markedly increased TSPO expression [27]. Batarseh and Papadopoulos [17] consider *TSPO* as a

highly conserved, housekeeping gene that is expected to remain permanently activated. Recently, *TSPO* gene has been suggested as a novel target for cancer chemotherapy [22]. It is possible that an altered regulation of the numerous cellular processes associated with mitochondria and cholesterol transport could partially be responsible for the unrestrained growth of tumors by mechanisms that remain unknown [17, 19, 23, 28–33].

While previous studies [32] have identified variable TSPO expression in adrenocortical and other tumors, our study represents the first description of TSPO expression in one AON. The present case is unusual and interesting because TSPO expression was paradoxically lost in the mitochondria of the tumor cells when assessed by immunofluorescence in comparison to the patient's normal adrenal gland. When these findings were further explored by direct semiquantification of the presence of protein by Western blot, up to a 77% decrease in expression was confirmed between the tumor and the patient's normal adrenal cells in both cytoplasm and nucleus. While our findings in this one particular case could represent a coincidence, we believe that the fact that a tissue section including the patient's normal adrenal gland adjacent to the tumor used to perform all tests argues otherwise, particularly, because deparaffinization, immunofluorescence, and Western blotting were performed on tumor and normal cells at the same time on the same slide in several occasions. Furthermore, preliminary results on the expression of TSPO in adrenocortical neoplasms in a study performed by our group employing immunohistochemistry demonstrated variable TSPO expression in tumors arising in the adrenal cortex, particularly adrenocortical carcinomas [27].

It is also possible that the increase in mitochondria could be a compensatory phenomenon that could be in part associated with tumor growth. While our findings could indicate that loss of TSPO expression could play a role in the tumorigenesis of this case of adrenocortical oncocytic neoplasm potentially related to defective steroid biosynthesis, additional studies including a larger number of cases of AON are necessary to validate these findings and to determine the role of TSPO in the pathogenesis of adrenocortical neoplasms including AON.

Acknowledgments

Arumugam R. Jayakumar was supported by Stanley J. Glaser Research Grant and AASLD/American Liver Foundation grants. Roberto Ruiz-Cordero was supported by an intradepartmental research grant sponsored by the Department of Pathology at the University of Miami/Jackson Memorial Hospital.

References

[1] M. Bisceglia, O. Ludovico, A. Di Mattia et al., "Adrenocortical oncocytic tumors: report of 10 cases and review of the literature,"

International Journal of Surgical Pathology, vol. 12, no. 3, pp. 231–243, 2004.

[2] A. Chang and S. J. Harawi, "Oncocytes, oncocytosis, and oncocytic tumors," *Pathology Annual*, vol. 27, part 1, pp. 263–304, 1992.

[3] L. J. Medeiros and L. M. Weiss, "New developments in the pathologic diagnosis of adrenal cortical neoplasms. A review," *American Journal of Clinical Pathology*, vol. 97, no. 1, pp. 73–83, 1992.

[4] L. Mearini, R. Del Sordo, E. Costantini, E. Nunzi, and M. Porena, "Adrenal oncocytic neoplasm: a systematic review," *Urologia Internationalis*, vol. 91, no. 2, pp. 125–133, 2013.

[5] R. Logasundaram, C. Parkinson, P. Donaldson, and P. E. Coode, "Co-secretion of testosterone and cortisol by a functional adrenocortical oncocytoma," *Histopathology*, vol. 51, no. 3, pp. 418–420, 2007.

[6] J. Fan, P. Lindemann, M. G. J. Feuilloley, and V. Papadopoulos, "Structural and functional evolution of the translocator protein (18 kDa)," *Current Molecular Medicine*, vol. 12, no. 4, pp. 369–386, 2012.

[7] V. Papadopoulos, M. Baraldi, T. R. Guilarte et al., "Translocator protein (18 kDa): new nomenclature for the peripheral-type benzodiazepine receptor based on its structure and molecular function," *Trends in Pharmacological Sciences*, vol. 27, no. 8, pp. 402–409, 2006.

[8] K. E. Krueger and V. Papadopoulos, "Peripheral-type benzodiazepine receptors mediate translocation of cholesterol from outer to inner mitochondrial membranes in adrenocortical cells," *The Journal of Biological Chemistry*, vol. 265, no. 25, pp. 15015–15022, 1990.

[9] V. Papadopoulos, Y. Aghazadeh, J. Fan, E. Campioli, B. Zirkin, and A. Midzak, "Translocator protein-mediated pharmacology of cholesterol transport and steroidogenesis," *Molecular and Cellular Endocrinology*, vol. 408, pp. 90–98, 2015.

[10] A. R. Jayakumar, X. Y. Tong, J. Ospel, and M. D. Norenberg, "Role of cerebral endothelial cells in the astrocyte swelling and brain edema associated with acute hepatic encephalopathy," *Neuroscience*, vol. 218, pp. 305–316, 2012.

[11] K. S. Panickar, A. R. Jayakumar, K. V. Rama Rao, and M. D. Norenberg, "Downregulation of the 18-kDa translocator protein: Effects on the ammonia-induced mitochondrial permeability transition and cell swelling in cultured astrocytes," *Glia*, vol. 55, no. 16, pp. 1720–1727, 2007.

[12] V. N. Shah, A. Premkumar, R. Walia et al., "Large but benign adrenal mass: adrenal oncocytoma," *Indian Journal of Endocrinology and Metabolism*, vol. 16, no. 3, pp. 469–471, 2012.

[13] T. Tirkes, T. Gokaslan, J. McCrea et al., "Oncocytic neoplasms of the adrenal gland," *American Journal of Roentgenology*, vol. 196, no. 3, pp. 592–596, 2011.

[14] S. S. In, J. D. Henley, and K.-W. Min, "Peculiar cytoplasmic inclusions in oncocytic adrenal cortical tumors: An electron microscopic observation," *Ultrastructural Pathology*, vol. 26, no. 4, pp. 229–235, 2002.

[15] M. P. Hoang, A. G. Ayala, and J. Albores-Saavedra, "Oncocytic adrenocortical carcinoma: A morphologic, immunohistochemical and ultrastructural study of four cases," *Modern Pathology*, vol. 15, no. 9, pp. 973–978, 2002.

[16] J. Schittenhelm, F. H. Ebner, P. Harter, and A. Bornemann, "Symptomatic intraspinal oncocytic adrenocortical adenoma," *Endocrine Pathology*, vol. 20, no. 1, pp. 73–77, 2009.

[17] A. Batarseh and V. Papadopoulos, "Regulation of translocator protein 18 kDa (TSPO) expression in health and disease states," *Molecular and Cellular Endocrinology*, vol. 327, no. 1-2, pp. 1–12, 2010.

[18] J.-J. Lacapère and V. Papadopoulos, "Peripheral-type benzodiazepine receptor: structure and function of a cholesterol-binding protein in steroid and bile acid biosynthesis," *Steroids*, vol. 68, no. 7-8, pp. 569–585, 2003.

[19] A. Fafalios, A. Akhavan, A. V. Parwani, R. R. Bies, K. J. McHugh, and B. R. Pflug, "Translocator protein blockade reduces prostate tumor growth," *Clinical Cancer Research*, vol. 15, no. 19, pp. 6177–6184, 2009.

[20] Y. Katz, A. Eitan, Z. Amiri, and M. Gavish, "Dramatic increase in peripheral benzodiazepine binding sites in human colonic adenocarcinoma as compared to normal colon," *European Journal of Pharmacology*, vol. 148, no. 3, pp. 483-484, 1988.

[21] S. Mukherjee and S. K. Das, "Translocator protein (TSPO) in breast cancer," *Current Molecular Medicine*, vol. 12, no. 4, pp. 443–457, 2012.

[22] C. J. D. Austin, J. Kahlert, M. Kassiou, and L. M. Rendina, "The translocator protein (TSPO): A novel target for cancer chemotherapy," *The International Journal of Biochemistry & Cell Biology*, vol. 45, no. 7, pp. 1212–1216, 2013.

[23] A. Batarseh, K. D. Barlow, D. B. Martinez-Arguelles, and V. Papadopoulos, "Functional characterization of the human translocator protein (18kDa) gene promoter in human breast cancer cell lines," *Biochimica et Biophysica Acta - Gene Regulatory Mechanisms*, vol. 1819, no. 1, pp. 38–56, 2012.

[24] Y. Katz, G. Ben-Baruch, Y. Kloog, J. Menczer, and M. Gavish, "Increased density of peripheral benzodiazepine-binding sites in ovarian carcinomas as compared with benign ovarian tumours and normal ovaries," *Clinical Science*, vol. 78, no. 2, pp. 155–158, 1990.

[25] L. Veenman, M. Gavish, and W. Kugler, "Apoptosis induction by erucylphosphohomocholine via the 18 kDa mitochondrial translocator protein: Implications for cancer treatment," *Anti-Cancer Agents in Medicinal Chemistry*, vol. 14, no. 4, pp. 559–577, 2014.

[26] N. Yasin, L. Veenman, S. Singh et al., "Classical and novel TSPO ligands for the mitochondrial TSPO can modulate nuclear gene expression: implications for mitochondrial retrograde signaling," *International Journal of Molecular Sciences*, vol. 18, no. 4, article 786, 35 pages, 2017.

[27] R. Ruiz-Cordero, M. A. Habra, A. Gupta et al., "Paradoxical decrease of TSPO expression in adrenocortical carcinomas confers a worse prognosis," *Modern Pathology*, vol. 29, p. 154a, 2016.

[28] J. Bode, L. Veenman, B. Caballero, M. Lakomek, W. Kugler, and M. Gavish, "The 18 kDa translocator protein influences angiogenesis, as well as aggressiveness, adhesion, migration, and proliferation of glioblastoma cells," *Pharmacogenetics and Genomics*, vol. 22, no. 7, pp. 538–550, 2012.

[29] J. Klubo-Gwiezdzinska, K. Jensen, A. Bauer et al., "The expression of translocator protein in human thyroid cancer and its role in the response of thyroid cancer cells to oxidative stress," *Journal of Endocrinology*, vol. 214, no. 2, pp. 207–216, 2012.

[30] K. Maaser, P. Grabowski, Y. Oezdem et al., "Up-regulation of the peripheral benzodiazepine receptor during human colorectal carcinogenesis and tumor spread," *Clinical Cancer Research*, vol. 11, no. 5, pp. 1751–1756, 2005.

27

The Biochemical Profile of Familial Hypocalciuric Hypercalcemia and Primary Hyperparathyroidism during Pregnancy and Lactation: Two Case Reports and Review of the Literature

S. A. Ghaznavi,[1] N. M. A. Saad,[1] and L. E. Donovan[1,2]

[1]Department of Medicine, Division of Endocrinology and Metabolism, University of Calgary, Calgary, AB, Canada
[2]Department of Obstetrics and Gynaecology, University of Calgary, Calgary, AB, Canada

Correspondence should be addressed to L. E. Donovan; lois.donovan@ahs.ca

Academic Editor: Takeshi Usui

Background. Primary hyperparathyroidism (PHPT) and Familial Hypocalciuric Hypercalcemia (FHH) result in different maternal and fetal complications in pregnancy. Calcium to creatinine clearance ratio (CCCR) is commonly used to help distinguish these two conditions. Physiological changes in calcium handling during pregnancy and lactation can alter CCCR, making it a less useful tool to distinguish PHPT from FHH. *Cases.* A 25-year-old female presented with hypercalcemia and an inappropriately normal PTH. Her CCCR was 0.79% before pregnancy and rose to 1.99% in her second trimester. The proband's mother and neonate had asymptomatic hypercalcemia. Genetic analysis revealed a CaSR mutation consistent with FHH. A 19-year-old female presented with a history of nephrolithiasis who underwent emergent caesarean section at 29 weeks of gestation for severe preeclampsia. At delivery, she was diagnosed with hypercalcemia with an inappropriately normal PTH and a CCCR of 2.67%, which fell to 0.88% during lactation. Parathyroidectomy cured her hypercalcemia. Pathology confirmed a parathyroid adenoma. *Conclusion.* These cases illustrate the influence of pregnancy and lactation on renal calcium indices, such as the CCCR. To avoid diagnostic error of women with hypercalcemia during pregnancy and lactation, calcium biochemistry of first-degree relatives and genetic testing of select patients are recommended.

1. Background

Primary hyperparathyroidism (PHPT) in pregnancy is associated with hyperemesis, nephrolithiasis, pancreatitis, and preeclampsia. In the fetus, maternal PHPT can result in fetal growth restriction, severe neonatal hypocalcemia, tetany, and death [1]. However, due to the increased availability of calcium testing, the majority of patients with PHPT are now asymptomatic and appear clinically similar to patients with Familial Hypocalciuric Hypercalcemia (FHH). FHH is associated with mild to moderate degrees of hypercalcemia and does not usually cause maternal pregnancy complications. Potential fetal complications include mild hypercalcemia, severe hypocalcemia, or neonatal severe hyperparathyroidism,

depending on the genotype of the fetus [1]. Parathyroidectomy is definitive therapy for patients with symptomatic PHPT but is inappropriate in those with FHH. This is because patients with FHH have a loss of function or inactivating mutation in the gene for the calcium sensing receptor (CaSR), leading to hypercalcemia starting in fetal life [2]. Although these patients have calcium levels above the reference range for the population, their degree of hypercalcemia reflects a higher set point for a physiological level of calcium; that is, they require a higher calcium level to maintain neurological, muscular, and other cellular functions. It is crucial for clinicians to differentiate sporadic PHPT from FHH in order to minimize the risk of symptomatic hypocalcemia and select the appropriate patients for parathyroidectomy.

We present two cases of women with hypercalcemia in pregnancy; patient 1 has genetically confirmed FHH, and patient 2 has histologically confirmed PHPT. The biochemistry in these two cases is summarized in Table 1. The cases reported here illustrate the effects of maternal calcium physiology on renal calcium indices including the calcium to creatinine clearance ratio (CCCR), calculated using the following formula:

$$\frac{[24\,\text{hr urinary calcium (mmol/L)} \times \text{serum creatinine } (\mu\text{mol/L})]}{[\text{serum calcium (mmol/L)} \times 24\,\text{hr urinary creatinine (mmol/L)}]}. \tag{1}$$

Due to the hypoalbuminemia of pregnancy, total serum calcium concentrations decline early in pregnancy, while ionized (physiologically active) calcium remains the same. Where available, we present albumin adjusted calcium using the following formula:

$$\text{Albumin adjusted Ca (mmol/L)}$$

$$= \text{Ca measured (mmol/L)} \tag{2}$$

$$+ [0.02 * (40 - \text{Albumin (g/L)})].$$

2. Case Presentations

2.1. Patient 1. A 25-year-old Caucasian woman with documented hypercalcemia since the age of 16 presented with concerns regarding the impact of hypercalcemia on pregnancy outcomes. The patient's biochemistry prior to pregnancy showed albumin adjusted calcium of 2.61 mmol/L (reference range: 2.10–2.55 mmol/L), albumin of 44 g/L (reference range: 33–48 g/L), PTH of 33 ng/L (reference range: 10–55 ng/L), and serum phosphate of 0.99 mmol/L (reference range: 0.80–1.50 mmol/L). A 25-hydroxyvitamin D level is unknown for the patient during pregnancy, but previous 25-hydroxyvitamin D was 58.1 nmol/L (reference range: 40–110 nmol/L). Her calcium to creatinine clearance ratio (CCCR) was 0.79% prior to pregnancy, which is consistent with FHH. The proband's mother was hypercalcemic (albumin adjusted calcium = 2.74 mmol/L, albumin 36 g/L).

During the second trimester of pregnancy the patient's albumin adjusted calcium was 2.59 mmol/L, albumin was 33 g/L, and her CCCR increased to 1.99%, a value more consistent with PHPT than FHH. She had an uncomplicated delivery at 40 weeks of gestational age. A healthy male was born with asymptomatic hypercalcemia (serum calcium = 2.79 mmol/L, reference range: 1.90–2.60 mmol/L), which persisted at two years of age. While breastfeeding, the patient's albumin adjusted calcium was 2.53 mmol/L. Subsequently, the patient had two first-trimester spontaneous abortions. She then carried a fourth pregnancy to term and gave birth to a healthy female who also had asymptomatic hypercalcemia (serum calcium = 2.75 mmol/L, reference range: 1.90–2.60 mmol/L) at birth. Ultimately, genetic analysis revealed a heterozygous mutation of the *R716 CE* gene on the calcium sensing receptor and the patient was diagnosed with Familial Hypocalciuric Hypercalcemia.

2.2. Patient 2. A 19-year-old woman of Mexican Mennonite descent underwent an emergency caesarean delivery at 29 weeks of gestation for severe preeclampsia. She had a history of recurrent nephrolithiasis since the age of 16, but there was no prior documentation of calcium levels. Her pregnancy was complicated by calcium oxalate kidney stones and pyelonephritis and intrauterine growth restriction. Due to severe preeclampsia, the baby was delivered at 29 weeks of gestation and was found to be normocalcemic (serum calcium = 2.21 mmol/L, reference range: 1.90–2.60 mmol/L) with a birth weight of 980 grams. Blood work on her at delivery revealed albumin adjusted calcium of 2.97 mmol/L (reference range: 2.10–2.55 mmol/L), albumin of 22 g/L, a 25-hydroxyvitamin D level of 36.5 nmol/L (reference range: 80–200 nmol/L), serum phosphate of 0.66 mmol/L (reference range: 0.80–1.50 mmol/L), an inappropriately normal PTH of 52 ng/L (13–54 ng/L), and a CCCR of 2.67%. Her albumin adjusted calcium was 2.76 mmol/L, 3.18 mmol/L, and 3.11 mmol/L on days 1, 3, and 5 postpartum. Investigations repeated one month postpartum during lactation revealed albumin adjusted calcium of 2.96 mmol/L, albumin of 33 g/L, a 25-hydroxyvitamin D level of 72 nmol/L on vitamin D supplementation, serum phosphate of 0.82 mmol/L, and a PTH of 54 ng/L. Her CCCR fell to 0.89% during lactation, suggestive of FHH. Calcium biochemistry from her family was unavailable.

Given her young age at presentation, she was investigated for genetic causes of PHPT including multiple endocrine neoplasia (MEN), jaw tumor syndrome, and FHH, which were all negative.

Plans for parathyroidectomy were deferred until she could be biochemically reevaluated after she completed lactation; however, the patient became pregnant again while still breastfeeding. Her pregnancy was discovered at nine-week gestational age, at which point she was both pregnant and lactating, and her biochemistry revealed albumin adjusted calcium of 2.76 mmol/L, albumin of 38 g/L, and vitamin D level of 77.4 nmol/L. Given her prior complicated pregnancy with severe preeclampsia, fetal growth restriction, and premature delivery, second-trimester parathyroidectomy was performed resulting in normalization of serum calcium. Surgical pathology confirmed a single parathyroid adenoma weighing 174 milligrams. Despite the surgical cure, her second pregnancy was also complicated by preeclampsia and fetal growth restriction. However, she progressed 6 weeks further in her second pregnancy and delivered by caesarean section at 35 weeks of gestational age. She gave birth to a healthy normocalcemic male (serum calcium of 2.38 mmol/L, reference range: 1.90–2.60 mmol/L) with a birth weight of 1900 grams.

TABLE 1: Summary of serum and urine biochemistry in patients 1 and 2 prior to pregnancy, during pregnancy, and during lactation.

	Patient 1 (FHH)	Patient 2 (PHPT)	Reference range*
Prior to pregnancy			
Albumin adjusted calcium (mmol/L)	2.61 mmol/L	n/a	2.10–2.55 mmol/L
PTH (ng/L)	33 ng/L	n/a	13–54 ng/L
CCCR (%)	0.79%	n/a	<2% = possible hypocalciuria <1% = hypocalciuria
Pregnancy			
Albumin adjusted calcium (mmol/L)	2.59 mmol/L	2.97 mmol/L	2.10–2.55 mmol/L
PTH (ng/L)	46 ng/L	52 ng/L	13–54 ng/L
CCCR (%)	1.99%	2.67%	n/d
Lactation			
Albumin adjusted calcium (mmol/L)	2.53 mmol/L	2.96 mmol/L	2.10–2.55 mmol/L
CCCR (%)	n/a	0.89%	n/d

n/a = not available.
n/d = not defined.
*=Reference ranges are for nonpregnant and nonlactating patients.

3. Discussion

3.1. Calcium Physiology during Pregnancy and Lactation. Maternal changes in calcium physiology occur during pregnancy in order to provide the growing fetal skeleton with adequate calcium. The dilutional hypoalbuminemia of pregnancy leads to a decline in total calcium measurements; however, the ionized calcium remains stable. Therefore, the ionized calcium is the preferred method of calcium measurement in pregnant women. A limitation of our paper is that the cases presented here were clinical cases and data has been gathered on a retrospective basis. Hence, ionized calcium measurements are not available, so albumin adjusted calcium measurements are provided.

The biochemical description of our cases is consistent with previous descriptions of "absorptive hypercalciuria" during pregnancy [3]. Absorptive hypercalciuria is a physiological change of pregnancy, defined as an elevated postprandial and 24-hour urine calcium excretion, due to increased intestinal calcium absorption of dietary calcium. In contrast, in the fasting state, the random urine calcium excretion should not be effected by absorptive hypercalciuria. The responsible physiological changes for absorptive hypercalciuria include placental production of PTHrP, a surge in the levels of 1,25 hydroxyvitamin D, and subsequent increase in the intestinal absorption of calcium and hence the increase in renal excretion of calcium [3]. In patient 1 with FHH, we saw a change in CCCR from 0.79% prepregnancy to 1.99% in the

second trimester, consistent with absorptive hypercalciuria of pregnancy.

At delivery, sudden loss of placental transfer of calcium to the fetus, in addition to increased bone resorption secondary to inactivity in the postpartum period, may lead to severe hypercalcemia [4]. Women with superimposed PHPT are particularly at risk for hypercalcemic crisis in the postpartum period, especially if lactating, although this was not seen in our patient with PHPT.

Lactation is a time of relative hypocalciuria. The major regulators of calcium during lactation are breast-derived PTHrP and, to a lesser degree, low estradiol levels. Postpartum estrogen deficiency together with rising PTHrP levels increases skeletal calcium resorption and renal calcium reabsorption, which lowers the renal calcium excretion [4]. Additionally, there is a rapid fall in 1,25 hydroxyvitamin D levels during puerperium, accompanied by a decline in the intestinal absorption of calcium and a reduction in renal calcium excretion [3]. In patient 2 with PHPT, we saw a change in CCCR from 2.67% in her first pregnancy to 0.89% while lactating and vitamin D replete, consistent with relative hypocalciuria of lactation.

When interpreting renal calcium indices in pregnancy and lactation, clinicians must take into account both the physiological changes in calcium homeostasis in these states and also the superimposed pathologic changes of FHH or PHPT on calcium handling. Moreover, the relative changes in calciuria during pregnancy and lactation are not absolutes, and varying degrees of hypercalciuria and hypocalciuria may be seen in either pregnancy or lactation, further adding to the difficulty in using renal calcium indices to aid in diagnosis during the reproductive window.

4. Diagnosis

Determining the etiology of hypercalcemia in pregnancy is necessary for appropriate management. A high or inappropriately normal PTH level suggests PTH mediated hypercalcemia and narrows the differential to Primary Hyperparathyroidism and Familial Hypocalciuric Hypercalcemia, provided vitamin D deficiency and/or very low calcium intake, renal insufficiency, and use of thiazides or lithium have been ruled out. Clinicians employ calcium biochemistry and genetic testing to distinguish PHPT from FHH.

4.1. Biochemical Testing in Hypercalcemia during Pregnancy. Guidelines cite a cutoff CCCR < 1% to suggest FHH and CCCR > 2% to suggest PHPT [5]. However, there is significant overlap of renal calcium indices such as the CCCR in normal, FHH, and PHPT patients [2]. Despite this, CCCR is used in conjunction with clinical features and genetic testing when required to distinguish between FHH and PHPT outside of pregnancy. In pregnant and lactating women, changes in maternal calcium handling as well as the individual effects of PHPT or FHH on renal calcium indices make CCCR an even less useful tool to distinguish between these two conditions.

The expected relative hypercalciuria of pregnancy may lead to an elevated CCCR, resulting in misdiagnosis of FHH as PHPT and subsequent inappropriate parathyroidectomy, as was seen in a recent case series [6].

4.2. Genetic Testing. The gold standard for diagnosis of FHH is molecular testing of the CaSR gene, which has identified over 100 mutations that result in reduced or inactive calcium sensing receptors [7]. However, analysis of the CaSR gene has many drawbacks that should be considered prior to its use in pregnancy. Due to the heterogeneity of CaSR mutations and the limitations of current genetic testing methods, a mutation is only detected in two-thirds of cases of FHH [8]. In addition, the cost, availability, and potential time delay in obtaining results are practical limitations in the use of genetic testing to definitely diagnose FHH during pregnancy. The urgency of a diagnosis of FHH versus PHPT is far greater in pregnant women than in nonpregnant women, as the safety of a curative parathyroidectomy for PHPT is considered highest in the second trimester [9]. Testing the serum and urine calcium of three first-degree relatives results in a lower false negative rate compared to DNA sequencing of that proband, and results of biochemistry are usually available much earlier than genetic testing [10].

5. Pregnancy Complications

Below are the known complications of PHPT and FHH in pregnancy.

5.1. Maternal Complications of PHPT. PHPT in pregnancy can lead to a number of serious maternal complications including hyperemesis, nephrolithiasis, pancreatitis, preeclampsia necessitating premature delivery, and postpartum hypercalcemic crisis [1, 4]. Rates of maternal complications in PHPT are quoted as up to 67% [3]. Evidence for reduction in maternal complications after parathyroidectomy is limited and largely derived from case studies of symptomatic PHPT patients in pregnancy [11]. Some studies suggest a benefit of second-trimester parathyroidectomy, while others show a persistent risk of preeclampsia despite surgical treatment of a parathyroid adenoma up to five years prior to delivery [9, 12].

PHPT, particularly in those of reproductive age or younger, may be the first clue that an individual has multiple endocrine neoplasia 2 (MEN2). Despite the fact that MEN2 is a rare cause of PHPT, undiagnosed pheochromocytoma during pregnancy carries a high risk of maternal and fetal mortality [13]. Proper detection and treatment for pheochromocytoma brings the mortality rate down from 50% to <5% and 15%, for mother and fetus, respectively [13].

Hence, we recommend considering screening for pheochromocytoma in patients with PHPT recognized before or during pregnancy, especially if there is a raised clinical suspicion of pheochromocytoma, such as a positive family history or severe hypertension. However, it should be noted that some patients with pheochromocytoma are normotensive in pregnancy, making the diagnosis more challenging in these cases [14].

5.2. Fetal Complications of PHPT. Based on old reports, offspring of mothers with untreated PHPT had an 80% chance of fetal or neonatal complications including fetal growth restriction, severe neonatal hypocalcemia, tetany, and death [1]. Neonatal hypocalcemia due to fetal parathyroid gland suppression in the setting of maternal hypercalcemia is usually transient (lasting 3–5 months after birth); however, it can be delayed in onset and prolonged in some cases, and permanent hypoparathyroidism has also been described [4]. Curative parathyroidectomy in mothers with PHPT has been associated with a fourfold reduction in fetal mortality, based on a review from 1976, which included 14 out of 21 mothers with symptomatic hypercalcemia during pregnancy [11].

Rates of maternal and fetal complications in PHPT are frequently quoted as up to 67% and 80%, respectively [1]. These numbers are derived from case reports and series of PHPT at a time when expense and availability of laboratory testing limited calcium measurements to symptomatic patients [11]. More widely available calcium testing has led to the predominance of milder forms of hypercalcemia in those with PHPT. Little data is available for pregnancy outcomes in women with mild PHPT, but these individuals likely carry a lower risk of pregnancy complications than previously stated [15]. Support for this comes from a recent retrospective cohort study of registry data from 1977 to 2010 that identified over 1000 women with PHPT [16]. Compared to age-matched controls, women with PHPT had no difference in most pregnancy outcomes, including stillbirths. Unfortunately this paper did not provide information on preeclampsia. Apgar scores and anthropometric measurements were generally similar in neonates of women with and without PHPT. Calcium levels were only available on a subset of case women and therefore the degree of hypercalcemia was unknown for most of the women. The women with PHPT who later underwent parathyroidectomy, possibly indicating more severe hypercalcemia, had more episodes of stillbirth compared to those that did not undergo surgery (1.6% versus 0.2%) [16]. Although not definitive, this observation supports the hypothesis that the degree of hypercalcemia correlates directly with the risk of adverse pregnancy outcomes.

5.3. Maternal Complications of FHH. Most pregnant women with FHH are asymptomatic, and the condition does not typically result in pregnancy complications. Murine models predict that lactating women with superimposed FHH are at risk of hypercalcemic crisis. Inactivating mutations of the CaSR receptor in murine models has been shown to lead to an increased production of mammary PTHrP, but with decreased excretion of calcium into breast milk. The end result is increased bone resorption, lower milk calcium content, and higher serum calcium concentration [4].

5.4. Fetal Complications of FHH. FHH is an autosomal dominant condition; accordingly, there are three genotypic possibilities for the fetus of a mother with FHH. Both unaffected and heterozygous fetuses (with 1 inactivating mutation of the CaSR gene) are at risk for transient or permanent hypoparathyroidism due to suppression of their parathyroid glands in the setting of maternal hypercalcemia in pregnancy [4]. In severe cases, neonates may experience seizures, tetany, and death [11]. Heterozygotes may eventually develop hypercalcemia with hypocalciuria in the neonatal period. A fetus may also inherit a second CaSR mutation from the father or through a spontaneous mutation, making them homozygously dominant. This situation classically results in neonatal severe hyperparathyroidism (NSHPT) necessitating parathyroidectomy in the neonatal period [1]. In rare cases, patients with NSHPT can have a heterozygous mutation, as is described in a case report of a heterozygous neonate with NSHPT who was successfully treated with cinacalcet monotherapy [17]. Given the range of possible neonatal outcomes, it is advisable to offer genetic counseling to all pregnant women with confirmed FHH. In addition, these neonates should undergo close monitoring of calcium in the neonatal period.

6. Conclusions

Given the significant overlap of renal calcium indices in normal, FHH, and PHPT patients [2] and the variable effect of changes in maternal calcium handling during pregnancy and lactation on renal calcium indices, the CCCR is even more difficult to interpret during these reproductive stages than outside pregnancy.

To distinguish between FHH and PHPT in pregnancy, we recommend testing of the proband's first-degree relatives, starting with the ionized calcium (or, if unavailable, albumin adjusted calcium) and, if elevated, progressing to 24-hour urine calcium corrected for creatinine. Genetic testing of the CaSR gene should be reserved for situations when the timely biochemical testing of family members is not possible and when parathyroidectomy cannot be delayed until the patient is biochemically reevaluated after completion of lactation. While parathyroidectomy appears to reduce pregnancy complications in the setting of symptomatic and severe hypercalcemia [11], the benefit of parathyroidectomy is less clear in women with asymptomatic hypercalcemia in pregnancy secondary to mild PHPT. In women with established FHH, we recommend offering genetic counseling to assess fetal risk. Active surveillance of neonatal serum calcium is recommended for both conditions. Further research is needed to better understand the true risk of complications in mother and fetus, as well as the benefit of parathyroidectomy in the setting of mild PHPT in pregnancy.

List of Abbreviations

CaSR: Calcium sensing receptor
CCCR: Calcium to creatinine clearance ratio
FHH: Familial Hypocalciuric Hypercalcemia
MEN: Multiple endocrine neoplasia
NSHPT: Neonatal severe hyperparathyroidism
PHPT: Primary hyperparathyroidism
PTHrP: Parathyroid hormone related peptide.

Acknowledgments

The authors would like to acknowledge the patients and their families for their contributions in providing them with their medical information and their consent to report this information.

References

[1] M. S. Cooper, "Disorders of calcium metabolism and parathyroid disease," *Best Practice and Research: Clinical Endocrinology and Metabolism*, vol. 25, no. 6, pp. 975–983, 2011.

[2] C. Kovacs, "Parathyroid Function and disease during pregnancy, lactation, and fetal/neonatal development," in *The Parathyroids*, J. Bilezikian, R. Marcus, C. Marcocci, S. Silverberg, and J. Potts, Eds., pp. 877–902, Elsevier, London, UK, 3rd edition, 2015.

[3] C. S. Kovacs, "Calcium and bone metabolism disorders during pregnancy and lactation," *Endocrinology and Metabolism Clinics of North America*, vol. 40, no. 4, pp. 795–826, 2011.

[4] G. E. Fuleihan and E. Brown, "Familial hypocalciuric hypercalcemia and neonatal severe hyperparathyroidism," in *The Parathyroids*, J. Bilezikian, R. Marcus, C. Marcocci, S. Silverberg, and J. Potts, Eds., pp. 365–387, Elsevier, London, UK, 3rd edition, 2015.

[5] J. P. Bilezikian, M. L. Brandi, R. Eastell et al., "Guidelines for the management of asymptomatic primary hyperparathyroidism: summary statement from the Fourth International Workshop," *The Journal of Clinical Endocrinology & Metabolism*, vol. 99, no. 10, pp. 3561–3569, 2014.

[6] A. Walker, J. Fraile, and J. Hubbard, "'Parathyroidectomy in pregnancy'—a single centre experience with review of evidence and proposal of treatment algorithm," *Gland Surgery*, vol. 3, pp. 158–164, 2014.

[7] G. N. Hendy, "CASRdb: Calcium-sensing receptor database," http://www.casrdb.mcgill.ca/.

[8] P. H. Nissen, S. E. Christensen, S. A. Ladefoged, K. Brixen, L. Heickendorff, and L. Mosekilde, "Identification of rare and frequent variants of the CASR gene by high-resolution melting," *International Journal of Clinical Chemistry*, vol. 413, no. 5-6, pp. 605–611, 2012.

[9] K. C. Kort, H. J. Schiller, and P. J. Numann, "Hyperparathyroidism and pregnancy," *The American Journal of Surgery*, vol. 177, no. 1, pp. 66–68, 1999.

[10] R. Eastell, A. Arnold, M. L. Brandi et al., "Diagnosis of asymptomatic primary hyperparathyroidism: proceedings of the third international workshop," *Journal of Clinical Endocrinology and Metabolism*, vol. 94, no. 2, pp. 340–350, 2009.

[11] F. L. Delmonico, R. M. Neer, A. B. Cosimi, A. B. Barnes, and P. S. Russell, "Hyperparathyroidism during pregnancy," *The American Journal of Surgery*, vol. 131, no. 3, pp. 328–337, 1976.

[12] H. Hultin, P. Hellman, E. Lundgren et al., "Association of parathyroid adenoma and pregnancy with preeclampsia," *Endocrine Care*, vol. 94, no. 9, pp. 3394–3399, 2009.

[13] J. W. Lenders, "Pheochromocytoma and pregnancy: a deceptive connection," *Endocrine Disorders in Pregnancy*, vol. 166, no. 2, pp. 143–150, 2012.

[14] A. Botchan, R. Hauser, M. Kupferminc, D. Grisaru, M. R. Peyser, and J. B. Lessing, "Pheochromocytoma in pregnancy: case report and review of the literature," *Obstetrical & Gynecological Survey*, vol. 50, no. 4, pp. 321–327, 1995.

28

Locally Advanced Thyroglossal Duct Cyst Carcinoma Presenting as a Neck Mass

Niranjan Tachamo,[1] Brian Le,[2] Jeffrey Driben,[3] and Vasudev Magaji[4]

[1]*Department of Internal Medicine, Reading Health System, West Reading, PA 19611, USA*
[2]*Department of Pathology, Reading Health System, West Reading, PA 19611, USA*
[3]*ENT Head & Neck Specialists, Wyomissing, PA 19610, USA*
[4]*Department of Endocrinology, Reading Health System, West Reading, PA 19611, USA*

Correspondence should be addressed to Niranjan Tachamo; niranjantachamo@gmail.com

Academic Editor: Eli Hershkovitz

Thyroglossal duct cyst carcinoma is rare and occurs in just 1% of cases with thyroglossal duct cysts. It is not always possible to distinguish a thyroglossal cyst harboring malignancy from its benign counterparts unless biopsied, thus posing the dilemma. Currently there is no clear consensus on the optimal management of thyroglossal duct cyst carcinoma. Here we present the case of a 69-year-old female who presented with a midline neck mass and dysphagia and was found to have papillary thyroid cancer in the biopsy specimen of the neck mass. She underwent excision of the mass and the thyroglossal duct cyst along with total thyroidectomy; however, the thyroidectomy specimen showed no malignancy. Her lymph node mapping was negative and she is awaiting radioactive iodine treatment.

1. Introduction

Thyroglossal duct cyst is a developmental anomaly arising from the failure of thyroglossal duct to involute during embryological development [1]. It is the most common congenital anomaly of the neck [1, 2] and is present in approximately 7% of the general population [1, 3]. Uncommonly, thyroglossal duct cyst carcinoma (TDCC) may be found in 1% of cases, the majority being papillary carcinoma [2, 4]. It may be difficult to ascertain the presence of thyroid carcinoma originating exclusively from a thyroglossal duct cyst as there is no way to distinguish the carcinoma from a benign cyst preoperatively [3]. There is no consensus regarding the optimal management of TDCC.

2. Case Presentation

A 69-year-old female was seen in the office for a neck lump and dysphagia for 1 year. She denied any fever, night sweats, dysphonia, dysarthria, palpitations, or weight loss. There was no history of radiation to the head and neck. There was no family history of thyroid cancer. The neck mass was 4 × 5 cm, soft to palpation, freely mobile, and located in the midline at the level of the thyroid cartilage. She was evaluated with an ultrasonogram (US) of the neck which revealed a right mid to superior lobe hyperechoic nodule measuring 7 × 3 × 4 mm, with mild increased vascularity, and a left inferior heterogeneous nodule measuring 1.5 × 0.7 × 0.7 cm, along with submandibular lymph nodes, measuring 1.7 × 0.9 × 1.3 cm on the right and measuring 2.1 × 0.9 × 1.1 cm on the left. Computed tomography (CT) of the neck revealed a lobulated soft tissue mass at the level of the left side of the hyoid bone measuring 1.8 × 2.9 cm with no evidence of erosion of the hyoid bone or thyroid cartilage (Figures 1 and 2). Fine needle aspiration biopsy of the neck mass revealed papillary thyroid cancer. The patient underwent excision of the mass and thyroglossal duct cyst via a Sistrunk procedure with total thyroidectomy.

On histologic examination, within the central neck soft tissue there is a cystic structure, within which is a proliferation of papillary fronds (Figure 3). The cyst is lined by respiratory-type epithelium, consistent with thyroglossal

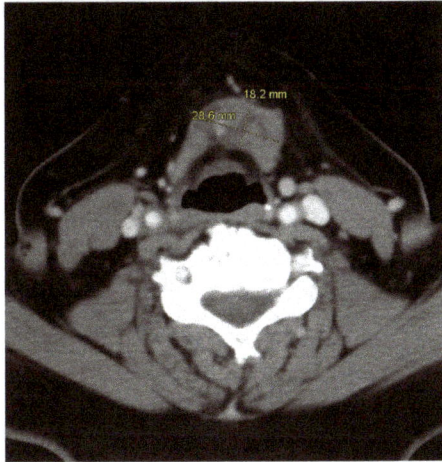

FIGURE 1: Transverse view of the CT neck that showed presence of a neck mass measuring 28.6 mm × 18.2 mm.

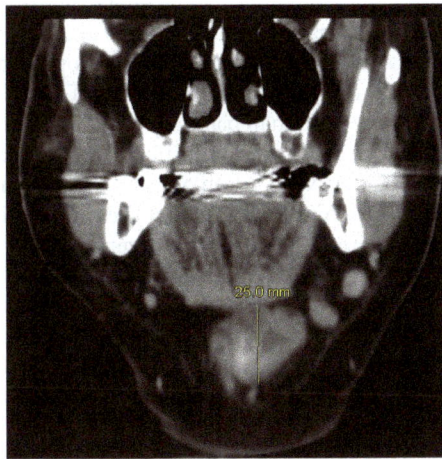

FIGURE 2: Axial view of the CT neck that showed presence of a neck mass measuring 25 mm in superior to inferior dimension.

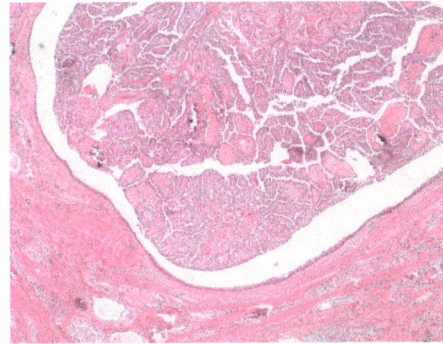

FIGURE 3: Central neck soft tissue demonstrating a cystic structure, within which is a proliferation of fibrovascular cores (H&E stain, 40x original magnification).

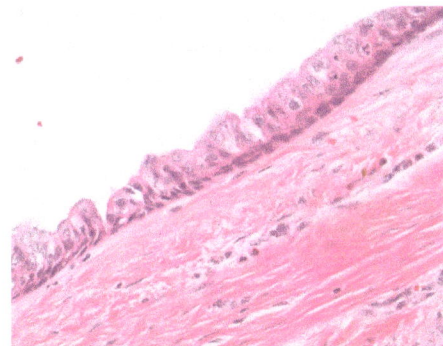

FIGURE 4: The cystic structure is lined by respiratory-type epithelium, consistent with thyroglossal duct cyst (H&E stain, 400x original magnification).

duct cyst (Figure 4), while the intraluminal proliferation, which extends into adjacent soft tissue, demonstrates complex and arborizing fibrovascular cores lined by epithelioid cells (Figure 5). These cells are characterized by nuclear grooves with pseudoinclusions, peripheralization of nuclear chromatin, and some prominence of nucleoli (Figure 6). The morphologic features are diagnostic of papillary thyroid carcinoma. As there is no demonstrable tumor in the total thyroidectomy specimen concurrently reviewed, the tumor is deemed to have arisen from the thyroglossal duct cyst. Her lymph node mapping was negative and she is planned for treatment with radioactive iodine.

3. Discussion

The thyroid gland develops from the endodermal thickening at the base of the tongue and descends via the thyroglossal tract into its final position in the anterior neck inferior to

the thyroid cartilage [2, 5, 6]. This thyroglossal tract usually disappears by 10th week of gestation [2, 5]. However, it fails to involute in 7% of cases [1, 4]. Cystic degeneration of this persistent duct forms a thyroglossal duct cyst, which is usually benign [5, 6]. So far, thyroglossal duct cyst is the most common congenital cause of neck swelling and accounts for more than 75% of midline neck swellings in childhood [6]. Between 1.5 and 45% of these cases show the presence of ectopic thyroid tissue [6].

Thyroglossal duct cyst carcinoma (TDCC) is a rare phenomenon and occurs in just 1% of cases of thyroglossal duct cysts [2, 4]. TDCC is more common in females than in males. The mean age of presentation is 6 years in the pediatric population and 38 years in the adult population [4]. Well differentiated thyroid carcinomas account for 95% of TDCC, with papillary cancer being the most common. However, anaplastic thyroid carcinoma and squamous cell carcinoma arising from the cyst have been reported [1].

The origin of TDCC is not entirely clear, whether it arises de novo from the native thyroid tissue in the cyst wall or as a metastasis from the thyroid gland [1, 5]. Interestingly, medullary carcinoma in thyroglossal cyst has never been reported in literature, suggesting a de novo origin of TDCC [5]. In our case, the presence of papillary carcinoma in the thyroglossal duct cyst despite normal thyroid tissue on

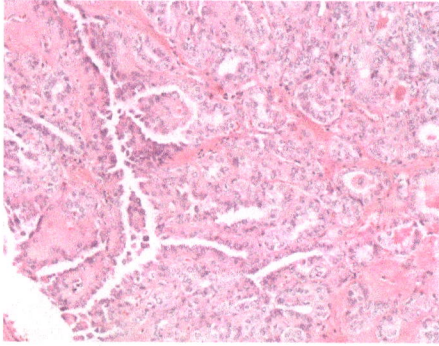

FIGURE 5: The proliferative tumor is characterized by complex and arborizing papillary fronds (H&E stain, 200x original magnification).

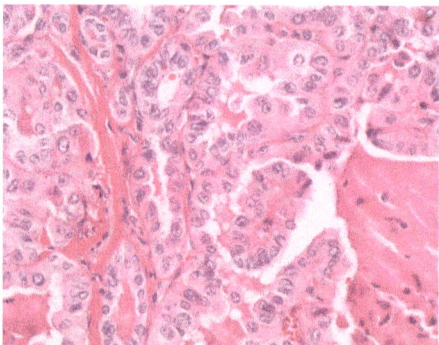

FIGURE 6: High-power view of the tumor, demonstrating cells with nuclear grooves, peripheralization of chromatin, and some prominence of nucleoli, diagnostic of papillary thyroid carcinoma (H&E stain, 400x original magnification).

surgical pathology supports the origin of the cancer from the thyroglossal duct remnant rather than metastasis. The most common papillary carcinomas have indolent growth and an excellent prognosis [1]. In one study, the 5- and 10-year survival rate were found to be 100% and 95.6%, respectively, with no disease-related deaths reported [7].

Most of the time, it is impossible to distinguish the thyroglossal duct cyst harboring malignancy from the benign counterparts [4–6]. Malignancy should be suspected if the thyroglossal duct cyst is hard, irregular, fixed, rapidly growing, and associated with palpable neck lymph nodes [2, 4]. Ultrasonogram (US) and fine needle aspiration cytology (FNAC) of the cyst may help diagnose TDCC preoperatively [5]. Calcifications within the cyst and/or regional calcifications suggest papillary carcinoma while a solid component suggests malignancy. However, TDCC may exist even with a normal US and FNAC [5].

The optimal management of TDCC is still controversial. In the study by de Tristan et al., TDCC was found to be present in just 1.4% (4 out of 352) of thyroglossal duct cysts, and all of them were papillary carcinoma. Three of the 4 patients underwent total thyroidectomy (TT) but none were found to have a second carcinoma in the thyroid suggesting that thyroidectomy was unnecessarily performed [8]. In this

regard, some authors suggest tailoring the surgical strategy as per the risk group stratification [5].

Accordingly, it is recommended that the Sistrunk procedure (SP) alone be performed in low risk situations with a clinical and radiologically normal thyroid gland [4, 5]. The low risk situation is defined as age < 45 years, size < 4 cm, no prior radiation exposure, no soft tissue invasion, no distant or lymphatic metastasis, and no aggressive tumor histology [4, 5]. The addition of total thyroidectomy and radioactive iodine ablation (RAI) is done in high risk patients and in cases with positive surgical margins [5]. The rationale is that there was no significant overall survival benefit of TT and RAI in low risk patients. However, Bakkar et al. in their studies found a high rate (62.3%) of concomitant thyroid cancer and recommend routine addition of TT to SP [5]. Moreover, coexisting thyroid cancers may go undetected in US thyroid and the size of a TDCC may not be a reliable predictor of coexisting thyroid carcinoma. In this context, routine TT and RAI would eliminate the latent or residual disease and would positively impact the disease-free survival [5]. This treatment strategy would further facilitate the detection of persistent or recurrent disease based on serum thyroglobulin measurement and RAI scan [5]. However, prophylactic neck dissection is not recommended for papillary TDCC as occult node positivity is common in papillary carcinomas of the thyroid gland, and it does not prognosticate disease recurrence or disease-specific survival [5]. In our case, the patient was an elderly female with muscle invasion at the time of diagnosis, necessitating the need for extensive surgery.

4. Conclusion

TDCC is uncommon and is usually diagnosed postoperatively. The majority of the cases are papillary carcinoma and have a good prognosis with long-term survival. However, controversy still exists regarding the optimal management of TDCC. Whether total thyroidectomy with radioactive ablation and lymph node dissection should be performed even in low risk cases is still not clear, necessitating the need for more prospective studies.

References

[1] D. W. Jang, A. G. Sikora, and A. Leytin, "Thyroglossal duct cyst carcinoma: case report and review of the literature," *Ear, Nose & Throat Journal*, vol. 92, no. 9, pp. E12–E14, 2013.

[2] N. Maleki, M. Iranparvar Alamdari, I. Feizi, and Z. Tavosi, "Papillary carcinoma of the thyroglossal duct cyst: case report," *Iranian Journal of Public Health*, vol. 43, no. 4, pp. 529–531, 2014.

[3] A. K. Lira Medina, E. Fernandez Berdeal, E. Bernal Cisneros, R. Betancourt Galindo, and P. Frigerio, "Incidental papillary thyroid carcinoma in thyroglossal duct cyst case report," *International Journal of Surgery Case Reports*, vol. 29, pp. 4–7, 2016.

[4] R. Akram, J. J. Wiltshire, J. Wadsley, and S. P. Balasubramanian, "Adult thyroglossal duct carcinoma of thyroid epithelial origin: a retrospective observational study," *Indian Journal of Otolaryngology and Head & Neck Surgery*, vol. 68, no. 4, pp. 522–527, 2016.

[5] S. Bakkar, M. Biricotti, G. Stefanini, C. E. Ambrosini, G. Materazzi, and P. Miccoli, "The extent of surgery in thyroglossal cyst carcinoma," *Langenbeck's Archives of Surgery*, pp. 1–6, 2016.

[6] L. Gordini, F. Podda, F. Medas et al., "Tall cell carcinoma arising in a thyroglossal duct cyst: a case report," *Annals of Medicine and Surgery*, vol. 4, no. 2, pp. 129–132, 2015.

[7] S. G. Patel, M. Escrig, A. R. Shaha, B. Singh, and J. P. Shah, "Management of well-differentiated thyroid carcinoma presenting within a thyroglossal duct cyst," *Journal of Surgical Oncology*, vol. 79, no. 3, pp. 134–141, 2002.

[8] J. de Tristan, J. Zenk, J. Künzel, G. Psychogios, and H. Iro, "Thyroglossal duct cysts: 20 years' experience (1992–2011)," *European Archives of Oto-Rhino-Laryngology*, vol. 272, no. 9, pp. 2513–2519, 2014.

29

Pituitary Apoplexy Presenting as Ophthalmoplegia and Altered Level of Consciousness without Headache

Nooshin Salehi ⓘ,[1] Anthony Firek,[2] and Iqbal Munir ⓘ[2]

[1]Department of Medicine, Riverside University Health System Medical Center, Moreno Valley, CA, USA
[2]Division of Endocrinology, Department of Medicine, Riverside University Health System Medical Center, Moreno Valley, CA, USA

Correspondence should be addressed to Iqbal Munir; i.munir@ruhealth.org

Academic Editor: Osamu Isozaki

Background. Pituitary apoplexy (PA) is a clinical syndrome caused by acute ischemic infarction or hemorrhage of the pituitary gland. The typical clinical presentation of PA includes acute onset of severe headache, visual disturbance, cranial nerve palsy, and altered level of consciousness. *Case Report*. A 78-year-old man presented to the emergency department with one-day history of ptosis and diplopia and an acute-onset episode of altered level of consciousness which was resolving. He denied having headache, nausea, or vomiting. Physical examination revealed third-cranial nerve palsy and fourth-cranial nerve palsy both on the right side. Noncontrast computed tomography (CT) scan of the head was unremarkable. Brain magnetic resonance imaging (MRI) showed a pituitary mass with hemorrhage (apoplexy) and extension to the right cavernous sinus. The patient developed another episode of altered level of consciousness in the hospital. Transsphenoidal resection of the tumor was done which resulted in complete recovery of the ophthalmoplegia and mental status. *Conclusion*. Pituitary apoplexy can present with ophthalmoplegia and altered level of consciousness without having headache, nausea, or vomiting. A CT scan of the head could be negative for hemorrhage. A high index of suspicion is needed for early diagnosis and timely management of pituitary apoplexy.

1. Background

Pituitary apoplexy (PA) is a potentially life-threatening disorder caused by acute ischemic infarction or hemorrhage of the pituitary gland [1]. Pituitary adenomas are prone to bleeding and necrosis, possibly because they outgrow their blood supply or because tumor expansion causes ischemia and resultant infarction by compressing the vessels against the sellar diaphragm [2]. The inherent fragility of tumor blood vessels may also explain the tendency to hemorrhage [2]. However, PA may also occur in nonadenomatous or even the normal pituitary gland, especially during pregnancy [1]. In one report, the prevalence of pituitary apoplexy among patients with nonfunctioning pituitary macroadenomas was 8 percent [3].

The clinical presentation of PA is highly variable and is largely determined by the extent of hemorrhage, necrosis, and edema. Headache of sudden and severe onset is the main symptom of PA and is present in more than 80% of the patients [2]. Patients can also present with visual disturbances, diplopia, hypopituitarism, and impaired

consciousness which, together with the radiological evidence of a pituitary lesion, establish the diagnosis [4]. In cases with severe, progressive visual, or neurological manifestations, surgical decompression is indicated [4], while the patients with mild stable clinical picture can be managed conservatively [4].

PA may present as isolated acute cranial nerve (CN) palsies [5–11], which usually indicates a milder disease [4] and possibly a more chronic onset. In the setting of PA, the third cranial nerve (CN III) is the most frequently affected cranial nerve [4–7, 10], but sixth-cranial nerve (CN VI) palsy [12], multiple CN palsies [8, 13], and even bilateral lesions [9, 14] have also been reported. CT scan of the head typically shows hemorrhage in the pituitary gland. Pituitary apoplexy presenting with ophthalmoplegia and recurrent brief episodes of altered level of consciousness, without demonstrating headache, nausea, or vomiting has not been previously described in the literature. The following is an illustrative case of an unusual presentation of PA in an elderly man and a focused review of the literature.

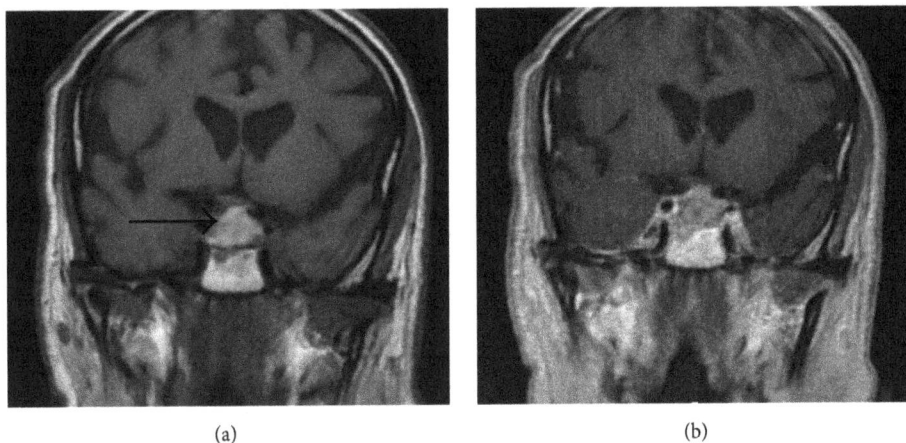

(a)   (b)

FIGURE 1: Brain MRI W/WO contrast 2 days before surgery. (a) Coronal T1-weighted image demonstrates a large sellar mass with suprasellar extension and slight mass effect on the optic chiasm. This mass exhibits marked hyperintense signal on T1-weighted image (arrow), which indicates blood products and recent hemorrhage. (b) Coronal T1-weighted postcontrast image shows normal enhancement of the cavernous sinus. No enhancing mass or nodule is evident in association with intrinsically T1 bright lesion. The mass abuts approximately 90 degrees of the right internal carotid artery contour. This abutment is less on the left side. The carotid arteries are patent and show normal caliber without any narrowing. No normal pituitary tissue is identified.

2. Case Report

A 78-year-old African American man with past medical history of hypertension and alveolar emphysema presented to the emergency department with altered level of consciousness (LOC). He was found unresponsive and drooling on the couch by a family member. The patient's family had noted drooping of the right eyelid that had started the day before the incident. No headache, head injury, chest pain, palpitation, or decreased vision was reported but it was noted that he possibly could not see well in his peripheral visual field. The emergency medical services (EMS) reported an initial Glasgow Coma Score (GCS) of 7/15 (Eye 1, Verbal 1, and Motor 5) that began to improve on the way to the hospital. According to the EMS report, the patient's vital signs were normal at the scene including a blood pressure of 118/82 mmHg, heart rate of 92 per minute, and respiratory rate of 12 per minute. His blood glucose level was at 155 mg/dL.

He was a smoker, using a quarter of pack of cigarettes a day. His medications included amlodipine, ipratropium nebulizer, and albuterol nebulizer. He did not use alcohol or illicit drugs.

Upon arrival to the hospital, the patient was lethargic and had poor attention but was oriented to the time, place, and person. He denied headache, nausea, or vomiting. Physical examination revealed a GCS of 14/15 and normal vital signs, including blood pressure of 115/76 mmHg, body temperature of 37°C, respiratory rate of 20 per minute, and a regular pulse rate of 83 beats per minute. Pupils were equal in size and both had normal direct and consensual responses to light. Visual acuity appeared to be reduced but full evaluation was not possible. Complete ptosis of the right eye was noted. The right eye was deviated to the right with severe limitation in supraduction, infraduction, and adduction consistent with pupil-sparing third-cranial nerve (CN III) palsy. Fourth-cranial nerve (CN IV) palsy was also present in the right

side. Extraocular eye movements were intact in the left eye. Sensation was intact over the face bilaterally. There were no other abnormal findings in the physical exam. Upon the admission, the plasma sodium level was slightly depressed at 130 mEq/L but the other initial lab findings were unremarkable (Table 1).

The patient was admitted to the internal medicine service for a stroke workup. Noncontrast computed tomography scan (CT scan) of the head showed only age related atrophic changes with no evidence of intracranial hemorrhage or mass effect. Brain magnetic resonance imaging (MRI) showed a sellar mass, and the pituitary MRI (Figure 1) revealed a large pituitary mass with extension to the right cavernous sinus. Intrinsic T1 hyperintensity suggested possible hemorrhage (pituitary apoplexy). Mild mass effect on the optic chiasm was noted. There were no evidence of extension of the mass beyond the lateral confines of the cavernous sinuses and no hydrocephalus or subarachnoid hemorrhage. The major intracranial flow voids were patent.

Lumbar puncture was performed and cerebrospinal fluid (CSF) analysis did not show any blood or xanthochromia. On his second hospital day, the patient developed an acute change in the mental status. He was noted to be lethargic and confused, not responding to his name, and having garbled speech. During that time, he had blood sugar of 98, blood pressure of 98/56 mmHg, and heart rate of 113 per minute. His acute confusional state resolved within an hour, but a clouding of consciousness continued to be present as was observed since admission. Electrocardiogram (EKG) and echocardiography were normal.

Based on the ophthalmoplegia, ptosis, altered mental status, visual symptom, and confirmatory findings in the MRI, the diagnosis of pituitary apoplexy was established. The hormonal profile (Table 1) included a low serum cortisol at baseline (1.1 mcg/dL) and low concurrent adreno-corticotropin hormone (ACTH). Cosyntropin stimulation

TABLE 1: Laboratory data findings.

Variable	Reference range	Day 1*	Day 2	Day 3	Day 4	Day 5	Day 6	Day 7	Day 8	Day 9	Day 10	3 months	6 months	9 months
Glucose, random (mg/dL)	74–106	103	90	83	84	89	115	118	107	109	84			84
Na, serum (mEq/L)	136–145	130		131	130									
K, serum (mEq/L)	3.6–5.0	4.0		4.3	4.3									
Thyroid stimulating hormone (mU/L)	0.40–4.50							0.114						1.68
Thyroxine (T4), free (ng/dL)	0.76–1.46			0.92							1.02	1.0		0.7
Triiodothyronine (T3), total (ng/dL)	76–181				61									
Follicular stimulating hormone (mIU/m)	1.6–8			6.4				4.8				3.1		
Luteinizing hormone (mIU/m)	1.6–15.2			2.8				3.2				1.3		1.3
Testosterone (ng/dL)	250–1100													14
Prolactin (ng/mL)	2.0–18.0			<1.0							<1.0	<1.0		<1.0
ACTH (pg/mL)	6–50			<5				<5				<5		<5
Serum osmolality (mosm)	274–309	273			288				298					
Urine osmolality (mosm)	281–1076				468				403	569				
AM Cortisol (mcg/dL)	4.0–22.0				1.1, 5.2, 11.6**									0.9***
Insulin growth factor-1 (ng/mL)	34–245				71			75				36		

*Day 1 is the first day of admission at our hospital. **Cortisol level was 1.1 mcg/dL at 8 am before stimulation. It was 5.2 mcg/dL and 11.6 mcg/dL after 30 minutes and 60 minutes of cosyntropin injection, respectively. ***The patient was told to skip the last two doses of steroid before this measurement.

increased the cortisol to 11.6 mcg/dL after 60 minutes. Free thyroxine (T4) and thyroid stimulating hormone (TSH) were normal but prolactin was below the normal range. Insulin-like growth factor 1 (IGF-1), follicular stimulating hormone (FSH), and luteinizing hormone (LH) were normal.

After the blood was collected for the endocrine workup, intravenous hydrocortisone was administered with the dose of 100 mg every 8 hours for 36 hours and then transitioned to oral hydrocortisone 20 mg in the morning and 10 mg at noon. On the fourth hospital day, transnasal transsphenoidal resection of the sellar mass was performed which was successful with no complications. Two days after the surgery, the patient reported that his vision was improving. Post-op MRI showed postsurgical changes with no definite residue and no acute complication (Figure 2). Histopathology exam showed pituitary gland tissue (most likely pituitary adenoma) with extensive necrosis and hemorrhage.

On the ophthalmologic exam 4 days after the surgery, visual acuity was 20/40 in both eyes which was at his baseline. There was no relative afferent pupillary defect. Extraocular movements were normal in both eyes. Ophthalmoscopy was bilaterally unremarkable with normal optic disc appearance. Visual field by confrontation technique was full in both eyes.

Postoperatively, the patient regained his normal mental status with no further episodes of confusion. Level of ACTH and endogenous cortisol remained low until the last follow-up, 9 months after the surgery (Table 1). The patient was found to be hypothyroid 9 months after the surgery. His testosterone level appeared to be low on 9 months, and his LH level dropped below the normal range, suggesting secondary hypogonadism. FSH and IGF-1 levels decreased to almost half while still being in the normal range (Table 1). The above-mentioned lab data indicates that the patient developed progressive hypopituitarism after the surgery.

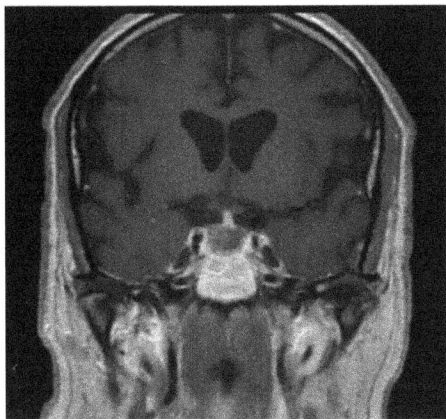

FIGURE 2: MRI (T1 weighted with contrast) one day after the surgery shows interval resection of the previously seen sellar mass/hemorrhage and resolution of mass effect on the optic chiasm.

3. Discussion

The clinical features of PA are typically sudden in onset and include headache, nausea/vomiting, visual disturbances, ophthalmoplegia, and altered consciousness [15].

Headache is present in more than 80% of the patients with pituitary apoplexy (PA) and is generally the initial manifestation [2]. PA typically causes an acute onset of severe frontal or retroorbital headache [16]. In a retrospective study on pituitary apoplexy cases, 95% of the patients presented with headache [17]. The potential mechanisms underlying headache in PA are meningeal irritation, duramater compression, enlargement of the sella turcica walls, or involvement of the superior division of the trigeminal nerve inside the cavernous sinus [1].

Visual disturbances are present in more than half of the patients with PA due to the compression of optic chiasm or optic nerves [2]. Variable degrees of visual-field impairment may be observed, but blindness is rare [2]. More than half of patients with PA have ocular motor palsy, due to functional impairment of CN III (the most affected), CN IV, and/or CN VI [2]. Nausea and vomiting may occur in PA due to meningeal irritation, adrenal insufficiency, hypothalamic dysfunction, or raised intracranial pressure [1].

Altered LOC is the most severe neurological finding in patients with pituitary apoplexy [18]. It is seen in around 20% of PA patients, and may range from mild lethargy to stupor and coma [19]. The mechanism of altered LOC remains elusive and might be related to subarachnoid hemorrhage, increased intracranial pressure, obstructive hydrocephalus, adrenal insufficiency leading to arterial hypotension and/or hypoglycemia, and hypothalamic compression [1].

Our patient developed recurrent brief episodes of altered LOC. Clouding of consciousness with transient brief episodes of confusion has not been previously described in cases of PA. The exact cause of the altered LOC could not be clearly determined in our patient but it could be possibly caused by a transient episode of increased intracranial pressure, cerebral vasospasm, or seizure episodes. Compression of the

vascular structures or vasospasm can rarely cause reversible or irreversible cerebral ischemia in pituitary apoplexy cases [20]; while MRI did not indicate a compressive effect on the vascular structures, vasospasm could have happened. Subarachnoid hemorrhage was ruled out in our case, based on the results of the CT scan and CSF analysis. Adrenal insufficiency would be less likely to cause episodes of altered LOC, as the episodes were not associated with hypotension or hypoglycemia, and hyponatremia was only mild.

In our case, CT scan, which was a conventional CT without coronal/sagittal reconstruction, did not show any findings suggestive of pituitary apoplexy while MRI demonstrated the pituitary mass and hemorrhage. Although CT scan may be used as a rapid screening test, in these patients, fine-cut CT scans, with and without contrast and with coronal and sagittal reconstructions, are necessary [16]. Compared to CT scan, MRI of the sella is superior in detecting tumor and hemorrhage/infarct [16]. MRI can also estimate the time of onset of hemorrhage and detect the superior and lateral extension of the tumor [16]. CT scan may show the intrasellar mass and hemorrhagic components in 80% of cases, but it is most useful in the acute setting (24–48 hours); after this time, blood intensity decreases and may be difficult to detect [2].

While bleeding inside the pituitary gland may occur without causing any symptoms [1], a typical pituitary apoplexy can have a catastrophic clinical manifestation. Based on what we observed in the present case and the review of the literature, the cases of pituitary apoplexy who initially present with ophthalmoplegia, as the only symptom or the main symptom, have a more chronic onset and probably a less dramatic clinical course. A relatively slower expansion of the mass may allow it to extend into the cavernous sinus and compress the elements inside it, without significant suprasellar extension and without causing acute neurologic events that would prompt immediate medical attention.

Common differential diagnoses of PA are subarachnoid hemorrhage and bacterial meningitis; other conditions include midbrain infarction, cavernous sinus thrombosis, migraine, hemorrhagic infarction in a Rathke's cleft cyst, and aneurysms [16, 21].

The first intervention after PA diagnosis is hemodynamic stabilization, correction of electrolyte disturbances, and corticosteroid administration [21]. After collecting blood sample for hematological, biochemistry, and hormonal analysis, glucocorticoids should be administered in supraphysiological doses not only to serve as replacement for endogenous hormone deficiency but also to help control the effect of edema [1].

Regarding endocrine deficiencies, signs and symptoms of hypocortisolism are generally observed in the early stage after apoplexy onset [22], as occurred in our patient. Hypothyroidism, hypogonadism, and growth hormone deficiency are extremely frequent and may occur progressively during weeks, months, or years [22]. Therefore, a periodic reevaluation of anterior pituitary function is recommended [22]. It has been suggested that pituitary deficiencies, once established, usually do not recover, regardless the treatment [2, 21]. Patients with low levels of prolactin exhibit a lower probability of pituitary function recovery after surgery [21, 23].

Hyponatremia, observed in 40% of cases, can be secondary to hypocortisolism or inappropriate antidiuretic hormone secretion [21].

This case report illustrates an unusual clinical presentations of PA: the patient had pupil-sparing CN III palsy, which is more characteristic of ischemic rather than compressive causes; CN IV palsy is not common in PA cases; and altered LOC in PA patients is usually associated with headache [24], nausea, vomiting, signs of meningismus, or evidence of subarachnoid hemorrhage none of which was present in our patient. There are some case reports that illustrated even more unusual or rare presentations of PA, such as PA presenting as bilateral anterior cerebral artery infarction [20] or diabetic ketoacidosis [25, 26]. The importance is to recognize these atypical presentations so that definitive therapy can be instituted.

Other than the wide variety of clinical presentations of PA, one should bear in mind that apoplexy is rare and can frequently develop before the diagnosis of pituitary adenoma is made. Moreover, CT scan cannot detect all the cases of pituitary apoplexy, especially if CT is obtained after the first 48 hours of the onset of hemorrhage, as happened in our case. Therefore, a high index of suspicion is needed for the early diagnosis of this condition. The timely diagnosis and management of PA can improve the visual outcome, relieve the bothersome symptoms, accelerate the recovery of ophthalmoplegia, and prevent the potentially severe consequences of hormonal disturbances or the mass effect. This can significantly improve the care of our patients.

4. Conclusions

Pituitary apoplexy can present with ophthalmoplegia and altered level of consciousness (LOC) without exhibiting any signs or symptoms of increased intracranial pressure, or any evidence of subarachnoid hemorrhage. In this case of pituitary apoplexy, we observed clouding of consciousness exacerbated by transient brief episodes of confusion for which we could not find any immediate cause. PA can present as various clinical pictures and therefore mimic different diseases or pathologies. A high index of suspicion is required for early diagnosis and appropriate treatment of this potentially fatal disease.

Disclosure

Work was done at Department of Medicine, Riverside University Health System Medical Center, Moreno Valley, CA, USA.

References

[1] C. V. Chang, A. C. Felicio, A. C. Toscanini, M. J. Teixeira, and M. B. C. Da Cunha-Neto, "Pituitary tumor apoplexy," *Arq Neuropsiquiatr*, vol. 67, pp. 328–333, 2009.

[2] C. Briet, S. Salenave, and P. Chanson, "Pituitary apoplexy," *Endocrinology and Metabolism Clinics of North America*, vol. 44, no. 1, pp. 199–209, 2015.

[3] G. Vargas, B. Gonzalez, G. Guinto et al., "Pituitary apoplexy in nonfunctioning pituitary macroadenomas: A case-control study," *Endocrine Practice*, vol. 20, no. 12, pp. 1274–1280, 2014.

[4] C. Capatina, W. Inder, N. Karavitaki, and J. A. H. Wass, "Management of endocrine disease: pituitary tumour apoplexy," *European Journal of Endocrinology*, vol. 172, no. 5, pp. R179–R190, 2015.

[5] M. Bahmani Kashkouli, M. R. Khalatbari, S. T. Yahyavi, H. Borghei-Razavi, and M. Soltan-Sanjari, "Pituitary apoplexy presenting as acute painful isolated unilateral third cranial nerve palsy," *Archives of Iranian Medicine*, vol. 11, no. 4, pp. 466–468, 2008.

[6] W. J. Cho, S. P. Joo, T. S. Kim, and B. R. Seo, "Pituitary apoplexy presenting as isolated third cranial nerve palsy with ptosis: Two case reports," *Journal of Korean Neurosurgical Society*, vol. 45, no. 2, pp. 118–121, 2009.

[7] R. Enatsu, M. Asahi, M. Matsumoto, and O. Hirai, "Pituitary apoplexy presenting atypical time course of ophthalmic symptoms," *The Tohoku Journal of Experimental Medicine*, vol. 227, no. 1, pp. 59–61, 2012.

[8] G. Famularo, C. Pozzessere, G. Piazza, and C. De Simone, "Abrupt-onset oculomotor paralysis: An endocrine emergency," *European Journal of Emergency Medicine*, vol. 8, no. 3, pp. 233–236, 2001.

[9] H. F. Komurcu, G. Ayberk, M. F. Ozveren, and O. Anlar, "Pituitary adenoma apoplexy presenting with bilateral third nerve palsy and bilateral proptosis: A case report," *Medical Principles and Practice*, vol. 21, no. 3, pp. 285–287, 2012.

[10] C. C. Lee, A. S. Cho, and W. A. Carter, "Emergency department presentation of pituitary apoplexy," *The American Journal of Emergency Medicine*, vol. 18, no. 3, pp. 328–331, 2000.

[11] A. I. Matti, A. K. Rudkin, A. W. Lee, and C. S. Chen, "Isolated unilateral abducens cranial nerve palsy: A rare presentation of pituitary apoplexy," *European Journal of Ophthalmology*, vol. 20, no. 1, pp. 234–236, 2010.

[12] R. Hage, S. R. Eshraghi, N. M. Oyesiku et al., "Third, Fourth, and Sixth Cranial Nerve Palsies in Pituitary Apoplexy," *World Neurosurgery*, vol. 94, pp. 447–452, 2016.

[13] R. E. Warwar, S. S. Bhullar, R. J. Pelstring, and R. J. Fadell, "Sudden death from pituitary apoplexy in a patient presenting with an isolated sixth cranial nerve palsy," *Journal of Neuro-Ophthalmology*, vol. 26, no. 2, pp. 95–97, 2006.

[14] F. Tanriverdi, Z. Karaca, A. Oner et al., "Complete surgical resolution of bilateral total opthalmoplegia without visual field defect in an acromegalic patient presented with pituitary apoplexy," *Endocrine Journal*, vol. 54, no. 5, pp. 681–684, 2007.

[15] J. Shavadia, S. Mwanzi, and K. Hameed, "Pituitary apoplexy: Report of two cases," *East African Medical Journal*, vol. 85, no. 3, pp. 142–144, 2008.

[16] P. C. Johnston, A. H. Hamrahian, R. J. Weil, and L. Kennedy, "Pituitary tumor apoplexy," *Journal of Clinical Neuroscience*, vol. 22, no. 6, pp. 939–944, 2015.

[17] D. C. Bills, F. B. Meyer, E. R. Laws et al., "A Retrospective Analysis of Pituitary Apoplexy," *Neurosurgery*, vol. 33, no. 4, pp. 602–609, 1993.

[18] R. N. Nawar, D. Abdelmannan, W. R. Selman, and B. M. Arafah, "Pituitary tumor apoplexy: a review," *Journal of Intensive Care Medicine*, vol. 23, no. 2, pp. 75–90, 2008.

[19] S. Ranabir and M. Baruah, "Pituitary apoplexy," *Indian Journal of Endocrinology and Metabolism*, vol. 15, 3, no. 7, p. 188, 2011.

[20] M. S. Abbas, M. N. Alberawi, I. Al Bozom, N. F. Shaikh, and K. Y. Salem, "Unusual complication of pituitary macroadenoma: A case report and review," *American Journal of Case Reports*, vol. 17, pp. 707–711, 2016.

[21] A. Glezer and M. D. Bronstein, "Pituitary apoplexy: pathophysiology, diagnosis and management," *Archives of Endocrinology and Metabolism*, vol. 59, no. 3, pp. 259–264, 2015.

[22] A. Albani, F. Ferraù, F. F. Angileri et al., "Multidisciplinary Management of Pituitary Apoplexy," *International Journal of Endocrinology*, vol. 2016, Article ID 7951536, 2016.

[23] D. H. Zayour, W. R. Selman, and B. M. Arafah, "Extreme elevation of intrasellar pressure in patients with pituitary tumor apoplexy: relation to pituitary function," *The Journal of Clinical Endocrinology & Metabolism*, vol. 89, no. 11, pp. 5649–5654, 2004.

[24] P. N. Elsasser Imboden, N. De Tribolet, A. Lobrinus et al., "Apoplexy in pituitary macroadenoma: eight patients presenting in 12 months," *Medicine*, vol. 84, no. 3, pp. 188–196, 2005.

[25] C. R. Camara-Lemarroy, A. Infante-Valenzuela, K. Rodriguez-Velver, R. Rodriguez-Gutiérrez, and H. J. Villareal-Velazquez, "Pituitary apoplexy presenting as diabetic ketoacidosis: A great simulator?" *Neuroendocrinology Letters*, vol. 37, no. 1, pp. 9–11, 2016.

[26] H.-J. Jiang, W.-W. Hung, and P. J. Hsiao, "A case of acromegaly complicated with diabetic ketoacidosis, pituitary apoplexy, and lymphoma," *Kaohsiung Journal of Medical Sciences*, vol. 29, no. 12, pp. 687–690, 2013.

30

Short Stature Homeobox-Containing Haploinsufficiency in Seven Siblings with Short Stature

Elizabeth S. Sandberg,[1] **Ali S. Calikoglu,**[1] **Karen J. Loechner,**[2] **and Lydia L. Snyder**[3]

[1]*Division of Endocrinology, Department of Pediatrics, University of North Carolina at Chapel Hill, Chapel Hill, NC, USA*
[2]*Division of Pediatric Endocrinology, Department of Pediatrics, Children's Healthcare of Atlanta, Atlanta, GA, USA*
[3]*Division of Pediatric Endocrinology, Department of Pediatrics, Nemours Children's Health System, Jacksonville, FL, USA*

Correspondence should be addressed to Elizabeth S. Sandberg; elizabeth.sandberg@unchealth.unc.edu

Academic Editor: Wayne V. Moore

Deficiency of the short stature homeobox-containing (SHOX) gene is a frequent cause of short stature in children (2–15%). Here, we report 7 siblings with SHOX deficiency due to a point mutation in the SHOX gene. Index case was a 3-year-old male who presented for evaluation of short stature. His past medical history and birth history were unremarkable. Family history was notable for multiple individuals with short stature. Physical exam revealed short stature, with height standard deviation score (SDS) of −2.98, as well as arm span 3 cm less than his height. His laboratory workup was noncontributory for common etiologies of short stature. Due to significant familial short stature and shortened arm span, SHOX gene analysis was performed and revealed patient is heterozygous for a novel SHOX gene mutation at nucleotide position c.582. This mutation is predicted to cause termination of the SHOX protein at codon 194, effectively causing haploinsufficiency. Six out of nine other siblings were later found to also be heterozygous for the same mutation. Growth hormone was initiated in all seven siblings upon diagnosis and they have demonstrated improved height SDS.

1. Background

Deficiency of the short stature homeobox-containing (SHOX) gene is a frequent cause of short stature in children [1]. Early studies indicated a gene or group of genes relating to short stature in the pseudoautosomal region (PAR) of the X and Y chromosomes [2]. In 1997, Rao et al. isolated the SHOX gene within a region in the pseudoautosomal region 1 (PAR1) that was deleted in multiple individuals with short stature, but not deleted in relatives with normal stature [3], at around the same time that Ellison et al. isolated a gene from the PAR region that was a candidate gene for the short stature of Turner syndrome [4]; both eventually would be identified as the SHOX gene. Ultimately, it was discovered that a dose-dependent relationship exists between an individual's height and the number of actives copies of the SHOX gene. Thus, SHOX haploinsufficiency is associated with short stature (as seen with Turner syndrome), and additional SHOX genes (as seen with sex-chromosome polyploidies such as Klinefelter syndrome, triple X syndrome, and XYY syndrome) are associated with tall stature [5]. SHOX deficiency is also the primary cause of short stature in most patients with Leri-Weill dyschondrosteosis. Loss of both SHOX alleles causes an extreme phenotype of osteodysplasia, which is also called Langer syndrome [1]. For children with idiopathic short stature, the prevalence of SHOX mutations is estimated to be within 2–15% [1].

The most common mutations involving the SHOX gene are deletions of various sizes which encompass either the SHOX gene itself or a regulatory enhancer region [1]. These deletions account for approximately two-thirds of all mutations, while point mutations are less common, making up approximately one-third of all mutations [6]. Here we present a family with short stature, of which 7 of 10 siblings were found to be heterozygous for a point mutation in the SHOX gene.

TABLE 1: Results of growth hormone (GH) treatment in seven siblings with short stature due to SHOX haploinsufficiency.

Case	Sex	Age at onset of GH (years)	Bone age at onset of GH (years)	Duration of GH treatment (years)	Height SDS at initiation of GH	Height SDS in June 2014	Change in Height SDS
1	M	3.8	3.5	9.3	−3.1	−1.06	+2.04
2	M	2.9	1.5	8.5	−2.71	−0.77	+1.94
3	F	9.3	8.8	4.5	−2.48	−1.42	+1.06
4	M	10.6	10	4.3	−2.42	−1.83	+0.59
5	F	1.8	2	4.3	−2.57	−2.23	+0.34
6	F	1.5	1.3	3.5	−3.00	−2.52	+0.48
7	M	1.8	2	2.1	−2.26	−1.41	+0.85

2. Case Presentation

2.1. Case 1. This Latino male is the third oldest child of a family originally from Mexico. He presented at the age of 3 years and 2 months for evaluation of short stature (Table 1).

He was born at full term, after an uncomplicated pregnancy and delivery, and his birth weight was near the 10th percentile. As an infant, his height initially was at the 10th percentile, then dropped below the 5th percentile at 22 months of life, and was far below the 3rd percentile by 33 months of life. He maintained his weight around the 10th percentile for the first 3 years of life. Family history is notable for maternal height of 143 cm (<3rd percentile) and paternal height of 156 cm (<3rd percentile), resulting in mid-parental target height of 156 cm. He also had five siblings with reported short stature and two siblings of normal stature.

On physical exam, his height was 85.4 cm (below 3rd percentile, height SDS −2.98), weight 11.8 kg (weight SDS −2.06). His arm span was 82.3 cm. He had no dysmorphic features. His testes were descended bilaterally, and he had a normal phallus.

Initial workup done for common etiologies for short stature revealed normal IGF-I, IGFBP-3, electrolytes, liver function tests, complete blood count, thyroid studies, sedimentation rate, and urinalysis. His bone age was congruent with his chronological age. No Madelung deformity was noted clinically or radiologically.

Because of his severe short stature, family history, and short arm span, a SHOX gene analysis was performed, which revealed a p.C194X sequence variant at nucleotide position c.582 in the SHOX gene, changing a nucleotide from C to A (c.582C>A) in codon 194. This creates a termination codon, which is predicted to cause truncation of the SHOX protein at codon 194. He was heterozygous for this nonsense mutation. The patient was started on growth hormone (GH) at 39 μg/kg/day, with resultant increased growth velocity (Figure 1). Height SDS improved to −1.06 after 9-year treatment (Table 1).

2.2. Cases 2–7. Six siblings of Case 1 subsequently presented for evaluation of short stature. The cases are listed in order of presentation to clinic, which occurred as they demonstrated

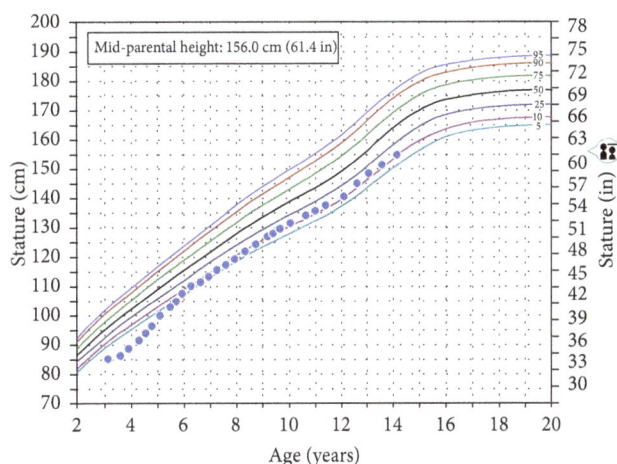

FIGURE 1: Height growth chart for Case 1.

decrease in growth velocity. Their clinical findings at presentation are summarized in Table 1.

All siblings were noted to have height SDS less than −2.0 at the time of presentation. None of the siblings were dysmorphic. Cases 2 and 3 were the only siblings to have any additional abnormal phenotypes diagnosed radiologically: a shortening of the ulna in Case 2, with short 4th and 5th metacarpals, and Madelung deformity of the radial epiphysis in Case 3. Bone ages were either normal or slightly delayed, and workup for other etiologies of short stature was negative in all individuals, as with Case 1. Due to the confirmed family history for SHOX mutation, the SHOX gene analysis was performed in all individuals, and all 6 siblings were found to be heterozygous for the same, novel mutation. Growth hormone treated was initiated in all cases (starting dose 36–45 μg/kg/day), leading to improved height SDS for all cases (Table 1). A representative growth chart is provided in Figure 2.

Case 3 was the eldest child, and her GH treatment was discontinued at age 13 years and 4 months as she neared completion of linear growth after menarche (Figure 3). At that time, her height SDS was −1.42, improved from −2.48 at

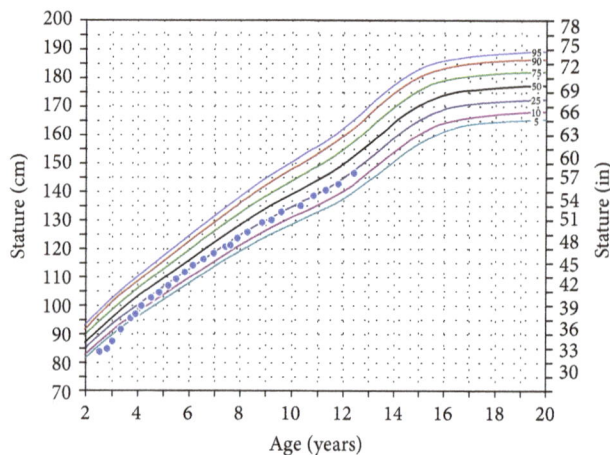

FIGURE 2: Height growth chart for Case 2.

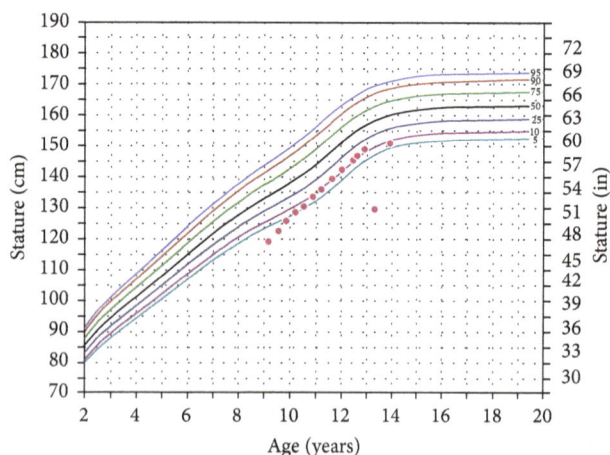

FIGURE 3: Height growth chart for Case 3.

the initiation of GH treatment. Otherwise, GH treatment is ongoing in all cases.

3. Conclusions

This report describes a family with seven siblings with severe short stature at presentation. All are heterozygous for a point mutation of the short stature homeobox-containing (SHOX) gene that was included in SHOX database (http:// grenada.lumc.nl/LOVD2/MR/home.php) but corresponding phenotype was not reported. The SHOX gene is located in the telomeric part of the pseudoautosomal region 1 (PAR1) region on the short arm of both sex chromosomes and does not undergo X inactivation [7]. Because of this, the SHOX gene is expressed on both X and Y chromosomes [1]. The SHOX gene encodes a transcription factor that appears to play a role in regulating chondrocyte differentiation and proliferation during early fetal life [7].

All cases had a mutation in exon 5, codon 194 (c.582C>A), that creates a termination codon. This results in a truncated protein and presumed haploinsufficiency. This truncated protein could potentially interfere with normal SHOX activity,

but, at this time, the true mechanism is unknown. There are reports of mutations in the SHOX gene homeodomain affecting nuclear translocation [8]; however, given the location of the mutation in the 5th exon, we believe effective haploinsufficiency is the most likely explanation in this family. Phenotypically, this haploinsufficiency resulted in short stature, as is seen with other patients with SHOX deficiency.

SHOX deficiency, in addition to short stature, has a wildly varying phenotype, some features of which can act as a clue to the diagnosis. The Madelung deformity is a "spontaneous subluxation of the distal ulna forward" which results in the hand and forearm resembling a dinner fork [1]. Additional, less-specific signs include shortened 4th and 5th metacarpals, highly arched palate, increased carrying angle of the elbow, scoliosis, micrognathia, and muscular hypertrophy [1]. Of note, the absence of any of these signs would not exclude a diagnosis of SHOX haploinsufficiency. Surprisingly in this family, only 2 individuals showed additional phenotypic changes, other than short stature, seen in individuals with SHOX deficiency: Case 3 has short 4th and 5th metacarpals and a Madelung deformity, and Case 2 has shortening of the ulna. It should be noted, however, that Case 3 is the oldest sibling and the severity of skeletal deformities tends to worsen with puberty [7], which may explain these skeletal deformities in the oldest sibling.

The decision to obtain genetic testing in Case 1 was made based on the combination of his severe short stature and shortened arm span. His siblings were subsequently tested based on their known family history and significant short stature. When deciding when to pursue testing for SHOX deletion, there are a variety of clinical features to consider. Binder et al. [9] demonstrated that patients with SHOX deletion have shortened arm span for age, as well as one characteristic radiological sign of Leri-Weill-dyschondrosteosis, and concluded that these would be reasonable features to trigger initial SHOX gene testing in a patient with idiopathic short stature. Rappold et al. [5] developed a phenotype scoring system to aid this decision making, based on 8 dysmorphic features and anthropometric measurements including elevated sitting height/height ratio. Malaquias et al. [10] demonstrated that an elevated sitting height/height ratio alone is a useful tool for selecting short children for SHOX analysis. Due to medical record limitations, these additional measurements are unavailable in these 7 cases.

Using the rationale that girls with Turner syndrome, whose short stature is believed to be due, at least in part, to SHOX haploinsufficiency, have had good response to GH treatment [8], GH was later evaluated in children with isolated SHOX deficiency. Blum et al. [7] evaluated the efficacy of GH therapy in children with short stature and SHOX deficiency in a randomized, controlled trial. The GH treatment, dosed at 50 μg/kg, resulted in significant increase in first- and second-year height velocities and in height SDS. Blum et al. [11] later found that GH treatment produces similar height gains for patients with SHOX deficiency when compared to girls with Turner syndrome. SHOX deficiency became an FDA approved indication for GH therapy in 2006 [9]. In this family, GH treatment was initiated upon diagnosis of SHOX deficiency related short stature, given the literature on the benefits on height gains in this patient population [11–13].

Consistent with previous observations, our patients all have a trend of improvement in their height SDS. In this family, there are a wide variety of ages at GH treatment onset as well as varied duration of GH treatment; however, we see that the two cases with the largest improvement in their SDS scores (Cases 1 and 2) also had the two longest durations of GH therapy. Based on the literature of girls with Turner syndrome, this is not surprising, as we would expect that the longer duration of treatment with GH would tend to lead to better improvement in height SDS [8]. This emphasizes the importance of early diagnosis of SHOX deficiency and early start of GH treatment before puberty triggers epiphyseal closure. In fact, Scalco et al. [14] demonstrated benefit of combining GH with GnRH therapy in children with SHOX defects who had just started puberty, to limit loss of growth potential triggered by puberty, and allow longer treatment duration.

Although there is known benefit of early initiation of GH therapy in older children, there is no precedent to direct the timing of GH initiation in a younger patient with known SHOX deficiency. Davenport et al. [15] showed that early GH treatment can correct growth failure and normalize height in infants and toddlers with Turner syndrome without significant adverse effect. Also, De Schepper et al. [16] studied the use of GH in very young children (<30 months) with failed catch-up growth after being born small for gestational age and found no significant negative impact mental or motor development in the very young children treated with GH, compared to the controls. Given these observations, three of the siblings (Cases 5, 6, and 7) were started on GH even before the age of 2, in an effort to maximize benefit of GH therapy on height.

In this family, the parents were never tested for SHOX deficiency. Presumably, one of the parents is heterozygous for this novel mutation and likely the proband for this mutation. Assuming the second parent is unaffected, a 50% inheritance rate would be anticipated, though in this family the inheritance rate was higher, at 70%, creating a unique opportunity to study 7 siblings from the same family.

In summary, SHOX deficiency should be considered in the differential diagnosis of children with severe short stature even in the absence of typical phenotypic features. A short parent, as well as other siblings with short stature, may increase the possibility of SHOX deficiency. Unfortunately, the diagnosis can be done only by genetic testing, which is costly and may not be available in many countries, and, as a result, testing should be reserved for children for whom there is a moderately high clinical suspicion for SHOX deficiency. GH treatment improves height with more favorable outcome when it is used for longer duration prior to epiphyseal fusion.

Abbreviations

SHOX: Short stature homeobox-containing
GH: Growth hormone.

Authors' Contributions

Elizabeth S. Sandberg acquired the clinical data, analyzed and interpreted the data, and drafted the manuscript. Lydia L. Snyder provided guidance to Elizabeth S. Sandberg in data acquisition, aided in analysis and interpretation of the data, and revised the manuscript. Karen J. Loechner diagnosed the index case, provided guidance in analysis and interpretation of the data, and revised the manuscript. Ali S. Calikoglu provided guidance to Elizabeth S. Sandberg in data acquisition, case report conception and design, analysis, and interpretation of data and revised the manuscript.

References

[1] G. Binder, "Short stature due to SHOX deficiency: Genotype, phenotype, and therapy," *Hormone Research in Paediatrics*, vol. 75, no. 2, pp. 81–89, 2011.

[2] V. A. Hamosh McKusick and A. Hamosh McKusick, "Short Stature Homeobox; SHOX," *Online Mendelian Inheritance in Man*, 2013, https://www.omim.org/entry/312865.

[3] E. Rao, B. Weiss, M. Fukami et al., "Pseudoautosomal deletions encompassing a novel homeobox gene cause growth failure in idiopathic short stature and Turner syndrome," *Nature Genetics*, vol. 16, no. 1, pp. 54–63, 1997.

[4] J. W. Ellison, Z. Wardak, M. F. Young, P. Gehron Robey, M. Laig-Webster, and W. Chiong, "PHOG, a candidate gene for involvement in the short stature of Turner syndrome," *Human Molecular Genetics*, vol. 6, no. 8, pp. 1341–1347, 1997.

[5] G. Rappold, W. F. Blum, E. P. Shavrikova et al., "Genotypes and phenotypes in children with short stature: Clinical indicators of SHOX haploinsufficiency," *Journal of Medical Genetics*, vol. 44, no. 5, pp. 306–313, 2007.

[6] C. Munns and I. Glass, "SHOX-related haploinsufficiency disorders," *GeneReviews*, 2005.

[7] W. F. Blum, B. J. Crowe, C. A. Quigley et al., "Growth hormone is effective in treatment of short stature associated with short stature homeobox-containing gene deficiency: Two-year results of a randomized, controlled, multicenter trial," *Journal of Clinical Endocrinology and Metabolism*, vol. 92, no. 1, pp. 219–228, 2007.

[8] N. Sabherwal, R. J. Blaschke, A. Marchini et al., "A novel point mutation A170P in the SHOX gene defines impaired nuclear translocation as a molecular cause for Léri-Weill dyschondrosteosis and Langer dysplasia.," *Journal of medical genetics*, vol. 41, no. 6, p. e83, 2004.

[9] G. Binder, M. B. Ranke, and D. D. Martin, "Auxology Is a Valuable Instrument for the Clinical Diagnosis of SHOX Haploinsufficiency in School-Age Children with Unexplained Short Stature," *Journal of Clinical Endocrinology and Metabolism*, vol. 88, no. 10, pp. 4891–4896, 2003.

[10] A. C. Malaquias, R. C. Scalco, E. G. P. Fontenele et al., "The sitting height/height ratio for age in healthy and short individuals and its potential role in selecting short children for SHOX analysis," *Hormone Research in Paediatrics*, vol. 80, no. 6, pp. 449–456, 2014.

[11] W. F. Blum, J. L. Ross, A. G. Zimmermann et al., "GH treatment to final height produces similar height gains in patients with SHOX deficiency and turner syndrome: Results of a multicenter trial," *Journal of Clinical Endocrinology and Metabolism*, vol. 98, no. 8, pp. E1383–E1392, 2013.

[12] C. J. Child, G. Kalifa, C. Jones et al., "Radiological features in patients with short stature homeobox-containing (SHOX) gene deficiency and turner syndrome before and after 2 years of gh treatment," *Hormone Research in Paediatrics*, vol. 84, no. 1, pp. 14–25, 2015.

[13] S. H. Donze, C. R. Meijer, S. G. Kant et al., "The growth response to GH treatment is greater in patients with SHOX enhancer deletions compared to SHOX defects," *European Journal of Endocrinology*, vol. 173, no. 5, pp. 611–621, 2015.

[14] R. C. Scalco, S. S. J. Melo, P. N. Pugliese-Pires et al., "Effectiveness of the combined recombinant human growth hormone and gonadotropin-releasing hormone analog therapy in pubertal patients with short stature due to SHOX deficiency," *Journal of Clinical Endocrinology and Metabolism*, vol. 95, no. 1, pp. 328–332, 2010.

[15] M. L. Davenport, B. J. Crowe, S. H. Travers et al., "Growth hormone treatment of early growth failure in toddlers with turner syndrome: A randomized, controlled, multicenter trial," *Journal of Clinical Endocrinology and Metabolism*, vol. 92, no. 9, pp. 3406–3416, 2007.

[16] J. De Schepper, J. Vanderfaeillie, P.-E. Mullis et al., "A 2-year multicentre, open-label, randomized, controlled study of growth hormone (Genotropin®) treatment in very young children born small for gestational age: Early Growth and Neurodevelopment (EGN) Study," *Clinical Endocrinology*, vol. 84, no. 3, pp. 353–360, 2016.

31

Artifactual Hypoglycaemia in Systemic Sclerosis and Raynaud's Phenomenon: A Clinical Case Report and Short Review

RH Bishay[1,2] and A. Suryawanshi[1,2]

[1]*Department of Endocrinology and Metabolism, Concord Repatriation General Hospital, Concord, Sydney, NSW 2139, Australia*
[2]*Sydney Medical School, University of Sydney, Sydney, NSW 2005, Australia*

Correspondence should be addressed to RH Bishay; ramy.bishay@gmail.com

Academic Editor: Wayne V. Moore

Background. Artifactual hypoglycaemia, defined as a discrepancy between glucometer (capillary) and plasma glucose levels, may lead to overtreatment and costly investigations. It is not infrequently observed in patients with Raynaud's phenomenon due to vascular capillary distortion, yet this is clinically underappreciated. *Case Report.* We report a 76-year-old woman with systemic sclerosis and Raynaud's phenomenon, who presented with upper gastrointestinal bleeding and found to have concomitant persistent hypoglycaemia (1.0–2.7 mmol/L) on a point-of-care glucometer in the absence hypoglycaemic symptoms. She underwent a 2-week hospital admission, repeated glucose monitoring, hydrocortisone replacement and dextrose infusions, with consequent hyperglycaemia on plasma measurements. Clinically, she did not satisfy *Whipple's* triad and radiological investigations failed to identify pituitary or pancreatic pathology. A 72-hour fast was negative for hyperinsulinaemia or exogenous insulin use and her sulphonylurea metabolite urinary screen was negative. *Discussion.* Treatment of low capillary blood glucose is usually met with clinical impetus to treat, even when hypoglycaemic symptoms are lacking. The correct diagnosis may have been achieved had there been an observation of her cold hands, scleroderma facies, and consideration of the likely distorted peripheral microvasculature. Early identification of this presumably rare clinical scenario may have prevented overtreatment, altered methods of monitoring, and avoided unnecessary investigations.

1. Background

Systemic sclerosis (previously known as scleroderma) is a multisystem disease with complex pathophysiology that results from extensive fibrosis, abnormal vascular tone, and autoimmunity to multiple cellular epitopes [1]. Raynaud's phenomenon, where there is an exaggerated vasoconstriction of peripheral blood vessels, can precede the diagnosis for many years [1]. With few exceptions, there are a limited number of reports in the literature of artifactual hypoglycaemia, also used interchangeably (albeit erroneously) with pseudohypoglycaemia, in patients with Raynaud's phenomenon and/or systemic sclerosis [2, 3] due to the abnormal blood transit time in peripheral capillaries. The following case illustrates the need for high clinical suspicion in patients with whom critically low glucose levels are obtained by capillary blood glucose measurements yet deny the classical symptoms of hypoglycaemia.

2. Case Report

A 76-year-old Caucasian female presented to the emergency department from home with a 1-day history of symptomatic anaemia and fatigue in the context of melaena. She denied respiratory or cardiac symptoms or a history of weight loss, painful defecation, obstruction, use of nonsteroidal anti-inflammatory medications, a history of upper gastrointestinal ulceration or *H. pylori* infection. Her past medical history was significant for centromere antibody positive systemic sclerosis with features of the CREST syndrome, inclusive of pulmonary fibrosis, severe pulmonary hypertension, Raynaud's phenomenon, gastric antral vascular ectasia, gastritis, and reflux oesophagitis; she also had postmenopausal osteoporosis exacerbated by corticosteroid use. Her medications included long-term prednisone 15 mg daily, bosentan 62.5 mg BD, furosemide 20 mg daily, esomeprazole 20 mg daily, denosumab 60 mg S/C six-monthly, cholecalciferol 1000 U daily,

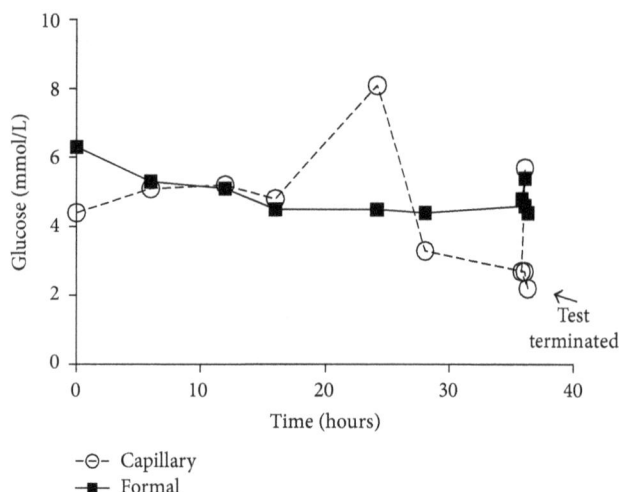

FIGURE 1: A seventy-two-hour fast protocol revealed a discrepancy between capillary (point-of-care glucometer) and venous blood glucose levels. The test was terminated early due to low capillary glucose levels (2.2 mmol/L).

and calcium carbonate 600 mg daily. She lived alone, is a life-long nonsmoker, and consumes 1-2 standard drinks of alcohol daily. She is independent of daily activities.

On examination, she appeared unwell and thin (body mass index 17.5 kg/m^2) with cool peripheries and scleroderma facies. Blood pressure was 70 mmHg systolic, heart rate was 70 beats per minute, and cardiorespiratory examination revealed fine, bibasal crackles consistent with pulmonary fibrosis. Gastrointestinal examination noted melaena on *per rectal* examination but no stigmata of chronic liver disease.

Initial point-of-care capillary glucometer readings revealed glucose levels of 1.7 mmol/L, 1.3 mmol/L, and then 1.0 mmol/L taken at 15-minute intervals. The patient denied sympathetic (i.e., palpitations, diaphoresis, and tremor) or neuroglycopenic (i.e., confusion, headache, visual changes, and nausea) symptoms associated with hypoglycaemia and denied a history of diabetes, exogenous use of insulin, or insulin secretagogues. Investigations revealed a formal glucose of 28.3 mmol/L. She also had normocytic anaemia (haemoglobin of 63 g/L [120–150]) with preserved renal function. Platelet count was normal with mildly deranged gamma-glutamyl transferase (130 U/L, [<35]), international normalised ratio (INR) (1.3), and reduced albumin (27 g/L [38–48]). Haemolytic anaemia screen was negative and iron studies revealed iron deficiency (transferrin saturation 13% [15–50], ferritin 41 ug/L [20–300]). C-reactive protein was 16.3. Thyroid function and lipase were within normal limits.

Acute management included two stat boluses of dextrose, with capillary blood glucose levels temporarily increasing from 1.0 mmol/L to 7.0 mmol/L and remaining unexpectedly low-normal (4.7 to 5.5 mmol/L). The patient was admitted to the high-dependency unit and, given her history of corticosteroid use and presumptive diagnosis of adrenal insufficiency, was given stress hydrocortisone doses, moderate fluid resuscitation, intravenous proton-pump inhibitor infusion, and several units of transfused packed red blood cells.

Her chest X-ray revealed longstanding ill-defined ground glass opacities. The patient underwent a gastroscopy which diagnosed severe ulcerative esophagitis as the cause of her bleeding. She had a 2-week admission with several medical review alerts for asymptomatic hypoglycaemia. Capillary glucose levels were consistently between 1.7 and 3.8 mmol/L. The patient eventually recovered well and was discharged on esomeprazole 20 mg BD without further melaena.

The patient underwent a 72-hour fast protocol that was terminated early due to hypoglycaemia (≤2.2 mmol/L) on capillary glucose monitoring (Figure 1). Her pituitary profile (adrenocorticotrophic hormone, morning cortisol, prolactin, growth hormone, insulin growth factor-1, and thyroid function) was within normal limits (not shown). Gonadotrophins were consistent with menopause. Given her anaemia, a computed tomographic imaging of her abdomen was performed to assess for malignancy, which was normal. Magnetic resonance imaging of her brain did not reveal pituitary apoplexy or other compressive sellar or suprasellar lesions.

3. Discussion

Artifactual hypoglycaemia has no clear definition but has been proposed to be defined as a discrepancy between capillary and plasma blood glucose levels, due to either differing laboratory techniques or other patient factors, as in our index patient. Pseudohypoglycaemia in contrast is defined as the presence of typical sympathetic or neuroglycopenic symptoms in the presence of a blood glucose level >3.9 mmol/L [4]. Artifactual hypoglycaemia in patients with systemic sclerosis is thought to be due to low capillary blood glucose levels due to reduced capillary flow, leading to deceleration of glucose transit and subsequent increased uptake of glucose by local tissues [5]. Patients with systemic sclerosis have vascular injury affecting primarily small vessels and arterioles that occurs early in the disease process, which can distort the integrity of the endothelial lining and results in progressive thinning of capillaries and loss of blood vessels [6, 7].

Confounding aspects contributing to her low capillary blood glucose levels included blood loss due to melaena and hypotension, which may have caused peripheral shunting of blood volume, as well as her long history of glucocorticoid use and possible adrenal insufficiency. However, even after correcting both of these conditions, the capillary hypoglycaemia persisted. In fact, relatively large volumes of dextrose and intravenous hydrocortisone may have precipitated worsening hyperglycaemia and the possible development of hyperosmolar hyperglycaemic state or diabetic ketoacidosis. Thus, the correct diagnosis is paramount to avoid further inpatient metabolic disturbance.

Previous case reports of patients with artifactual hypoglycaemia in the context of systemic sclerosis with Raynaud's phenomenon all seemingly had very low fasting and random capillary, point-of-care measurements using a glucometer, ranging between 0.61 mmol/L and 3 mmol/L [2, 3, 8, 9]. In all cases, blood samples taken from either the forearm or a vein from the cubital fossa were normal however. The majority of patients underwent screening for hypopituitarism with a tetracosactide test as well as 72-hour fast to exclude endogenous hyperinsulinaemia, as in our index patient. Obtaining symptoms from history is critical as most patients will deny the classic sympathetic and neuroglycopenic symptoms of hypoglycaemia and therefore do not satisfy *Whipple's* triad. *Whipple's* triad confirms true hypoglycaemia secondary to endogenous hyperinsulinaemia and includes the following criteria: (i) typical symptoms of hypoglycaemia with (ii) a low plasma glucose measured at the time of the symptoms and (iii) relief of these symptoms when the glucose is raised to normal; none of these criteria were met by the patient. *Whipple's* triad is also a necessary to establish grounds for a 72-hour fast to exclude the presence of an insulinoma, the commonest functioning neuroendocrine tumour arising from the pancreas. In some cases, however, symptoms alone cannot be relied upon as many patients may falsely attribute nonspecific complaints to hypoglycaemia [8]. Other investigations including insulin, proinsulin, glucagon, cortisol, growth hormone, and hydroxybutyrate (a surrogate marker of starvation and inversely related to insulin secretion) are expectedly normal. All patients however should be assessed for surreptitious insulin or sulphonylurea use, the latter with a urinary sulphonylurea metabolite analysis.

Although the terms artifactual hypoglycaemia (coined in the 1960s) and pseudohypoglycaemia continue to be used interchangeably, there is a potential for some confusion since the American Diabetes Association and the Endocrine Society workgroup favoured the use of the term pseudohypoglycaemia in 2013 [4]. Its definition is problematic in at least three scenarios: (1) it does not differentiate between pseudohypoglycaemia from patients with symptoms attributable to other causes and falsely low glucose readings from a point-of-care glucometer, as in our index patient; (2) patients who are chronically hyperglycaemic who have sudden correction of their glucose to normal levels may have similar symptoms in the presence of normal capillary glucose levels; and (3) patients with poor glycaemic control may, in the context of a condition or a medication that affects capillary glucose readings, be falsely reassured of optimal glycaemic control. Therefore, the authors support the distinction between pseudohypoglycaemia and artifactual hypoglycaemia, the latter being better suited to our case.

It is notable to mention other causes of pseudohypoglycaemia, which are summarised in Table 1, such as disorders that lead to impaired capillary blood flow, increased glycolysis, hyperviscosity and medications [10] as well as preanalytic factors. Leukemia, in particular, can lead to artifactual hypoglycaemia due to the increased glucose metabolism by a large number of leukocytes.

In summary, clinicians should be mindful of the limitations of point-of-care blood glucose measurements (i.e., glucometer). In general, low capillary glucose levels (e.g., <3 mmol/L) without associated sympathetic or neuroglycopenic symptoms should prompt formal blood glucose testing concomitant with a capillary glucose level to assess for a difference, as well as a reasonable search for other possible causes. Artifactual hypoglycaemia is inadvertently common in patients with systemic sclerosis due to abnormal capillary blood flow; hence heightened vigilance is required in interpreting capillary glucose values. Currently, there is no

TABLE 1: Causes of pseudohypoglycaemia or artifactual hypoglycaemia.

Mechanism	Examples
Impaired capillary blood flow	Raynaud's phenomenon, acrocyanosis, peripheral vascular disease, Eisenmenger syndrome, circulatory shock, hypothermia
Increased glycolysis	Leukemia, polycythemia vera
Hyperviscosity	Plasma cell dyscrasias, for example, multiple myeloma, monoclonal gammopathy of unknown significance, Waldenstrom macroglobulinaemia
Medication	Ascorbic acid, dopamine, mannitol, acetaminophen
Preanalytic factors	Delay in separation of plasma from formed blood contents

consensus on establishing a distinction between pseudohypoglycaemia and artifactual hypoglycaemia, though confirmation of the latter can help alleviate the unnecessary burden of multiple investigations, taxing healthcare expenditure, and provocation of patient anxiety that often accompanies these seemingly well patients.

Additional Points

Novelty Statement. (i) Artifactual hypoglycaemia has real clinical implications, that is, when point-of-care glucometer readings are incorrect or misleading. (ii) Patients with Raynaud's phenomenon may display persistent artifactual hypoglycaemia due to distorted peripheral vasculature; this observation however is underrecognised in clinical practise and scarcely reported in literature. (iii) Costly monitoring, aggressive management, and radiological examinations often accompany the finding of persistent capillary hypoglycaemia in patients with Raynaud's phenomenon; this should be replaced with high clinical suspicion and consideration of a secondary cause of hypoglycaemia. (iv) In general, secondary causes of hypoglycaemia should be considered if the hypoglycaemia is persistent, symptoms are lacking, or conventional treatment is ineffective.

Authors' Contributions

RH Bishay provided substantial contributions to conception and design, drafted the article and revised it critically, and approved the final version to be published. A. Suryawanshi was clinically involved in the care of the patient, provided substantial critical review of the case report, and also approved the final version.

References

[1] A. Gabrielli, E. V. Avvedimento, and T. Krieg, "Mechanisms of disease: scleroderma," *New England Journal of Medicine*, vol. 360, no. 19, pp. 1989–2003, 2009.

[2] M. El Khoury, F. Yousuf, V. Martin, and R. M. Cohen, "Pseudohypoglycemia: a cause for unreliable finger-stick glucose measurements," *Endocrine Practice*, vol. 14, no. 3, pp. 337–339, 2008.

[3] V. D. Tarasova, M. Zena, and M. Rendell, "Artifactual hypoglycemia: an old term for a new classification," *Diabetes Care*, vol. 37, no. 5, pp. e85–e86, 2014.

[4] E. R. Seaquist, J. Anderson, B. Childs et al., "Hypoglycaemia and diabetes: a report of a workgroup of the American Diabetes Association and the Endocrine Society," *Diabetes Care*, vol. 36, no. 5, pp. 1384–1395, 2013.

[5] E. A. H. McGuire, J. H. Helderman, J. D. Tobin, R. Andres, and M. Berman, "Effects of arterial versus venous sampling on analysis of glucose kinetics in man," *Journal of Applied Physiology*, vol. 41, no. 4, pp. 565–573, 1976.

[6] R. J. Prescott, A. J. Freemont, C. J. P. Jones, J. Hoyland, and P. Fielding, "Sequential dermal microvascular and perivascular changes in the development of scleroderma," *Journal of Pathology*, vol. 166, no. 3, pp. 255–263, 1992.

[7] R. Fleischmajer and J. S. Perlish, "Capillary alterations in scleroderma," *Journal of the American Academy of Dermatology*, vol. 2, no. 2, pp. 161–170, 1980.

[8] F. R. Kaufman, L. C. Gibson, M. Halvorson, S. Carpenter, L. K. Fisher, and P. Pitukcheewanont, "A pilot study off the continuous glucose monitoring system: clinical decisions and glycemic control after its use in pediatric type 1 diabetic subjects," *Diabetes Care*, vol. 24, no. 12, pp. 2030–2034, 2001.

[9] "Abstracts of the Society of Hospital Medicine Annual Meeting. April 1–4, 2012. San Diego, California, USA," *Journal of Hospital Medicine*, vol. 7, supplement 2, pp. S1–S323, 2012.

[10] Z. Tang, X. Du, R. F. Louie, and G. J. Kost, "Effects of drugs on glucose measurements with handheld glucose meters and a portable glucose analyzer," *American Journal of Clinical Pathology*, vol. 113, no. 1, pp. 75–86, 2000.

32

Syndrome of Reduced Sensitivity to Thyroid Hormones: Two Case Reports and a Literature Review

Anastasios Anyfantakis,[1] Dimitrios Anyfantakis,[2] and Irene Vourliotaki[1]

[1]*Department of Endocrinology, Venizeleio General Hospital, Heraklion, Crete, Greece*
[2]*Primary Health Care Centre of Kissamos, Chania, Crete, Greece*

Correspondence should be addressed to Dimitrios Anyfantakis; danyfantakis@med.uoc.gr

Academic Editor: Thomas Grüning

Resistance to thyroid hormone (RTH) is an extremely rare dominantly inherited condition of impaired tissue responsiveness to thyroid hormone (TH). Most patients with RTH have mutations in the gene that encodes the β isoform of the receptor of thyroid hormone (*THR-β* gene). Mutant receptors are unable to activate or repress target genes. The majority of them are asymptomatic or rarely have hypo- or hyperthyroidism. RTH is suspected by the finding of persistent elevation of serum levels of free T3 (FT3) and free T4 (FT4) and nonsuppressed TSH. We present two cases of RTH diagnosed after total thyroidectomy. The first patient was initially diagnosed with primary hyperthyroidism due to toxic multinodular goiter. The second patient had undergone thyroidectomy for multinodular goiter 16 years before diagnosis of RTH. After thyroidectomy, although on relatively high doses of levothyroxine, both of them presented with the laboratory findings of RTH. Genetic analysis revealed RTH.

1. Introduction

RTH is an unusual dominantly inherited condition of impaired tissue responsiveness to TH, expressed clinically by the persistent elevation of serum levels of FT3 and FT4 and inappropriate high levels of TSH. These hormone levels reflect a compensated endocrine state in which increased levels of TH are required to establish normal levels of TSH. Despite the high TH levels, TSH responds to stimulation with TSH releasing hormone (TRH) and the levels of TH required to suppress TSH and produce metabolic effects on peripheral tissues are higher than normal [1]. The incidence of RTH is probably 1 case per 50000 live births [2]. Syndrome of RTH is rarely suspected due to its heterogenous presentation and atypical symptoms at onset. Goiter is the principal clinical finding which is usually further investigated [3]. In most cases the elevated TH levels compensate for the tissue resistance, so the individuals are euthyroid. However, not rarely, the compensation appears to be incomplete and hypothyroidism is produced. Rarely, high endogenous thyroid hormone levels can produce toxic effects on peripheral tissues. Here we present two cases with RTH. A literature review on the diagnosis and management of the condition is also performed.

2. Case Presentation

2.1. 1st Patient. A 58-year-old male was referred by his general practitioner to the Endocrinology Department of the Venizeleio General Hospital of Heraklion, Crete, Greece, due to frequent episodes of sinoatrial tachycardia. His personal medical history was free, with no known thyroid disease in his family. His weight and height were 79 kg and 175 cm, respectively (BMI 26). Clinically, his thyroid was enlarged with multinodular consistency at palpation. Laboratory investigation disclosed suppressed TSH with FT3 and FT4 levels higher than the upper normal limits (Table 1). AntiTg and antiTPO autoantibodies were negative. Thyroid ultrasound revealed multinodular goiter with a dominant nodule of 1.8 cm maximum diameter. Increased uptake was found on the Tc99 thyroid scan. Whole blood count, erythrocyte sedimentation rate, liver and renal function, and the rest of biochemical parameters were all normal, except for triglycerides, which were found elevated (230 mg/dL). The patient was diagnosed to have multinodular toxic goiter and was prescribed carbimazole at a starting dose of 45 mg/d, which was gradually tapered. Three months later, while on carbimazole 15 mg/d, he became euthyroid (TSH, FT3

TABLE 1: TSH, FT3, and FT4 levels and antithyroid medication in the first patient, before thyroidectomy.

TSH (μUI/mL)	FT3 (pg/mL)	FT4 (ng/dL)	Medication
0.06	7.85	2.42	None: prescribed carbimazole 45 mg/d
5.16	4.8	1.92	Carbimazole 25 mg/d
0.94	3.83	2.39	Carbimazole 15 mg/d

Normal values: TSH = 0.4–4 μUI/mL.
FT3 = 1.8–4.2 pg/mL.
FT4 = 0.8–1.9 ng/dL.

TABLE 2: TSH, FT3, and FT4 levels and levothyroxine therapy in both patients, after thyroidectomy.

	TSH (μUI/mL)	FT3 (pg/mL)	FT4 (ng/dL)	Medication (levothyroxine)
1st patient	65.6	1.59	0.81	100 μg/d
	22.7	3.51	2.4	200 μg/d
	14.3	3.17	2.59	300 μg/d
	5.5	4.3	2.91	325 μg/d
2nd patient	32	4	1.87	150 μg/d
	20.8	4.5	2.05	200
	10.3	4.3	3.16	250
	5.3	5	3.50	300

normal), although FT4 was marginally elevated. This finding was not considered at that time. It should be mentioned that, after 3 months, while he was on carbimazole 15 mg/d, high levels of FT3 and FT4 did not suppress TSH, as expected; on the contrary, TSH was found to be a little elevated (Table 1). This finding was not considered at that time. Five months later he underwent near total thyroidectomy. Biopsy showed multinodular goiter with no signs of malignancy. There were no complications after surgery but it proved difficult to treat his postsurgical hypothyroidism, with levothyroxine at doses higher than usual.

While he was on levothyroxine 300 μg/d, TSH remained elevated with FT4 and FT3 above the upper normal limits (Table 2). Differential diagnosis included either a TSH-producing pituitary adenoma or RTH, in which tissue insensitivity to the action of TH is compensated by elevated levels of these hormones without suppression of TSH. In order to discriminate between these two conditions, the patient had a TRH test while on levothyroxine 300 μg/d. TSH increased from basal levels of 14.3 μUI/mL to peak levels of 70 μUI/mL thirty minutes after the i.v. administration of 200 μg TRH.

The diagnosis of RTH was even more suspected, as MRI of the pituitary was negative for any lesion and the rest of the pituitary hormones were found normal. Next diagnostic test was genetic analysis for RTH, which proved to be positive. In terms of further investigation of RTH, metabolic markers affected by TH, such as cholesterol and triglycerides, were found elevated. Ferritin and liver enzymes were normal and Sex Hormone Binding Globulin (SHBG) was low normal (Table 3). Finally, the dose of levothyroxine was increased to 325 μg/d. It was well tolerated and the patient presented with tissue euthyroidism, as it was evidenced by metabolic markers (Table 3). TH profile was the optimum until that time (Table 2).

2.2. 2nd Patient. A 32-year-old woman was referred by her general practitioner to our Department for post thyroidectomy hypothyroidism, resistant to usual doses of levothyroxine. She had had near total thyroidectomy at the age of 16 because of multinodular goiter with a dominant cold nodule. No malignancy was found on biopsy. Clinical examination was normal. Her weight was 70 kg and her height was 160 cm (BMI 28). Her personal medical history was free and no thyroid disease was reported in her family. At the time of referral and while on levothyroxine 150 μg/d, her TSH was high, with FT3 and FT4 unexpectedly normal (Table 2). Liver and renal function tests were normal (Table 3). Thyroid ultrasound showed a small remnant with no nodules. The dose of levothyroxine was increased to 200 and then to 250 μg/d, but TSH levels remained high, despite the fact that FT3 and FT4 were above the upper limits of the normal range (Table 2). Taking levothyroxine 250 μg/d the patient complained of palpitations and at that time she did not try any higher dose. As in the first patient, in order to clarify the possibility of RTH, we performed a TRH test, while the patient was on levothyroxine 250 μg/d. Her serum TSH increased from basal levels of 11 μUI/mL to peak levels of 110 μUI/mL thirty minutes after the i.v. administration of 200 μg TRH. Consequently, the diagnosis of RTH was highly suspected. MRI of the pituitary did not show any lesion and the rest of the pituitary hormones were found normal.

Metabolic markers, such as cholesterol and triglycerides, were normal, ferritin was low normal, and SHBG was found low. Liver enzymes were within normal limits, except for Alkaline Phosphatase (ALP), which was high (Table 3). Genetic analysis revealed RTH syndrome. Finally, on levothyroxine 300 μg/d the patient's TSH was decreased to just above the upper normal limits, FT3 and FT4 were marginally elevated, and metabolic markers remained within normal limits (Tables 2 and 3).

TABLE 3: Markers of metabolism on increasing doses of levothyroxine, in both patients.

	SHBG (nmol/L)	ALP (U/I)	Ferritin (ng/mL)	Cholesterol (mg/dL)	Triglycerides (mg/dL)	SGOT (U/I)	SGPT (U/I)	Medication (levothyroxine) (μg/d)
1st patient	—	74	—	310	198	21	20	100
	18.7	81	—	—	—	20	18	200
	19.4	68	59.7	250	173	14	15	250
	21.7	80	46.5	247	165	12	15	300
	18	65	40	200	149	13	14	325
2nd patient	—	110	—	—	—	12	17	150
	8.17	125	21.1	190	55	14	16	200
	22.7	111	35.16	188	63	14	21	300

Normal values:

SHBG (sex hormone binding globulin): 18–114 nmol/L females, 13–71 nmol/L males.

ALP (alkaline phosphatase): 42–98 U/I.

Ferritin: 17–293 ng/mL males, 7–283 ng/mL females.

SGOT: 10–40 U/I.

SGPT: 10–35 U/I.

Concomitant administration of atenolol 25 mg/d controlled tachycardia.

3. Genetic Analysis

Genetic analysis was performed in both index cases by using high-molecular-weight DNA isolated from white blood cells [4]. Exons 7, 8, 9, and 10 of the *THRβ* gene were amplified by PCR using specific primers [5]. For sequencing, unwanted dNTPs and primers were removed from PCR products using ExoSAP-IT (# 78201, USB, Cleveland, USA). In brief, $2\,\mu L$ of ExoSAP-IT was added to $5\,\mu L$ of PCR product and was incubated at 37°C for 20 min and 80°C for 10 min. After that, we added $0.5\,\mu L$ (20 pmol) of specific primer and $2\,\mu L$ of sequencing Mix (BigDye® Terminator v3.1 cycle sequencing kit # 4336911, Applied Biosystems, Foster City, CA). Reactions were run in a 3100 automated DNA sequencer (Applied Biosystems, Foster City, CA). Sequence analysis of exon 10 in the 1st patient showed a heterozygous single base pair substitution of C to T at codon 383 resulting in a change from arginine to cytosine (R383C). This mutation has been previously described [6]. Sequence analysis of exon 10 in the 2nd patient showed single base pair substitution of C to T at codon 448 to the end (codon 461) increasing the polypeptide chain length by two aminoacids. This mutation has also been described previously [7].

4. Discussion

Both of our patients were found to have mutations on the exon 10 of the *THRβ* gene.

Exons 8–10 in the carboxyterminus of the *THRβ* gene are the most common spots of mutations described in RTH [8]. Codon 453 is the most frequent site of mutations. RTH is generally inherited in the autosomal dominant manner. A total of about 150 different *THRβ* gene mutations have been identified so far [9, 10]. No mutation has been found to date in the *THRα* gene. Thyroid hormone receptors

(THRs) are encoded by two genes (*THRα*, *THRβ*) located on chromosomes 17 and 3, respectively. There are 4 *THR* isoforms: *THRβ1* and *THRβ2* derived from the *THRβ* gene and *THRα1* and *THRα2* from the *THRa* gene. They have in common a DNA binding domain (DBD) at their aminoterminus and, with the exception of the *THRα2* isoform, a TH (ligand) binding domain (LBD) at their carboxyterminus. The THRs associate with specific DNA sequences termed thyroid response elements (TREs). The THRs associated with TREs usually become functional only after binding of T3 on LBD. This produces a modulation in the rate of transcription of the target gene [11]. In the absence of T3, THR homodimers and heterodimers are associated with corepressors (NCoR and SMRT) that repress or silence the transcription of genes positively regulated by the ligand.

Binding of T3 to THRs releases the corepressors and recruits nuclear coactivators which stimulate gene transcription. Mutant THRβs interfere with the function of the wild type THRs, a phenomenon termed dominant negative effect (DNE). The DNE involves the occupation of a TRE by a mutant THR that cannot bind T3 or has reduced affinity for it, *tighter affinity* for the corepressors, or reduced ability to recruit coactivators necessary to enhance gene transcription. In some patients, mutations in the LBD are reported to maintain TH binding and yet cause RTH in certain tissues, due probably to selective impairment of TH-mediated gene repression [12].

Mutations in the *THRβ* gene were not found in a subgroup of patients with RTH. In the absence of *THRβ* mutations, an RTH phenotype could be caused by abnormal corepressors that fail to dissociate from THRs or defective coactivators that do not associate with THRs upon T3 binding [13–16]. There have also been reported cases of mosaicism, with the *THRβ* mutation present in some cell lineages, but not in others [17]. Most RTH patients undergo thyroidectomy for multinodular goiters. Goiter is a very common finding in RTH and is attributed to the continuously high levels of TSH. Additionally, in this syndrome TSH is reported to be of enhanced bioactivity. This could explain the relatively high percentage of RTH patients with goiter in the presence of normal levels of TSH and elevated TH levels [18].

There are no pathognomonic symptoms associated with RTH.

Its presentation is heterogenous [19]. The majority of individuals are completely asymptomatic, achieving normal growth and mental development, because the elevated thyroid hormone levels compensate for the tissue resistance.

In asymptomatic patients, Pulcrano et al., although, report the presence of echocardiographic signs similar to those reported in hypothyroid patients [20].

Diagnosis of the syndrome in asymptomatic patients is usually made on routine laboratory investigation in which "inappropriately high" TSH is discovered. In contrast, some patients with TH levels not necessarily elevated appear to be hypermetabolic with rapid heart rate [21]. More rarely, when RTH is not compensated, patients may present hypothyroid, especially in the rare cases where autoimmune thyroiditis coexists [22–24].

A possible reason for the variability in symptoms could be that not all the individuals express the same levels of normal and mutant THRs in their tissues [25]. Furthermore, not all mutations have the same effect on T3 binding [26]. Another factor could be the different tissue distribution of THRs' isoforms. For instance the heart is a predominantly THRα tissue. As the THRα is normal in RTH patients but their FT3 levels are high, it can be expected that they will react to the extra amount of T3 in a hyperthyroid manner, as far as heart is concerned [27]. Furthermore, not every individual will express the same amount of THRs or corepressors/coactivators in a particular tissue, leading to differences between patients.

For the diagnosis to be confirmed, the demonstration of reduced sensitivity of peripheral tissues to endogenous or exogenous TH is required. The degree of central resistance is assessed by the response of TSH to the TRH stimulation test. Usually, in RTH the TSH response to TRH is either normal or slightly exaggerated. In both of our patients, TSH showed a rather exaggerated response to TRH, while they received relatively high doses of levothyroxine. This is in accordance with RTH and also ameliorates the possibility of a TSH secreting pituitary adenoma. The majority of such adenomas are characterized by autonomous secretion of TSH [28], which neither responds to TRH nor is suppressed by increasing doses of administered T3 or T4. Peripheral resistance is estimated by metabolic markers such as serum SGOT, SGPT, ferritin, SHBG, cholesterol, and triglycerides. They are measured to determine the effect of TH on metabolism and hepatic function. CK and ankle jerk relaxation time are assessed to determine the effect of TH on neuromuscular system. Basal cardiac status is assessed with an echocardiogram and heart rate measurement.

Administration of TH in individuals without RTH causes alteration of these indexes, demonstrating a sensitivity to the rising T3 levels. In contrast, patients with RTH respond only to high doses of levothyroxine. The degree of sensitivity varies among tissues. Heart rate alone is a poor indicator of RTH status [29]. Such tests lack sufficient specificity and sensitivity to discriminate normal subjects from individuals with RTH. Lack of specificity is due to genetic and dietary factors, as well as alterations produced by age and sex. For these reasons the value of tests estimating the effects of TH on peripheral tissues is enhanced if determinations are obtained before and after the administration of TH with the subject serving as its own control [29]. In most patients, RTH appears to be adequately compensated (TSH near normal) by the increased endogenous supply of thyroid hormone. The 2nd patient seemed to belong to this category, as she was eumetabolic before thyroidectomy. Treatment should not be given to such individuals. Treatment with TH is reserved for those who, due to misdiagnosis, have received ablative therapy and have limited thyroid reserve and for subjects in whom the compensation appears to be incomplete due to the concomitant presence of autoimmune thyroid disease [1].

When RTH is not compensated, thyroid hormone should be given in incremental doses and parameters that are directly linked to TH action should be followed. Large goiters, a relatively common finding in RTH, are reported to regress with supraphysiological doses of TH [3]. In this direction as shown in Table 3, our patients did not become hypercatabolic, despite being treated with high doses of levothyroxine, which proved enough to bring TSH down almost to normal. The presence of tachycardia should not be a reason to detract treatment. It is best managed by the concomitant administration of atenolol. This β-adrenergic blocker is preferred, since it has the least inhibitory effect on the conversion of T4 to T3 [11]. The optimal dose of TH varies among individuals. Reduction of the serum TSH concentration to normal is a guide to therapy.

The 1st patient required levothyroxine 325 μg/d and the 2nd 300 μg/d. The dose of T3 or T4 required to achieve a beneficial effect is reported to be as high as 1000 μg/d and 500 μg/d, respectively. Triac is an acetic acid derivative of T4 and plays a minor role in normal thyroid physiology. However, it can be useful in the treatment of RTH, because it binds preferentially to the beta receptor [30]. Thus, adequate binding to certain mutated beta receptor can be achieved, without excessive stimulation of alpha receptors which predominate in the heart.

In conclusion, as the clinical presentation of RTH is atypical [31], the syndrome should be suspected whenever an individual presents with a high serum FT4 level, accompanied by a normal or even elevated TSH level. Despite the rarity of the condition, primary care physicians and endocrinologists should be alert when they encounter patients with these findings and a previous history of thyroidectomy receiving substitution therapy.

References

[1] R. E. Weiss and S. Refetoff, "Treatment of resistance to thyroid hormone—primum non nocere," *Journal of Clinical Endocrinology and Metabolism*, vol. 84, no. 2, pp. 401–404, 1999.

[2] D. Snyder, D. Sesser, M. Skeels, G. Nelson, and S. LaFrancis, "Thyroid disorders in newborn infants with elevated screening T4," *Thyroid*, vol. 7, supplement 1, pp. S1–S29, 1997.

[3] J. Anselmo and S. Refetoff, "Regression of a large goiter in a patient with resistance to thyroid hormone by every other day treatment with triiodothyronine," *Thyroid*, vol. 14, no. 1, pp. 71–74, 2004.

[4] S. A. Miller, D. D. Dykes, and H. F. Polesky, "A simple salting out procedure for extracting DNA from human nucleated cells," *Nucleic Acids Research*, vol. 16, no. 3, p. 1215, 1988.

[5] M. Adams, C. Matthews, T. N. Collingwood, Y. Tone, P. Beck-Peccoz, and K. K. Chatterjee, "Genetic analysis of 29 kindreds with generalized and pituitary resistance to thyroid hormone. Identification of thirteen novel mutations in the thyroid hormone receptor beta gene," *The Journal of Clinical Investigation*, vol. 94, no. 2, pp. 506–515, 1994.

[6] A. Margotat, G. Sarkissian, C. Malezet-Desmoulins et al., "Identification of eight new mutations in the c-erb AB gene of patients with resistance to thyroid hormone," *Annals of Endocrinology*, vol. 62, pp. 220–225, 2001.

[7] R. Parrilla, A. J. Mixson, J. A. McPherson, J. H. McClaskey, and B. D. Weintraub, "Characterization of seven novel mutations of the c-erbAβ gene in unrelated kindreds with generalized thyroid hormone resistance: evidence for two 'hot spot' regions of the ligand binding domain," *Journal of Clinical Investigation*, vol. 88, no. 6, pp. 2123–2130, 1991.

[8] S. Refetoff and A. M. Dumitrescu, "Syndromes of reduced sensitivity to thyroid hormone: genetic defects in hormone receptors, cell transporters and deiodination," *Best Practice & Research: Clinical Endocrinology & Metabolism*, vol. 21, no. 2, pp. 277–305, 2007.

[9] J. Lado-Abeal, A. M. Dumitrescu, X.-H. Liao et al., "A de novo mutation in an already mutant nucleotide of the thyroid hormone receptor β gene perpetuates resistance to thyroid hormone," *Journal of Clinical Endocrinology and Metabolism*, vol. 90, no. 3, pp. 1760–1767, 2005.

[10] C. M. Rivolta, M. C. Olcese, F. S. Belforte et al., "Genotyping of resistance to thyroid hormone in South American population. Identification of seven novel missense mutations in the human thyroid hormone receptor β gene," *Molecular and Cellular Probes*, vol. 23, no. 3-4, pp. 148–153, 2009.

[11] S. Refetoff, R. E. Weiss, and S. J. Usala, "The syndromes of resistance to thyroid hormone," *Endocrine Reviews*, vol. 14, no. 3, pp. 348–399, 1993.

[12] D. S. Machado, A. Sabet, L. A. Santiago et al., "A thyroid hormone receptor mutation that dissociates thyroid hormone regulation of gene expression in vivo," *Proceedings of the National Academy of Sciences of the United States of America*, vol. 106, no. 23, pp. 9441–9446, 2009.

[13] S. Reutrakul, P. M. Sadow, S. Pannain et al., "Search for abnormalities of nuclear corepressors, coactivators, and a coregulator in families with resistance to thyroid hormone without mutations in thyroid hormone receptor β or α genes," *Journal of Clinical Endocrinology and Metabolism*, vol. 85, no. 10, pp. 3609–3617, 2000.

[14] S. Romeo, C. Menzaghi, R. Bruno et al., "Search for genetic variants in the retinoid X receptor-γ gene by polymerase chain reaction-single-strand conformation polymorphism in patients with resistance to thyroid hormone without mutations in thyroid hormone receptor β gene," *Thyroid*, vol. 14, no. 5, pp. 355–358, 2004.

[15] P. Beck-Peccoz, L. Persani, D. Calebiro, M. Bonomi, D. Mannavola, and I. Campi, "Syndromes of hormone resistance in the hypothalamic-pituitary-thyroid axis," *Best Practice & Research: Clinical Endocrinology & Metabolism*, vol. 20, no. 4, pp. 529–546, 2006.

[16] Y. Bottcher, T. Paufler, T. Stehr, F. L. Bertschat, R. Paschke, and C. A. Koch, "Thyroid hormone resistance without mutations in thyroid hormone receptor beta," *Medical Science Monitor*, vol. 13, no. 6, pp. CS67–CS70, 2007.

[17] S. Mamanasiri, S. Yesil, A. M. Dumitrescu et al., "Mosaicism of a thyroid hormone receptor-β gene mutation in resistance to thyroid hormone," *The Journal of Clinical Endocrinology & Metabolism*, vol. 91, no. 9, pp. 3471–3477, 2006.

[18] L. Persani, C. Asteria, M. Tonacchera et al., "Evidence for the secretion of thyrotropin with enhanced bioactivity in syndromes of thyroid hormone resistance," *The Journal of Clinical Endocrinology & Metabolism*, vol. 78, pp. 1034–1039, 1994.

[19] P. Beck-Peccoz and V. K. K. Chatterjee, "The variable clinical phenotype in thyroid hormone resistance syndrome," *Thyroid*, vol. 4, no. 2, pp. 225–232, 1994.

[20] M. Pulcrano, E. A. Palmieri, D. Mannavola et al., "Impact of resistance to thyroid hormone on the cardiovascular system in adults," *The Journal of Clinical Endocrinology & Metabolism*, vol. 94, no. 8, pp. 2812–2816, 2009.

[21] T. Bayraktaroglu, J. Noel, F. Alagol, N. Colak, N. M. Mukaddes, and S. Refetoff, "Thyroid hormone receptor beta gene mutation (P453A) in a family producing resistance to thyroid hormone," *Experimental and Clinical Endocrinology & Diabetes*, vol. 117, no. 1, pp. 34–37, 2009.

[22] H. Sato and H. Sakai, "A family showing resistance to thyroid hormone associated with chronic thyroiditis and its clinical features: a case report," *Endocrine Journal*, vol. 53, no. 3, pp. 421–425, 2006.

[23] H. Sato, Y. Koike, M. Honma, M. Yagame, and K. Ito, "Evaluation of thyroid hormone action in a case of generalized resistance to thyroid hormone with chronic thyroiditis: discovery of a novel heterozygous missense mutation (G347A)," *Endocrine Journal*, vol. 54, no. 5, pp. 727–732, 2007.

[24] D. Y. Aksoy, A. Gurlek, U. Ringkananont, R. E. Weiss, and S. Refetoff, "Resistance to thyroid hormone associated with autoimmune thyroid disease in a Turkish family," *Journal of Endocrinological Investigation*, vol. 28, no. 4, pp. 379–383, 2005.

[25] A. J. Mixson, P. Hauser, G. Tennyson, J. C. Renault, D. L. Bodenner, and B. D. Weintraub, "Differential expression of mutant and normal beta T3 receptor alleles in kindreds with generalized resistance to thyroid hormone," *The Journal of Clinical Investigation*, vol. 91, no. 5, pp. 2296–2300, 1993.

[26] Y. Hayashi, R. E. Weiss, D. H. Sarne et al., "Do clinical manifestations of resistance to thyroid hormone correlate with the functional alteration of the corresponding mutant thyroid hormone-beta receptors?" *Journal of Clinical Endocrinology and Metabolism*, vol. 80, no. 11, pp. 3246–3256, 1995.

[27] G. J. Kahaly, C. H. Matthews, S. Mohr-Kahaly, C. A. Richards, and V. K. K. Chatterjee, "Cardiac involvement in thyroid hormone resistance," *Journal of Clinical Endocrinology and Metabolism*, vol. 87, no. 1, pp. 204–212, 2002.

[28] P. Caron, "Thyrotropin-secreting pituitary adenomas," *Presse Medicale*, vol. 38, no. 1, pp. 107–111, 2009.

[29] J. D. Safer, M. G. O'Connor, S. D. Colan, S. Srinivasan, S. R. Tollin, and F. E. Wondisford, "The thyroid hormone receptor-β gene mutation R383H is associated with isolated central resistance to thyroid hormone," *Journal of Clinical Endocrinology and Metabolism*, vol. 84, no. 9, pp. 3099–3109, 1999.

[30] S.-Y. Wu, W. L. Green, W.-S. Huang, M. T. Hays, and I. J. Chopra, "Alternate pathways of thyroid hormone metabolism," *Thyroid*, vol. 15, no. 8, pp. 943–958, 2005.

[31] A. J. Amor, I. Halperin, R. Alfayate et al., "Identification of four novel mutations in the thyroid hormone receptor-β gene in 164 Spanish and 2 Greek patients with resistance to thyroid hormone," *Hormones*, vol. 13, no. 1, pp. 74–78, 2014.

33

Primary Bone Marrow B-Cell Lymphoma Undetected by Multiple Imaging Modalities That Initially Presented with Hypercalcemia

Jin Sae Yoo,[1] Juwon Kim [ID],[2] Hyeong Ju Kwon,[3] and Jung Soo Lim [ID][1,4]

[1]Department of Internal Medicine, Wonju Severance Christian Hospital, Yonsei University Wonju College of Medicine, Wonju, Republic of Korea
[2]Department of Laboratory Medicine, Wonju Severance Christian Hospital, Yonsei University Wonju College of Medicine, Wonju, Republic of Korea
[3]Department of Pathology, Wonju Severance Christian Hospital, Yonsei University Wonju College of Medicine, Wonju, Republic of Korea
[4]Institute of Evidence Based Medicine, Wonju Severance Christian Hospital, Yonsei University Wonju College of Medicine, Wonju, Republic of Korea

Correspondence should be addressed to Jung Soo Lim; isiss21@yonsei.ac.kr

Academic Editor: Lucy Mastrandrea

Purpose. We report a rare case of severe hypercalcemia that was ultimately diagnosed as primary bone marrow diffuse large B-cell lymphoma (BCL). *Case Report.* A 74-year-old male patient visited our hospital complaining of tenderness and swelling of the left knee caused by supracondylar fracture of the left distal femur. His initial blood tests showed a serum calcium level of 13.9 mg/dL, inorganic phosphorus of 4.34 mg/dL, and a serum creatinine level of 1.54 mg/dL. A serum assay of intact parathyroid hormone showed 5.24 pg/mL, and the patient's serum 25(OH)D level was 22.33 ng/mL. To exclude malignancy, we performed imaging studies, including abdomen or chest computed tomography and positron emission tomography-computed tomography; however, no suspicious lesion was found, although the serum PTH-related peptide level was elevated at 4.0 pmol/L. A bone marrow biopsy was performed to identify any hidden hematologic malignancy. As a result, the pathology of bone marrow confirmed the presence of atypical lymphocytes that stained positive for the CD20 marker, which is consistent with BCL involving the bone marrow. *Conclusion.* This case highlights the importance of pursuing a thorough workup for rare underlying causes of hypercalcemia when parathyroid-related etiologies can be excluded.

1. Introduction

Hypercalcemia is a frequent finding in patients presenting to both outpatient clinics and emergency departments. While mild hypercalcemia is usually asymptomatic, patients with more severe hypercalcemia may present with a wide range of symptoms and signs, ranging from nausea, lethargy, and altered consciousness to life-threatening renal failure and cardiac arrhythmia that may lead to mortality if left unmanaged [1, 2].

Common causes of hypercalcemia are parathyroid-related diseases and malignancy [1]; one study investigated patients who visited the emergency department of a single hospital for hypercalcemia and found that 44% of cases were caused by malignancies [3]. In addition, malignancy accompanied by hypercalcemia is usually associated with a poor prognosis. Therefore, an aggressive, thorough investigation into the etiology of hypercalcemia is warranted whenever it is encountered [1].

We report a case of a 74-year-old male patient who presented with hypercalcemia and was ultimately diagnosed with primary bone marrow diffuse large B-cell lymphoma (DLBCL).

2. Case Report

A 74-year-old male patient visited the emergency department of our hospital for tenderness and swelling of the left knee. He had a past history of hypertension, spinal stenosis, benign prostate hypertrophy, and unruptured aneurysm of the right carotid artery. He also had visited an orthopedic surgery clinic due to an old fracture of the right tibial tuberosity six weeks previously. Initial physical examination found tenderness and crepitus of the left knee. Radiographs of both knee joints confirmed the diagnosis of supracondylar fracture of the left distal femur. His initial vital signs were as follows: blood pressure 164/81 mmHg; heart rate: 66 beats per minute; respiratory rate: 18/min; and body temperature: 36.0°C.

The results of an initial complete blood cell count were within the normal range: white blood cell count 8.66×10^9/L with 70.3% neutrophils, hemoglobin 14.1 g/dL, hematocrit 40.7%, and platelet count 173×10^9/L. Serum blood urea nitrogen and creatinine were 15.2 mg/dL and 1.07 mg/dL, respectively. In addition, serum calcium and alkaline phosphatase levels were elevated at 13.9 mg/dL and 152 U/L, respectively; inorganic phosphorus and serum albumin levels were within the normal ranges (4.34 mg/dL and 3.9 g/dL, respectively). Thyroid function test was also normal. The patient underwent a successful closed reduction and retrograde intramedullary nailing of the fractured joint the following day. However, he soon began to complain of general weakness, nausea, vomiting, and anorexia. His serum creatinine level was increased to 2.37 mg/dL on postoperative day 7, while the hemoglobin level decreased to 8.2 g/dL on postoperative day 9. On postoperative day 10, the patient's right distal femur fractured when rising from a wheelchair. Whole-body radionuclide bone scan with technetium-99 found multiple focal activities at bilateral femoral shafts, both knee joints, and left tibia (data not shown).

He was referred to our endocrinology department for evaluation of hypercalcemia. A serum assay of intact parathyroid hormone (iPTH) was 5.24 pg/mL (range: 15-65), and the serum 25(OH)D level was 22.33 ng/mL. In addition, a workup for anemia was concurrently carried out: serum iron of 77 μg/dL (range: 65-175), total iron binding capacity of 296 μg/dL (range: 250-425), ferritin of 761.91 ng/mL (range: 22-322), and serum lactate dehydrogenase of 258 U/L (range: <290 U/L). The peripheral blood smear was unremarkable, except for moderate toxic changes in neutrophils. His reticulocyte index was 0.6%, which implied inadequate red blood cell production despite the presence of anemia. Also, β2-microglobulin was elevated to 7.33 mg/L (range: 0.81-2.19). Due to the combination of persistent hypercalcemia, renal failure, anemia, and bone lesions, serum and urine electrophoresis were performed to rule out the possibility of multiple myeloma, both of which were negative. However, serum PTH-related peptide (PTHrP) assay showed a level elevated to 4.0 pmol/L (range: <1.1).

The patient underwent a complete diagnostic workup to find any hidden malignancy. Serum tumor biomarkers were all within normal ranges (carcinoembryonic antigen: < 2 ng/mL, cancer antigen 19-9: 7.3 U/mL, alpha-fetoprotein: 3.71 ng/mL, and prostate specific antigen: 0.17 ng/mL). A

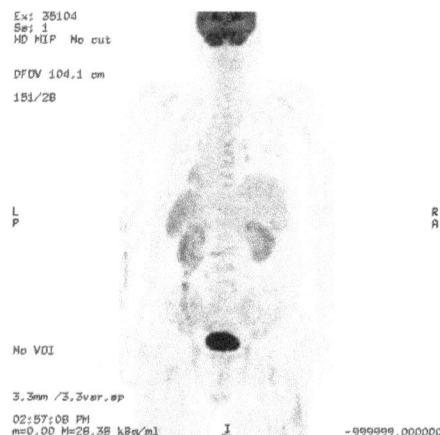

FIGURE 1: Torso positron emission tomography-computed tomography scan demonstrated no abnormal FDG uptake.

thin-slice (1 mm) chest CT and abdominopelvic CT scans were unremarkable (data not shown). A torso positron emission tomography-computed tomography (PET-CT) scan also showed no abnormal FDG uptake (Figure 1). To exclude hematologic malignancy, a bone marrow biopsy at the left iliac crest was performed. The bone marrow smear revealed several large atypical lymphocytes with a high nucleus-to-cytoplasm ratio and prominent nucleoli. Initial chromosomal karyotyping revealed both aneuploidy and multiple deletions and translocations across a number of chromosomes, including 73 chromosomes, XXY, del(1)(p22), and (q21;q26.2). Pathology of the bone marrow confirmed the presence of atypical lymphocytes that stained positive for the CD20 marker, which is consistent with B-cell lymphoma (BCL) involving the bone marrow. Immunophenotyping of bone marrow cells further supported the diagnosis of BCL, with the population testing positive for CD45, CD19, CD20, CD79a, and HLA-DR (Figures 2 and 3); however, terminal deoxynucleotidyl transferase expression in bone marrow cells was negative. This case was confirmed to be a rare case of primary bone marrow DLBCL.

3. Discussion

This case emphasizes the importance of detecting less common causes of hypercalcemia if the clinical presentation of other causes of hypercalcemia is not definite when performing diagnostic workups. Besides primary hyperparathyroidism and malignancy, there are other numerous conditions associated with hypercalcemia: granulomatous diseases such as sarcoidosis and tuberculosis; drugs like lithium carbonate and thiazide diuretics; prolonged immobilization; endocrine disorders including thyrotoxicosis and adrenal insufficiency [1]. The first step for evaluating the cause of hypercalcemia is the measurement of iPTH; then, the possibility of cancer should be considered in the setting of low serum iPTH concentration [1]. PTHrP is often measured to screen for malignancy-induced hypercalcemia [1]; however,

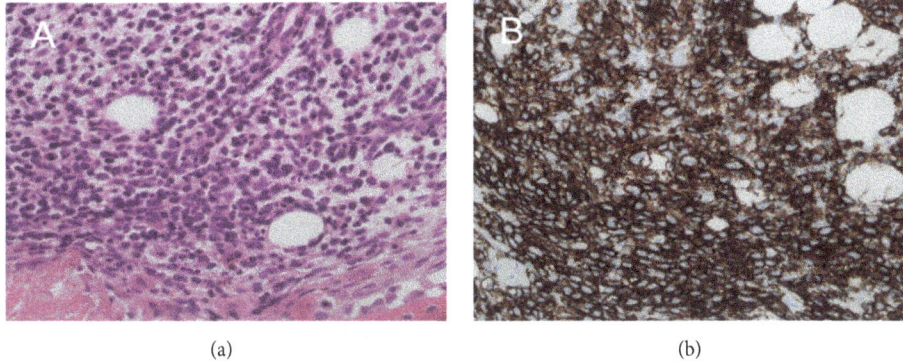

FIGURE 2: Histopathology of bone marrow biopsy specimen. (a) Bone marrow biopsy (hematoxylin-eosin stain, x200) shows infiltration of large atypical cells. (b) The immunohistochemical staining for CD20 (x100) is diffusely positive in large atypical cells.

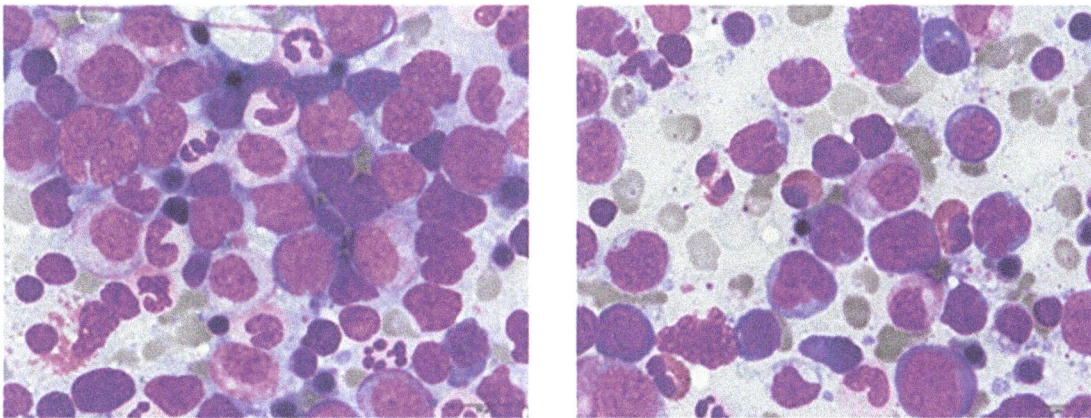

FIGURE 3: Bone marrow aspiration (Wright-Giemsa stain, x1000) shows infiltration of diffuse large B-cell lymphoma. Large, atypical cells with irregularly shaped nuclei and basophilic cytoplasm are noted in clusters.

PTHrP elevation can be observed in various benign conditions such as systemic lupus erythematosus with multiple organ involvement [4]. Therefore, caution is necessary when interpreting laboratory or radiographic findings in patients with hypercalcemia who showed PTHrP elevation.

Several case reports on lymphomas that initially presented with severe, unexplained hypercalcemia have been published [5–7]. Ha et al. [5] reported a case of intravascular large BCL in a 68-year-old male who presented with lethargy and weight loss. Similar to our case, their patient also showed hypercalcemia with decreased serum iPTH and elevated PTHrP levels. However, his PET-CT scan demonstrated strong, diffuse uptake in the bones and spleen. Kapur and Levin [8] also described a 69-year-old female who presented with worsening confusion and weight loss; in their case, multiple large intra-abdominal and pelvic masses were visible on abdominopelvic CT and PET-CT scans. However, the malignancy-associated hypercalcemia described in our case was unique in that lesions suggestive of malignancy were not found across several imaging modalities.

Furthermore, primary bone marrow BCL is a very rare disease in itself. Bhagat et al. [9] described a case series of primary bone marrow lymphoma from a single tertiary care center, which reported a total of four cases over the past 15

years. The median age was 52 years, and chief complaints included general weakness, fatigue, and dyspnea on exertion. All patients presented with a moderate degree of anemia and showed hypercalcemia, as in our case. The prognosis was generally poor; two patients died while receiving standard chemotherapy, and two additional patients experienced a relapse despite achieving remission after completion of the first round of chemotherapy.

Unfortunately, no bone tissue was obtained during the surgery, because this patient was referred to our department for the workup for hypercalcemia after the surgery. In addition, the bone scintigraphy was performed 1 month after the surgery, and in such clinical setting, the focal activities may reflect postsurgical inflammation or healing process at and around the site of injury instead of malignancy. Recently, Zhang X et al. [10] demonstrated clinical characterization and outcome of 61 patients with primary bone lymphoma (PBL); their mean age was 45 years, and patients aged less than 60 years accounted for approximately 75%. Those with PBL commonly showed soft tissue invasion (68.9%), lymph node involvement (44.3%), and B symptoms (31.1%), and the most common sites in all patients with PBL were the spine and pelvic bones [10]. Furthermore, a majority of PBL patients had a localized disease rather than multifocal disease [11, 12].

In contrast, our patient was very much older than that of previous reports regarding PBL. He had no associated signs or symptoms, including nerve compression, local mass, soft tissue invasion, lymph node involvement, and B symptoms. Furthermore, there were no signs of hemophagocytosis, such as high fever, liver failure, or coagulopathy; clear evidence of intravascular lymphoma in the pathology was also not found. Moreover, the bone scintigraphy showed unremarkable skeletal activities in spine or pelvic bones, which are the most common sites of PBL. Particularly, ^{18}F-PET-CT is known to play important roles in the decision making of diagnosis and treatment response as well as the determination of recurrence and residual disease in patients with PBL [13], because PBL is usually presented as a hypermetabolic lesion on FDG-PET [14]. In this case, the PET-CT demonstrated no abnormally hypermetabolic lesion throughout skeletal systems, which makes the possibility of PBL unlikely, even though this image did not show the entire body.

According to Stewart [15], the mechanisms behind hypercalcemia associated with cancer can be divided into four categories: (1) humoral hypercalcemia of malignancy (HHM), which accounts for approximately 80% of cases; (2) local osteoclastic hypercalcemia consisting of 20% of cases; (3) 1,25(OH)$_2$-dihydroxyvitamin D (1,25(OH)$_2$D) secreting lymphomas (<1%); and (4) ectopic hyperparathyroidism (<1%). HHM involves the overproduction of PTHrP by malignant tissues (most often squamous-cell cancer, breast cancer, and non-Hodgkin's lymphoma), which circulates throughout the body and ultimately stimulates bone resorption and calcium storage release [15]. Osteoclastic hypercalcemia is predominantly found in breast cancer and multiple myeloma due to extensive bone involvement of the malignancies [15]. Active secretion of 1,25(OH)$_2$D by certain lymphomas enhances osteoclastic bone resorption and intestinal calcium absorption, causing hypercalcemia [15]. In this case, HHM appears to be the most likely mechanism behind the hypercalcemia as the PTHrP was elevated, although the possibility of 1,25(OH)$_2$D secreting lymphoma could not be completely ruled out.

In conclusion, this rare case of primary bone marrow DLBCL suggests that hypercalcemia should not be overlooked. A thorough workup of rare underlying causes of hypercalcemia should always be considered when parathyroid-related causes can be excluded.

Disclosure

The authors declare that they presented this case at a seminar organized by the Korean Endocrine Society held in Wonju, South Korea, in May 2018.

Authors' Contributions

Jin Sae Yoo and Jung Soo Lim contributed to conceptualization. Juwon Kim, Hyeong Ju Kwon, and Jung Soo Lim contributed to data curation. Jin Sae Yoo was responsible for writing and original draft. Jin Sae Yoo, Juwon Kim, and Jung Soo Lim were responsible for writing, review, and editing.

References

[1] S. Minisola, J. Pepe, S. Piemonte, and C. Cipriani, "The diagnosis and management of hypercalcaemia," *British Medical Journal (Clinical Research)*, vol. 350, no. 1, Article ID h2723, 2015.

[2] I. R. Reid, S. M. Bristow, and M. J. Bolland, "Calcium and cardiovascular disease," *Endocrinology and Metabolism*, vol. 32, no. 3, pp. 339–349, 2017.

[3] G. Lindner, R. Felber, C. Schwarz et al., "Hypercalcemia in the ED: Prevalence, etiology, and outcome," *The American Journal of Emergency Medicine*, vol. 31, no. 4, pp. 657–660, 2013.

[4] L. J. Deftos, D. W. Burton, S. M. Baird, and R. A. Terkeltaub, "Hypercalcemia and systemic lupus erythematosus," *Arthritis & Rheumatology*, vol. 39, no. 12, pp. 2066–2069, 1996.

[5] J. M. Ha, E. Kim, W. J. Lee et al., "Unusual manifestation of intravascular large B-cell lymphoma: Severe hypercalcemia with parathyroid hormone-related protein," *Cancer Research and Treatment*, vol. 46, no. 3, pp. 307–311, 2014.

[6] H. Hong, T. Hayashi, K. Hagiwara et al., "Hypercalcemia associated with parathyroid hormone-related protein (PTHrP) in a patient with diffuse large-type B-cell lymphoma (DLBCL)," *Gan to Kagaku Ryoho*, vol. 38, no. 11, pp. 1881–1884, 2011.

[7] T. Iida, S. Satoh, H. Kaneto et al., "A case of hypercalcemia associated with parathyroid hormone-related protein produced by the recurrence of B-cell lymphoma of the pancreas," *Nihon Shokakibyo Gakkai Zasshi*, vol. 111, no. 11, pp. 2163–2173, 2014.

[8] S. Kapur and M. B. Levin, "Transformation of follicular lymphoma to double hit b-cell lymphoma causing hypercalcemia in a 69-year-old female: a case report and review of the literature," *Case Reports in Hematology*, vol. 2014, Article ID 619760, 8 pages, 2014.

[9] P. Bhagat, M. U. S. Sachdeva, P. Sharma et al., "Primary bone marrow lymphoma is a rare neoplasm with poor outcome: Case series from single tertiary care centre and review of literature," *Hematological Oncology*, vol. 34, no. 1, pp. 42–48, 2016.

[10] X. Zhang, J. Zhu, Y. Song, L. Ping, and W. Zheng, "Clinical characterization and outcome of primary bone lymphoma: a retrospective study of 61 Chinese patients," *Scientific Reports*, vol. 6, no. 1, 2016.

[11] A. Alencar, D. Pitcher, G. Byrne, and I. S. Lossos, "Primary bone lymphoma—the University of Miami experience," *Leukemia & Lymphoma*, vol. 51, no. 1, pp. 39–49, 2010.

[12] K. Beal, L. Allen, and J. Yahalom, "Primary bone lymphoma: treatment results and prognostic factors with long-term follow-up of 82 patients," *Cancer*, vol. 106, no. 12, pp. 2652–2656, 2006.

[13] A. Çirakli, M. Elli, N. Dabak, F. C. Tosun, A. Dağdemir, and S. Çirakli, "Evaluation of primary bone lymphoma and the importance of positron emission tomography," *Acta Orthopaedica et Traumatologica Turcica*, vol. 48, no. 3, pp. 371–378, 2014.

[14] H.-Y. Zhou, F. Gao, B. Bu et al., "Primary bone lymphoma: A case report and review of the literature," *Oncology Letters*, vol. 8, no. 4, pp. 1551–1556, 2014.

[15] A. F. Stewart, "Clinical practice. Hypercalcemia associated with cancer," *The New England Journal of Medicine*, vol. 352, no. 4, pp. 373–379, 2005.

34

Anterior Pituitary Aplasia in an Infant with Ring Chromosome 18p Deletion

Edward J. Bellfield,[1] Jacqueline Chan,[1] Sarah Durrin,[2] Valerie Lindgren,[3] Zohra Shad,[4] and Claudia Boucher-Berry[1]

[1]*Division of Pediatric Endocrinology, University of Illinois College of Medicine, Chicago, IL 60612, USA*
[2]*University of Illinois College of Medicine, Chicago, IL 60612, USA*
[3]*Department of Pathology, University of Illinois College of Medicine, Chicago, IL 60612, USA*
[4]*Division of Genetics, University of Illinois College of Medicine, Chicago, IL 60612, USA*

Correspondence should be addressed to Edward J. Bellfield; ejbellf1@uic.edu

Academic Editor: Lucy Mastrandrea

We present the first reported case of an infant with 18p deletion syndrome with anterior pituitary aplasia secondary to a ring chromosome. Endocrine workup soon after birth was reassuring; however, repeat testing months later confirmed central hypopituitarism. While MRI reading initially indicated no midline defects, subsequent review of the images confirmed anterior pituitary aplasia with ectopic posterior pituitary. This case demonstrates how deletion of genetic material, even if resulting in a chromosomal ring, still results in a severe syndromic phenotype. Furthermore, it demonstrates the necessity of close follow-up in the first year of life for children with 18p deletion syndrome and emphasizes the need to verify radiology impressions if there is any doubt as to the radiologic findings.

1. Introduction

18p deletion syndrome is caused by loss of all or parts of the short arm of chromosome 18 and is estimated to occur in approximately 1 in 50,000 live births [1]. The resultant syndrome has high phenotypic variability but is generally characterized by dysmorphic facies as well as congenital heart defects, isolated growth hormone (GH) deficiency, hypopituitarism, autoimmune conditions, and holoprosencephaly (HPE) [2]. While many of these cases are due to terminal deletions of the chromosome, other reported cases include unbalanced translocations, malsegregation of a balanced parental translocation, or a ring chromosome [1, 3, 4]. Here we present the first reported case of a patient with 18p deletion due to a ring chromosome with anterior pituitary aplasia.

2. Case Presentation

We present a female infant born at term to a 28-year-old G7P2 mother. The patient was prenatally diagnosed with a cystic hygroma and pleural effusions but the mother declined amniocentesis. At delivery, the patient was noted to have multiple dysmorphic features including round face, hypotelorism, unilateral ptosis, flattened midface, small nose, low set ears, and generalized hypotonia. Her features are shown at 3 months of age (Figures 1(a) and 1(b)). She also had mild coarctation of the aorta and persistent patent ductus arteriosus (PDA) despite indomethacin therapy. Her birth was complicated by respiratory distress requiring oxygen support, as well as unconjugated hyperbilirubinemia, which responded well to triple phototherapy. The presence of so many physical abnormalities leads to suspicion of a genetic syndrome. A chromosome analysis was then performed, which demonstrated a ring chromosome 18 (Figure 2).

Single nucleotide polymorphism (SNP) chromosome microarray analysis confirmed copy loss of ~13.93 Mb of 18p11.21p11.32—the entire short (p) arm of chromosome 18 (Figure 3). No single copy sequences were deleted from the long arm. Therefore, this finding is equivalent to simple deletion of 18p with respect to gene content. A subsequent brain

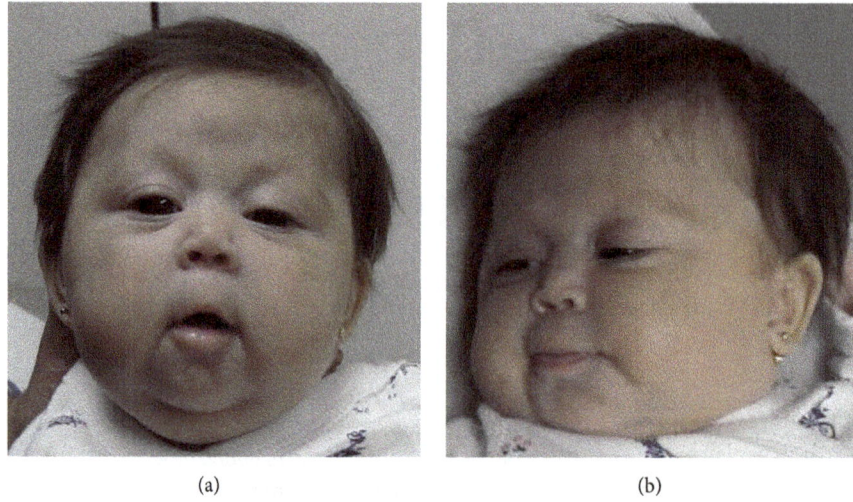

(a)   (b)

FIGURE 1: (a) Demonstration of round face, hypotelorism, and left-sided ptosis. (b) Demonstration of low set ear and flattened midface.

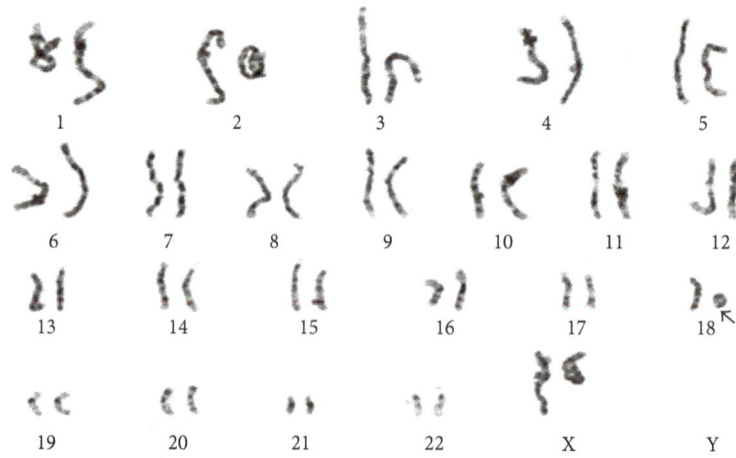

FIGURE 2: The patient's karyogram demonstrates a ring chromosome 18.

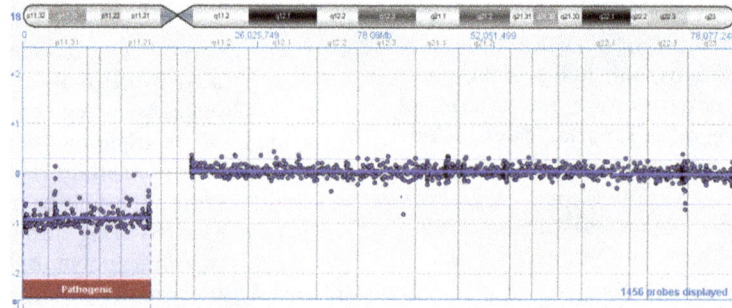

FIGURE 3: SNP based chromosome microarray confirmed a copy loss of ~13.93 Mb of 18p11.21p11.32, the entire short (p) arm of chromosome 18.

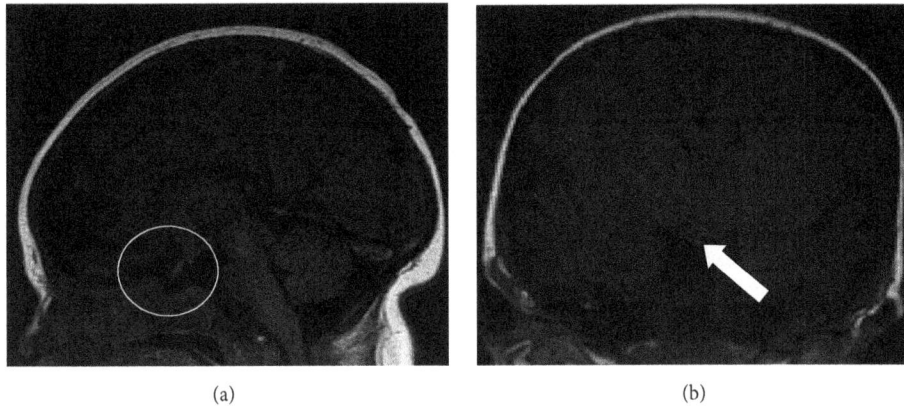

(a) (b)

FIGURE 4: (a) MRI. Sagittal view demonstrates no evidence of the sella turcica and no pituitary soft tissue within the presumed area of the sella. (b) MRI. Coronal view demonstrates a superiorly displaced T1 bright spot consistent with an ectopic posterior pituitary.

TABLE 1: Endocrinology workup obtained at day of life 22, compared with that obtained at day of life 100 (3 months of age).

Lab test	DOL 22	DOL 100	Reference values
IGF-1	16	<1	56–124 ng/mL
IGF-BP3	—	<500	1039–3169 ng/mL
Cortisol	3.2 (random)	8 (post-ACTH)	≥18 μg/dL (post-ACTH)
TSH	6	2.2	0.35–10 μIU/mL
FT4	0.7	0.5	0.6–1.7 ng/mL

MRI was performed to evaluate for presence of associated HPE and was initially read as having no midline structural defect.

Endocrinopathies are known to be associated with 18p deletion syndrome, so initial lab workup was done at birth which demonstrated low insulin-like growth factor-1 (IGF-1) without hypoglycemia and normal thyroid function tests. The patient's feeding status continued to progressively decline leading to suboptimal weight gain. In part due to patient's worsening energy level, endocrine workup was repeated at 3 months of age.

These labs demonstrated undetectable IGF-1 and insulin-like growth factor-binding protein 3 (IGF-BP3), low free thyroxine (T4) with an inappropriately normal thyroid stimulating hormone (TSH), weak cortisol response post-1 hour adrenocorticotropic hormone (ACTH) stimulation test, and normal electrolytes without polyuria (Table 1). These findings were consistent with growth hormone deficiency, central thyroid deficiency, and secondary adrenal insufficiency, respectively—the hallmarks of anterior panhypopituitarism. She was started on hydrocortisone and later on somatropin and levothyroxine. It is highly likely that she will also exhibit gonadotropin deficiency, requiring hormonal supplementation to induce and maintain pubertal development.

A gastrostomy tube was placed to supplement oral feeds. Only after demonstrating appropriate weight gain did she undergo an uncomplicated PDA repair. Upon review of the initial imaging studies months later, it was concluded that she in fact did have an undeveloped sella turcica with no evidence of an anterior pituitary. The posterior pituitary bright spot was visible but displaced superiorly, which was expected due to a lack of symptoms of diabetes insipidus (Figures 4(a) and 4(b)).

3. Discussion

We present a patient with an 18p deletion syndrome secondary to ring chromosome, who exhibited phenotypic features similar to those described straightforward deletions of chromosome 18p. To our knowledge, there have been relatively few cases of isolated 18p deletion syndrome due to ring chromosome 18 described in the literature [3, 5, 6]. One significant aspect in which our patient differs from previously reported 18p deletion syndrome due to ring chromosome is the presence of anterior pituitary aplasia with posterior pituitary ectopy.

Since 18p deletion syndrome was first described by de Grouchy and colleagues in 1963 [7], a fairly comprehensive set of phenotypic effects due to breaks occurring in the short arm have been described. The most common features include neonatal complications (jaundice, respiratory distress, and feeding difficulties), hypotonia, and dystonia. Also frequently noted are facial dysmorphisms, ptosis, refractive errors, strabismus, and conductive hearing loss. HPE and its microforms have been observed in approximately 12% of these patients [8]. Interestingly, HPE has been linked to GH deficiency and there is evidence that isolated pituitary hypoplasia and pituitary stalk interruption syndrome are milder forms of HPE [6, 9]. Reports have varied on the developmental and behavioral manifestations, although recent reviews estimate an average IQ of 69, with patients ranging from mild impairment to normal functioning [2]. However regardless of IQ, many studies have noted that these individuals have difficulty with communication skills, activities of daily living, and management of social and occupational activities [2, 10].

Isolated hormone deficiencies and hypopituitarism have all been described as a feature of 18p deletion syndrome. Approximately 50% of breaks on chromosome 18 occur at the centromere, and while there are reports of direct parent-to-child transmission, approximately 70–85% of cases are due to de novo mutations [1, 2]. The remaining 50% of cases are due to an assortment of insults along the short arm of chromosome 18, adding to the phenotypic variability of this syndrome [3].

While GH deficiency has been previously described in both isolated 18p deletion syndrome and ring chromosome 18, the presentation is variable. Of the case reports describing GH deficiency associated with isolated 18p deletion syndrome, 2 of 3 patients had normal brain MRI [10, 11]. The third case report presented a patient with only partial GH deficiency and empty sella with rudimentary pituitary stalk [12]. Reported cases of GH deficiency in patients with ring 18 chromosome reveal inconsistent brain imaging results [5, 11, 13]. Additionally, a female with a ring 18 chromosome, GH deficiency, hypothyroidism, and ectopic posterior pituitary (but normal cortisol) has been described [14].

The most recent review of 18p deletion syndrome [2] cited that approximately 23% of patients had isolated GH deficiency, while 13% had hypopituitarism or panhypopituitarism. In the authors' own cohort of 54 patients, 6 had pituitary abnormalities, including hypoplastic pituitary or pituitary stalk, absent posterior pituitary, or complete pituitary absence. Additionally, 5 of these 54 had hypothyroidism without structural abnormalities. Another recent review of patients with ring chromosome 18 described similar findings: 93% of patients had isolated GH deficiency, 41% had hypothyroidism, and 13% had a spectrum of HPE [15].

Current research in 18p deletion syndrome is aimed at establishing gene-specific phenotypic correlations and determining the penetrance of these phenotypes in order to provide genotype-specific anticipatory guidance for these patients and their families [2]. While there is a clear association between 18p deletion syndrome and endocrinopathies and structural pituitary abnormalities, the specific genes responsible for these phenotypes have yet to be identified. Our hope is that case reports such as this in addition to further molecular characterization of 18p deletion genotypes will help to further elucidate the mechanism behind this condition and allow for improved care and treatment.

4. Conclusion

This is the first reported case of an infant with an 18p deletion syndrome secondary to a ring chromosome with anterior pituitary aplasia and ectopic posterior pituitary. Although endocrinology labs soon after birth were reassuring, repeat testing months later identified central endocrinopathy and review of the imaging confirmed the diagnosis. This case demonstrates the necessity of close follow-up in the first year of life for children with 18p deletion syndrome but also emphasizes the need to verify radiology impressions if there is any doubt as to the radiologic findings.

Acknowledgments

The authors thank the family for allowing them to share their story. They also thank the Division of Genetics for providing them with pictures of the patient, the Department of Radiology for providing MRI images, and Kayesha Cobb of the UIC Cytogenetic Laboratory for expert technical assistance. They also thank the Research Open Access Publishing (ROAAP) Fund of the University of Illinois at Chicago for financial support towards the open access publishing fee for this article.

References

[1] C. Turleau, "Monosomy 18p," *Orphanet Journal of Rare Diseases*, vol. 3, no. 1, article 4, 2008.

[2] M. Hasi-Zogaj, C. Sebold, P. Heard et al., "A review of 18p deletions," *American Journal of Medical Genetics, Part C: Seminars in Medical Genetics*, vol. 169, no. 3, pp. 251–264, 2015.

[3] P. Stankiewicz, I. Brozek, Z. Hélias-Rodzewicz et al., "Clinical and molecular-cytogenetic studies in seven patients with ring chromosome 18," *American Journal of Medical Genetics*, vol. 101, no. 3, pp. 226–239, 2001.

[4] J.-C. C. Wang, L. Nemana, S. Y. Kou, R. Habibian, and M. J. Hajianpour, "Molecular cytogenetic characterization of 18;21 whole arm translocation associated with monosomy 18p," *American Journal of Medical Genetics*, vol. 71, no. 4, pp. 463–466, 1997.

[5] S. S. Abusrewil, A. McDermott, and D. C. L. Savage, "Growth hormone, suspected gonadotrophin deficiency, and ring 18 chromosome," *Archives of Disease in Childhood*, vol. 63, no. 9, pp. 1090–1091, 1988.

[6] H. G. Artman, C. A. Morris, and A. D. Stock, "18p-syndrome and hypopituitarism," *Journal of Medical Genetics*, vol. 29, no. 9, pp. 671–672, 1992.

[7] J. de Grouchy, M. Lamy, S. Thieffry, M. Arthuis, and C. H. Salmon, "Dysmorphie complexe avec oligophrenie: deletion des bras courts d'un chromosome 17-18," *Comptes Rendus de l'Académie des Sciences*, vol. 258, pp. 1028–1029, 1963.

[8] K. L. Jones, *Smith's Recognizable Patterns of Human Malformation*, Elsevier Saunders, Philadelphia, Pa, USA, 6th edition, 2006.

[9] C. Tatsi, A. Sertedaki, A. Voutetakis et al., "Pituitary stalk interruption syndrome and isolated pituitary hypoplasia may be caused by mutations in holoprosencephaly-related genes," *The Journal of Clinical Endocrinology & Metabolism*, vol. 98, no. 4, pp. E779–E784, 2013.

[10] C. Sebold, B. Soileau, P. Heard et al., "Whole arm deletions of 18p: medical and developmental effects," *American Journal of Medical Genetics, Part A*, vol. 167, no. 2, pp. 313–323, 2015.

[11] A. Meloni, L. Boccone, L. Angius, S. Loche, A. M. Falchi, and A. Cao, "Hypothalamic growth hormone deficiency in a patient with ring chromosome 18," *European Journal of Pediatrics*, vol. 153, no. 2, pp. 110–112, 1994.

[12] E. Schober, S. Scheibenreiter, and H. Frisch, "18p monosomy with GH-deficiency and empty sella: good response to GH-treatment," *Clinical Genetics*, vol. 47, no. 5, pp. 254–256, 1995.

[13] S. Aritaki, A. Takagi, H. Someya, and L. I. Jun, "Growth hormone neurosecretory dysfunction associated with ring chromosome 18," *Acta Paediatrica Japonica*, vol. 38, no. 5, pp. 544–548, 1996.

[14] J. V. Thomas, D. F. C. Mezzasalma, A. M. Teixeira et al., "Growth hormone deficiency, hypothyroidism and ring chromosome 18—case report," *Arquivos Brasileiros de Endocrinologia e Metabologia*, vol. 50, no. 5, pp. 951–956, 2006.

35

Moyamoya Disease with Coexistent Hypertriglyceridemia in Pediatric Patient

Jacqueline Chan, Fabiola D'Ambrosio Rodriguez, Deepank Sahni, and Claudia Boucher-Berry

Department of Pediatric, Children's Hospital of the University of Illinois, Chicago, IL, USA

Correspondence should be addressed to Jacqueline Chan; jtchan@uic.edu

Academic Editor: Osamu Isozaki

Moyamoya disease is a rare chronic and progressive cerebrovascular disease of the arteries of the circle of Willis that can affect children and adults. It has been associated with multiple diseases, including immunologic, like Graves' disease, diabetes mellitus, and SLE. Hyperlipidemia has been recognized in patients with Moyamoya disease with an incidence of 27–37%. However, no case in pediatric patients has been reported of the coexistence of Moyamoya disease and hyperlipidemia. Here we present a case of a 9-year-old female diagnosed with Moyamoya disease after a stroke with incidental finding of familial hypercholesterolemia. This finding will make our patient a very unique case, since there has not been any reporting of Moyamoya disease and hypercholesterolemia association.

1. Introduction

Moyamoya disease (MMD) is a rare idiopathic chronic and progressive steno-occlusion of bilateral intracranial arteries of the circle of Willis that develop in children and adults. It is characterized by collateral vessels seen on cerebral angiography. An immunologic basis has been suggested for this disease and recent reports have noted an association between Moyamoya and autoimmune diseases including Graves' disease, diabetes mellitus, and Systemic Lupus Erythematosus. Analysis of the comorbidities may be helpful in determining the pathogenesis of Moyamoya [1]. Usual age of onset of MMD in pediatric is after 5 years and progresses more rapidly than in adults [2].

MMD is mainly found in East Asia, especially in Japan and South Korea [3–6]. Because MMD is extremely uncommon in the western countries, no systemic surveys have been conducted in either Europe or North America although there have been some sporadic reports [7, 8].

Familial combined hyperlipidemia (FCHL) is a dominantly inherited hyperlipidemia that occurs in at least 1% of the adult population and is responsible for 10% of premature coronary artery disease. Several metabolic defects apparently are associated with the FCHL phenotype. Most commonly, excess production of very low density lipoprotein apolipoprotein B can be demonstrated [1, 9].

Hyperlipidemia has been recognized in patients with Moyamoya disease with an incidence of 27.7% in a study done in Mayo Clinic Minnesota 1979–2011 and 37.3% in a study done in Japan 2001–2011 [1, 10]. However, no study has been documented in a pediatric patient with abnormal lipid profile with concurrent Moyamoya disease. We report a case of a 9-year-old female with Moyamoya disease and coexistent hyperlipidemia.

2. Case Presentation

Patient is a 9-year-old previously healthy Caucasian female. She was adopted at 3 weeks of age and the family history is unknown. She has a past medical history of gross motor delay, followed closely by Neurology and Physical Therapy and was well by 3 years of age. The patient presented to the Emergency Department with an acute onset of right arm weakness, described as inability to move her arm and write. No history of recent trauma or illness. On arrival to the Emergency Department, vital signs obtained were BP 113/67, pulse 106, and temp. 36.7. Her weight was 26 kg (20% ile), height was 122 cm (3% cile), and BMI was 17 (70% ile).

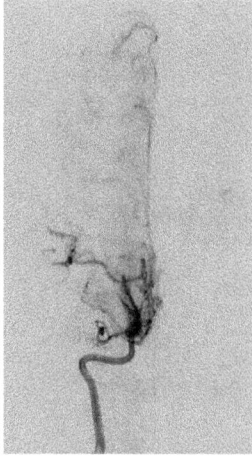

FIGURE 1: Right internal cerebral artery in cerebral angiogram.

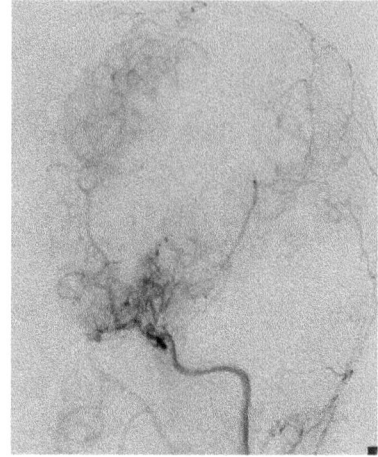

FIGURE 2: Left internal cerebral artery in cerebral angiogram.

Physical exam is only significant for right arm motor weakness 3/5. No sensory deficit was noted. MRI done for stroke protocol revealed small occlusion of the distal internal carotid arteries and numerous small collateral vessels projecting from the circle of Willis region, and MRA was consistent with Moyamoya disease. Six-vessel angiogram confirmed the diagnosis with bilateral internal carotid arteries occlusion as shown in Figures 1 and 2. Baseline fasting lipid profile was abnormal: elevated fasting triglyceride (870 mg/dL, $n <$ 150 mg/dL), elevated total cholesterol (427 mg/dL, $n <$ 200 mg/dL), normal HDL 48 mg/dL, and LDL not measurable due to elevated triglycerides. Apolipoprotein B was elevated at 219 mg/dL (55 mg/dL–125 mg/dL). Thyroid function test was done and revealed slightly elevated TSH of 5.7 mcIU/mL (n 0.35 mcIU/mL–4.0 mcIU/mL) which was not considered clinically significant. She was placed on a pediatric low fat/low cholesterol diet based on nutrition recommendation. She was started on Pravastatin 20 mg daily. Seven days after initial presentation, she developed slurring of speech. MRI demonstrated new acute ischemic infarct involving the left frontal lobe, in the vascular territory of the anterior left middle cerebral artery. Prompt evaluation and revascularization were scheduled. Total cholesterol and triglyceride level decreased to 267 mg/dL and 433 mg/dL, respectively, after fourteen days of Pravastatin therapy, as demonstrated in Figure 3. Patient underwent bilateral superficial temporal artery-middle cerebral artery bypass (STA-MCA) with no complications.

3. Discussion

Moyamoya disease is an uncommon cerebrovascular disease characterized by progressive steno-occlusive changes in the terminal internal carotid arteries (ICA) and their main branches. A bimodal age distribution has been reported for Moyamoya, with a high peak at 5 years and at 40 years [3, 10, 11]. The clinical features of Moyamoya disease differ between children and adults. Moyamoya disease often presents in children initially as a stroke often accompanied by muscular weakness. This is in contrast to adults who typically present with subarachnoid or intraparenchymal hemorrhage

[11, 12]. The predominance of ischemic events in childhood, but hemorrhagic strokes in adulthood, has been noted in Taiwanese with MMD [13] Diagnosis is usually possible with a magnetic resonance imaging (MRI) scan to look at the brain and a magnetic resonance angiogram (MRA) to look at the blood vessels of the brain. Although a genetic role has been postulated particularly due to higher incidence of Moyamoya and familial Moyamoya among Asians and Asian-Americans, the pathogenesis underlying this condition among other ethnicities and within North American populations is still unclear. Immunologic basis has been a study of interest due to association of Moyamoya with autoimmune diseases such as Graves' disease and Systemic Lupus Erythematous (SLE). Atherosclerosis and thyroid disease are the most frequent concurrent diseases with MMD especially on the adult population [1, 10].

Long-term prognosis for patients with nonsurgically treated MMD is not fully understood. However, some reports have described its natural clinical course and the results of conservative treatment. Kuroda et al. [14] reported a disease progression rate of approximately 20% over 6 years. Being female was identified as an independent risk factor for disease progression by multivariate analysis. Other investigations on the progression rate of the unaffected side of surgically treated unilateral MMD reported that six of the 41 cases (14.6%) exhibited contralateral progression during the mean follow-up of 34 months [15]. Considering these reports, MMD seems to have a progressive nature. Among many studies examining risk factors for MMD progression, the presence of thyroid disease such as Graves' disease has been a well-known medical condition linked to rapid progression of MMD [16, 17]. Recently, the RNF213 variant was suggested as a possible causative genetic alteration leading to the development as well as progression of MMD [18]. Because surgical revascularization has been recommended for symptomatic patients with impaired hemodynamics, some studies have described the outcomes of conservative treatment among asymptomatic or hemodynamically stable patients with MMD. A multicenter, nationwide survey for conservative treatment results was conducted in 2007 in Japan. The authors reported the annual

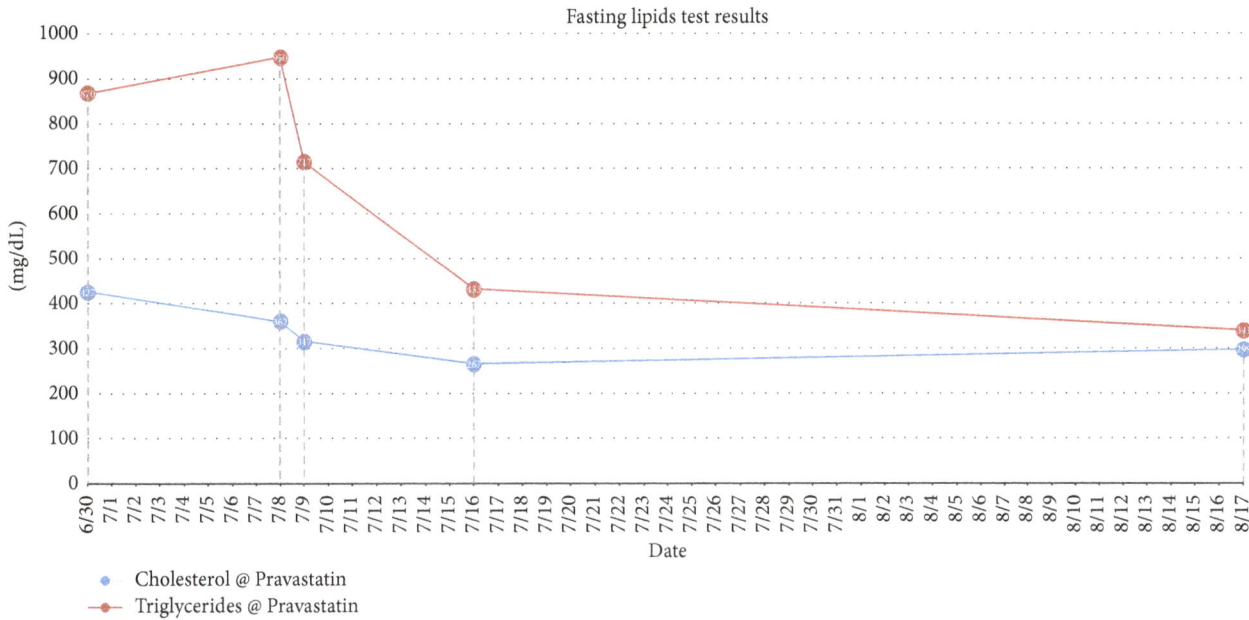

FIGURE 3: Graph showing decrease in cholesterol and triglycerides with Pravastatin treatment.

stroke rate as 3.2% from the observation of 34 asymptomatic patients conservatively followed over 44 months. Hemodynamic disturbance was revealed to be a risk factor for newly developed stroke [19]. In a North American series, the rates of annual ischemic and hemorrhagic stroke rate were reported as 13.3% and 1.7%, respectively. Being female and smoking were risk factors for stroke development [20]. Cho et al. reported an annual stroke rate of 4.5% among 241 hemodynamically stable patients with MMD over 83 months. The annual stroke rate was higher in the hemorrhagic presentation group (5.7%) than the ischemic presentation group (4.2%) or the asymptomatic group (3.4%). They found familial disease and thyroid disease to be risk factors affecting stroke occurrence [21]. As for ischemic presenting MMD, 5.6% of the annual ischemic stroke rate also reported that posterior circulation involvement was a strong risk factor for ischemic stroke [22]. Antiplatelet treatment for preventing stroke in patients with MMD had been utilized by many physicians, especially in non-Asian areas. According to the reports of a worldwide survey, 31% of responders agreed to use long-term acetylsalicylic acid [23]. However, the evidence for antiplatelet treatment is lacking. Recently, the efficacy of antiplatelet therapy for preventing stroke was investigated in a cohort study with a large sample size. According to the authors, antiplatelet therapy could not prevent recurrent cerebral infarction for ischemic presenting patients with MMD. The nature of the ischemic insult in patients with MMD is not an embolic infarction, but instead it is mainly a hemodynamic infarction. The pathologic changes of the MMD vessels near the ICA bifurcation are not a type of endothelial damage, which is prone to platelet adhesion. Therefore, theoretically, antiplatelet drugs will not be effective for preventing ischemic stroke in patients with MMD. Although antiplatelet users are subject to hemorrhagic complications, the therapy was not

associated with an increase in cerebral hemorrhage among patients with MMD [24]. Thus, prescribing antiplatelet agents for symptomatic patients with MMD should not yet be considered as an alternative treatment.

Pathologic analysis has demonstrated that affected vessels generally do not exhibit arteriosclerotic or inflammatory changes, even though there may be minimal lipid deposition seen in the intima with fibrous thickening [25, 26]. Rather, vessel occlusion results from a combination of both hyperplasia of smooth muscle cells and luminal thrombosis [10]. The Moyamoya collaterals are dilated perforating arteries believed to be a combination of preexisting and newly developed vessels [26, 27]. A number of growth factors, enzymes, and other peptides have been reported in association with Moyamoya, including basic fibroblast growth factor, transforming growth factor-β1, hepatocyte growth factor, vascular endothelial growth factor, matrix metalloproteinases, intracellular adhesion molecules, and hypoxia-inducing factor-1α, among others [27–34].

In children with primary hyperlipidemia, familial combined hyperlipidemia (FCHL) is expressed three times more commonly than familial hypercholesterolemia and half of the siblings are affected. In our patient, family history is not available. However, FCHL can be defined as elevated fasting cholesterol and triglycerides, with Apo B level of >120 mg/dL, which is consistent with the level seen in our patient. Prognosis includes development of cerebrovascular disease and insulin resistance leading to type 2 diabetes, which itself is a risk factor for atherosclerosis. Long-term prognosis of FCHL in a pediatric patient is not yet well understood as limited pediatric patients with FCHL have been followed through adulthood. Mainstay of treatment of any form of hypertriglyceridemia includes risk-factor control and diet. Children older than 2 years are usually managed with weight control and step-one diet, that is, less than or equal to 30% of total calories being fat [35]. One of the leading comorbidities documented in patients with Moyamoya is hyperlipidemia. However, no study has been reported regarding incidence of Moyamoya coexistent with hypertriglyceridemia on a pediatric patient. Recent case reports and meta-analysis involving patients with Moyamoya and concurrent hyperlipidemia all included patients over 30 years of age. These patients were not diagnosed to have familial hypercholesterolemia (FHC) nor familial combined hyperlipidemia (FCHL). Reasons for elevated cholesterol levels were not clear and were sometimes attributed to other occlusive vascular diseases, as well as untreated hypothyroidism, which is uncommon in the pediatric age group. Our patient by far is the first pediatric patient to have Moyamoya disease and concurrent FCHL, being well managed with Pravastatin.

Acknowledgments

The authors acknowledge the Research Open Access Publishing (ROAAP) Fund of the University of Illinois at Chicago for financial support towards the open access publishing fee for this article.

References

[1] N. E. El Tecle, T. Y. El Ahmadieh, A. M. Bohnen, A. D. Nanney, and B. R. Bendok, "Are hyperlipidemia and autoimmune diseases synergistic in moyamoya disease pathophysiology? Insight from the midwest," World Neurosurgery, vol. 82, no. 1-2, p. e398, 2014.

[2] G. M. Burke, A. M. Burke, A. K. Sherma, M. C. Hurley, H. H. Batjer, and B. R. Bendok, "Moyamoya disease: a summary," Neurosurgical Focus, vol. 26, no. 4, pp. 1–10, 2009.

[3] W. Miao, P.-L. Zhao, Y.-S. Zhang et al., "Epidemiological and clinical features of Moyamoya disease in Nanjing, China," Clinical Neurology and Neurosurgery, vol. 112, no. 3, pp. 199–203, 2010.

[4] R. S. Bower, G. W. Mallory, M. Nwojo, Y. C. Kudva, K. D. Flemming, and F. B. Meyer, "Moyamoya disease in a primarily white, Midwestern us population: increased prevalence of autoimmune disease," Stroke, vol. 44, no. 7, pp. 1997–1999, 2013.

[5] L. Berglund, J. D. Brunzell, A. C. Goldberg et al., "Evaluation and treatment of hypertriglyceridemia: an endocrine society clinical practice guideline," Journal of Clinical Endocrinology and Metabolism, vol. 97, no. 9, pp. 2969–2989, 2012.

[6] C.-C. Hung, Y.-K. Tu, C.-F. Su, L.-S. Lin, and C.-J. Shih, "Epidemiological study of Moyamoya disease in Taiwan," Clinical Neurology and Neurosurgery, vol. 99, no. 2, pp. S23–S25, 1997.

[7] Y. Yonekawa, J. Fandino, M. Hug, M. Wiesli, M. Fujioka, and N. Khan, Moyamoya Angiopathy in Europe. Moyamoya Disease Update, Springer, Tokyo, Japan, 2010.

[8] H. Fodstad, M. Bodosi, A. Forssell, and D. Perricone, "Moyamoya disease in patients of Finno-Ugric origin," British Journal of Neurosurgery, vol. 10, no. 2, pp. 179–186, 1996.

[9] A. V. Gaddi, A. F. G. Cicero, F. O. Odoo, A. Poli, and R. Paoletti, "Practical recommendations for familial combined hyperlipidemia diagnosis and management: an update," Vascular Disease Prevention, vol. 4, no. 3, pp. 229–236, 2007.

[10] Y.-C. Wei, C.-H. Liu, T.-Y. Chang et al., "Coexisting diseases of moyamoya vasculopathy," Journal of Stroke and Cerebrovascular Diseases, vol. 23, no. 6, pp. 1344–1350, 2014.

[11] R. M. Scott and E. R. Smith, "Moyamoya disease and moyamoya syndrome," The New England Journal of Medicine, vol. 360, no. 12, pp. 1226–1237, 2009.

[12] J.-I. Takanishi, Moyamoyan Disease in Children, Brain and Development, Elsevier, 2011.

[13] C.-C. Hung, Y.-K. Tu, C.-F. Su, L.-S. Lin, and C.-J. Shih, "Epidemiological study of moyamoya disease in Taiwan," Clinical Neurology and Neurosurgery, vol. 99, supplement 2, pp. S23–S25, 1997.

[14] S. Kuroda, T. Ishikawa, K. Houkin, R. Nanba, M. Hokari, and Y. Iwasaki, "Incidence and clinical features of disease progression in adult moyamoya disease," Stroke, vol. 36, no. 10, pp. 2148–2153, 2005.

[15] S. C. Lee, J. S. Jeon, J. E. Kim et al., "Contralateral progression and its risk factor in surgically treated unilateral adult moyamoya disease with a review of pertinent literature," Acta Neurochirurgica, vol. 156, no. 1, pp. 103–111, 2014.

[16] S. J. Kim, K. G. Heo, H. Y. Shin et al., "Association of thyroid autoantibodies with moyamoya-type cerebrovascular disease: a prospective study," Stroke, vol. 41, no. 1, pp. 173–176, 2010.

[17] S.-H. Im, C. W. Oh, O. K. Kwon, J. E. Kim, and D. H. Han, "Moyamoya disease associated with Graves disease: special considerations regarding clinical significance and management," Journal of Neurosurgery, vol. 102, no. 6, pp. 1013–1017, 2005.

[18] Y. Mineharu, Y. Takagi, J. C. Takahashi et al., "Rapid progression of unilateral moyamoya disease in a patient with a family history and an RNF213 risk variant," Cerebrovascular Diseases, vol. 36, no. 2, pp. 155–157, 2013.

[19] S. Kuroda, N. Hashimoto, T. Yoshimoto, Y. Iwasaki, and Research Committee on Moyamoya Disease in Japan, "Radiological findings, clinical course, and outcome in asymptomatic moyamoya disease: results of multicenter survey in Japan," Stroke, vol. 38, pp. 1430–1435, 2007.

[20] B. A. Gross and R. Du, "The natural history of Moyamoya in a North American adult cohort," Journal of Clinical Neuroscience, vol. 20, no. 1, pp. 44–48, 2013.

[21] W.-S. Cho, Y. S. E. Chung, J. E. U. Kim et al., "The natural clinical course of hemodynamically stable adult moyamoya disease," Journal of Neurosurgery, vol. 122, no. 1, pp. 82–89, 2015.

[22] H. J. Noh, S. J. Kim, J. S. Kim et al., "Long term outcome and predictors of ischemic stroke recurrence in adult moyamoya disease," Journal of the Neurological Sciences, vol. 359, no. 1-2, pp. 381–388, 2015.

[23] M. Kraemer, P. Berlit, F. Diesner, and N. Khan, "What is the expert's option on antiplatelet therapy in moyamoya disease? Results of a worldwide Survey," European Journal of Neurology, vol. 19, no. 1, pp. 163–167, 2012.

[24] S. Yamada, K. Oki, Y. Itoh et al., "Effects of surgery and antiplatelet therapy in ten-year follow-up from the registry study of research committee on moyamoya disease in Japan," Journal of Stroke and Cerebrovascular Diseases, vol. 25, no. 2, pp. 340–349, 2016.

[25] M. Fukui, S. Kono, K. Sueishi, and K. Ikezaki, "Moyamoya disease," *Neuropathology*, vol. 20, supplement 1, pp. S61–S64, 2000.

[26] A. M. I. Andeejani, M. A. M. Salih, T. Kolawole et al., "Moyamoya syndrome with unusual angiographic findings and protein C deficiency: review of the literature," *Journal of the Neurological Sciences*, vol. 159, no. 1, pp. 11–16, 1998.

[27] P. Cerrato, M. Grasso, A. Lentini et al., "Atherosclerotic adult Moya-Moya disease in a patient with hyperhomocysteinaemia," *Neurological Sciences*, vol. 28, no. 1, pp. 45–47, 2007.

[28] F. Booth, R. Yanofsky, I. B. Ross, P. Lawrence, and K. Oen, "Primary antiphospholipid syndrome with moyamoya-like vascular changes," *Pediatric Neurosurgery*, vol. 31, no. 1, pp. 45–48, 1999.

[29] H. Tsuda, S. Hattori, S. Tanabe et al., "Thrombophilia found in patients with Moyamoya disease," *Clinical Neurology and Neurosurgery*, vol. 99, supplement 2, pp. S229–S233, 1997.

[30] H. C. Jeong, Y. J. Kim, W. Yoon, S. P. Joo, S. S. Lee, and Y. W. Park, "Moyamoya syndrome associated with systemic lupus erythematosus," *Lupus*, vol. 17, no. 7, pp. 679–682, 2008.

[31] T. Czartoski, D. Hallam, J. M. Lacy, M. R. Chun, and K. Becker, "Postinfectious vasculopathy with evolution to moyamoya syndrome," *Journal of Neurology, Neurosurgery and Psychiatry*, vol. 76, no. 2, pp. 256–259, 2005.

[32] N. J. Ullrich, R. Robertson, D. D. Kinnamon et al., "Moyamoya following cranial irradiation for primary brain tumors in children," *Neurology*, vol. 68, no. 12, pp. 932–938, 2007.

[33] S. R. Levine, J. E. Knake, and A. B. Young, "Atypical progressive stroke syndrome associated with oral contraceptives and cigarette use," *Stroke*, vol. 18, no. 2, pp. 519–523, 1987.

[34] J. C. Drees, J. A. Stone, and A. H. B. Wu, "Morbidity involving the hallucinogenic designer amines MDA and 2C-I," *Journal of Forensic Sciences*, vol. 54, no. 6, pp. 1485–1487, 2009.

[35] M. S. Tullu, A. V. Advirkar, R. G. Ghildiyal, and S. Tambe, "Familial hypertriglyceridemia," *Indian Journal of Pediatrics*, vol. 75, no. 12, pp. 1257–1258, 2008.

36

Severe Symptomatic Hypocalcemia from HIV Related Hypoparathyroidism

Sartaj Sandhu ⓘ,[1] **Akshata Desai,**[2] **Manav Batra ⓘ,**[2] **Robin Girdhar,**[2] **Kaushik Chatterjee,**[2]
E. Helen Kemp ⓘ,[3] **Antoine Makdissi,**[2] **and Ajay Chaudhuri**[2]

[1]*Advocare DelGiorno Endocrinology, Sewell, New Jersey, USA*
[2]*Department of Endocrinology, Diabetes and Metabolism, State University of New York, Buffalo, New York, USA*
[3]*Department of Oncology and Metabolism, University of Sheffield, Sheffield, UK*

Correspondence should be addressed to Sartaj Sandhu; sandhusartaj@yahoo.com

Academic Editor: Wayne V. Moore

We report the case of a 54-year-old Caucasian female who presented with a two-year history of persistent hypocalcemia requiring multiple hospitalizations. Her medical history was significant for HIV diagnosed four years ago. She denied any history of prior neck surgery or radiation. Her vital signs were stable with an unremarkable physical exam. Pertinent medications included calcium carbonate, vitamin D3, calcitriol, efavirenz, emtricitabine, tenofovir disoproxil, hydrochlorothiazide, and inhaled budesonide/formoterol. Laboratory testing showed total calcium of 5.7 mg/dL (normal range: 8.4-10.2 mg/dL), ionized calcium of 2.7 mg/dL (normal range: 4.5-5.5 mg/dL), serum phosphate of 6.3 mg/dL (normal range: 2.7-4.5 mg/dL), and intact PTH of 7.6 pg/mL (normal range: 15-65 pg/mL). She was diagnosed with primary hypoparathyroidism. Anti-calcium-sensing receptor antibodies and NALP5 antibodies were tested and found to be negative. During subsequent clinic visits, doses of calcium supplements and calcitriol were titrated. Last corrected serum calcium level was 9.18 mg/dL. She was subsequently lost to follow-up. This case gives insight into severe symptomatic hypocalcemia from primary hypoparathyroidism attributed to HIV infection. We suggest that calcium levels should be closely monitored in patients with HIV infection.

1. Introduction

Endocrine involvement is frequent in HIV infected patients, although it rarely involves the parathyroid glands [1]. Hypocalcemia is an infrequent phenomenon in HIV infection and it is mostly attributed to Vitamin D deficiency, hypoalbuminemia, or pharmacotherapy. We report a rare case of severe symptomatic hypocalcemia from primary hypoparathyroidism attributed to HIV infection.

2. Case Presentation

A 54-year-old Caucasian female presented to our clinic with a two-year history of persistent hypocalcemia requiring multiple hospitalizations. Her symptoms included muscle cramps, tingling and perioral paresthesias. Her medical history was significant for HIV diagnosed four years ago, gastric bypass surgery done 15 years ago, hypertension, and COPD. She denied any history of prior neck surgery or radiation. She denied any history of hearing loss. She had no family history of autoimmune disease.

Her vital signs were stable with an unremarkable physical exam. Chvostek's and Trousseau's signs were negative. Pertinent medications included calcium carbonate, vitamin D3, calcitriol, atripla (efavirenz/emtricitabine/tenofovir disoproxil), hydrochlorothiazide, and inhaled budesonide/formoterol.

Laboratory testing showed total calcium of 5.7 mg/dL (normal range: 8.4-10.2 mg/dL), serum albumin 3.9 mg/dL, ionized calcium 2.7 mg/dL (normal range: 4.5-5.5 mg/dL), serum magnesium 1.7 mg/dL (normal range: 1.7-2.7 mg/dL), serum phosphate 6.3 mg/dL (normal range: 2.7-4.5 mg/dL), and intact PTH 7.6 pg/mL (normal range: 15-65 pg/mL). She had normal 25-hydroxy vitamin D 32 ng/mL (normal range: 30-100 ng/mL), 1,25 dihydroxy vitamin D 23 pg/mL (normal range: 18-72 pg/mL), TSH 1.2 μIU/L (normal range:

TABLE 1: Clinical course showing laboratory studies and treatment regimen.

Date	Corrected total calcium (normal range, 8.4–10.2 mg/dL)	Ionized calcium (normal range, 4.5-5.5 mg/dL)	Serum phosphate (normal range, 2.7–4.5 mg/dL)	Medications
11/2012	6.9	3.0	5.9	Calcitriol 0.25 mcg daily Total elemental calcium 1440 mg daily (as calcium carbonate 3600 mg daily in divided doses) Vitamin D 50,000 units weekly
12/2012	7.0	3.5	5.9	Calcitriol 0.25 mcg twice daily Total elemental calcium 2400 mg daily (as calcium carbonate 6000 mg daily in divided doses) Vitamin D 50,000 units weekly
3/2013	7.2	3.5	5.7	Calcitriol 0.25 mcg three times daily Total elemental calcium 1800 mg daily (as calcium carbonate 4500 mg daily in divided doses) Vitamin D 50,000 units weekly
6/2013	7.0	3.2	5.4	Calcitriol 0.5 mcg twice daily Total elemental calcium 2000 mg daily (as calcium carbonate 5000 mg daily in divided doses) Vitamin D 50,000 units weekly
8/2013	7.9	-	-	Calcitriol 0.5 mcg three times daily Total elemental calcium 3600 mg daily (as calcium carbonate 7500 mg daily and calcium citrate 2850 mg daily in divided doses) Vitamin D 50,000 units weekly
11/2013	9.2	4.8	-	Calcitriol 0.5 mcg three times daily Total elemental calcium 3800 mg daily (as calcium carbonate 7500 mg daily and calcium citrate 3800 mg daily in divided doses) Vitamin D 50,000 units weekly

0.40-4.5 μIU/L), and creatinine 0.98 mg/dL (normal range: 0.5 -1.1 mg/dL). Absolute CD4 count was 629 cells/μL (normal range: 185-2273 cells/μL) with undetectable HIV-1 RNA viral load.

She was diagnosed with primary hypoparathyroidism. A serum sample was tested for anti-calcium sensing receptor (CaSR) antibodies [2] and NALP5 antibodies [2] to rule out autoimmune hypoparathyroidism and it was found to be negative; the CaSR antibody index was 1.09 (normal range: 0.57-1.38; upper limit of normal, 1.73) and the NALP5 antibody index was 1.12 (normal range: 0.62-1.93; upper limit of normal, 2.17). During subsequent clinic visits, doses of calcium supplements and calcitriol were titrated and she was started on magnesium oxide. She required calcium carbonate 2500 mg three times per day, calcium citrate 1900 mg twice per day, and calcitriol 0.5 mcg three times per day (Table 1). Her last corrected serum calcium level was 9.18 mg/dL. She was considered for treatment with recombinant human PTH but subsequently she was lost to follow-up.

3. Discussion

Hypocalcemia is defined as low albumin corrected total serum calcium or low ionized serum calcium levels. It is a relatively common condition. Broadly, the causes of hypocalcemia are divided into disorders associated with low

or high PTH levels, drugs, and hypomagnesemia [3], as shown in Table 2.

Increased prevalence of hypocalcemia has been reported in HIV positive individuals, but it was mostly related to vitamin D deficiency [4]. A retrospective review reported greater frequency of parathyroid hyperplasia in autopsy specimens of HIV infected African American patients, which could be result of high prevalence of vitamin D deficiency in HIV infected patients [5].

Other causes of hypocalcemia in HIV infected patients are attributed to hypoalbuminemia [6], medications like foscarnet [7] and Fanconi's syndrome related to antiretroviral medications [8]. Tenofovir can rarely cause hypocalcemia as part of Fanconi's syndrome, along with hypophosphatemia and normal or slightly elevated PTH levels [9].

Our patient had hypocalcemia, hyperphosphatemia with low PTH levels, consistent with primary hypoparathyroidism. With the absence of neck surgery and an unlikely autoimmune etiology (negative antibody testing, late onset, absence of family history, hearing loss, and associated conditions), HIV infection was considered as the principal etiology causing hypoparathyroidism leading to hypocalcemia. This has been very rarely reported in literature [10].

The cause of hypoparathyroidism in HIV infected individuals is thought to be related to impaired parathyroid hormone release and altered parathyroid function [11, 12].

TABLE 2: Pathogenesis and differential diagnosis of hypocalcemia.

Hypocalcemia associated with	Disorders
Low PTH	Abnormal PTH synthesis; Abnormal parathyroid gland development; Post-surgical hypoparathyroidism; Autoimmune polyglandular syndrome type 1; Activating mutations of the calcium-sensing receptor; Infiltration of parathyroid gland; Radiation-induced hypoparathyroidism; HIV infection; Hungry bone syndrome
High PTH	Vitamin D deficiency or resistance; PTH resistance (pseudohypoparathyroidism); Loss of calcium in circulation (tumor lysis syndrome, acute pancreatitis, sepsis, osteoblastic metastases, hyperphosphatemia); Renal disease
Drugs	Inhibitors of bone resorption (bisphosphonates, calcitonin, denosumab); Cinacalcet; Calcium chelators (EDTA, citrate, phosphate); Foscarnet; Phenytoin; Fluoride poisoning
Disorders of magnesium metabolism	Hypomagnesemia causing functional hypoparathyroidism

Mechanisms explaining hypoparathyroidism in HIV infected patients are not well described. There is suggestion of expression of a CD4 like molecule by the parathyroid cells making them a potential target of HIV, leading to impaired PTH secretion [13].

Further, our patient was unique and challenging to manage due to requirement of high doses of calcium, calcitriol, and Vitamin D. It may be in part due to previous history of gastric bypass surgery which may impair calcium and Vitamin D absorption.

4. Conclusion

Although rare, primary hypoparathyroidism should be considered in the differential diagnosis of hypocalcemia in HIV infected patients. We suggest that calcium levels, PTH levels, and 25(OH) vitamin D levels should be monitored regularly in those patients.

Disclosure

The case abstract and poster was presented at the 23rd Annual American Association of Clinical Endocrinologists (AACE) meeting held in 2014.

References

[1] S. K. Grinspoon and J. P. Bilezikian, "HIV disease and the endocrine system," *The New England Journal of Medicine*, vol. 327, no. 19, pp. 1360–1365, 1992.

[2] E. H. Kemp, M. Habibullah, N. Kluger et al., "Prevalence and clinical associations of calcium-sensing receptor and NALP5 autoantibodies in finnish APECED patients," *The Journal of*

Clinical Endocrinology & Metabolism, vol. 99, no. 3, pp. 1064–1071, 2014.

[3] R. V. Thakker, "Hypocalcemia: Pathogenesis, differential diagnosis, and management," in *Primer on the Metabolic Bone Diseases and Disorders of Mineral Metabolism*, American Society of Bone and Mineral Research, Washington, DC, USA, 6th edition, 2006.

[4] E. W. Kuehn, H. J. Anders, J. R. Bogner, J. Obermaier, F. D. Goebel, and D. Schlöndorff, "Hypocalcaemia in HIV infection and AIDS," *Journal of Internal Medicine*, vol. 245, no. 1, pp. 69–73, 1999.

[5] R. Cherqaoui, K. M. M. Shakir, B. Shokrani, S. Madduri, F. Farhat, and V. Mody, "Histopathological changes of the thyroid and parathyroid glands in HIV-infected patients," *Journal of Thyroid Research*, vol. 2014, 2014.

[6] M. A. Perazella and E. Brown, "Electrolyte and acid-base disorders associated with AIDS - An etiologic review," *Journal of General Internal Medicine*, vol. 9, no. 4, pp. 232–236, 1994.

[7] M. A. Jacobson, J. G. Gambertoglio, F. T. Aweeka, D. M. Causey, and A. A. Portale, "Foscarnet-induced hypocalcemia and effects of foscarnet on calcium metabolism," *The Journal of Clinical Endocrinology & Metabolism*, vol. 72, no. 5, pp. 1130–1135, 1991.

[8] K. E. Earle, T. Seneviratne, J. Shaker, and D. Shoback, "Fanconi's syndrome in HIV+ adults: Report of three cases and literature review," *Journal of Bone and Mineral Research*, vol. 19, no. 5, pp. 714–721, 2004.

[9] D. Quimby and M. O. Brito, "Fanconi syndrome associated with use of tenofovir in HIV-infected patients: A case report and review of the literature," *The AIDS Reader*, vol. 15, no. 7, pp. 357–364, 2005.

[10] R. Lehmann, B. Leuzinger, and F. Salomon, "Symptomatic hypoparathyroidism in acquired immunodeficiency syndrome," *Hormone Research in Paediatrics*, vol. 42, no. 6, pp. 295–299, 1994.

[11] P. Hellman, J. Albert, M. Gidlund et al., "Impaired Parathyroid Hormone Release in Human Immunodeficiency Virus Infection," *AIDS Research and Human Retroviruses*, vol. 10, no. 4, pp. 391–394, 1994.

37

Persistent Primary Hyperparathyroidism, Severe Vitamin D Deficiency, and Multiple Pathological Fractures

Victoria Mendoza-Zubieta,[1] Mauricio Carvallo-Venegas,[2] Jorge Alberto Vargas-Castilla,[2] Nicolás Ducoing-Sisto,[2] Alfredo Alejandro Páramo-Lovera,[2] Lourdes Josefina Balcázar-Hernández,[1] and Julián Malcolm Mac Gregor-Gooch[3]

[1]*Endocrinology Department, Hospital de Especialidades, Centro Médico Nacional Siglo XXI, IMSS, 06720 Mexico City, DF, Mexico*
[2]*Faculty of Medicine, Universidad Nacional Autónoma de México (UNAM), 04510 Mexico City, DF, Mexico*
[3]*Division of Medicine, Hospital de Especialidades, Centro Médico Nacional Siglo XXI, IMSS, 06720 Mexico City, DF, Mexico*

Correspondence should be addressed to Victoria Mendoza-Zubieta; vmendozazu@yahoo.com

Academic Editor: Michael P. Kane

Persistent primary hyperparathyroidism (PHPT) refers to the sustained hypercalcemia state detected within the first six months following parathyroidectomy. When it coexists with severe vitamin D deficiency, the effects on bone can be devastating. We report the case of a 56-year-old woman who was sent to this center because of persistent hyperparathyroidism. Her disease had over 3 years of evolution with nephrolithiasis and hip fracture. Parathyroidectomy was performed in her local unit; however, she continued with hypercalcemia, bone pain, and pathological fractures. On admission, the patient was bedridden with multiple deformations by fractures in thoracic and pelvic members. Blood pressure was 100/80, heart rate was 86 per minute, and body mass index was 19 kg/m². Calcium was 14 mg/dL, parathormone 1648 pg/mL, phosphorus 2.3 mg/dL, creatinine 2.4 mg/dL, urea 59 mg/dL, alkaline phosphatase 1580 U/L, and vitamin D 4 ng/mL. She received parenteral treatment of hypercalcemia and replenishment of vitamin D. The second surgical exploration was radioguided by gamma probe. A retroesophageal adenoma of 4 cm was resected. *Conclusion.* Persistent hyperparathyroidism with severe vitamin D deficiency can cause catastrophic skeletal bone softening and fractures.

1. Introduction

The classic manifestation of PHPT bone disease is cystic fibrous osteitis, which is clinically characterized by bone pain and radiographically by subperiosteal bone resorption, cysts, and brown tumors [1–3]. The severe deficiency of vitamin D (25-hydroxyvitamin D < 10 ng/dL or <25 nmol/L) produces a lack of mineralization of bone matrix resulting in bone softening and deformities, also called osteomalacia. Persistent PHTP, when coexisting with severe vitamin D deficiency, can have devastating consequences on the skeleton [4–6].

The persistent PHPT is mainly due to delayed diagnosis, lack of localization of ectopic adenomas, and inadequate tumor resection, which prolong the illness and complicate the clinical course [7–10]. First-line treatment and the only one that may be curative in primary hyperparathyroidism (PHPT) is surgery. However, cure rates depend on the experience of the multidisciplinary team; therefore it is important to refer patients to specialized centers with radiologists, surgeons, endocrinologists, and pathologists experienced in the diagnosis and treatment of primary hyperparathyroidism [11–13].

The case presented is a postmenopausal woman with persistent PHPT by ectopic adenoma with multiple atypical fractures due to cystic fibrous osteitis associated with possible osteomalacia.

2. Case Report

A 56-year-old woman was referred to a High Specialized Medical Unit with a diagnosis of persistent primary hyperparathyroidism and multiple pathologic fractures.

The patient had no familial history of bone disease or any other chronic-degenerative disease. She had no diabetes, hypertension, or other pathological antecedents. There was no tobacco or alcohol consumption. She presented 3 years earlier with nephrolithiasis and hip fracture due to a fall from her own height that conditioned prostration and limitation of daily living activities. In her local hospital, she fulfilled biochemical criteria for PHPT. No localization studies were performed. She underwent parathyroidectomy with resection of left superior parathyroid and biopsy of left inferior parathyroid; final histopathology reported hyperplasia (the slides of the first histology could not be revised). The surgery was made in another state with surgeons and pathologists inexperienced in parathyroid surgery. The patient persisted with hypercalcemia and elevated levels of PTH during the first 6 months of clinical follow-up; thus, she was sent to our Medical Unit for additional evaluation.

During the first visit to our center, the patient was found with generalized bone pain. On the physical examination, she had normal vital signs including blood pressure 100/80 mmHg, heart rate 86 per minute, and body mass index (BMI) 19 kg/m^2; she was bedridden and with multiple bone deformities and contractures due to pathologic fractures in thoracic and pelvic extremities.

Laboratory tests reported elevated levels of calcium (14 mg/dL; reference range: 8.4–10.2 mg/dL), low serum phosphorus (2.3 mg/dL; reference range: 2.7–4.5 mg/dL), normal levels of magnesium (2.2 mg/dL; reference range: 1.6–2.6 mg/dL), azotemia with elevated creatinine (2.4 mg/dL; reference range: 0.4–1.2 mg/dL) and urea (59 mg/dL; reference range: 10–50 mg/dL), elevation levels of Intact PTH (iPTH) (1648 pg/mL; reference range: 10–65 pg/mL), severe vitamin D deficiency (<5 ng/mL; sufficiency 30 ng/mL and deficiency < 10 mg/dL), and elevated levels in alkaline phosphatase (1580 UI/L, reference range: 40–129 UI/L) (Table 1). Gonadotropins, thyroid function test, cortisol, and IGF-1 levels were normal for the age of the patient. We corroborated biochemical persistence of PHPT.

Radiographically, chest and pelvis X-ray showed severe widespread cortical bone loss, cysts, brown tumors, and multiple pathological fractures because of severe cystic fibrous osteitis (Figures 1 and 2). No localization studies for parathyroid pathologies could not be performed due to the duration of the studies and the pain induced by the position required to perform them.

We initiated treatment with aggressive intravenous hydration with 0.9% sodium chloride solutions, loop diuretics, and intravenous calcitonin 48 hours before surgery. An experienced head and neck surgeon performed the second surgical bilateral neck exploration with radioguided minimally invasive parathyroidectomy using hand-held gamma probe, evidencing an ectopic adenoma approximately 4 cm in larger diameter (Figure 3).

Postoperatively, the patient presented symptomatic hypocalcemia, with a nadir of 6.8 mg/dL and biochemical evidence of hungry bone syndrome, requiring treatment with intravenous calcium up to 2 mg/kg/min, intravenous magnesium, and oral calcitriol replacement. Despite intensive multidisciplinary approach, the patient had a torpid clinical evolution and died a month later from respiratory complications due to nosocomial pneumonia.

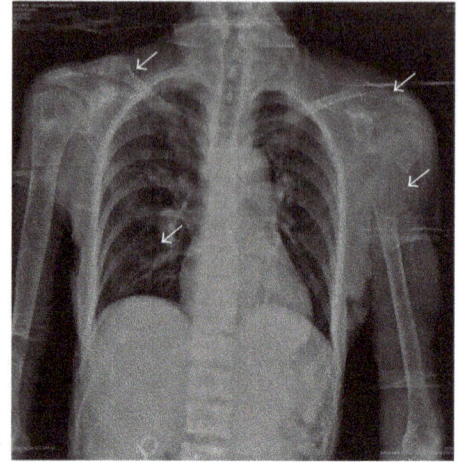

FIGURE 1: Chest X-ray with severe widespread cortical bone loss, cysts, and brown tumors (arrows) in ribs, distal third of the clavicle, and humerus for severe cystic fibrous osteitis due to prolonged PHPT.

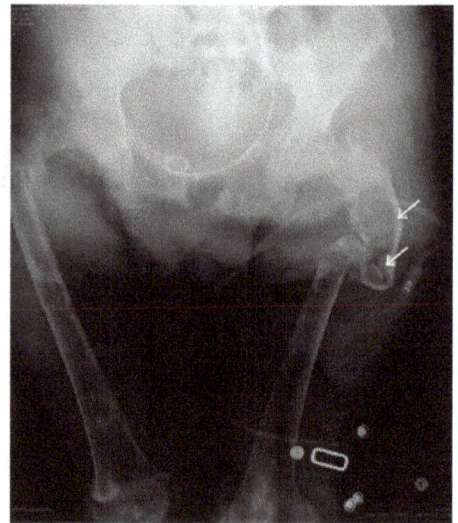

FIGURE 2: Pelvis X-ray with diffuse demineralization, marked decrease in cortical long bone, cysts, and brown tumors (arrows) and multiple pathological fractures for severe osteitis fibrous cystic.

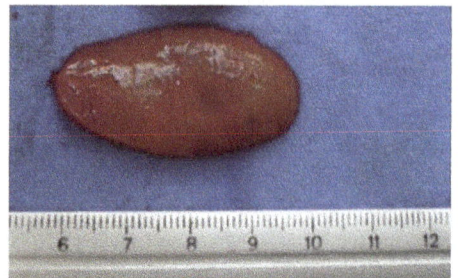

FIGURE 3: Ectopic parathyroid adenoma with approximately 4 cm dimension in the larger diameter.

Table 1: Laboratory test at hospitalization and follow-up after surgery.

Laboratory test	Reference range	Baseline	8 days after surgery	One month after surgery
Urea (mg/dL)	10.0–50.0 mg/dL	59	93	96
Creatinine (mg/dL)	0.4–1.2 mg/dL	2.4	1.27	1.49
Calcium (mg/dL)	8.4–10.2 mg/dL	14	6.8	8.2
Phosphorus (mg/dL)	2.7–4.5 mg/dL	2.3	2.1	3.5
Magnesium (mg/dL)	1.6–2.6 mg/dL	2.2	1.1	1.8
Alkaline phosphatase (UI/L)	40–129 UI/L	1580	1297	910
PTH (pg/mL)	10–65 pg/mL	1648	37.3	37.6
Vitamin D (ng/mL)	Deficiency < 10 mg/mL Insufficiency 10–30 mg/dL, Sufficiency 30–100 mg/dL Toxicity > 100 mg/dL	4	15	17

PTH, parathyroid hormone.

3. Discussion

The PHPT is a common endocrine disease with the highest incidence in postmenopausal women. It is characterized by hypercalcemia and elevated levels of PTH [1]. In the last few years, the most common presentation of PHPT has been the asymptomatic form with incidental findings of hypercalcemia in screening laboratories or during the evaluation of patients with nephrolithiasis, osteoporosis, or pathologic fractures [1–3].

Persistent PHPT refers to a sustained hypercalcemia state detected within the first six months following parathyroidectomy, and recurrent PHPT is applicable when the patient has been normocalcemic for at least six months after surgery and then hypercalcemia reappears [8], the most common cause of persistent PHPT in the presence of an ectopic gland that was not identified in the first intervention. One frequent cause of persistent PHPT is surgeon inexperience in locating and adequately excising a parathyroid adenoma. Other causes include a previously unnoticed multiglandular disease (multiple adenomas or hyperplasia) or carcinoma [7–10].

Ectopic adenomas are infrequent; the incidence reported is 5 to 20% cases with a variable localization. The ectopic localization of adenomas is related to abnormal cell migration in the embryogenesis that determines the presence of parathyroid gland from the submandibular region to mediastinum [7–9]. It has also been suggested that, during the development of adenomas, the progressive increase in size and weight of the tumor can produce a gradual descent due to gravity as the parathyroid glands are attached to adjacent tissue by a lax fibroconnective tissue [10]. Udelsman and Donovan described that the most frequent sites of ectopic adenomas are the retroesophageal space, thymus, intrathyroidal, carotid sheath, submandibular region, and the aortic window [14].

The definitive treatment of PHPT is surgery [11, 12]. A frequent factor in the persistence of HTP is the surgeon's lack of experience. The experienced surgeon must have extensive knowledge of the anatomy, embryology, biochemistry, and physiology of parathyroid glands and the pathophysiology of their diseases. In the first surgical neck exploration, when there is a suspicion of ectopic adenoma, the experienced surgeon can find and resect the ectopic tissue in 90% of cases [13]. Thus, the parathyroid surgery must always be made by a multidisciplinary team expert in parathyroid diseases.

In a series of PHPT, the ectopic glands were associated with high calcium levels, larger adenoma, and more frequent cystic fibrous osteitis compared with hyperparathyroidism with eutopic gland location [15].

Bone manifestations of severe PHPT have been increasingly rare due to early detection and treatment. The most emblematic manifestation of PHPT is the cystic fibrous osteitis, which is characterized clinically by bone pain and radiographically by subperiosteal bone resorption principally in the phalanges, distal third of the clavicles, and radiological appearance of "salt and pepper" in the skull. Although bone cysts and brown tumors can occur anywhere in the skeleton, they mainly affect the ribs, humerus, and jaw. Brown tumors result from excessive osteoclast activity and by an accumulation of osteoclasts interspersed with fibrous tissue in an area with poor mineralization. The brown color is due to hemosiderin deposits. Brown tumors can form real tumors with extrinsic destructive compression that can cause pathological fractures in long bones. The fibrous cystic osteitis is very rare in developed countries and mainly occurs in patients with hyperparathyroidism with prolonged evolution or aggressive behavior [2, 6, 16, 17].

Vitamin D deficiency in PHPT patients is related to higher PTH levels, larger adenomas, and severe clinical evolution, including fibrous cystic osteitis and hungry bone syndrome in postsurgery [4, 5, 18]. Vitamin D, through its receptor, has essential actions in the parathyroid cells. It participates in the regulation of PTH secretion and inhibits cell proliferation. The effect of vitamin D deficiency in the pathogenesis of secondary hyperparathyroidism and parathyroid hyperplasia in elderly, renal insufficiency, and intestinal malabsorption syndromes is well established. With the prolonged evolution of PHPT and severe deficiency of vitamin D, adenomas can grow and secrete greater levels of parathyroid hormone causing greater hypercalcemia and greater target organ damage, mainly bone and kidney [2, 4, 5].

The present case report describes a patient with prolonged and severe PHPT with a devastating effect on bone and multiple pathological fractures in hips, pelvic, and thoracic members that conditioned prostration and limitation in daily living activities. Our patient had multiple risk factors like age, prolonged evolution of HPTP, and vitamin D deficiency that contributed to the severe bone affection in a rare presentation of persistent PHPT.

References

[1] W. D. Fraser, "Hyperparathyroidism," *The Lancet*, vol. 374, no. 9684, pp. 145–158, 2009.

[2] S. J. Silverberg, E. Shane, T. P. Jacobs et al., "Nephrolithiasis and bone involvement in primary hyperparathyroidism," *The American Journal of Medicine*, vol. 89, no. 3, pp. 327–334, 1990.

[3] S. J. Mark, "Hyperparathyroidism and hypoparathyroid disorders," *The New England Journal of Medicine*, vol. 89, no. 3, pp. 327–334, 2000.

[4] D. S. Rao, M. Honasoge, G. W. Divine et al., "Effect of vitamin D nutrition on parathyroid adenoma weight: pathogenetic and clinical implications," *The Journal of Clinical Endocrinology and Metabolism*, vol. 85, no. 3, pp. 1054–1058, 2000.

[5] R. Nuti, D. Merlotti, and L. Gennari, "Vitamin D deficiency and primary hyperparathyroidism," *Journal of Endocrinological Investigation*, vol. 34, no. 7, supplement, pp. 45–49, 2011.

[6] K. Ağbaht, A. Aytaç, and S. Güllü, "Catastrophic bone deformities associated with primary hyperparathyroidism in a middle-aged man," *The Journal of Clinical Endocrinology & Metabolism*, vol. 98, no. 9, pp. 3529–3531, 2013.

[7] G. Åkerström, C. Rudberg, L. Grimelius, H. Johansson, B. Lundström, and J. Rastad, "Causes of failed primary exploration and technical aspects of re-operation in primary hyperparathyroidism," *World Journal of Surgery*, vol. 16, no. 4, pp. 562–568, 1992.

[8] R. Udelsman, "Approach to the patient with persistent or recurrent primary hyperparathyroidism," *The Journal of Clinical Endocrinology & Metabolism*, vol. 96, no. 10, pp. 2950–2958, 2011.

[9] C. A. Wang, "Parathyroid re-exploration A clinical and pathological study of 112 cases," *Annals of Surgery*, vol. 186, no. 2, pp. 140–145, 1977.

[10] G. G. Callender, E. G. Grubbs, T. Vu et al., "The fallen one: the inferior parathyroid gland that descends into the mediastinum," *Journal of the American College of Surgeons*, vol. 208, no. 5, pp. 887–893, 2009.

[11] R. Udelsman, G. Åkerström, C. Biagini et al., "The surgical management of asymptomatic primary hyperparathyroidism: Proceedings of the Fourth International Workshop," *The Journal of Clinical Endocrinology and Metabolism*, vol. 99, no. 10, pp. 3595–3606, 2014.

[12] G. G. Callender and R. Udelsman, "Surgery for primary hyperparathyroidism," *Cancer*, vol. 120, no. 23, pp. 3602–3616, 2014.

[13] B. Zarebczan and H. Chen, "Influence of surgical volume on operative failures for hyperparathyroidism," *Advances in Surgery*, vol. 45, no. 1, pp. 237–248, 2011.

[14] R. Udelsman and P. I. Donovan, "Remedial parathyroid surgery: changing trends in 130 consecutive cases," *Annals of Surgery*, vol. 244, no. 3, pp. 471–479, 2006.

[15] V. Mendoza, C. Ramírez, A. E. Espinoza et al., "Characteristics of ectopic parathyroid glands in 145 cases of primary hyperparathyroidism," *Endocrine Practice*, vol. 16, no. 6, pp. 977–981, 2010.

[16] A. Khan and J. P. Bilezikian, "Primary hyperparathyroidism: pathophysiology and impact on bone," *Canadian Medical Association Journal*, vol. 163, no. 2, pp. 184–187, 2000.

[17] T. D. T. Vu, X. F. Wang, Q. Wang et al., "New insights into the effects of primary hyperparathyroidism on the cortical and trabecular compartments of bone," *Bone*, vol. 55, no. 1, pp. 57–63, 2013.

[18] J. E. Witteveen, S. van Thiel, J. A. Romijn, and N. A. Hamdy, "Hungry bone syndrome: still a challenge in the post-operative management of primary hyperparathyroidism: a systematic review of the literature," *European Journal of Endocrinology*, vol. 168, no. 3, pp. R45–R53, 2013.

38

Diabetes Mellitus Secondary to Acute Pancreatitis in a Child with Wolf-Hirschhorn Syndrome

Asma Deeb

Paediatric Endocrinology Department, Mafraq Hospital, P.O. Box 2951, Abu Dhabi, UAE

Correspondence should be addressed to Asma Deeb; adeeb@seha.ae

Academic Editor: Toshihiro Kita

Wolf-Hirschhorn Syndrome (WHS) is a rare genetic disease caused by deletion in the short arm of chromosome 4. It is characterized by typical fascial features and a varying degree of intellectual disabilities and multiple systemic involvement. Epidemiological studies confirmed the association of acute pancreatitis with the development of diabetes. However, this association has not been reported in WHS. We report an 18-year-old girl with WHS who presented acutely with nonketotic Hyperglycemic Hyperosmolar Status (HHS) in association with severe acute pancreatitis. Her presentation was preceded by febrile illness with preauricular abscess. She was treated with fluids and insulin infusion and remained on insulin 18 months after presentation. Her parents are cousins and the mother was diagnosed with type 2 diabetes. She had negative autoantibodies and no signs of insulin resistance and her monogenic diabetes genetic testing was negative. Microarray study using WHS probe confirmed deletion of 4p chromosome. Acute pancreatitis is uncommon in children and development of diabetes following pancreatitis has not been reported in WHS. HHS is considerably less frequent than diabetes ketoacidosis in children. We highlight the complex presentation with HHS and acute pancreatitis leading to diabetes that required long term of insulin treatment.

1. Introduction

Cooper and Hirschhorn first documented Wolf-Hirschhorn syndrome (WHS) in 1961. The syndrome is caused by a molecular deletion in the short arm of chromosome 4 (4p). It is characterized by the typical fascial features of the Greek warrior helmet appearance of the nose and forehead. Patients with WHS have a varying degree of intellectual disabilities and systemic involvement [1].

The American Diabetes Association classified diabetes resulting from exocrine damage as type 3c. The exocrine damage can be related to pancreatitis, cystic fibrosis, hemochromatosis, pancreatic cancer, pancreatectomy, and pancreatic agenesis [2].

A meta-analysis highlighted the risk of diabetes following pancreatitis. 24 prospective studies of 1,102 patients with pancreatitis were studied. 37% developed prediabetes or diabetes. 16% who developed diabetes needed insulin. It was shown that a diagnosis of acute pancreatitis increases the risk of developing diabetes by over twofold over 5 years [3]. Pooled prevalence of newly diagnosed diabetes within 1 year was 15% and increased to 40% after 5 years of the acute pancreatitis.

A population-based study examined the risk of diabetes after pancreatitis. The study included 2996 patients. Incidence of diabetes was 60.8 per 1000 indicating a twofold increase of developing diabetes [4]. The study showed that the risk of developing diabetes is higher in young males of under 45 years.

To the best of our knowledge, this is the first report of a child with WHS who developed diabetes following acute pancreatitis.

2. Clinical Presentation

The patient is an 18-year-old girl who presented acutely with severe abdominal pain, diarrhea, and vomiting. She was dehydrated and had acidotic breathing. She had hyperglycemia (glucose of 40 mmol/720 mg) and hypernatremia (sodium of 176 mmol). Inflammatory markers were high: procalcitonin 7.550 ng/ml and CRP of 179. Her white cell count was 24.2 × 10^9/l (NR 4–11) with 65.3% neutrophilia and 8.4% monocytosis. She had severe acidosis (pH of 6.95) with no ketosis. Her serum amylase was 354 IU/L (NR 28–100)

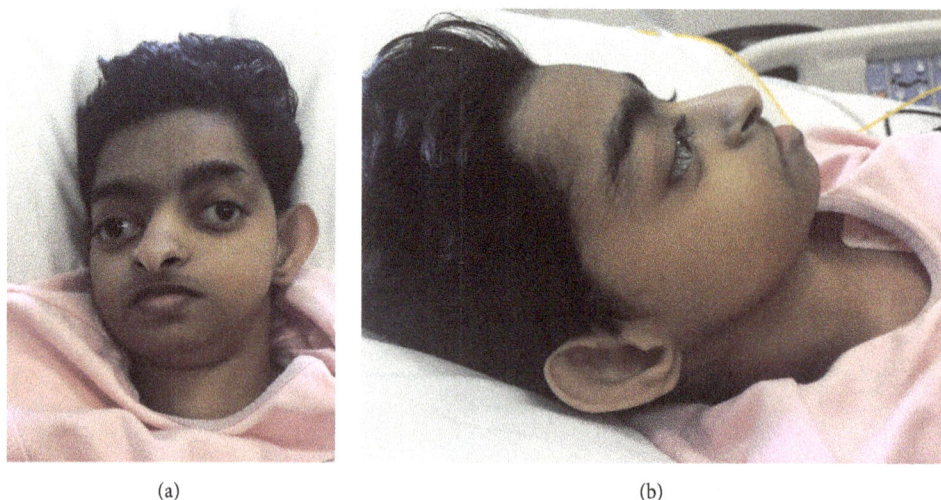

(a)   (b)

FIGURE 1: Front and side fascial photo of the patient showing characteristic features of WHS (Roman helmet appearance, microcephaly, proptosis, short philtrum, high-arched eyebrows, and big ears with minimal creases).

and serum lipase was 5739 IU/L (NR 13–60). LDH was high at 502 (NR 135–225). Her urea was high at 20.9 mmol/L (NR < 8.3), creatinine 269 μmol/L (NR 45–84), and GFR 15 ml/min/1.73 m^2. Liver function tests were normal as was the triglyceride level. Blood, stool, and urine cultures were negative. CT abdomen excluded intra-abdominal abscesses. Chest X-ray showed blunting of both costophrenic angles with no other pulmonary features suggestive of inflammation or pneumonia. Chest CT confirmed bilateral pleural effusion. The diagnosis was reached as severe acute pancreatitis complicated by HHS.

2.1. Past Medical History. The patient was diagnosed clinically with WHS. She has the typical fascial features of the syndrome (Figures 1(a) and 1(b)) and had severe learning disability and global developmental delay. She has microcephaly with marked brain atrophy and ventricular dilatation and suffered from epilepsy. Her seizures were well-controlled on valproic acid and levetiracetam. She has a solitary ectopic kidney with nephrocalcinosis and chronic renal failure (Figure 2). Six weeks prior to the acute presentation, she was febrile with a preauricular abscess. The abscess was drained and she was started on antibiotics. Inflammatory markers were high but her abscess fluid showed no bacterial growth. She remained unwell for about 6 weeks until she presented with the acute illness.

2.2. Family History. Parents are second-degree cousins of Yemeni origin. The mother, who is 52 years, was diagnosed with type 2 diabetes at the age of 45 and is on multiple oral hypoglycemic agents. Her BMI is 28 kg/m^2 and her HbA1c is 9%. She has 4 healthy siblings.

2.3. Treatment. On the acute presentation, she was treated for the HHS. She was rehydrated with normal saline and put on insulin infusion initially at 0.05 unit/kg/day. Her clinical status improved, glucose normalized, and she was shifted to

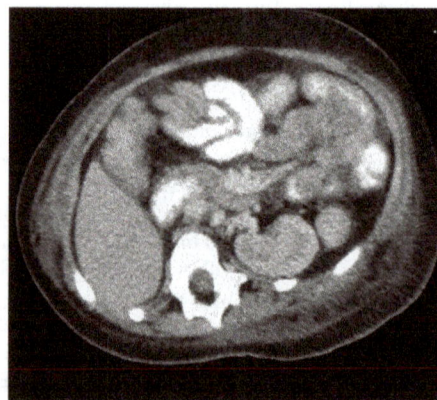

FIGURE 2: Abdominal CT scan showing solitary left kidney with kidney cyst and nephrocalcinosis.

subcutaneous insulin as basal bolus regime with an insulin requirement of 0.3 unit/kg. She was treated conservatively for acute pancreatitis and showed progressive clinical improvement. Her insulin requirement continued to drop and she started having hypoglycaemia. Insulin was stopped and she was discharged home off insulin.

2.4. Progress. Three weeks after discharge, she presented acutely with HHS. She was readmitted and restarted on insulin. After recovery, she was discharged home on insulin glargine and insulin aspart. Her fasting glucose ranged between 90 and 127 mg and postprandial glucose between 110 and 138 mg. She experienced no hypoglycaemia and remained on 0.3 units/kg/day of insulin.

3. Further Investigations

3.1. Biochemistry. Initial HbA1c was 8.4%. Following treatment, it went down to 6.9% in 3 months and to 5.4% in 6 months. Her latest HbA1c (18 months after the initial presentation) is 6.5%. Her initial C-peptide was 0.11 nmol (NR 0.37–1.47). After 6 months, it was 0.3 nmol. Her autoantibodies to GAD, IA2, and insulin were negative.

3.2. Microarray Analysis. Microarray analysis was performed using the critical region probe (WHSCR). FISH analysis on the metaphase spreads and the interphase nuclei showed abnormal signal pattern for the WHSCR probe with deletion in all cells examined (100 cells). These results are diagnostic for WHS.

3.3. Genetic Test for Monogenic Diabetes. Analysis of all coding regions and exon/intron boundaries of the *HNF1β* gene by Sagner sequencing was done. Dosage analysis of *GCK, HNF4A, and HNF1B* by MLPA using MRC-Holland kit P241-D1 was performed. Analyses did not identify a pathogenic mutation or partial/whole gene deletion.

4. Discussion

The patient presentation was complex. In addition to her underlying WHS and chronic renal failure, she has a picture of severe acute pancreatitis. The underlying cause of the pancreatitis was not established. However, her preceding presentation with preauricular sterile abscess suggested viral parotitis with possible pancreatic involvement. Her extreme elevation in glucose and hyperosmolality without ketosis are characteristic of HHS. HHS is considerably less frequent in children than diabetes ketoacidosis [5]. Unlike HHS in adults, where comorbidity conditions are seen, paediatric HHS occurs most often in otherwise healthy children and adolescents with type 2 diabetes particularly obese males [5]. These known facts about HHS added complexity to her presentation and diagnosis.

On the initial presentation, her hyperglycemia was thought to be "stress hyperglycemia" due to the severity of pancreatitis. However, glucose was very high and associated with acidosis requiring insulin infusion. As her HbA1c was high and she remained requiring insulin, it became apparent that she had diabetes rather than transient stress hyperglycemia.

High glucose has been integrated in the scoring to assess the severity of acute pancreatitis. Elevated pancreatic enzymes can be seen in decompensated diabetes; however, only 11% of cases with diabetes ketoacidosis display elevated enzymes and the radiological features of pancreatitis in imaging [6].

The ideal fluid choice in acute pancreatitis management is debatable. Our patient was resuscitated with normal saline fluid boluses. Some references suggest using Ringer lactate solution might be superior in acute pancreatitis [7]. The rationale for using Ringer lactate is its anti-inflammatory effect that can be beneficial in pancreatitis.

The link between acute pancreatitis and development of diabetes is debatable. Studies showed that patients who had surgery for acute pancreatitis have a 28–100% chance of developing diabetes [8] while the risk is lower with conservative treatment (6.2–15.7%) [9]. These observations

suggested that acquiring diabetes is secondary to surgical intervention. However, Das et al. showed that neither the treatment modality nor the severity is detrimental in developing diabetes [3]. Over 30% of patient who had an episode of pancreatitis develop glucose intolerance, impaired β-cell function, and insulin resistance even after mild pancreatitis [10].

Developing diabetes concurrently or shortly after severe pancreatitis can be explained by the extensive necrosis of the pancreas with severe acute pancreatitis which is the case in our patient. However, developing diabetes shortly after mild pancreatitis might be less plausible.

Das et al. proposed that pancreatitis might not be causative but a triggering insult with certain predisposing factors including autoimmunity, genetic susceptibility, or certain metabolic factors such as obesity and dyslipidemia. Our patient had a negative autoimmune screen; her BMI was 16.33 kg/m^2 (−2.66 SDS) with no clinical features of insulin resistance and normal lipid profile. These, collectively, make the diagnosis of type 1 and type 2 diabetes unlikely. Due to lack of autoimmune markers and the history of consanguinity, monogenic diabetes was considered. As she has a kidney cyst, the possibility of MODY 5 (renal cyst and diabetes syndrome) was raised. However, testing for genetic causes of monogenic diabetes, including HNF1β, was negative. Accordingly, we postulate that the pancreatitis was causal of the diabetes. On presentation, her HbA1c was 8.4% indicating that her glucose intolerance was existing prior to her presentation. She was unwell for few weeks prior to presentation and we presume that she could have had subacute pancreatitis which was not picked up considering the severity of the child disability and lack of communication.

An additional thought about the link of diabetes and WHS is related to the C4orf48 which is a gene located in the locus of WHS. C4orf48 is important for cell differentiation. High level of this gene is expressed in the pancreatic tissue postnatally [11]. It is intriguing whether deletion of the WHS locus might be related to dysfunction of pancreatic cell differentiation and causation (or predisposition) of diabetes.

Additional Points

(i) This is the first case report of a patient with WHS who developed diabetes mellitus following acute pancreatitis. (ii) Diabetes can present as HHS in adolescents following severe pancreatitis. (iii) Establishing the cause of diabetes is important for proper treatment and follow-up.

Acknowledgments

The author thanks Professor John Sayer for facilitating the genetic testing for monogenic diabetes.

References

[1] K. Hirschhorn, H. L. Cooper, and I. L. Firschein, "Deletion of short arms of chromosome 4-5 in a child with defects of midline fusion," *Human Genetics*, vol. 1, no. 5, pp. 479–482, 1965.

[2] ADA, "Diagnosis and classification of diabetes mellitus," *Diabetes Care*, vol. 35, supplement 1, pp. S64–S71, 2012.

[3] S. L. M. Das, P. P. Singh, A. R. J. Phillips, R. Murphy, J. A. Windsor, and M. S. Petrov, "Newly diagnosed diabetes mellitus after acute pancreatitis: a systematic review and meta-analysis," *Gut*, vol. 63, no. 5, pp. 818–831, 2014.

[4] H.-N. Shen, C.-C. Yang, Y.-H. Chang, C.-L. Lu, and C.-Y. Li, "Risk of diabetes mellitus after first-attack acute pancreatitis: a national population-based study," *American Journal of Gastroenterology*, vol. 110, no. 12, pp. 1698–1706, 2015.

[5] A. L. Rosenbloom, "Hyperglycemic hyperosmolar state: an emerging pediatric problem," *Journal of Pediatrics*, vol. 156, no. 2, pp. 180–184, 2010.

[6] S. Nair, D. Yadav, and C. S. Pitchumoni, "Association of diabetic ketoacidosis and acute pancreatitis: observations in 100 consecutive episodes of DKA," *American Journal of Gastroenterology*, vol. 95, no. 10, pp. 2795–2800, 2000.

[7] E. de-Madaria, I. Herrera-Marante, V. González-Camacho et al., "Fluid resuscitation with lactated Ringer's solution vs normal saline in acute pancreatitis: A triple-blind, randomized, controlled trial," *United European Gastroenterology Journal*, p. 205064061770786, 2017.

[8] S. Connor, N. Alexakis, M. G. T. Raraty et al., "Early and late complications after pancreatic necrosectomy," *Surgery*, vol. 137, no. 5, pp. 499–505, 2005.

[9] D. Wu, Y. Xu, Y. Zeng, and X. Wang, "Endocrine pancreatic function changes after acute pancreatitis," *Pancreas*, vol. 40, no. 7, pp. 1006–1011, 2011.

[10] T. Symersky, B. van Hoorn, and A. A. Masclee, "The outcome of a long-term follow-up of pancreatic function aft er recovery from acute pancreatitis," *JOP. Journal of the Pancreas*, pp. 447-53, 2006.

[11] M. C. H Wreschner, "C4orf48, a gene related to the Wolf-Hirschhorn contiguous gene syndrome, codes for a novel secreted protein linked to cell differentiation processes," *Journal of Proteomics & Bioinformatics*, vol. 10, no. 05, 2017.

39

Hypoglycemia Secondary to Sulfonylurea Ingestion in a Patient with End Stage Renal Disease: Results from a 72-Hour Fast

Alice Abraham, Mishaela Rubin, Domenico Accili, John P. Bilezikian, and Utpal B. Pajvani

Division of Endocrinology, Department of Medicine, Columbia University College of Physicians and Surgeons, New York, NY 10032, USA

Correspondence should be addressed to Alice Abraham; draliceabraham@gmail.com

Academic Editor: Najmul Islam

Insulin, proinsulin, and C-peptide levels increase with sulfonylurea exposure but the acuity of increase has not been described in dialysis patients. We present a case of a dialysis patient who presented with hypoglycemia and was found to have accidental sulfonylurea ingestion. This is a 73-year-old man with ESRD on peritoneal dialysis, without history of diabetes, who presented with hypoglycemia. Past medical history includes multiple myeloma, congestive heart failure, and hypertension. At initial presentation, his blood glucose was 47 mg/dL, with concomitant elevations in the following: C-peptide 30.5 (nl: 0.8–3.5 ng/mL), insulin 76 (nl: 3–19 μIU/mL), and proinsulin 83.3 (nl: $\leq$8.0 pmol/L). During the 72-hour fast, which he completed without hypoglycemia, insulin declined to be within normal limits (to 12 μIU/mL); proinsulin (to 12.1 pmol/L) and C-peptide (to 7.2 ng/mL) levels decreased but remained elevated. The sulfonylurea screen ultimately returned positive for glipizide, clinching the diagnosis. This is the first reported case which characterizes the chronic elevation of proinsulin in a patient with ESRD, as well as its dramatic increase after a presumed solitary exposure to sulfonylurea. The 72-hour fast conducted gives insight into the clearance of insulin, proinsulin, and C-peptide after sulfonylurea ingestion in ESRD.

1. Introduction

Insulin, proinsulin, and C-peptide levels increase with sulfonylurea exposure but the degree and acuity of increase are not known in dialysis patients. We describe a man with end stage renal disease (ESRD) on peritoneal dialysis with no previous history of diabetes who presented with unexplained hypoglycemia. To determine the source of his protracted hypoglycemia, he underwent a 72-hour fast in which we observed progressive declines in insulin, proinsulin, and C-peptide levels. Sulfonylurea screen returned positive for glipizide. The 72-hour fast gives insight into the rate of C-peptide, proinsulin, and insulin clearance in ESRD after sulfonylurea ingestion, which, to our knowledge, has not yet been described in the literature.

2. Case Report

We describe a 73-year-old man with ESRD on peritoneal dialysis, without history of diabetes, who presented to the emergency department (ED) with hypoglycemia. Past medical history was notable for multiple myeloma, congestive heart failure, and hypertension. His ESRD was the result of long-standing hypertension and was diagnosed years before the multiple myeloma. Nine months prior to presentation, the patient received three cycles of thalidomide for multiple myeloma in his native Dominican Republic, but no recent or new chemotherapeutic agents were added prior to admission. In the ED, he was diaphoretic and found to have fingerstick glucose of 43 mg/dL; his symptoms resolved immediately upon normalization of blood glucose. His hypoglycemia was recurrent with fingerstick glucose persistently in the 30–40 mg/dL range prior to initiation of a dextrose 10% (D10) drip. He required a D10 infusion for forty-eight hours before it could be safely titrated off.

The patient denied prior neuroglycopenic symptoms. He denied recent changes to his dialysate or symptoms of infection or adrenal insufficiency. His medications include a beta-adrenergic blocker, folic acid, nephrovite vitamin B complex, and omeprazole. Two weeks prior to presentation, his beta-adrenergic blocker dosage was increased; otherwise

TABLE 1: Results of C-peptide, proinsulin, insulin, and glucose obtained during 72-hour fast.

Time (hours)	C-peptide (normal 0.8–3.5 ng/mL)	Proinsulin (normal ≤ 8 pmol/L)	Insulin (normal 3–19 μIU/mL)	Glucose (mg/dL)
0	21.2	26.5	34	115
6	14.7	15.2	20	101
12	11.2	11.8	22	104
18	9.9	12.6	25	107
24	7.4	10.5	10	108
30	8	10.7		104
36	6.8	7.8	9	100
42		10.1		90
48	5	8.6	8	80
54	6.4	10.2	11	95
60	5.3	9.1	9	82
66	5.7	9.9	9	106
68	5.4	9.6	9	67
72	7.2	12.1	12	95

there were no changes to his medication regimen. He lives with two family members who both have Type 2 Diabetes on sulfonylurea (glipizide), but he denied accidental or intentional ingestion. His family members were unable to recall the dose and frequency of their glipizide medications. The patient performs nightly peritoneal dialysis. Throughout his hospitalization, he performed peritoneal dialysis using 1.5/2.5% Dianeal PD solution every 6 hours with a 2 L fill.

Physical exam was notable for normal vital signs [blood pressure 113/74, pulse 64, temperature 37.2 degrees Celsius, and respiratory rate 20]. He was overweight with a BMI of 26.6 kg/m^2. He was a well appearing Hispanic elderly gentleman with acanthosis nigricans present over his posterior neck. Serum electrolytes were within normal limits (potassium 4.5 mmol/L [3.6–5.0], sodium 138.0 mmol/L [136–146], and chloride 101 mmol/L [97–107]). Creatinine and blood urea nitrogen (BUN) concentrations were both elevated at 10.00 mg/dL [0.60–1.20 mg/dL] and 48 mg/dL [7–20 mg/dL], respectively, but unchanged from baseline values (creatinine 9.48–12.82 mg/dL and BUN 48–83 mg/dL). The serum albumin concentration was mildly reduced at 3.1 [3.5–5.5 g/dL], attributed to malnutrition and chronic inflammation. The INR 1.1 [0.9–1.2] and transaminases (AST 15 [12–38 U/L] and ALT 11 [7–41 U/L]) were normal.

The hypoglycemia prompted measurement of serum fructosamine which was normal, 186 [170–285 umol/L], but interpretation is potentially confounded by his low albumin and multiple myeloma history. Similarly, the hemoglobin A1C was normal at 5.7 but was also difficult to interpret in ESRD. Additional laboratory evaluation included normal cosyntropin stimulation testing (36.7 μg/dL before cosyntropin to 42.7 μg/dL 1 hour after cosyntropin administration) and negative infectious disease workup, including urine, blood, and peritoneal dialysate fluid cultures. CT scan of the abdomen with intravenous contrast performed six months prior to admission for abdominal pain revealed a normal pancreas.

At the time of admission, the blood glucose was 47 mg/dL, with concomitant elevations in the following: C-peptide 30.5

(nl: 0.8–3.5 ng/mL), insulin 76 (nl: 3–19 μIU/mL), and proinsulin 83.3 (nl: ≤8.0 pmol/L). C-peptide, insulin, and proinsulin were measured by ARUP laboratories using quantitative chemiluminescent immunoassays. Our differential diagnosis for hyperinsulinemic hypoglycemia included insulinoma versus exposure to an oral hypoglycemic agent. We entertained the possibility of an insulin antibody mediated hypoglycemia in light of his multiple myeloma history [1]; however, insulin antibody was not detectable. As it would take days to receive the results from his sulfonylurea screen and we could not entirely eliminate insulinoma from the differential, he underwent a 72-hour fast to determine whether the source of the hypoglycemia was exogenous or endogenous.

During the 72-hour fast, insulin levels rapidly declined within 24 hours to normal; proinsulin and C-peptide levels fell in parallel but remained abnormally high (Table 1 and Figure 1). The patient completed the fast without developing further hypoglycemia or neuroglycopenic symptoms. The sulfonylurea screen, obtained at the time of admission, was positive for glipizide (performed by ARUP laboratories, positive at concentrations greater than 5 ng/mL). The patient and family denied inadvertent use of glipizide. The patient was discharged with new prescriptions in case there was a pharmacy error. When the patient returned for outpatient laboratory testing 1 week later, the repeated values were similar to those obtained at the end of the fast, with persistently elevated fasting C-peptide (8.8 ng/mL) and proinsulin (10.7 pmol/L) but normal insulin (14 μIU/mL) levels. He denied any recurrent hypoglycemia symptoms one week after hospital discharge. Furthermore, during subsequent admissions for worsening congestive heart failure, he exhibited no further signs or symptoms of hypoglycemia.

3. Discussion

Sulfonylurea ingestion is a well-recognized cause of hyperinsulinemic hypoglycemia. In this case, we believe this was our patient's first exposure to sulfonylurea, as he had no

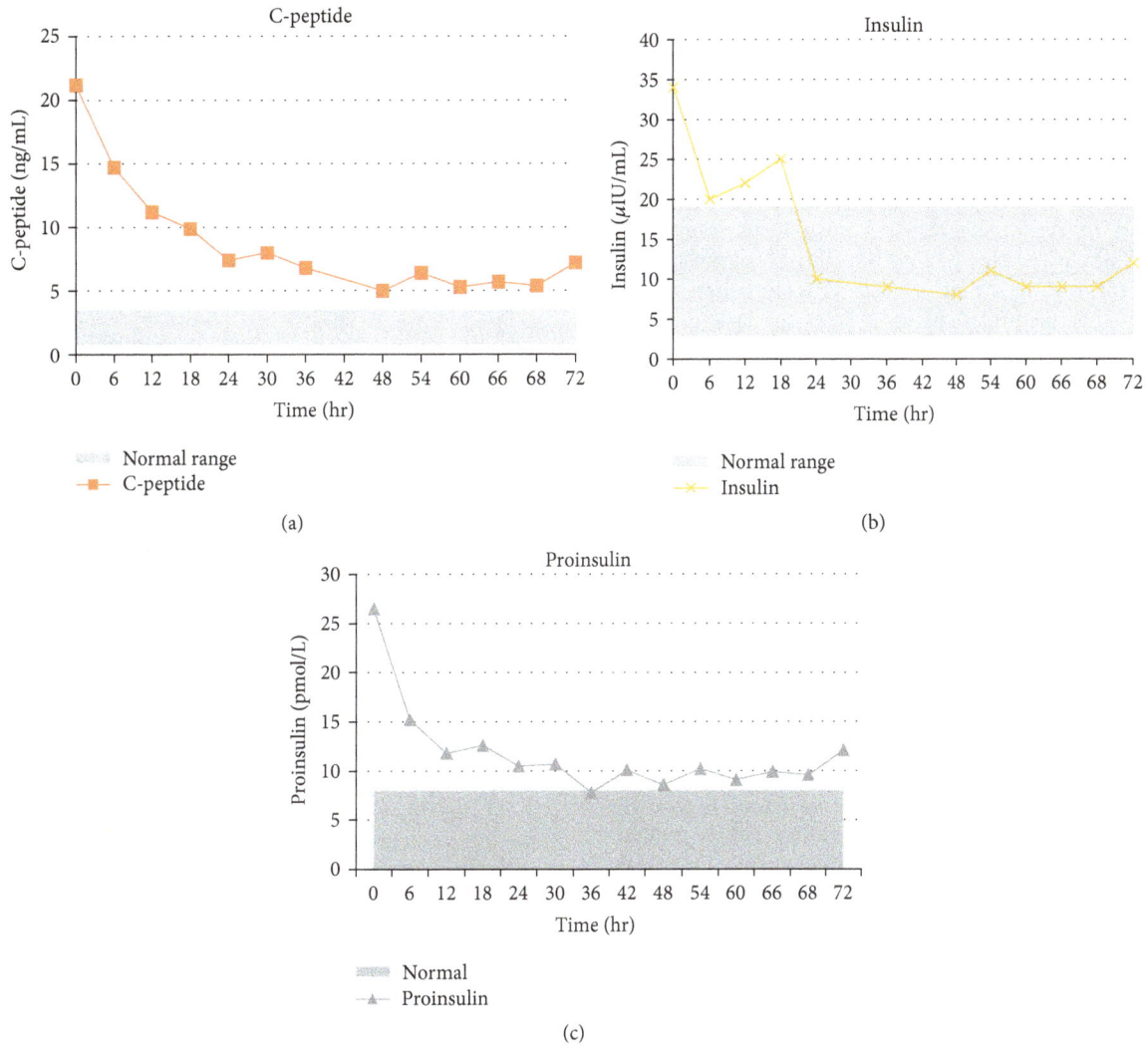

FIGURE 1: Decline of C-peptide, insulin, and proinsulin observed during 72-hour fast.

neuroglycopenic symptoms until shortly prior to admission. Although some medications such as H2 receptor blockers, salicylates, and trimethoprim-sulfamethoxazole are known to prolong the hypoglycemic effects of sulfonylureas [2, 3], this patient was not taking any of them. Thus, the data may well represent rates of recovery in proinsulin, C-peptide, and insulin levels after endogenous stimulation by sulfonylurea ingestion in renal failure.

Glipizide is a potent, second generation sulfonylurea, and, in patients with normal renal and liver function, it has an elimination half-time of about 7 hours and duration of action of 12 to 24 hours. Glipizide undergoes extensive enterohepatic metabolism and is converted in the liver to several inactive metabolites. Thus, in patients with cirrhosis, glipizide has a prolonged half-life [4]. Less than 5 percent is excreted in the urine as intact glipizide, with the majority excreted as inactive metabolites (60 percent as 4-hydroxyglipizide, 15 percent as 3-hydroxyglipizide, and 2 percent as N-(β-acetyl-aminoethyl-benzene-sulfonyl)-N-cyclohexylurea) [5]. Unlike sulfonylureas such as acetohexamide and

glyburide which are metabolized to active metabolites [6], one would not expect accumulation of glipizide metabolites to have a significant clinical impact in renal insufficiency. In fact, the package insert for glipizide suggests caution but no dose adjustment in renal impairment. Some, however, have recommended a 50% reduction in dose in patients with GFR ≤ 50 mL/minute [7].

The biochemical markers of endogenous hyperinsulinism documented in this case suggest unique rates of disappearance of insulin and its precursors in patients with ESRD. We found a marked relative increase in proinsulin and C-peptide (8–10x ULN) as compared to insulin (4x ULN) levels. Assuming an equivalent production rate, the disproportionate elevation of insulin precursors is most likely related to the relatively faster clearance of insulin (60–70% by liver, with the remainder by other insulin-responsive tissues) and proinsulin/C-peptide (by kidneys) [8, 9]. This estimate is substantiated by the progressive reduction in insulin levels to normal, whereas proinsulin and C-peptide levels declined but remained high, even after completion of the 72-hour fast

(Table 1 and Figure 1). Elevations of C-peptide in renal insufficiency are thought secondary to impaired renal degradation and excretion into urine, exacerbated by insulin resistance induced by uremia [9]; the effects of renal failure on proinsulin are known to be similar [10, 11] although the mechanism was not as clearly understood.

One of the more surprising aspects of this case is the rapid and marked increase in proinsulin in response to acute sulfonylurea exposure. Proinsulin is synthesized in the endoplasmic reticulum of beta cells and then cleaved to mature insulin and C-peptide prior to packaging into secretory vesicles [12]. It is known that, in Type 2 Diabetes (T2D), proinsulin levels are mildly elevated and that there is a further 30% increase with chronic sulfonylurea therapy [13], but why this precursor appears in serum at all is unclear. Two theories are worth considering: (1) excessive secretory demand of beta cells and (2) impaired proinsulin processing in the face of chronic hyperglycemia in T2D patients. Our results suggest that even after acute exposure in a nondiabetic patient, proinsulin levels can rise by 3-fold over baseline, suggesting that hyperproinsulinemia in response to sulfonylureas is likely caused by excessive secretory demand of an "unprepared" beta cell. In this patient, hyperproinsulinemia was likely further enhanced by an element of insulin resistance, as evidenced by acanthosis nigricans on the physical examination. Thus, he may have been "primed" by underlying insulin resistance and baseline chronic elevation of his insulin secretion machinery which together exacerbated sulfonylurea-induced hypoglycemia. One of the unavoidable limitations of this case was the fact that the patient's peritoneal dialysis solution contained a low amount of glucose, but this does not invalidate the results described.

Although C-peptide levels are known to increase with ESRD and sulfonylurea therapy, to our knowledge, this is the first reported case which characterizes the acute and chronic increase in proinsulin after a first and presumed solitary exposure to a sulfonylurea in an ESRD patient.

References

[1] B. Redmon, K. L. Pyzdrowski, M. K. Elson, N. E. Kay, A. P. Dalmasso, and F. Q. Nuttall, "Hypoglycemia due to a monoclonal insulin-binding antibody in multiple myeloma," *The New England Journal of Medicine*, vol. 326, no. 15, pp. 994–998, 1992.

[2] A. J. Scheen and P. J. Lefebvre, "Antihyperglycaemic agents. Drug interactions of clinical importance," *Drug Safety*, vol. 12, no. 1, pp. 32–45, 1995.

[3] P. Marchetti and R. Navalesi, "Pharmacokinetic-pharmacodynamic relationships of oral hypoglycaemic agents. An update," *Clinical Pharmacokinetics*, vol. 16, no. 2, pp. 100–128, 1989.

[4] R. A. Harrigan, M. S. Nathan, and P. Beattie, "Oral agents for the treatment of type 2 diabetes mellitus: pharmacology, toxicity, and treatment," *Annals of Emergency Medicine*, vol. 38, no. 1, pp. 68–78, 2001.

[5] J. E. Gerich, "Oral hypoglycemic agents," *The New England Journal of Medicine*, vol. 321, no. 18, pp. 1231–1245, 1989.

[6] P. M. Thulé and G. Umpierrez, "Sulfonylureas: a new look at old therapy," *Current Diabetes Reports*, vol. 14, no. 4, article 473, 2014.

[7] G. A. Aronoff, W. M. Bennett, J. S. Berns et al., *Drug Prescribing in Renal Failure: Dosing Guidelines for Adults and Children*, American College of Physicians, Philadelphia, Pa, USA, 5th edition, 2007.

[8] T.-E. Wideroe, L. C. Smeby, and O. L. Myking, "Plasma concentrations and transperitoneal transport of native insulin and C-peptide in patients on continuous ambulatory peritoneal dialysis," *Kidney International*, vol. 25, no. 1, pp. 82–87, 1984.

[9] H. T. S. Kajinuma, K. Ishiwata, and N. Kuzuya, "Urinary excretion of C-peptide in relation to renal function," in *Symposium on Proinsulin, Insulin and C-Peptide*, pp. 183–189, Excerpta Medica, Tokushima, Japan, 1978.

[10] J. H. Henriksen, B. Tronier, and J. B. Bülow, "Kinetics of circulating endogenous insulin, C-peptide, and proinsulin in fasting nondiabetic man," *Metabolism*, vol. 36, no. 5, pp. 463–468, 1987.

[11] Y. Imamura, K. Yokono, K. Shii, J. Hari, H. Sakai, and S. Baba, "Plasma levels of proinsulin, insulin and C-peptide in chronic renal, hepatic and muscular disorders," *Japanese Journal of Medicine*, vol. 23, no. 1, pp. 3–8, 1984.

[12] A. E. Kitabchi, "Proinsulin and C-peptide: a review," *Metabolism: Clinical and Experimental*, vol. 26, no. 5, pp. 547–587, 1977.

[13] T. Inoguchi, P. Li, F. Umeda et al., "High glucose level and free fatty acid stimulate reactive oxygen species production through protein kinase C—dependent activation of NAD(P)H oxidase in cultured vascular cells," *Diabetes*, vol. 49, no. 11, pp. 1939–1945, 2000.

40

Congenital Bands with Intestinal Malrotation after Propylthiouracil Exposure in Early Pregnancy

Alexander A. Leung,[1] Jennifer Yamamoto,[1] Paola Luca,[2] Paul Beaudry,[3] and Julie McKeen[1]

[1]*Division of Endocrinology and Metabolism, Department of Medicine, University of Calgary, Calgary, AB, Canada T2T 5C7*
[2]*Division of Endocrinology and Metabolism, Department of Pediatrics, University of Calgary, Calgary, AB, Canada T3B 6A9*
[3]*Division of Pediatric Surgery, Department of Surgery, University of Calgary, Calgary, AB, Canada T3B 6A9*

Correspondence should be addressed to Julie McKeen; julie.mckeen@albertahealthservices.ca

Academic Editor: Yuji Moriwaki

Exposure to propylthiouracil in early pregnancy may be associated with an increased risk of birth defects. But the spectrum of associated congenital anomalies is not yet well defined. While preliminary reports suggest that most cases of propylthiouracil-associated birth defects are restricted to the preauricular and urinary systems, careful consideration should be given to other possible manifestations of teratogenicity. We propose that congenital bands may potentially represent a rare yet serious complication of propylthiouracil exposure in early pregnancy, possibly arising from an early mesenteric developmental anomaly. We report a case of a 17-day-old girl that presented with acute small bowel obstruction associated with intestinal malrotation arising from several anomalous congenital bands. Her mother was treated for Graves' disease during pregnancy with first trimester exposure to propylthiouracil but remained clinically and biochemically euthyroid at conception and throughout the duration of pregnancy. This case suggests that the use of propylthiouracil in early pregnancy may be associated with congenital bands and intestinal malrotation. More reports are needed to further support this association.

1. Introduction

Antithyroid drugs, such as propylthiouracil (PTU) and methimazole (MMI), are widely considered to be first line therapy in the treatment of hyperthyroidism in pregnancy [1–3]. Still, treatment is not without potential risk. The use of MMI in pregnancy has been associated with an increased risk of congenital anomalies [4–6]. PTU, on the other hand, may rarely cause severe maternal hepatotoxicity [3, 7]. In order to balance these risks, a number of expert panels, such as the American Thyroid Association and the Endocrine Society, have recommended treatment of hyperthyroidism during the first trimester of pregnancy with PTU to reduce the risk of teratogenicity to the fetus but recommended switching to MMI for the remainder of pregnancy to minimize unnecessary PTU exposure for the mother [1, 2].

Notably, these recommendations were initially formed in response to studies linking MMI (but not PTU) exposure to a variety of birth defects. However, emerging evidence now suggests that PTU may not be as safe to fetal development as previously believed and may actually pose an increased risk of malformations as well [4, 8–10]. Preliminary data suggest that the congenital anomalies associated with PTU appear to be rare, less severe, and of a different spectrum compared to those associated with MMI and as such may be easily overlooked. Accordingly, there has been a call for more reports of possible cases of PTU-associated birth defects to better characterize this condition [8]. Herein, we report the first case of congenital bands resulting in intestinal malrotation in a neonatal girl following PTU exposure in early pregnancy.

2. Case Presentation

A 17-day-old girl presented to hospital with irritability, decreased appetite, and repeated bilious vomiting for a day. Examination revealed a tender and distended abdomen. A subsequent computed tomography scan of the abdomen with contrast revealed the presence of a high-grade small bowel obstruction with multiple dilated, fluid-filled loops of bowel in the proximal ileum, characterized by muscosal hypoenhancement. There also appeared to be a reversal of the relationship between the superior mesenteric artery and superior mesenteric vein, suggestive of an underlying rotational abnormality.

An emergency laparotomy was then performed. Upon entering the abdomen, the cecum and ascending colon were found to be loose without any obvious lateral attachments in keeping with a rotational abnormality. Further exploration revealed a necrotic, closed loop obstruction at the distal jejunum. Using gentle traction, this twisted segment was exteriorized and several congenital bands were noted. Ligation of the bands was performed and the bowel was detorted. The segment of necrotic bowel was then resected and a primary end-to-end anastomosis was performed. The remaining bowel was examined and no other anatomical abnormalities were found. The postoperative course was uneventful.

The patient is the first child of nonconsanguineous Sri Lankan parents, born at term by elective cesarean section, and was initially discharged home two days after birth in stable condition without any perinatal complications. Incidentally, a small (3 mm) ventricular septal defect was discovered on routine newborn examination and managed expectantly. She was initially breastfed and remained well until she eventually presented with a small bowel obstruction on day 17 of life, as described. Prior to this, she had no surgeries.

Notably, during pregnancy, the child's mother, who was 29 years old, was treated for hyperthyroidism. She was diagnosed with Graves' disease 5 months before pregnancy and was initially treated with PTU 100 mg p.o. t.i.d. The dosage was reduced to 50 mg p.o. t.i.d. a month before conception; she continued on this same dose at conception and for the duration of the first trimester until the 14th week of gestation. Afterwards, MMI 5 mg p.o. q.d. was prescribed. She was clinically and biochemically euthyroid at the time of conception and thyroid function tests remained normal for the entire pregnancy. Immediately after birth, the patient's thyroid function was monitored closely because of her maternal history of Graves' disease. On the newborn screen (collected on the second day of life), her thyroid stimulating hormone (TSH) level was modestly elevated at 41 mIU/L. After two weeks, her TSH level remained elevated at 27.84 mIU/L but with a normal free T4 of 19.8 pmol/L. Although she remained well (and clinically euthyroid), levothyroxine replacement was initiated as a precaution with subsequent normalization of thyroid function tests soon thereafter.

There were no other significant maternal illnesses or medication exposures during pregnancy. The child had no other past medical history. There was no family history of any significant congenital birth defects.

3. Discussion

Concerns of potential teratogenicity of antithyroid drugs were initially raised in 1972 when the first report of aplasia cutis was noted in children born to mothers treated with MMI during pregnancy [11]. Since then, numerous reports and several large studies have emerged, confirming this association, as well as noting a number of other related birth defects (i.e., choanal atresia, esophageal atresia, and omphalocele), now collectively referred to as "methimazole embryopathy" [4–6]. Up until recently though, PTU was widely believed to pose no major threat to fetal development and was therefore recommended as the preferred therapy during the first trimester of pregnancy [1, 2]. However, this notion was challenged by a large Danish cohort study, which reported a higher prevalence of congenital malformations of the face, neck, and urinary systems in children exposed to PTU in early pregnancy [4]. When compared to the birth defects associated with MMI exposure, however, those associated with PTU appeared to largely involve different organ systems, tended to be less severe, and sometimes remained undiagnosed for longer periods of time [8].

Indeed, both MMI and PTU freely cross the placenta and likely pose the greatest risk to fetal development during the first trimester of pregnancy (i.e., during the critical period of organogenesis) [3]. A recent review of 91 case reports of potential birth defects associated with antithyroid drug exposure in utero found that, with the exception of only two cases, nearly all the reports claimed antithyroid drug exposure between the 6th week and 10th week of gestation [9]. While the timing of medication exposure appears to be crucial, there has been no detectable association between the dose of antithyroid drug and the subsequent risk of malformation [6, 9]. Therefore, the most important considerations in identifying potential cases of PTU-associated birth defects are exposure to PTU during early pregnancy as well as biological plausibility.

We propose that congenital bands may potentially represent a rare yet serious complication of PTU exposure in early pregnancy. While most cases of intestinal obstruction in the pediatric population are from postoperative adhesions or stenosis, other causes should be considered in those without prior history of abdominal surgery [12]. Uncommonly, intestinal obstruction may be secondary to embryological remnants of the vitelline vessels, omphalomesenteric ducts, or mesourachus; these are typically recognized by their anatomical location [13]. Rarely, obstruction may be caused by anomalous congenital bands without apparent embryogenic origin [14–17]. While their etiology is not well understood, it has been suggested that these fibrous bands of tissue arise from a mesenteric anomaly occurring around the 4th week of gestation and are later associated with malrotation, anomalous intestinal fixation, and obstruction [14, 17]. In our case, we also found evidence of several anomalous congenital bands associated with an intestinal rotational abnormality resulting in complete obstruction, therefore raising the suspicion of an early mesenteric developmental abnormality. To date, no teratogen has yet been implicated in the development of congenital bands. Although hypothyroidism may rarely result in intestinal pseudoobstruction (i.e., paralytic ileus) [18], this did not appear to be a contributing factor in our patient, as she was euthyroid at the time and had a demonstrable anatomic reason for her obstruction.

Of note, our patient was also incidentally found to have a small ventricular septal defect shortly after birth. Normally, the major septa of the heart are formed by the 5th week of fetal development. Incomplete closure of the interventricular septum may result in an isolated ventricular septal defect [19]. This condition is common and is estimated to be present in up to 5% of all newborns, and the vast majority close spontaneously without intervention [20]. Accordingly, multiple large studies have reported that the prevalence of ventricular septal defects among children exposed to PTU appears similar to those never exposed to any antithyroid drugs in utero [4, 7]. As such, it is unclear whether the presence of an incidental ventricular septal defect in our patient had any causal relationship with her prior exposure to PTU in early pregnancy at all.

It should be pointed out that thyrotoxicosis itself may be teratogenic [21]. Indeed, critics have raised concern that most of the previous large-scale studies showing an association between antithyroid drugs and congenital malformations have not consistently reported on maternal thyroid function [22–24]. As such, some have proposed that poorly controlled hyperthyroidism may be the underlying reason for the increased rate of congenital malformations rather than treatment itself [25]. However, the striking differences in the spectrum of birth defects associated with MMI compared to PTU argue that these congenital anomalies are more likely mediated by antithyroid drug exposure rather than abnormal maternal thyroid hormone levels [4]. In our case, specifically, we can confirm that maternal thyroid function was checked at least once each trimester and was normal at the time of conception and throughout the duration of the pregnancy.

The potential teratogenicity of PTU remains to be elucidated. While preliminary reports have suggested that most cases are mild in nature and are restricted to preauricular and urinary system malformations [4, 8, 9], careful consideration should also be given to other manifestations of disease that may potentially be more severe and possibly involve other organ systems too. Congenital bands may potentially represent a rare yet serious complication of PTU exposure in early pregnancy. More reports are needed to further support this association. This case report serves to alert clinicians of a potential new teratogenic association of PTU, thus prompting further confirmatory reports and future definitive studies.

Authors' Contribution

All listed authors consented to the submission of this paper and meet criteria for authorship through conception (Alexander A. Leung and Julie McKeen), acquisition of data (Paul Beaudry, Paola Luca, and Julie McKeen), drafting of initial paper (Alexander A. Leung), critical revision for important intellectual content (Alexander A. Leung, Jennifer Yamamoto, Paola Luca, Paul Beaudry, and Julie McKeen), and supervision (Julie McKeen).

References

[1] L. De Groot, M. Abalovich, E. K. Alexander et al., "Management of thyroid dysfunction during pregnancy and postpartum: an Endocrine Society clinical practice guideline," Journal of Clinical Endocrinology and Metabolism, vol. 97, no. 8, pp. 2543–2565, 2012.

[2] A. Stagnaro-Green, M. Abalovich, E. Alexander et al., "Guidelines of the American Thyroid Association for the diagnosis and management of thyroid disease during pregnancy and postpartum," Thyroid, vol. 21, no. 10, pp. 1081–1125, 2011.

[3] D. S. Cooper and P. Laurberg, "Hyperthyroidism in pregnancy," The Lancet Diabetes and Endocrinology, vol. 1, no. 3, pp. 238–249, 2013.

[4] S. L. Andersen, J. Olsen, C. S. Wu, and P. Laurberg, "Birth defects after early pregnancy use of antithyroid drugs: a Danish nationwide study," Journal of Clinical Endocrinology and Metabolism, vol. 98, no. 11, pp. 4373–4381, 2013.

[5] M. Clementi, E. Di Gianantonio, M. Cassina et al., "Treatment of hyperthyroidism in pregnancy and birth defects," Journal of Clinical Endocrinology and Metabolism, vol. 95, no. 11, pp. E337–E341, 2010.

[6] A. Yoshihara, J. Y. Noh, T. Yamaguchi et al., "Treatment of graves' disease with antithyroid drugs in the first trimester of pregnancy and the prevalence of congenital malformation," Journal of Clinical Endocrinology and Metabolism, vol. 97, no. 7, pp. 2396–2403, 2012.

[7] J. C. Lo, S. A. Rivkees, M. Chandra, J. R. Gonzalez, J. J. Korelitz, and M. W. Kuzniewicz, "Gestational thyrotoxicosis, antithyroid drug use and neonatal outcomes within an integrated healthcare delivery system," Thyroid, vol. 25, no. 6, pp. 698–705, 2015.

[8] S. L. Andersen, J. Olsen, C. S. Wu, and P. Laurberg, "Severity of birth defects after propylthiouracil exposure in early pregnancy," Thyroid, vol. 24, no. 10, pp. 1533–1540, 2014.

[9] P. Laurberg and S. L. Andersen, "Therapy of endocrine disease: antithyroid drug use in early pregnancy and birth defects: time windows of relative safety and high risk?" European Journal of Endocrinology, vol. 171, no. 1, pp. R13–R20, 2014.

[10] S. A. Rivkees, "Propylthiouracil versus methimazole during pregnancy: an evolving tale of difficult choices," Journal of Clinical Endocrinology and Metabolism, vol. 98, no. 11, pp. 4332–4335, 2013.

[11] S. Milham and W. Elledge, "Maternal methimazole and congenital defects in children," Teratology, vol. 5, no. 1, pp. 125–125, 1972.

[12] C. A. Hajivassiliou, "Intestinal obstruction in neonatal/pediatric surgery," Seminars in Pediatric Surgery, vol. 12, no. 4, pp. 241–253, 2003.

[13] A. T. Michopoulou, S. S. Germanos, A. P. Ninos, and S. K. Pierrakakis, "Vitelline artery remnant causing intestinal obstruction in an adult," Surgery, vol. 154, no. 5, pp. 1137–1138, 2013.

[14] F. M. Akgür, F. C. Tanyel, N. Büyükpamukçu, and A. Hiçsönmez, "Anomalous congenital bands causing intestinal obstruction in children," Journal of Pediatric Surgery, vol. 27, no. 4, pp. 471–473, 1992.

[15] D.-S. Lin, N.-L. Wang, F.-Y. Huang, and S.-L. Shih, "Sigmoid adhesion caused by a congenital mesocolic band," Journal of Gastroenterology, vol. 34, no. 5, pp. 626–628, 1999.

[16] C. Liu, T.-C. Wu, H.-L. Tsai, T. Chin, and C. Wei, "Obstruction of the proximal jejunum by an anomalous congenital band—a case report," *Journal of Pediatric Surgery*, vol. 40, no. 3, pp. E27–E29, 2005.

[17] D. Sarkar, P. Gongidi, T. Presenza, and E. Scattergood, "Intestinal obstruction from congenital bands at the proximal jejunum: a case report and literature review," *Journal of Clinical Imaging Science*, vol. 2, article 78, 2012.

[18] C. Chua, S. Gurnurkar, Y. Rodriguez-Prado, and V. Niklas, "Prolonged ileus in an infant presenting with primary congenital hypothyroidism," *Case Reports in Pediatrics*, vol. 2015, Article ID 584735, 4 pages, 2015.

[19] T. W. Sadler, *Langman's Medical Embryology*, Lippincott Williams & Wilkins, Philadelphia, Pa, USA, 12th edition, 2011.

[20] J. I. E. Hoffman and S. Kaplan, "The incidence of congenital heart disease," *Journal of the American College of Cardiology*, vol. 39, no. 12, pp. 1890–1900, 2002.

[21] N. Momotani, K. Ito, N. Hamada, Y. Ban, Y. Nishikawa, and T. Mimura, "Maternal hyperthyroidism and congenital malformation in the offspring," *Clinical Endocrinology*, vol. 20, no. 6, pp. 695–700, 1984.

[22] R. Hackmon, M. Blichowski, and G. Koren, "The safety of methimazole and propylthiouracil in pregnancy: a systematic review," *Journal of Obstetrics and Gynaecology Canada*, vol. 34, no. 11, pp. 1077–1086, 2012.

[23] H. Li, J. Zheng, J. Luo et al., "Congenital anomalies in children exposed to antithyroid drugs in-utero: a meta-analysis of cohort studies," *PLoS ONE*, vol. 10, no. 5, Article ID e0126610, 2015.

[24] X. Li, G. Y. Liu, J. L. Ma, and L. Zhou, "Risk of congenital anomalies associated with antithyroid treatment during pregnancy: a meta-analysis," *Clinics*, vol. 70, no. 6, pp. 453–459, 2015.

[25] E. Gianetti, L. Russo, F. Orlandi et al., "Pregnancy outcome in women treated with methimazole or propylthiouracil during pregnancy," *Journal of Endocrinological Investigation*, vol. 38, no. 9, pp. 977–985, 2015.

41

Thyroid Sporadic Goiter with Adult Heterotopic Bone Formation

Adriana Handra-Luca,[1] **Marie-Laure Dumuis-Gimenez,**[2]
Mouna Bendib,[1] **and Panagiotis Anagnostis**[3]

[1]*Service d'Anatomie Pathologique, APHP GHU Avicenne, UFR Médecine, Université Paris Nord Sorbonne Cité,
125 rue Stalingrad, 93009 Bobigny, France*
[2]*Service Medecine Nucleaire, APHP GHU Avicenne, 93009 Bobigny, France*
[3]*Division of Endocrinology, Police Medical Centre, Monastiriou 326, 54627 Thessaloniki, Greece*

Correspondence should be addressed to Adriana Handra-Luca; adriana.handra-luca@hotmail.com

Academic Editor: Osamu Isozaki

Thyroid heterotopic bone formation (HBF) in goiter is a rare finding. Five thyroid resection specimens were analyzed for HBF. The results were correlated with clinicomorphological features. All patients were women (33–82 years). The preoperative diagnosis was thyroid goiter or nodule. Treatment consisted in thyroidectomy and lobectomy (3 and 2, resp.). Microscopy showed sporadic nodular goiter. Malformative blood vessels and vascular calcifications were seen in intra- and extrathyroid location (5 and 3, resp.). The number and size of HBFs (total: 28) ranged between 1 and 23/thyroid gland (one bilateral) and 1 and 10 mm, respectively. Twelve HBFs were in contact with the thyroid capsule. Most were extranodular (21, versus 6 intranodular). The medical history was positive for dyslipidemia, hyperglycemia, renal dysfunction, and hyperuricemia (2, 3, and 3 cases and 1 case, resp.) without any parathyroid abnormality. In conclusion, thyroid HBF may be characterized by subcapsular or extranodular location, various size (usually ≥2 mm), and vascular calcifications and malformations. Features of metabolic syndrome and renal dysfunction may be present, but their exact role in the pathogenesis of HBFs remains to be elucidated.

1. Introduction

Heterotopic bone formation (HBF) is defined as extraskeletal bone formation. Thyroid HBF, frequently designated as bone metaplasia, occurs rarely in the thyroid, being reported both in goiter and in tumors such as adenomas and carcinosarcomas [1–10]. To our knowledge, seven cases of thyroid sporadic goiter with complete, adult HBF are reported in the English medical literature [2, 4, 7–10]. Here we report five additional cases of complete, adult HBF occurring in the context of sporadic thyroid nodular goiter.

2. Methods

Five thyroid resection specimens were analyzed for HBF as defined by the presence of lamellar bone trabeculae delimiting fat or fibrofat tissue with hematopoietic elements and capillaries. The number, size, and location of HBF foci (subcapsular or not, intranodular or not) were tabulated. Foci of ossification consisting only of bone trabeculae were considered separately. Thyroid parenchyma was also analyzed for nodules (hyperplastic, adenoma-type, or carcinoma), atrophy, necrosis, fibrosis, calcifications, inflammation, and vascular lesions (pseudoangioma lesions or vascular conglomerates, thrombosis, intima/media fibrosis and hyperplasia, and calcifications). Two thyroids were sampled quasi-entirely (Cases 1 and 2). Serial and/or multistep tissue sections were analyzed for the HBFs. The results were analyzed with regard to clinicomorphological features. The rank correlation Kendall test was used for evaluating the statistical significance of correlations (Medcalc v14, Belgium). A P value of less than 0.05 indicated statistical significance.

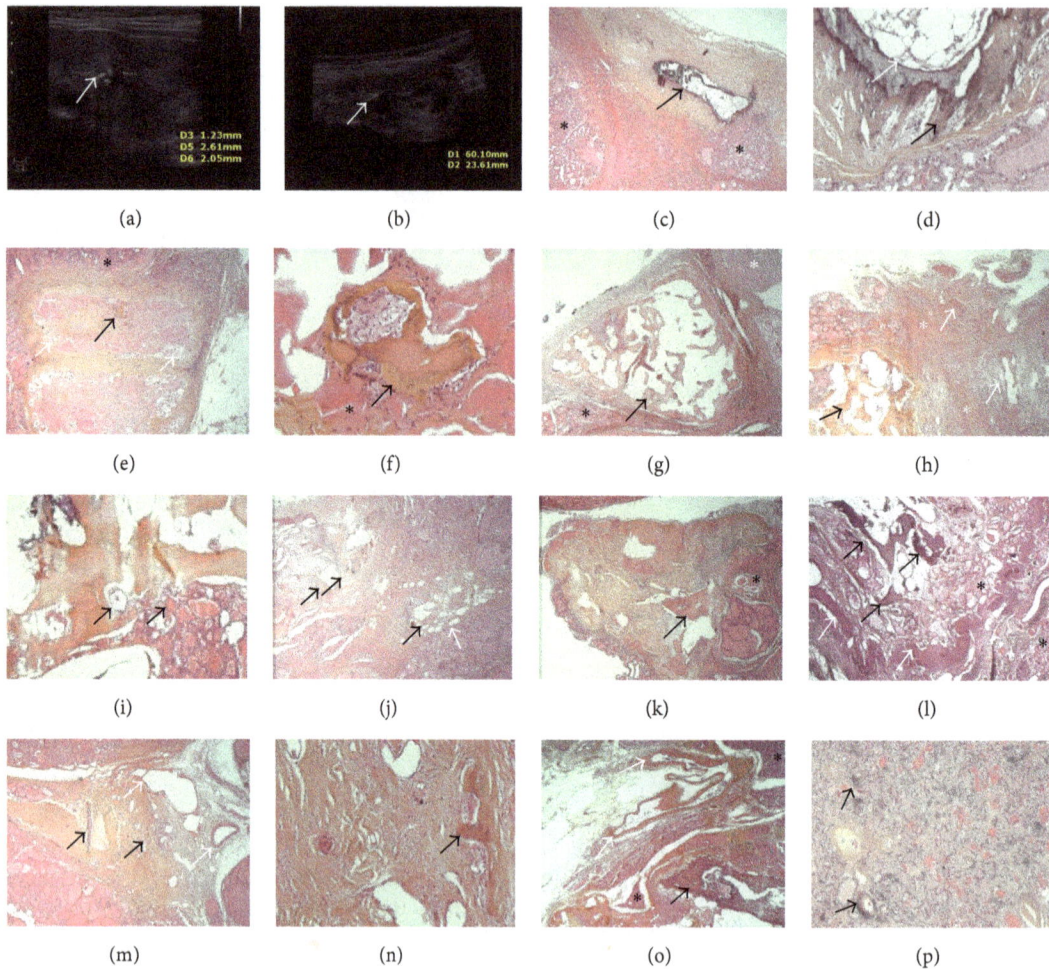

FIGURE 1: At ultrasound examination the thyroid showed several nodules and micro- and macrocalcifications (a, b: white arrows, Case 1). Microscopy showed in this case a HBF (heterotopic bone formation) focus in a thick rim of dense fibrosis (c, d: black arrow/HBF, asterisks/thyroid vesicles, and white arrow/intertrabecular fat with hematopoietic elements). Several HBFs were seen in Case 2 (e–k). A subcapsular nodule, largely fibrotic and atrophic, contained an infracentimetric HBF (e-f: black arrow/HBF, white arrow/nodular atrophic vesicles, and asterisk/reactive thyroid follicles). Another subcapsular HBF showed triangular shape and was situated in contact with an atrophic goiter nodule (g: black arrow/HBF, asterisk/thyroid vesicles, atrophic for some). A 3rd HBF was situated in contact with sheet-patterned fibrosis which contained large malformative vessels (h: black arrow/HBF, asterisks/thyroid vesicles, and white arrows/vessels). For this HBF, vesicles were at proximity and contact of bone trabeculae (i: black arrows). A 4th HBF was situated at proximity of intrathyroid adipose cells englobed in fibrosis (j: black arrow/HBF, white arrow/adipose cells). A 5th HBF was situated in a triangular-shaped zone of fibrosis, focally undulated, with an atrophic follicular nodule at contact (k: black arrow/HBF, asterisk/atrophic nodule). In Case 3 (l) a vaguely nodular zone, containing the HBF and thyroid vesicles, was delimited by undulated connective tissue (black arrows/HBF, asterisk/thyroid vesicles, and white arrows/undulated fibrosis with large vessels at contact). In Case 4 (m-n), the thyroid contained sheet-like fibrosis with large, malformative vessels at proximity and with ossification foci (m, n: black arrows/ossifications, white arrows/abnormal vessels). In Case 5 (o-p) the HBF was located in the subcapsular thyroid, at proximity to large malformative vessels (intra- and perithyroid) (o: black arrow/HBF, white arrow/malformative vessels, and asterisks/thyroid vesicles). The follicular nodule, situated at distance from the HBF, contained intervesicular disperse calcifications, some in the perivascular hyaline (p: black arrows).

3. Results

The main features of the cases are demonstrated in Tables 1 and 2.

Case 1. The patient (51-year-old woman) had undergone a total thyroidectomy for toxic goiter. The patient was treated with carbimazole and thyroxine for 1.5 years. The medical history was positive for arterial hypertension and tachycardia as well as for cardiomegaly. There was no evidence of anemia. Foci of micro- and macrocalcifications were observed on thyroid ultrasound examination (Figure 1). Postsurgical hypocalcemia occurred and was treated with calcium supplementation. The patient was well at postsurgical consultation (after 3 months of follow-up).

Microscopy showed sporadic multinodular goiter with malformative, large, and tortuous blood vessels (intra- and extrathyroidal) intermingled with rare nerves. There were no

TABLE 1: Clinical features of the 5 patients with adult bone metaplasia.

Case number	Age (years)	Gender	Euthyroid	Punction	Presurgical diagnosis	Cardiovascular disease	Dyslipidemia	Diabetes	Osteoarticular disease	Impaired renal function	BMI	Type of thyroid surgery	Morphological diagnosis	Postsurgical hypocalcemia
1	51	W	No	No	Toxic goiter	AHT, tachycardia cardiomegaly	NA	No	Odontoid chondrocalcinosis, C4-C7 arthrosis	No	31.3	Right and left thyroid lobectomies	Sporadic goiter	Yes
2	33	W	Yes	No	Multinodular goiter (trachea deviation)	No	NA	No	No	Yes	32	Total thyroidectomy	Sporadic goiter	No
3	63	W	Yes	No	Multinodular goiter	AHT, mitral stenosis	Yes	Yes	No	Yes	22.5	Total thyroidectomy	Sporadic goiter	Yes
4	83	W	No	No	Left cystic nodule (trachea deviation)	AHT	NA	No	Osteoporosis	Yes	26.4	Left thyroid lobectomy	Goiter with adenoma-like nodule	No
5	71	W	Yes	Yes*	Compressive cyst	AHT	Yes	No	Arthrosis, serum vitamin D OH 25D1 D3 insufficiency, and hyperuricemia	No	41.9	Right thyroidectomy	Follicular adenoma, cystic change	Yes

BMI: body mass index, NA: nonavailable, W: woman, and AHT: arterial hypertension.

*The punction was performed for evacuating the cyst (65 mL); no cytological analysis was performed (Case 5).

Hyperthyroidism was diagnosed in Cases 1 and 4 and treated by carbimazole and thyroxin for 1.5 years in Case 1 and by carbimazole only in Case 4 (for 15 days due to temporary drug unavailability).

Decreased serum creatinine was diagnosed in Case 2, hypocalcemia and hypoalbuminemia were diagnosed in Case 3, and renal failure was diagnosed in Case 4. The type of dyslipidemia was not available in Case 3 and consisted in hypercholesterolemia and hyper-LDL-emia in Case 5. Cases 4 and 5 showed fluctuant hyperglycemia. Case 3 diabetes was type II.

Case 4 showed a history of sigmoidectomy for diverticulosis (date NA), gastric resection for gastrointestinal stromal tumor (date NA), and breast cancer (treated by surgery, radiotherapy, and hormonotherapy). Case 5 showed a history of appendectomy and skin papillomas. Case 3 showed hypoacusia (prosthesis).

There was no alcohol abuse in any of the cases; smoking habits (10 PA) were noted in Case 2. A treatment with propranolol was known for Case 1 and with atorvastatin, metformin, Lectil, beta-histidine chlorhydrate, metformin, glimepiride, hydroxyzine (allergy to penicillin and cetirizine), alendronic acid, spironolactone, atenolol, and zolpidem for Case 4. Allergy to fish and amoxicillin was known in Case 5, to penicillin and cetirizine in Case 3, and to penicillin and aspirin in Case 4.

TABLE 2: Main morphological characteristics of the 5 thyroidectomy specimens.

Number	Thyroid weight (grams)	Thyroid volume (mm^3)	Number of HBF foci (size, mm)	Number of ossification foci	Thyroid calcifications	Thyroid fibrosis	Thyroid inflammation	Vascular calcifications	Thyroid adipose involution
1	48	93.75	1 (2.5 mm)	0	1	Severe	Moderate	No	Multifocal
2	32	72	27 (2–10 mm)	11	1	Severe	Moderate	No	Multifocal
3	38	51	1 (10)	0	1*	Mild	Mild	Intra-, perithyroid	No
4	115	195	2 (1 and 9.5 mm)	14	1*	Mild	Moderate	Intra-, perithyroid	No
5	43	180	1 (8 mm)	0	1*	Mild	Mild to moderate	Intra-, perithyroid	Multifocal

*Cases 3, 4, and 5 showed also reticular and perivascular calcifications in hyperplastic nodules.
Normal parathyroid tissue was seen in the perithyroid adipose tissue in Case 1.

vascular thromboses. Parenchymal nodules, several encapsulated, were hyperplastic and adenoma-like. Inflammation was moderate. Fibrosis was severe and extensive with a band-like pattern without extrathyroid extension. One HBF was identified (2.5 mm) with no ossification foci. Multifocal adipose involution was seen.

Case 2. The patient (33-year-old woman) had undergone a total thyroidectomy for goiter with trachea deviation. She was euthyroid. Smoking of 10 packs/year was noted. There was no evidence of anemia. Thyroid ultrasound examination showed foci of micro- and macrocalcifications (Figure 1). The patient was well at postsurgical consultation (after 0.5 months of follow-up).

Microscopy showed sporadic multinodular goiter with malformative, large, and tortuous blood vessels (intra- and extrathyroidal) intermingled with rare nerves. Vascular cavities with tuft-like projections were associated. There were no vascular thromboses. Parenchymal nodules, several encapsulated, were hyperplastic and adenoma-like. Several atrophic nodules, some with intranodular fibrocollagen, were also seen. Inflammation was moderate. Fibrosis was severe and extensive with a band-like pattern, containing or being at proximity of large blood vessels (intra- or extrathyroid), without extrathyroid extension. Twenty-three HBFs (2–10 mm) were identified with 11 ossification foci. Three extranodular HBFs were in direct contact with the capsule of fibroatrophic nodules. For two HBFs, band-like fibrosis connected malformative vessels to the HBF. On serial sections, two ossification foci revealed intertrabecular spaces and were thus diagnosed as HBFs. Multifocal adipose involution was seen as well as intrathyroid muscle tissue (the closest at 6.5 mm from the HBF).

Case 3. The patient (63-year-old woman) had undergone a thyroidectomy for goiter. The patient was euthyroid and was diagnosed with arterial hypertension and mitral stenosis. There was no evidence of anemia. Postsurgical hypocalcemia was treated with calcium. The patient was well at postsurgical consultation (after 1 month of follow-up).

Microscopy showed sporadic multinodular goiter with malformative, large, and tortuous blood vessels (intra- and extrathyroid) intermingled with rare nerves. There were no

vascular thromboses. Parenchymal nodules, several encapsulated, were hyperplastic and adenoma-like. Calcifications of the internal elastic lamina and media (von Monckeberg sclerosis-type) were observed in the vessel wall, in peri- and intrathyroid locations [11]. Perivascular calcifications of calcipheresis-type were seen in hyperplastic nodules. Inflammation was mild as well as fibrosis. One HBF (10 mm) was identified. Abnormal blood vessels were seen around the HBF.

Case 4. The patient (83-year-old woman) had undergone left thyroidectomy for a cystic nodule with trachea deviation. The patient had been treated with carbimazole and thyroxine (15 days). The medical history was positive for arterial hypertension and osteoporosis. There was no evidence of anemia. The patient was well at postsurgical consultation (after 2 months of follow-up).

Microscopy showed sporadic multinodular goiter with malformative, large, and tortuous blood vessels (intra- and extrathyroidal) intermingled with rare nerves. Vascular cavities with tuft-like projections were associated. There were no thromboses. Parenchymal nodules, several encapsulated, were hyperplastic and adenoma-like. Calcifications of the internal elastic lamina and media (von Monckeberg sclerosis-type) were observed in the vessel wall. Perivascular calcifications of calcipheresis-type were also seen. Thyroid inflammation was moderate and fibrosis mild. Two HBFs were identified (1 and 9.5 mm) with 14 ossification foci. Abnormal blood vessels were seen around the largest HBF.

Case 5. The patient (71-year-old woman) had undergone right thyroidectomy for compressive cyst. The patient was euthyroid. The medical history was positive for arterial hypertension. The patient also showed vitamin D deficiency (10.1 ng/mL) as well as hyperuricemia and arthrosis and did not show anemia. An evacuatory punction was followed by reincrease in size of the nodule (3 months afterwards). Postsurgical hypocalcemia occurred and was treated with calcium supplementation. The patient was well at postsurgical consultation (after 3 weeks of follow-up).

Microscopy showed sporadic multinodular goiter with malformative, large, and tortuous blood vessels (intra- and extrathyroidal) intermingled with rare nerves. There were no vascular thromboses. Parenchymal nodules, several encapsulated, were hyperplastic and adenoma-like. Calcifications of the internal elastic lamina and media (von Monckeberg sclerosis-type) were observed in the vessel wall. Perivascular calcifications of calcipheresis-type were seen in hyperplastic nodules. There were no vascular thromboses. Inflammation was mild to moderate and fibrosis was mild. One HBF (8 mm) was identified. Abnormal blood vessels were seen around the HBF. Adipose involution was multifocal.

3.1. Heterotopic Bone Formation Foci Feature Analysis. The total number of HBF foci was 28. The number varied between 1 and 23 foci/thyroid specimen (bilateral: one) and size ranged from inframillimetric to 10 mm. Eighteen (64%) HBFs were ≥2 mm and six (21%) ≥5 mm. The shape varied: triangular ($n = 2$), oval ($n = 7$), or rounded ($n = 19$) with a trend for triangular HBF to correlate with increased size ($P = 0.08$, tau = 0.233). Twelve HBFs were subcapsular in the thyroid and six occurred in nodules (hyperplastic adenoma-like and one entirely fibroatrophic). When extranodular, HBFs were situated in or in contact with band-patterned fibrosis. Thyroid vesicles, atrophic or not, were in contact with three intranodular and five extranodular HBFs. The intertrabecular tissue was adipose or fibroadipose (seven and 21 HBFs, resp.), with osteoblast-rimming and megakaryocytes (in two HBFs each). Adipose involution foci were close to some HBFs in Case 2. Intranodular HBFs were more frequently ≥2 mm (4 versus 2 intranodular HBFs of <2 mm). Size correlated with subcapsular location ($P = 0.02$, tau = 0.308), presence of adipose intertrabecular spaces (as compared to fibroadipose spaces, $P < 0.01$, tau = 0.385), contact with thyroid vesicles ($P = 0.01$, tau = 0.320), and presence of adjacent dysmorphic/ malformative vessels ($P = 0.01$, tau = 0.435).

4. Discussion

Here we report five cases of thyroid HBF occurring in the context of sporadic goiter in euthyroid or hyperthyroid patients. The diagnosis of such lesions was microscopic. The imaging diagnosis was difficult; both micro- and macro-calcifications occurred. Although the HBFs were frequently extranodular and more than 2 mm in size when intranodular, the imaging features do not allow the precise diagnosis of HBF-type lesions. Whether the subcapsular location, seen in approximately one-third of the HBFs, might be useful remains to be further studied. The main relevance of intrathyroid HBFs is morphological, microscopical. Unlike on ultrasound examination, a misdiagnosis of carcinoma may be made on frozen-section examinations due to the presence of osteoclast-like elements [12].

The histogenesis of such lesions remains a matter of debate. The various thyroid topography, intraparenchymal or subcapsular, of the HBF foci we have seen, occurring in sheet-like fibrosis, more frequently extranodular, suggests a nonneoplastic origin. The presence of multiple, bilateral foci, round to oval more frequently, suggests a dysmetabolic rather than an ectopic nature. The most plausible hypothesis is that of degenerative changes, similar to those reported in

the femoral arteries and, less frequently in the carotid, at ages above 60 [13]. Although we have noted von Monckeberg sclerosis-type calcifications both in the media and in the internal elastic lamina in three thyroids, including in intrathyroid location, the morphological aspects we have seen do not indicate a direct vascular origin, as no direct transition zones from blood vessel calcifications to HBF foci were detected on the different serial and multistep tissue sections. Moreover, malformative vessels lacked within the HBFs and were rare at contact. However, von Monckeberg sclerosis-type calcifications were seen in a perithyroid large vessel at 5 mm from the HBF in Case 5. An abnormal blood perfusion in the context of enlarged, plunging, goiter-thyroids with modified thyroid-vessel reports, possibly resulting in hypoxia/ischemia might be a favoring factor, as suggested by the presence of sheet-like patterned fibrosis connecting the large malformative tortuous vessels with the HBF foci. The presence of several fibroatrophic vesicular nodules in contact with some HBFs was also highly suggestive of an ischemic nature. Clotting abnormalities were not detected, neither anemia nor hematological disease. Of interest would be the relatively increased frequency of reported cases with intrathyroid hematopoiesis (associated with myelofibrosis or anemia or not) as compared to that of thyroid bone metaplasia [10]. The extensive study of the quasi-totality of thyroidectomy specimens revealed numerous ossification foci (more than 10) in two of the cases, while hematopoietic elements without bone formation lacked. However no hematologic disease was detected in the cases we report. Dysmetabolic factors such as dyslipidemia, diabetes, or fluctuant hyperglycemia and hyperuricemia as well were diagnosed in our cases, younger or older, and could be incriminated in the histogenesis of HBF. Multifocal thyroid adipose involution was seen in three thyroids, the patients' body mass index being above 30. However these lesions were rarely in direct contact with the adipose intertrabecular spaces of the HBFs to explain a possible participation to the HBF genesis.

HBF in the context of abnormal parathyroid functioning has been reported recently in one case [8]. Although we have detected fibroadipose intertrabecular spaces and osteoblast-rimming in some HBFs, the patterns of these lesions were not specific neither for hyperthyroid bone formation and resorption nor for hyperparathyroidism-bone modelling [14]. We did not encounter parathyroid function abnormality and the parathyroids were normal preoperatively and during perioperative examination.

Interestingly, the intranodular perivascular or intervesicular pattern of some calcifications observed in some of the nodules suggests a relationship with renal dysfunction, at least for early/initial lesions. Thyroid inflammatory disease may be also incriminated although there was no significant inflammation at the time of surgery. Riedel thyroiditis was ruled out based on microscopic features of the lesions: fibrosis, although focally extensive in two thyroids, remained intrathyroid [15]. Extensive fibrotic scarring may follow the fine-needle aspiration procedure. This hypothesis was ruled out in the cases we report since the punctured nodule was at distance from the HBF. Postradiotherapy fibrosis may be incriminated in the HBF genesis in Case 4, the patient's breast carcinoma being treated with radiotherapy, however, nine years before the thyroid surgery. Other causative agents of extensive fibrosis, such as radioactive iodine treatment, were not identified in any of the cases. The rarity of thyroid HBF in thyroid goiters rules out also a possible abnormal iodine metabolism. In animals, bone abnormalities are reported to relate to a possible iodine uptake [16]. Interestingly, iodine deficiency can also result in growth abnormalities with destructive alterations in bone and bone marrow, with decrease in hydroxyproline, hexosamines, and phosphomonoesterase-I activities, as well as in disorders of phosphate-calcium metabolism [16]. Whether systemic relationships, possibly indirect, exist between the thyroid HBFs and systemic osteoarticular conditions (diagnosed in three of the cases) such as osteoporosis, chondrocalcinosis, dorsal or lumbar arthrosis, hyperuricemia, and vitamin D deficiency remains to be further investigated. Of note would be the fact that in experimental models on guinea pigs thyroid hormones may result in bone (without cartilage) formation when injected intramuscularly, by a possible osteoblast transportation in muscle fibroblasts [17]. This hypothesis requires further explorations, particularly in humans, despite the simplicity of our observations of thyroid vesicles in contact with HBFs as well as of intrathyroid muscle, however not in direct contact with the HBF.

In conclusion, HBF may occur in sporadic thyroid goiter. A subcapsular or extranodular location and size ≥2 mm may be useful for the imaging diagnosis. Histogenesis is multifactorial, dysmetabolic conditions, renal dysfunction or vascular abnormalities being possibly involved, without associated parathyroid pathologies. Whether a disturbed iodine metabolism can also be involved requires further investigation.

Acknowledgments

The authors thank I. Alexandre, V. Ipotesi, N. Akdim, J. Raleche, L. Delagarde, A. Meloni, Professor A. Sapino, Dr. C. Westhoff, Dr. E. Dragoescu, Dr. I. Keller, Dr. SA Polyzos, Dr. T. Leger, MC Portenier, S. Chambris, P. Pausicles, the BIUM, CMDP/APHP, and NCA/Avicenne teams.

References

[1] S. Akbulut, R. Yavuz, B. Akansu, N. Sogutcu, Z. Arikanoglu, and M. Basbug, "Ectopic bone formation and extramedullary hematopoiesis in the thyroid gland: report of a case and literature review," *International Surgery*, vol. 96, no. 3, pp. 260–265, 2011.

[2] G. Ardito, G. Fadda, L. Revelli et al., "Follicular adenoma of the thyroid gland with extensive bone metaplasia," *Journal of Experimental & Clinical Cancer Research*, vol. 20, no. 3, pp. 443–445, 2001.

[3] M. Basbug, R. Yavuz, M. Dablan, and B. Akansu, "Extensive osseous metaplasia with mature bone formation of thyroid gland," *Journal of Clinical Endocrinology & Metabolism*, vol. 2, no. 2, pp. 99–101, 2012.

[4] J. S. Chun, R. Hong, and J. A. Kim, "Osseous metaplasia with mature bone formation of the thyroid gland: three case reports," *Oncology Letters*, vol. 6, no. 4, pp. 977–979, 2013.

[5] K. Cooper and E. M. Barker, "Thyroid carcinosarcoma. A case report," *South African Journal of Surgery*, vol. 27, no. 5, pp. 192–193, 1989.

[6] M. Harsh, P. Dimri, and N. M. Nagarkar, "Osseous metaplasia and mature bone formation with extramedullary hematopoiesis in follicular adenoma of thyroid gland," *Indian Journal of Pathology and Microbiology*, vol. 52, no. 3, pp. 377–378, 2009.

[7] N. Pontikides, D. Botsios, E. Kariki, K. Vassiliadis, and G. E. Krassas, "Extramedullary hemopoiesis in a thyroid nodule with extensive bone metaplasia and mature bone formation," *Thyroid*, vol. 13, no. 9, pp. 877–880, 2003.

[8] I. Sayar, A. Isik, E. M. Akbas, H. Eken, and L. Demirtas, "Bone marrow metaplasia in multinodular goiter with primary hyperparathyroidism," *The American Journal of the Medical Sciences*, vol. 348, no. 6, pp. 530–531, 2014.

[9] G. N. Tzanakakis, C. D. Scopa, M. P. Vezeridis, and A. Vagenakis, "Ectopic bone in multinodular goiter," *Rhode Island Medical Journal*, vol. 72, no. 5, pp. 171–172, 1989.

[10] C. C. Westhoff, E. Karakas, C. Dietz, and P. J. Barth, "Intrathyroidal hematopoiesis: a rare histological finding in an otherwise healthy patient and review of the literature," *Langenbeck's Archives of Surgery*, vol. 393, no. 5, pp. 745–749, 2008.

[11] R. G. Micheletti, G. A. Fishbein, J. S. Currier, and M. C. Fishbein, "Mönckeberg sclerosis revisited: a clarification of the histologic definition of Mönckeberg sclerosis," *Archives of Pathology & Laboratory Medicine*, vol. 132, pp. 43–47, 2008.

[12] F. Leoni, R. Fabbri, A. Pascarella et al., "Extramedullary haematopoiesis in thyroid multinodular goitre preceding clinical evidence of agnogenic myeloid metaplasia," *Histopathology*, vol. 28, no. 6, pp. 559–561, 1996.

[13] F. Herisson, M. F. Heymann, M. Chétiveaux et al., "Carotid and femoral atherosclerotic plaques show different morphology," *Atherosclerosis*, vol. 216, no. 2, pp. 348–354, 2011.

[14] F. Melsen and L. Mosekilde, "Morphometric and dynamic studies of bone changes in hyperthyroidism," *Acta Pathologica et Microbiologica Scandinavica, Section A: Pathology*, vol. 85, no. 2, pp. 141–150, 1977.

[15] G. Papi and V. A. LiVolsi, "Current concepts on Riedel thyroiditis," *American Journal of Clinical Pathology*, vol. 121, supplement, pp. S50–S63, 2004.

[16] V. I. Smoliar, "Effect of iodine deficiency on the growth and formation of the bone tissue," *Voprosy Pitaniia*, vol. 2, pp. 38–42, 1983 (Russian).

[17] K. Zarrin, "The bone inducing capacity of syngeneic thyroid tissue in guinea-pig muscle," *The Journal of Pathology*, vol. 125, no. 2, pp. 99–102, 1978.

42

Measurement of Serum Free Thyroxine Index May Provide Additional Case Detection Compared to Free Thyroxine in the Diagnosis of Central Hypothyroidism

Kevin M. Pantalone,[1] **Betul Hatipoglu,**[1] **Manjula K. Gupta,**[2]
Laurence Kennedy,[1] **and Amir H. Hamrahian**[1,3]

[1]*Endocrinology and Metabolism Institute, Cleveland Clinic, Desk F-20, 9500 Euclid Avenue, Cleveland, OH 44195, USA*
[2]*Pathology and Laboratory Medicine Institute, Cleveland Clinic, Desk LL3-140, 9500 Euclid Avenue, Cleveland, OH 44195, USA*
[3]*Department of Endocrinology, Cleveland Clinic Abu Dhabi, Abu Dhabi, UAE*

Correspondence should be addressed to Kevin M. Pantalone; pantalk@ccf.org

Academic Editor: Suat Simsek

The diagnosis of central hypothyroidism is often suspected in patients with hypothalamic/pituitary pathology, in the setting of low, normal, or even slightly elevated serum TSH and low free thyroxine (FT4). We present four cases of central hypothyroidism (three had known pituitary pathology) in whom central hypothyroidism was diagnosed after the serum free thyroxine index (FTI) was found to be low. All had normal range serum TSH and free thyroxine levels. This report illustrates that the assessment of the serum FTI may be helpful in making the diagnosis of central hypothyroidism in the appropriate clinical setting and when free T4 is in the low-normal range, particularly in patients with multiple anterior pituitary hormone deficiencies and/or with symptoms suggestive of hypothyroidism.

1. Background

Central hypothyroidism is a rare cause of hypothyroidism in the general population, estimated to occur in 1 : 20,000 to 1 : 80,000 [1]. However, in patients with pituitary pathology, it is observed much more frequently, particularly in patients with other pituitary hormone deficiencies. The diagnosis of central hypothyroidism is often suspected in patients with hypothalamic/pituitary pathology, in the setting of low free thyroxine (FT4). Most clinicians measure serum free thyroxine rather than total T4 or free thyroxine index to avoid problems with thyroid binding proteins. Pituitary mass lesions are the most common cause of central hypothyroidism. In cases of central hypothyroidism, serum TSH can be low, within the normal reference range, or even slightly elevated since TSH may have reduced biologic activity but normal immunoactivity [2–4]. In cases where FT4 is frankly low, making the diagnosis of central hypothyroidism is usually straightforward. However, in cases where free T4 is

within the normal reference range, especially in the setting of normal serum TSH, making the diagnosis of central hypothyroidism can be challenging. We present four cases of central hypothyroidism that were diagnosed via the assessment of serum FTI, in cases where patients had serum TSH and FT4 values within their respective reference ranges.

2. Methods

A retrospective chart review was completed on four subjects seen in our pituitary clinics with suspected central hypothyroidism, with serum TSH and free T4 measures within their respective reference ranges, in the setting of low serum FTI. All of the reported laboratory tests were performed at our institution's reference laboratory.

Total T4 and T-uptake both were measured on Roche Elecsys electrochemiluminescence immunoassay analyzer. Total T4 is measured by competitive inhibition assay using specific T4 antibody labeled with ruthenium complex. Serum T4, released from binding proteins by the action of 8-anilino-1-naphthalene sulfonic acid, competes with the added biotinylated T4 for the binding sites on the antibodies. Percent coefficient of variation for interassay precision was <5%. The reference range for adults is 5–11 ng/dL.

Thyroxine binding capacity (TBC) is measured by T-uptake immunoassay. For this patient, serum is first incubated with exogenous T4 and biotinylated T4 polyhapten that binds to the free binding sites in the serum. Labeled T4 specific antibody (ruthenium) was added which complexes with the biotinylated T4 polyhapten. This antibody-T4 biotin complex is then separated by addition of streptavidin coated microparticles and chemiluminescence is measured which is inversely proportional to the exogenous T4 concentration. Results are generated by 2-point calibration curve and the analyzer automatically calculates the T-uptake as thyroxine binding index (TBI). Free thyroxine index is calculated by dividing the total T4 by the TBI value (T-uptake ratio). Interassay precision (CV) is <5%. Reference range for T-uptake ratio is 0.7–1.2 and for FTI is 6–11.00 μg/dL.

Free T4 was also measured with the use of specific anti-T4 antibody labeled with a ruthenium complex which binds the free T4 in the serum in the first incubation. This is followed by the addition of biotinylated T4 that binds to the remaining free binding sites on the T4 antibody. The antibody complexes are then removed by addition of streptavidin coated microparticles and chemiluminescence is measured.

TSH was measured by two-site electrochemiluminescence immunoassay on cobas immunoassay analyzer from Roche Diagnostics. Lower limit of detection is 0.005 and interassay precision [CV] at two levels is <5%.

3. Results and Discussion

3.1. Case Reports

Case 1. A 55-year-old woman presented to endocrinology for management of type 2 diabetes (T2D). During her evaluation, multinodular goiter was appreciated on physical exam. A thyroid ultrasound noted a 5.9 × 4.4 × 4.0 cm complex nodule occupying the left lobe. Her TSH was 1.49 (0.4–5.5 μU/mL). The nodule underwent fine-needle aspiration and was found to be benign. The patient reported chronic fatigue, weight gain, constipation, and hair thinning. Her TSH had been measured multiple times and always reported within the normal range. She asked for additional evaluation of her thyroid function, so her TSH was repeated and an assessment of free thyroxine (FT4) was conducted: TSH 1.06 (0.4–5.5 μU/mL) and FT4 0.7 (0.7–1.8 ng/dL). The thyroid function tests were repeated in six weeks and were as follows: TSH 0.80 (0.4–5.5 μU/mL), FT4 0.7 (0.7–1.8 ng/dL), and FT3 2.2 (1.8–4.6 pg/mL). Because the free thyroid hormone levels were on the lower side of the normal reference range, a complete assessment of pituitary function was performed and was notable for undetectable gonadotropins and a prolactin level of 1775.2 (2.0–17.4 ng/mL). An ACTH stimulation test demonstrated a normal cortisol response and serum IGF-1

was within normal limits. A 1.8 cm sellar mass (prolactinoma) was subsequently found on computed tomography (CT). Her thyroid function tests were repeated, this time with an assessment of serum FTI and total T4 and T3; the results were as follows: TSH 0.92 (0.4–5.5 μU/mL), FT4 0.7 (0.7–1.8 ng/dL), FT3 2.1 (1.8–4.6 pg/mL), FTI 3.8 (6–11 μg/dL), T4 4.0 (5.0–11 μg/dL), and T3 88 (94–170 ng/dL). Cabergoline (0.5 mg twice per week) and levothyroxine 100 mcg daily were initiated and subsequently her prolactin and thyroid function tests after three months of therapy were as follows: prolactin 1.1 (2.0–17.4 ng/mL), FTI 9.2 (6–11 μg/dL), free T4 1.4 (0.7–1.8 ng/dL), and TSH 0.466 (0.4–5.5 μU/mL). The patient reported a significant improvement in her symptoms and has experienced a modest weight loss since the initiation of therapy.

Case 2. A 36-year-old male presented for a second opinion regarding the management of acromegaly. He underwent craniotomy for the management of a prolactin and GH secreting tumor six years ago. Subsequently, his prolactin and IGF-1 levels improved, but residual tumor and persistent hormone elevations were noted. He was initiated on octreotide LAR and bromocriptine; however, his tumor continued to increase in size. The second surgery was not successful to normalize IGF-1 and prolactin levels. During his evaluation, he reported fatigue and erectile dysfunction. He developed secondary hypogonadism and adrenal insufficiency after his initial surgery. During his initial hormone assessment postoperatively, he was noted to have slightly low TSH 0.32 (0.4–5.5 μU/mL), on one occasion, but with a normal range serum FT4 1.1 (0.7–1.8 ng/dL). All subsequent TSH and FT4 assessments were within the normal reference range; levothyroxine therapy was never initiated. Repeat assessment of his thyroid function tests, at the time of his initial encounter at our institution, showed the following: TSH 0.85 (0.4–5.5 μU/mL), FT4 0.9 (0.7–1.8 ng/dL), FT3 3.0 (1.8–4.6 pg/mL), FTI 4.9 (6–11 μg/dL), T4 4.4 (5.0–11 μg/dL), and T3 81 (94–170 ng/dL). Initiation of levothyroxine therapy resulted in improvement in his fatigue. Subsequent thyroid function tests, while taking 150 mcg of levothyroxine daily, were as follows: FTI 7.5 (6–11 μg/dL), TSH 0.120 (0.4–5.5 μU/mL), FT4 1.3 (0.7–1.8 ng/dL), and FT3 3.3 (1.8–4.6 pg/mL).

Case 3. A 60-year-old male presented with the complaints of blurry vision (left > right) and profound fatigue. Evaluation led to the discovery of a visual field deficit (left > right) and a large sellar mass (3.0 cm) with suprasellar extension and bilateral cavernous sinus invasion. Magnetic resonance imaging characteristics were suggestive of pituitary macroadenoma. His labs were consistent with secondary hypogonadism, but his remaining pituitary function tests were within their respective reference ranges: IGF-1 110 (60–211 ng/mL), random cortisol 20.9 μg/dL, TSH 4.06 (0.4–5.5 μU/mL), and FT4 0.7 (0.7–1.8 ng/dL). Given the notion that the FT4 level was on the lower side of the reference range and our experience with similar cases in the past, he underwent further assessment of his thyroid function: TSH 3.56 (0.4–5.5 μU/mL), FT4 0.8 (0.7–1.8 ng/dL), FTI 4.2 (6–11 μg/dL), T4 5.6 (5.0–11 μg/dL), and T3 100 (94–170 ng/dL). Levothyroxine

50 mcg daily was initiated, and follow-up thyroid function tests were as follows: TSH 0.936 (0.4–5.5 μU/mL) and FTI 7.7 (6–11 μg/dL). He noted an improvement in his fatigue. The patient subsequently underwent subtotal surgical resection of the nonfunctional mass followed by gamma knife stereotactic radiosurgery. His visual field deficit improved. Repeat thyroid function tests, while taking 50 mcg of levothyroxine, 1 month and 5 months postoperatively, revealed slightly low TSH and midnormal range serum FTI. His levothyroxine was increased to 75 mcg.

Case 4. A 62-year-old male presented to an outside hospital emergency department with symptoms of stroke. The evaluation of his right-sided hemiparesis included a CT scan of the brain, which showed an incidental sellar mass (3.5 cm). MRI characteristics were consistent with macroadenoma. A full assessment of his pituitary function tests showed hypopituitarism: testosterone < 12 (220–1000 ng/dL), LH 2.0 (1.0–7.0 mU/mL), FSH 2.7 (1.0–10.0 mU/mL), IGF-1 13 (39–231 ng/mL), peak cortisol level after cosyntropin stimulation 6.7 mg/dL (>18 μ/dL), TSH 5.44 (0.4–5.5 μU/mL), FT4 0.7 (0.7–1.8 ng/dL), FTI 4.3 (6–11 μg/dL), T4 5.5 (5.0–11 μg/dL), and prolactin 44.1 (2.0–14.0 ng/mL). He was initiated on hydrocortisone (20 mg per day) and levothyroxine therapy 75 mcg daily; subsequent thyroid function tests were as follows: TSH 3.6 (0.4–5.5 μU/mL) and FTI 6.7 (6–11 μg/dL). The patient underwent surgical resection of the mass; pathology was consistent with a nonfunctional pituitary adenoma.

Please see Table 1 for a complete summary of the lab data provided.

Our report highlights the utility of assessing serum FTI in making the diagnosis of central hypothyroidism, particularly when the serum TSH value is within the normal reference range and free T4 is in the lower part of the normal range. As it was the situation in the cases discussed, free T4 in the low-normal range failed to prompt the appropriate diagnosis and initiation of thyroxine in most cases. T3 values (total or free) are usually not helpful in making the diagnosis of central hypothyroidism, as both are frequently within the normal range in patients with mild hypothyroidism due to increased 5'-deiodinase activity [5–7]. Gupta et al. have previously reported that free T4 assessment is less sensitive for detecting hypothyroidism as compared to FTI [8]. In all four cases, the FTI was clearly low and was consistent with the presence of partial central hypothyroidism in the context of the clinical presentation and other pituitary function studies. Based on our experience over the years and in the appropriate clinical setting, we use serum FTI < 5 (6–11 μg/dL) to diagnose central hypothyroidism.

In certain cases, a TRH stimulation test may be useful in the evaluation of suspected cases of central hypothyroidism. Baseline TSH is obtained, and then 200 mcg of TRH is administered as an IV bolus. TSH values are subsequently obtained at 20 and 60 minutes after TRH administration. The normal increment in TSH at 20 min is 5–30 (mean 15) IU/mL with slight diminution at 60 min (http://www.pathology .leedsth.nhs.uk/dnn_bilm/Investigationprotocols/Pituitary-protocols/TRHTest.aspx). TRH is not commercially available in the U.S. Future studies comparing the results of FTI and

TRH stimulation test, in patients with suspected central hypothyroidism, would be of great interest and will hopefully be the subject of future research in areas of the world where TRH is commercially available.

One patient (Case 2) was receiving octreotide LAR therapy when the diagnosis of central hypothyroidism was made. A reduction in TSH secretion with somatostatin analogue therapy has been reported in the literature [9, 10]. While this is usually not clinically relevant (i.e., it does not usually cause overt central hypothyroidism), certainly it is possible that the therapy may have played a role in the development of central hypothyroidism in this patient.

It is unclear why measurement of serum FTI compared to FT4 may provide additional case detection in patients with central hypothyroidism. One may speculate that the normal reference range for serum FT4 may need to be reexamined in a larger reference population. It is important to note that while measurement of FTI may provide us with a better tool to identify additional cases of central hypothyroidism (higher sensitivity), in our experience it is not uncommon to get low FTI values between 5 and 6 (normal range: 6–11 μg/dL) in patients without pituitary disorders (lower specificity). Therefore, it is very important to interpret thyroid function studies in the appropriate clinical context, taking into consideration the presence of symptoms and the status of other pituitary axes. This report documents our personal experience and may be assay dependent and needs to be further evaluated in future studies. Moreover, one must consider that free thyroxine assays have low precision at the lower end of the reference range and high interassay variability [11]. Clinicians should be familiar with the specific assay being utilized at their institution.

While this study reports an interesting observation, it is not without limitation. It is a retrospective study that only includes 4 subjects. Further prospective studies are needed to compare the two tests (FTI versus FT4). The goal of this report is to alert clinicians about the limitation of FT4 measurements in evaluating suspected cases of partial secondary hypothyroidism and that assessment of serum FTI may better allow for identification of such cases. Certainly one may argue that instead of measuring FTI the possibility of secondary hypothyroidism in the presence of low-normal free T4 in the appropriate clinical context should be taken into account and a trial of hormone replacement be considered. It is unknown whether the measurement of free T4 by some other method, such as equilibrium dialysis, would have assisted in identifying these patients as having central hypothyroidism. Future studies assessing serum FTI and FT4 in patients with new-onset central hypothyroidism and primary hypothyroidism would be helpful in further evaluating our observations.

It is also important to note that there are multiple ways of assessing the free thyroxine index, using T-uptake and T4, as was the case in our subjects, or using T4/TBG. Gupta et al. [8] compared these two methods, and the results of the regression analysis were similar, $r = 0.94$ for hypothyroid patients (primary hypothyroidism) and $r = 0.89$ for all patients. This high correlation indicates that the T4/TBG index may not provide any additional value over the standard

TABLE 1

Pituitary disorder	TSH (0.4–5.5 µU/mL)	T4 (5–11 mcg/dL)	T4 uptake (0.7–1.2)	FTI (6–11 mcg/dL)	FT4 (0.7–1.8 ng/dL)	FT3 (1.8–4.6 pg/dL)	T3 (94–170 ng/dL)	Albumin (3.5–5.0 g/dL)	Hormone deficiencies
Prolactinoma	0.922	4	1.06	3.8	0.7	2.1	88	4.2	Hypogonadism
Acromegaly	0.85	4.4	0.89	4.9	0.9	3	81	4.2	Panhypopituitarism
Macroadenoma (NF*)	4.06	5.6	1.34	4.2	0.7	N/A	93	4.7	Hypogonadism
Macroadenoma (NF)	5.44	5.5	1.28	4.3	0.7	N/A	N/A	4.3	Panhypopituitarism

*NF: nonfunctional.

FTI (T-uptake and T4) assessment; thus it is not normally used and will only increase the cost of testing. As TBG levels were not obtained on the subjects of this report, comparing these two methods in our subjects is not possible. Future research including assessment of the T4/TBG index in the evaluation of suspected cases of central hypothyroidism and a comparison of these values to that of the FTI (T-uptake and T4) would be of great interest.

Lastly, it is important to note that the reference ranges for the thyroid function studies included in this report were derived from the general population. It is possible that some of the subjects included in our report may have had circulating anti-TPO antibodies, and this could theoretically explain why the FT4 values were in the low-normal reference range (i.e., they may have an underlying recent-onset primary thyroid disorder). Unfortunately, as we were not suspecting a primary thyroid disorder in these subjects, given their clinical presentation, the anti-TPO status of the subjects was not assessed.

4. Conclusion

In the appropriate clinical setting, the measurement of serum FTI may provide additional case detection of central hypothyroidism when free T4 is in the low-normal range. Further prospective studies are needed to compare the use of FTI and FT4 in the evaluation of TSH axis in patients with pituitary disorders.

Authors' Contribution

Kevin M. Pantalone wrote the paper. Betul Hatipoglu, Manjula K. Gupta, Laurence Kennedy, and Amir H. Hamrahian reviewed and edited the paper and contributed to the discussion.

References

[1] L. Persani, "Clinical review: central hypothyroidism: pathogenic, diagnostic, and therapeutic challenges," *Journal of Clinical Endocrinology and Metabolism*, vol. 97, no. 9, pp. 3068–3078, 2012.

[2] P. Beck-Peccoz, S. Amr, M. Menezes-Ferreira, G. Faglia, and B. D. Weintraub, "Decreased receptor binding of biologically inactive thyrotropin in central hypothyroidism. Effect of treatment with thyrotropin-releasing hormone," *The New England Journal of Medicine*, vol. 312, no. 17, pp. 1085–1090, 1985.

[3] G. Faglia, L. Bitensky, A. Pinchera et al., "Thyrotropin secretion in patients with central hypothyroidism: evidence for reduced biological activity of immunoreactive thyrotropin," *Journal of Clinical Endocrinology and Metabolism*, vol. 48, no. 6, pp. 989–998, 1979.

[4] L. Persani, E. Ferretti, S. Borgato, G. Faglia, and P. Beck-Peccoz, "Circulating thyrotropin bioactivity in sporadic central hypothyroidism," *Journal of Clinical Endocrinology and Metabolism*, vol. 85, no. 10, pp. 3631–3635, 2000.

[5] O. Alexopoulou, C. Belguin, P. De Nayer, and D. Maiter, "Clinical and hormonal characteristics of central hypothyroidism at diagnosis and during follow-up in adult patients," *European Journal of Endocrinology*, vol. 150, no. 1, pp. 1–8, 2004.

[6] E. Ferretti, L. Persani, M.-L. Jaffrain-Rea, S. Giambona, G. Tamburrano, and P. Beck-Peccoz, "Evaluation of the adequacy of levothyroxine replacement therapy in patients with central hypothyroidism," *Journal of Clinical Endocrinology and Metabolism*, vol. 84, no. 3, pp. 924–929, 1999.

[7] J. L. Leonard, C. A. Siegrist-Kaiser, and C. J. Zuckerman, "Regulation of type II iodothyronine 5′-deiodinase by thyroid hormone. Inhibition of actin polymerization blocks enzyme inactivation in cAMP-stimulated glial cells," *The Journal of Biological Chemistry*, vol. 265, no. 2, pp. 940–946, 1990.

[8] M. K. Gupta, R. Salazar, and O. P. Schumacher, "A solid phase radioimmunoassay for the measurement of free thyroxine. A new screening test for thyroid function?" *American Journal of Clinical Pathology*, vol. 79, no. 3, pp. 334–340, 1983.

[9] S. L. Lightman, P. Fox, and M. J. Dunne, "The effect of SMS 201–995, a long-acting somatostatin analogue, on anterior pituitary function in healthy male volunteers," *Scandinavian Journal of Gastroenterology*, vol. 21, no. 119, pp. 84–95, 1986.

[10] R. D. Murray, K. Kim, S.-G. Ren et al., "The novel somatostatin ligand (SOM230) regulates human and rat anterior pituitary hormone secretion," *Journal of Clinical Endocrinology and Metabolism*, vol. 89, no. 6, pp. 3027–3032, 2004.

[11] L. M. Thienpont, K. Van Uytfanghe, S. Van Houcke et al., "A progress report of the IFCC committee for standardization of thyroid function tests," *European Thyroid Journal*, vol. 3, no. 2, pp. 109–116, 2014.

43

Diabetic Myonecrosis: A Diagnostic and Treatment Challenge in Longstanding Diabetes

Lima Lawrence (ID),[1] **Oscar Tovar-Camargo,**[2] **M. Cecilia Lansang** (ID),[1] and **Vinni Makin**[1]

[1]*Cleveland Clinic, Department of Endocrinology and Metabolism, Cleveland, OH, USA*
[2]*Cleveland Clinic, Department of Anesthesiology, Cleveland, OH, USA*

Correspondence should be addressed to Lima Lawrence; lawrenl4@ccf.org

Academic Editor: John Broom

Objective. Diabetes mellitus is associated with microvascular and macrovascular complications; the most commonly recognized ones include diabetic nephropathy, retinopathy, and neuropathy. Less well-known complications are equally important, as timely recognition and treatment are essential to decrease short- and long-term morbidity. *Methods.* Herein, we describe a case of a 41-year-old female with longstanding, uncontrolled type 2 diabetes, who presented with classical findings of diabetic myonecrosis. *Results.* Our patient underwent extensive laboratory and imaging studies prior to diagnosis due to its rarity and similarity in presentation with other commonly noted musculoskeletal conditions. We emphasize the clinical presentation, laboratory and imaging findings, treatment regimen, and prognosis associated with diabetic myonecrosis. *Conclusion.* Diabetic myonecrosis is a rare complication of longstanding, poorly controlled diabetes mellitus. The diagnosis requires a high index of suspicion in the right clinical setting: acute onset nontraumatic muscular pain with associated findings on clinical exam, laboratory studies, and imaging. While the short-term prognosis is good, the recurrence rate remains high and long-term prognosis is poor given underlying uncontrolled diabetes and associated sequelae.

1. Introduction

Diabetic myonecrosis, also known as diabetic muscle infarction, causes spontaneous ischemic necrosis of skeletal muscle most commonly in the thigh or calf. It is a rare complication seen in patients with longstanding, uncontrolled diabetes mellitus. It was first described in 1965 by Angervall and Sterner as "tumoriform focal muscular degeneration" [1]. Patients present with acute pain, swelling, and tenderness of the affected muscle group [2]. As diabetic myonecrosis is infrequently seen, heightened awareness of the condition is necessary to exclude similarly presenting muscular and vascular pathology and promptly initiate treatment.

2. Clinical Case

A 41-year-old African American woman presented to the emergency department (ED) with right leg pain for 2 weeks. She had a past medical history of type 2 diabetes mellitus diagnosed more than 10 years ago, end-stage renal disease (ESRD) on hemodialysis, hypertension, congestive heart failure, and recently resolved left lower extremity cellulitis. She described her right leg pain as constant, aching, stabbing pain in the right posterior mid-thigh with radiation distally to the calf. She denied any trauma or falls and reported worsening pain with weight-bearing and ambulation. She had already presented to 2 other EDs and had X-ray of the right knee and lumbar spine, venous Doppler of the right lower extremity, CT femur and right ankle-brachial index, which were normal. She had been taking oxycodone-acetaminophen without significant relief. During the current visit, she had CT angiogram of the abdomen and pelvis with lower extremity runoff, which found no vessel stenosis, but noted soft tissue and fascial edema in the right thigh. She was discharged home with analgesics and recommended follow-up with orthopedics.

The following month, patient presented to the ED again with excruciating right thigh pain. Laboratory studies were remarkable for leukocytosis 12.77 k/uL (3.7–11.0 k/uL), elevated creatinine kinase (CK) 683 U/L (42–196 U/L),

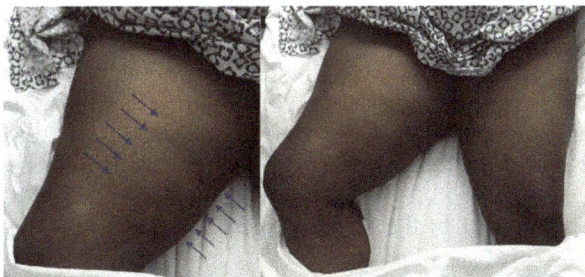

FIGURE 1: Diabetic myonecrosis involving the right thigh with overlying palpable skin induration (arrows). Enlargement of right thigh compared to left. Right leg was kept externally rotated.

C-reactive protein (CRP) 3.7 mg/dL (<0.9 mg/dL), and erythrocyte sedimentation rate (ESR) 68 mm/hr (0–20 mm/hr). Additionally, poor glycemic control was confirmed with random blood glucose of 569 mg/dL and hemoglobin A1c 13.8%. MRI of the right leg revealed diffuse subcutaneous edema in the right thigh, extending to the level of the knee, with diffusely increased T2 signal in the mid and distal thigh. Intramuscular fascial edema around the proximal hamstring muscles was noted, without any findings of abscess or osteomyelitis. Patient received analgesics, with optimization of glycemia, and was discharged home after physical therapy evaluation.

One week later, patient was readmitted after a fall. Endocrinology was consulted to address hyperglycemia. Physical examination revealed an obese woman in mild distress due to pain. She had a swollen right thigh, exquisitely tender to palpation and noticeably larger than the left. The overlying skin was palpably indurated without warmth, erythema, bullae, greyish hue, or crepitus (Figure 1). Passive and active movements at the right hip and knee were limited due to pain and patient kept the right leg externally rotated. No visible cord or joint effusions at the knee or hip were noted and lower extremity pulses were palpable bilaterally. Laboratory studies were notable for persistent leukocytosis 13.60 k/uL, elevated CRP 8.4 mg/dL, ESR 117 mm/hr, and CK 714 U/L. As the inflammatory markers doubled in a short interval, repeat lower extremity MRI was obtained to rule out abscess or infectious myositis. T1-weighted imaging on MRI noted diffuse swelling and edema-like signal involving the right thigh musculature with fluid-like signal at the fascial planes without any focal fluid collection (Figure 2). Altogether, these findings were suggestive of ischemic changes in the right thigh musculature. Based on the clinical history as well as labs and imaging findings, a diagnosis of diabetic myonecrosis was made. Patient was prescribed aspirin 81 mg daily, analgesics including acetaminophen and oxycodone as needed (with avoidance of NSAIDs due to ESRD), and lidocaine patch. Patient's blood glucose was targeted from 140 to 180 mg/dL with adjustments of insulin glargine and lispro. She was evaluated by physical therapy and discharged home shortly with endocrine follow-up.

3. Discussion

Diabetic myonecrosis is infrequently observed in patients with diabetes. The pathogenesis of diabetic muscle

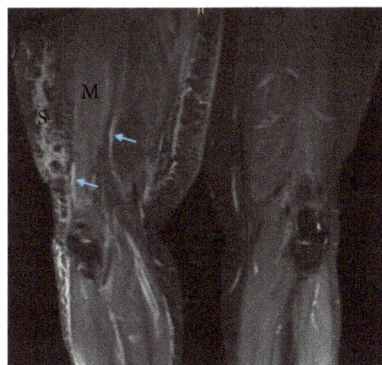

FIGURE 2: **MRI leg without contrast.** Right thigh musculature (M) and subcutaneous tissues (S) with diffuse swelling and edema-like signal on T1-weighted imaging. Fluid-like signal is noted at the fascial planes (arrows).

infarction is poorly understood, but various theories have been proposed including vasculopathic changes from longstanding, poorly controlled diabetes, vasculitic changes, hypercoagulability, or ischemia-reperfusion injury. Microvascular endothelial damage leads to tissue ischemia, triggering the inflammatory cascade leading to ischemic necrosis. Reperfusion of necrotic tissues leads to generation of reactive oxygen species and production of inflammatory mediators including tumor necrosis factor and platelet-activating factor, which mediate vasculopathic changes [2]. Additionally, alterations in the coagulation-fibrinolysis system have been implicated in diabetic myonecrosis by causing hypercoagulability and vascular endothelial damage [2].

Diabetic myonecrosis should be suspected in any patient with diabetes who presents with sudden-onset muscle swelling and pain, particularly of the proximal lower extremities. A higher index of suspicion should be reserved for poorly controlled, longstanding diabetes patients with coexisting complications. Diabetic myonecrosis is more commonly seen in women (53.7–61.5%) with a mean age at presentation around 42.6 to 44.5 years [2–4]. A systematic review examined 126 cases of diabetic myonecrosis and observed that the mean diabetes duration at the time of diagnosis was 18.9 years in type 1 diabetes and 11.0 years in type 2 diabetes. Additionally, mean hemoglobin A1c at the time of diagnosis was

9.34%. Similarly, an examination of diabetic myonecrosis in 41 patients with ESRD found that more than 60% of patients had hemoglobin A1c above 7.0% [3]. Coexisting diabetes complications are frequently noted, with nephropathy in 75% of patients, two other macrovascular complications in 65.8% of patients, and 46.6% with nephropathy, neuropathy, and retinopathy related to diabetes [2].

Initial symptoms most commonly present in the thigh and calf, followed by upper extremity sites. The most commonly affected muscle groups are found in the anterior thigh, followed by the calf and posterior thigh [2]. Painful swelling may be acute or evolve over days to weeks. There is usually no preceding trauma and bilateral involvement is uncommon [4]. Although there are no specific markers, a common pattern is noted with elevation of CK, ESR, and CRP. Leukocytosis may be noted, although most patients are afebrile on presentation. Diagnosis is based on clinical presentation, labs, and imaging, for which MRI is the modality of choice. Characteristic features on MRI include increased signal intensity in the affected intramuscular and subcutaneous tissues, hyperintense signal on T2-weighted imaging, and isointense to hypointense signal on T1-weighted images associated with inflammatory changes and edema [5]. Doppler ultrasound is commonly performed to exclude underlying deep venous thrombus (DVT) or abscess and may visualize subcutaneous or muscle edema. Additional imaging is not necessary but may be performed to exclude other diagnoses as appropriate. Differential diagnoses include DVT, pyomyositis, necrotizing fasciitis, soft tissue abscess, ruptured Baker's cyst, osteomyelitis, and benign tumors or muscle sarcomas [6]. Muscle biopsy must be reserved for atypical presentation, uncertain diagnosis, or when treatment fails to improve symptoms. On biopsy, gross findings include non-hemorrhagic and pale muscle tissue. Under light microscopy, initial stages of diabetic myonecrosis reveal areas of muscle necrosis and edema, with replacement of necrotic muscle fibers by fibrous tissue, lymphocytic infiltration, and muscle regeneration in later stages [3, 5].

Rest, analgesia, and intense glycemic control are the cornerstones of diabetic myonecrosis therapy. As no randomized trials are available comparing specific treatment regimens, recommendations are based on case reports and case series. Initially, bed rest is advised as patients receiving physical therapy were noted to have the longest mean time to symptom resolution [2]. Low-dose aspirin and NSAIDs are recommended for those without contraindication; however, it is important to note that a large majority have concomitant renal disease, necessitating evaluation of NSAID therapy on a case-by-case basis. The benefits of antiplatelet and anti-inflammatory agents in diabetic myonecrosis may be attributed to its antithrombotic effects and amelioration of endothelial dysfunction. Surgical intervention is not routinely recommended as recovery time and recurrence rate were highest in this group [2]. With timely diagnosis and initiation of treatment, diabetic myonecrosis resolves spontaneously over a few weeks to months. Average recovery times were 5.5 weeks with aspirin and/or NSAID use, 8 weeks with bed rest and analgesics, and 13 weeks with surgical resection [7]. Even with treatment, diabetic myonecrosis carries a high recurrence rate of 34.9 to 47.8% usually involving a contralateral limb within 6 months [2, 3, 5]. Additionally, the long-term outlook remains poor with high morbidity and mortality, given underlying diabetes complicated by severe end-organ disease. A 25-year Mayo Clinic experience review revealed that out of 5 patients with diabetic myonecrosis, one required kidney transplantation, and a second patient died 2 years after diagnosis of myonecrosis [8].

4. Conclusion

Diabetic myonecrosis is a rare complication of longstanding, poorly controlled diabetes mellitus. Diagnosis requires a high index of suspicion in the right clinical setting: acute onset nontraumatic muscular pain with associated findings on clinical exam, labs, and imaging. Muscle biopsy is not routinely indicated and treatment is mainly conservative with good short-term prognosis and resolution of symptoms. However, the recurrence rate remains high, and long-term prognosis is poor given underlying uncontrolled diabetes and its associated sequelae.

Disclosure

This article does not contain any studies with human or animal subjects.

References

[1] L. Angervall and B. Stener, "Tumoriform focal muscular degeneration in two diabetic patients," *Diabetologia*, vol. 1, no. 1, pp. 39–42, 1965.

[2] W. Horton, J. Taylor, T. Ragland et al., "Diabetic muscle infarction: a systematic review," *BMJ Open Diabetes Research & Care*, vol. 3, no. 1, 2015.

[3] T. Yong and K. Khow, "Diabetic muscle infarction in end-stage renal disease: A scoping review on epidemiology, diagnosis and treatment," *World Journal of Nephrology*, vol. 7, no. 2, pp. 58–64, 2018.

[4] T. Joshi, E. D'Almeida, and J. Luu, "Diabetes myonecrosis - A rare complication," *Diabetes Research and Clinical Practice*, vol. 109, no. 3, pp. e18–e20, 2015.

[5] A. J. Trujillo-Santos, "Diabetic muscle infarction: an underdiagnosed complication of long-standing diabetes," *Diabetes Care*, vol. 26, no. 1, pp. 211–215, 2003.

[6] A. Chawla, N. Dubey, K. M. Chew, D. Singh, V. Gaikwad, and W. C. Peh, "Magnetic resonance imaging of painful swollen legs in the emergency department: a pictorial essay," *Emergency Radiology*, vol. 24, no. 5, pp. 577–584, 2017.

[7] S. Kapur, J. Brunet, and R. McKendry, "Diabetic muscle infarction: case report and review," *The Journal of Rheumatology*, vol. 31, pp. 190–194, 2004.

[8] T. J. Bunch, L. M. Birskovich, and P. W. Eiken, "Diabetic myonecrosis in a previously healthy woman and review of a 25-year Mayo clinic experience," *Endocrine Practice*, vol. 8, no. 5, pp. 343–346, 2002.

44

Effects of Mifepristone on Nonalcoholic Fatty Liver Disease in a Patient with a Cortisol-Secreting Adrenal Adenoma

Enzo Ragucci,[1] Dat Nguyen,[2] Michele Lamerson,[2] and Andreas G. Moraitis[2]

[1]*Diabetes and Endocrinology Consultants, 2 Crosfield Ave, No. 204, West Nyack, NY 10994, USA*
[2]*Corcept Therapeutics, 149 Commonwealth Drive, Menlo Park, CA 94025, USA*

Correspondence should be addressed to Andreas G. Moraitis; amoraitis@corcept.com

Academic Editor: John Broom

Cushing syndrome (CS), a complex, multisystemic condition resulting from prolonged exposure to cortisol, is frequently associated with nonalcoholic fatty liver disease (NAFLD). In patients with adrenal adenoma(s) and NAFLD, it is essential to rule out coexisting endocrine disorders like CS, so that the underlying condition can be properly addressed. We report a case of a 49-year-old woman with a history of hypertension, prediabetes, dyslipidemia, biopsy-confirmed steatohepatitis, and benign adrenal adenoma, who was referred for endocrine work-up for persistent weight gain. Overt Cushing features were absent. Biochemical evaluation revealed nonsuppressed cortisol on multiple 1-mg dexamethasone suppression tests, suppressed adrenocorticotropic hormone, and low dehydroepiandrosterone sulfate. The patient initially declined surgery and was treated with mifepristone, a competitive glucocorticoid receptor antagonist. In addition to improvements in weight and hypertension, substantial reductions in her liver enzymes were noted, with complete normalization by 20 weeks of therapy. This case suggests that autonomous cortisol secretion from adrenal adenoma(s) could contribute to the metabolic and liver abnormalities in patients with NAFLD. In conclusion, successful management of CS with mifepristone led to marked improvement in the liver enzymes of a patient with long-standing NAFLD.

1. Introduction

Nonalcoholic fatty liver disease (NAFLD) is a common cause of chronic liver disease in westernized countries, affecting 17% to 30% of the population [1]. Defined histologically as the accumulation of fat within the hepatocytes that exceeds 5% of liver weight [1, 2], NAFLD is generally considered the hepatic manifestation of metabolic syndrome [3]. Liver damage associated with NAFLD can range from simple steatosis to nonalcoholic steatohepatitis (NASH), which may progress to cirrhosis, liver failure, and hepatocellular carcinoma [1, 2]. NAFLD is strongly associated with risk factors including obesity, insulin resistance, type 2 diabetes, hypertension, and dyslipidemia. Although secondary causes of NAFLD (e.g., lipid metabolism disorders, medications, and other diseases) occur in the minority of cases [1], it is important to exclude them during the differential diagnosis, especially in patients with coexisting adrenal adenoma(s).

Both hypercortisolism from exogenous sources and that from endogenous sources are recognized causes of NAFLD [3]. For instance, NAFLD is frequently seen in patients with Cushing syndrome (CS) [4], a complex, multisystemic condition resulting from prolonged exposure to cortisol. A computed tomography- (CT-) based study found hepatic steatosis in 20% of CS patients with active disease [4].

The mechanisms by which cortisol impacts lipid metabolism are complex [5, 6] and not yet fully elucidated. Here we report a case of autonomous cortisol secretion due to an adrenal adenoma in which medical therapy with the competitive glucocorticoid receptor antagonist mifepristone resulted in biochemical remission of NAFLD.

2. Case Presentation

A 49-year-old woman with a medical history of hypertension, prediabetes, dyslipidemia, and histologically confirmed

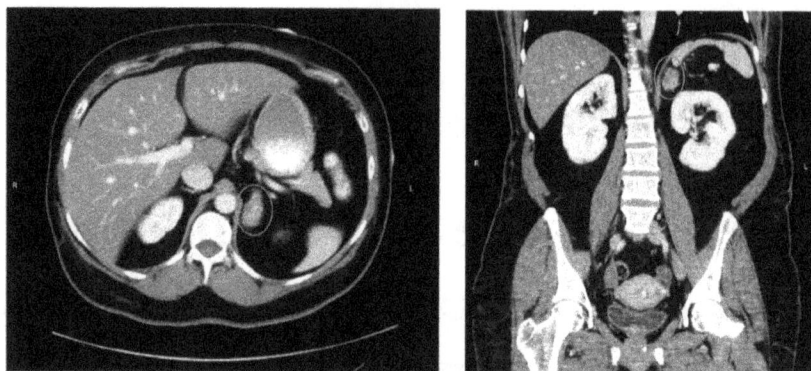

FIGURE 1: Images showing left adrenal adenoma measuring $2.9 \times 1.9 \times 2.5$ cm (shown in circles).

NASH (80% diffused steatosis with pericellular inflammation) was referred by her primary care provider for endocrine evaluation for complaint of persistent weight gain with central obesity. Two years prior to the referral she was discovered to have a left adrenal adenoma on a routine abdominal CT scan for evaluation of nephrolithiasis. Phenotypic features of overt CS (i.e., moon face, striae, buffalo hump, etc.) were not present, and biochemical evaluation of the adenoma was not performed at that time. At referral, the patient still did not have overt phenotypic features of CS. A follow-up scan revealed a stable benign left adrenal adenoma ($2.9 \times 1.9 \times 2.5$ cm) measuring 14 Hounsfield units on noncontrast CT (Figure 1). The adenoma was described as lobulated with a high fat content. Baseline clinical characteristics and laboratory findings are listed in Table 1.

Results of hormonal testing were negative for pheochromocytoma and primary aldosteronism. Testing for autonomous cortisol secretion showed mildly elevated urinary free cortisol (UFC), failure to suppress cortisol on multiple 1-mg overnight dexamethasone suppression tests (DSTs), elevated late-night salivary cortisol, suppressed adrenocorticotropic hormone (ACTH) on multiple tests, and low dehydroepiandrosterone sulfate (DHEA-S) (Table 1).

The patient declined adrenalectomy. Ketoconazole was not considered because of the patient's fatty liver and elevated liver enzymes. Medical therapy with mifepristone (Korlym®, Corcept Therapeutics, Menlo Park, CA) was initiated at 300 mg per day and increased to 900 mg during the 34 weeks of treatment. After 4 weeks, her antihypertensive medication (amlodipine/olmesartan medoxomil 10/20 mg) was discontinued and her blood pressure remained stable (Figure 2). During the course of mifepristone treatment, she lost 16 lbs and marked improvement in her liver enzymes was noted, with complete normalization by week 20 (Figure 3).

At week 20 she complained of vaginal spotting, and a pelvic ultrasound showed multiple uterine fibroids. Subsequently she elected to undergo a hysterectomy and a left adrenalectomy. Mifepristone was discontinued 2 weeks prior to the adrenalectomy. Her prediabetes remained stable during mifepristone treatment; HbA1c was 40 mmol/mol before surgery.

TABLE 1: Baseline patient characteristics and laboratory findings.

Parameter	Result
Age, years	49
BMI, kg/m^2	30.6
BP, mmHg	142/90
HbA1c, mmol/mol	41
Lipids, mmol/L	
Total cholesterol	7.1
LDL	5.3
TG	1.5
Liver function	
AST, U/L (normal 2–40)	110
ALT, U/L (normal 2–60)	232
Endocrine evaluation	
UFC, nmol/d (normal 11–138)	172.8
1-mg DST, nmol/L (normal < 49.5)	364.3; 345.0
Late night salivary cortisol, nmol/L (normal < 2.5)	5.2
ACTH, pmol/L (normal 1.1–9.9)	<1.1 × 2
DHEA-S, μmol/L (normal 1.1–7.9)	0.54

ACTH, adrenocorticotropic hormone; ALT, alanine transaminase; AST, aspartate transaminase; BMI, body mass index; BP, blood pressure; DHEA-S, dehydroepiandrosterone sulfate; DST, dexamethasone suppression test; HbA1c, glycated hemoglobin A1c; LDL, low-density lipoprotein; TG, triglyceride; UFC, urinary free cortisol.

During the 34-week course of medical therapy with mifepristone, the patient's hypothalamic-pituitary-adrenal (HPA) axis recovered, as indicated by increases in ACTH levels from undetectable at baseline and week 16 to 2.4 pmol/L at week 24 (Figure 4). She was treated postoperatively with glucocorticoid replacement (hydrocortisone 50 mg), which was tapered and discontinued within 6 weeks. Her liver enzymes remained within the normal range and there were no further changes in blood pressure and weight 1 year postoperatively. Her most recent HbA1c was 33 mmol/mol (5.2%).

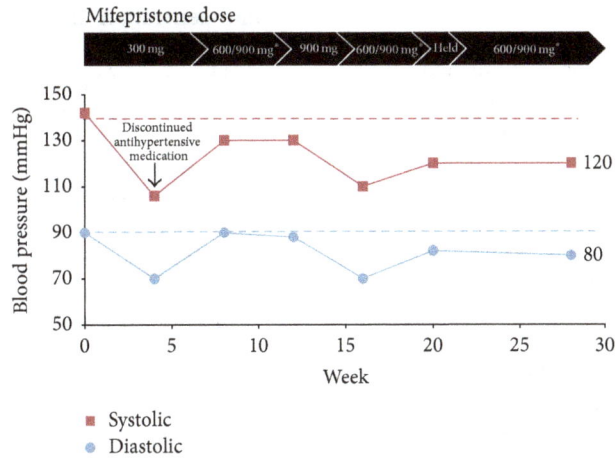

FIGURE 2: Change in blood pressure over time after initiating mifepristone treatment. *Alternating daily doses of 600 and 900 mg.

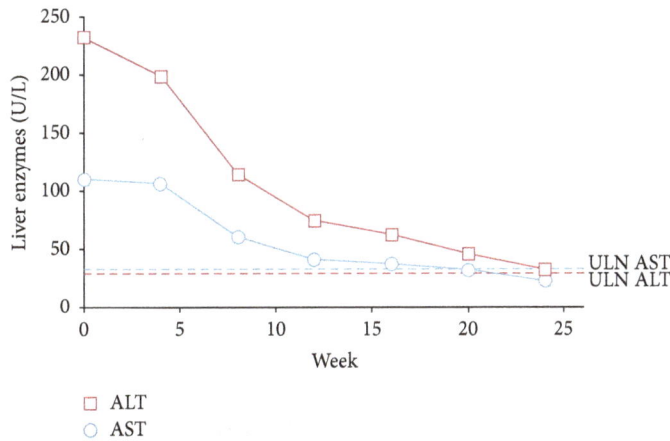

FIGURE 3: Change in liver enzymes over time after initiating mifepristone treatment. ALT, alanine transaminase; AST, aspartate transaminase; ULN, upper limit of normal.

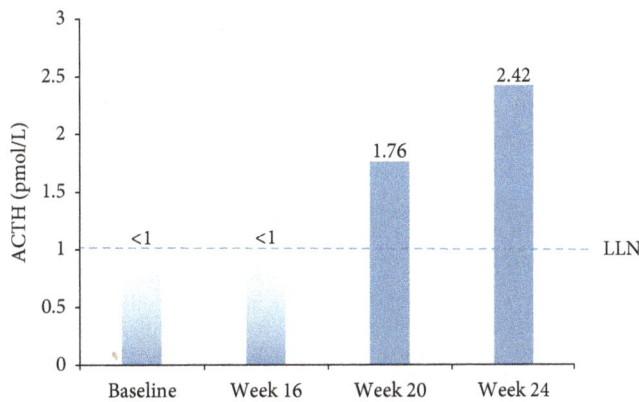

FIGURE 4: Change in ACTH over time after initiating mifepristone treatment. ACTH, adrenocorticotropic hormone; LLN, lower limit of normal.

3. Discussion

We have described a case of hypercortisolism due to an adrenal adenoma associated with biopsy-confirmed NASH. The patient was treated medically with mifepristone therapy for 34 weeks. In addition to improvement in cardiometabolic parameters associated with hypercortisolism, we also noted marked improvement in her liver function tests (LFTs) during treatment.

NAFLD is associated with cardiometabolic risk factors (obesity, diabetes, dyslipidemia, and hypertension) and is diagnosed by hepatic steatosis on imaging or histology and exclusion of other causes of liver disease [7]. Although LFTs are a good surrogate biomarker for NAFLD, a substantial portion of patients, 79% according to one study [8], may have normal LFTs. Thus, liver biopsy, while being costly and invasive, remains the only definitive method for diagnosis.

NAFLD is frequently seen in patients with CS [4], which is not surprising as metabolic derangements are also common in CS. In fact, one study found a higher prevalence and greater severity of NAFLD among patients with CS when compared to matched cohorts of nonfunctioning adrenal adenomas and controls [9]. A high prevalence of metabolic syndrome features and cardiometabolic risk factors has also been reported in patients with adrenal adenoma(s) [10–12]. Other studies have shown HPA axis dysfunction among patients with NAFLD [13–15]. In overweight/obese NAFLD patients, HPA axis dysfunction was correlated with the severity of NAFLD [16]. Together, these studies suggest that subtle and chronic activation of the HPA axis can contribute to the development and progression of NAFLD.

Hypercortisolism without classically described features of overt CS occurs in up to 30% of patients with adrenal adenomas [17]. Clinical assessment for signs and symptoms of hypercortisolism, as well as biochemical evaluation using the 1-mg overnight DST, is recommended as part of the work-up for patients with newly discovered adrenal adenomas [18]. In our case, the patient was not referred for endocrine evaluation until 2 years after the adenoma was discovered and her comorbidities had worsened. This case underscores the need for greater awareness among primary care providers of the importance of cortisol evaluation for benign adrenal adenomas, regardless of clinical symptomology.

Mifepristone, a competitive glucocorticoid receptor antagonist, is an effective medical therapy for patients with endogenous CS [19]. Patients from the SEISMIC trial demonstrated significant improvement in glucose abnormalities (assessed by oral glucose tolerance test), significant reductions in fasting plasma glucose and HbA1c, and a rapid and significant decrease in mean area under the curve insulin levels [19]. Together, these suggest improved insulin sensitivity.

The effects of mifepristone on metabolic parameters in patient populations outside of CS have also been explored. In a small study of patients with type 2 diabetes and fatty liver, short-term doses of mifepristone and metyrapone, a cortisol biosynthesis inhibitor, appeared to improve insulin sensitivity [10]. Two other clinical studies conducted in healthy men demonstrated that mifepristone significantly attenuated not only the side effect of weight gain caused by second-generation antipsychotic medications, but also the increases in fasting plasma insulin and triglyceride levels caused by their use [20, 21].

In our patient with hypercortisolism and biopsy-confirmed NASH, mifepristone treatment was associated with dramatic improvement in LFTs, as well as improvements in weight and hypertension leading to discontinuation of her antihypertensive medication. Follow-up liver imaging was not available for comparison; however, the overall improved functional and metabolic status of the patient, along with no signs or symptoms of deteriorating liver function (cirrhosis), support the LFT findings. The effect of mifepristone on LFTs was a novel finding and suggests that mifepristone may offer an alternative treatment to surgery in patients with hypercortisolism and NAFLD. It also may provide a useful method to assess the contribution of autonomous cortisol secretion of an adrenal adenoma to the cardiometabolic profile and liver abnormalities in patients with NAFLD. Larger prospective studies are needed to determine whether mifepristone use in patients with NAFLD and adrenal adenoma(s) can be used as a screening tool to select patients who will benefit from adrenalectomy.

Disclosure

Data from this case report were presented at the annual ENDO meeting in San Diego, CA, on March 5–8, 2015.

Acknowledgments

The authors wish to thank Sarah Mizne, PharmD, of MedVal Scientific Information Services, LLC, for providing professional editorial assistance. Funding to support the preparation of this manuscript was provided to MedVal by Corcept Therapeutics. This manuscript was prepared according to the International Society for Medical Publication Professionals' "Good Publication Practice for Communicating Company-Sponsored Medical Research: the GPP3 Guidelines" and the International Committee of Medical Journal Editors' "Uniform Requirements for Manuscripts Submitted to Biomedical Journals."

References

[1] J. M. Kneeman, J. Misdraji, and K. E. Corey, "Secondary causes of nonalcoholic fatty liver disease," *Therapeutic Advances in Gastroenterology*, vol. 5, no. 3, pp. 199–207, 2012.

[2] P. Angulo, "GI epidemiology: nonalcoholic fatty liver disease," *Alimentary Pharmacology & Therapeutics*, vol. 25, no. 8, pp. 883–889, 2007.

[3] F. Ferraù and M. Korbonits, "Metabolic comorbidities in Cushing's syndrome," *European Journal of Endocrinology*, vol. 173, no. 4, pp. M133–M157, 2015.

[4] A. G. Rockall, S. A. Sohaib, D. Evans et al., "Hepatic steatosis in Cushing's syndrome: a radiological assessment using computed tomography," *European Journal of Endocrinology*, vol. 149, no. 6, pp. 543–548, 2003.

[5] C. P. Woods, J. M. Hazlehurst, and J. W. Tomlinson, "Glucocorticoids and non-alcoholic fatty liver disease," *The Journal of Steroid Biochemistry and Molecular Biology*, vol. 154, article no. 4458, pp. 94–103, 2015.

[6] L. L. Gathercole, S. A. Morgan, I. J. Bujalska, D. Hauton, P. M. Stewart, and J. W. Tomlinson, "Regulation of lipogenesis by glucocorticoids and insulin in human adipose tissue," *PLoS ONE*, vol. 6, no. 10, Article ID e26223, 2011.

[7] N. Chalasani, Z. Younossi, and J. E. Lavine, "The diagnosis and management of non-alcoholic fatty liver disease: practice guideline by the American Association for the Study of Liver Diseases, American College of Gastroenterology, and the American Gastroenterological Association," *Hepatology*, vol. 55, no. 6, pp. 2005–2023, 2012.

[8] J. D. Browning, L. S. Szczepaniak, R. Dobbins et al., "Prevalence of hepatic steatosis in an urban population in the United States: impact of ethnicity," *Hepatology*, vol. 40, no. 6, pp. 1387–1395, 2004.

[9] S. Yener, A. Comlekci, S. Ertilav, M. Secil, M. Akarsu, and S. Yesilli, "Non-alcoholic fatty liver disease in subjects with nonfunctioning adrenal adenomas," *Turkish Journal of Endocrinology and Metabolism*, vol. 15, pp. 116–120, 2011.

[10] D. P. Macfarlane, P. J. Raubenheimer, T. Preston et al., "Effects of acute glucocorticoid blockade on metabolic dysfunction in patients with type 2 diabetes with and without fatty liver," *American Journal of Physiology-Gastrointestinal and Liver Physiology*, vol. 307, no. 7, pp. G760–G768, 2014.

[11] R. Rossi, L. Tauchmanova, A. Luciano et al., "Subclinical Cushing's syndrome in patients with adrenal incidentaloma: clinical and biochemical features," *The Journal of Clinical Endocrinology & Metabolism*, vol. 85, no. 4, pp. 1440–1448, 2000.

[12] M. Terzolo, A. Pia, A. Alì et al., "Adrenal incidentaloma: a new cause of the metabolic syndrome?" *The Journal of Clinical Endocrinology & Metabolism*, vol. 87, no. 3, pp. 998–1003, 2002.

[13] G. Zoppini, G. Targher, C. Venturi, C. Zamboni, and M. Muggeo, "Relationship of nonalcoholic hepatic steatosis to overnight low-dose dexamethasone suppression test in obese individuals," *Clinical Endocrinology*, vol. 61, no. 6, pp. 711–715, 2004.

[14] J. Westerbacka, H. Yki-Järvinen, S. Vehkavaara et al., "Body fat distribution and cortisol metabolism in healthy men: enhanced 5β-reductase and lower cortisol/cortisone metabolite ratios in men with fatty liver," *The Journal of Clinical Endocrinology & Metabolism*, vol. 88, no. 10, pp. 4924–4931, 2003.

[15] G. Targher, L. Bertolini, G. Zoppini, L. Zenari, and G. Falezza, "Relationship of non-alcoholic hepatic steatosis to cortisol secretion in diet-controlled Type 2 diabetic patients," *Diabetic Medicine*, vol. 22, no. 9, pp. 1146–1150, 2005.

[16] G. Targher, L. Bertolini, S. Rodella, G. Zoppini, L. Zenari, and G. Falezza, "Associations between liver histology and cortisol secretion in subjects with nonalcoholic fatty liver disease," *Clinical Endocrinology*, vol. 64, no. 3, pp. 337–341, 2006.

[17] I. Chiodini, "Clinical review: diagnosis and treatment of subclinical hypercortisolism," *The Journal of Clinical Endocrinology & Metabolism*, vol. 96, no. 5, pp. 1223–1236, 2011.

[18] M. Fassnacht, W. Arlt, I. Bancos et al., "Management of adrenal incidentalomas: European Society of Endocrinology Clinical Practice Guideline in collaboration with the European Network for the Study of Adrenal Tumors," *European Journal of Endocrinology*, vol. 175, no. 2, pp. G1–G34, 2016.

[19] M. Fleseriu, B. M. K. Biller, J. W. Findling, M. E. Molitch, D. E. Schteingart, and C. Gross, "Mifepristone, a glucocorticoid receptor antagonist, produces clinical and metabolic benefits in patients with Cushing's syndrome," *The Journal of Clinical Endocrinology & Metabolism*, vol. 97, no. 6, pp. 2039–2049, 2012.

[20] C. Gross, C. M. Blasey, R. L. Roe, K. Allen, T. S. Block, and J. K. Belanoff, "Mifepristone treatment of olanzapine-induced weight gain in healthy men," *Advances in Therapy*, vol. 26, no. 10, pp. 959–969, 2009.

[21] C. Gross, C. M. Blasey, R. L. Roe, and J. K. Belanoff, "Mifepristone reduces weight gain and improves metabolic abnormalities associated with risperidone treatment in normal men," *Obesity*, vol. 18, no. 12, pp. 2295–2300, 2010.

45

Short-Term PTH(1-34) Therapy in Children to Correct Severe Hypocalcemia and Hyperphosphatemia due to Hypoparathyroidism: Two Case Studies

Pooja E. Mishra,[1] **Betsy L. Schwartz,**[2] **Kyriakie Sarafoglou,**[3] **Kristen Hook,**[4] **Youngki Kim,**[5] **and Anna Petryk**[3]

[1]*St John's Medical College, Bangalore, India*
[2]*Pediatric Endocrinology, Park Nicollet, Minneapolis, MN, USA*
[3]*Pediatric Endocrinology, University of Minnesota, Minneapolis, MN, USA*
[4]*Pediatric Dermatology, University of Minnesota, Minneapolis, MN, USA*
[5]*Pediatric Nephrology, University of Minnesota, Minneapolis, MN, USA*

Correspondence should be addressed to Anna Petryk; petry005@umn.edu

Academic Editor: Osamu Isozaki

The standard treatment of hypoparathyroidism is to control hypocalcemia using calcitriol and calcium supplementation. However, in severe cases this approach is insufficient, and the risks of intravenous (i.v.) calcium administration and prolonged hospitalization must be considered. While the use of recombinant human parathyroid hormone 1-34 [rhPTH(1-34)] for long-term control of hypocalcemia has been established, the benefits of short-term rhPTH(1-34) treatment in children have not been explored. We report two patients with hypoparathyroidism treated with rhPTH(1-34). Patient 1 is a 10-year-old female with polyglandular autoimmune syndrome type 1. Patient 2 is a 12-year-old female with hypoparathyroidism after total thyroidectomy. Both patients showed poor response to i.v. and oral calcium and calcitriol, and patient 1 did not respond to phosphate binders. Patient 1 had rapid increase in serum calcium with a decrease in serum phosphate after a 3-day course of subcutaneous rhPTH(1-34). Patient 2 had normalization of calcium and phosphate levels after a 7-day course of rhPTH(1-34). These cases support a role for rhPTH(1-34) in the acute management of hypoparathyroidism in hospitalized patients to more rapidly correct hypocalcemia and hyperphosphatemia, shorten hospitalization, and reduce the need for frequent i.v. calcium boluses.

1. Introduction

Hypoparathyroidism may be due to a number of causes, including autoimmune destruction of parathyroid glands, accidental removal of or damage to the parathyroid glands following thyroid surgery, or genetic disorders such as 22q11.2 deletion. Hypoparathyroidism manifests as hypocalcemia and hyperphosphatemia with a low serum parathyroid hormone (PTH) level. Acute hypocalcemia is typically controlled with calcium and calcitriol supplementation. However, in some children these standard measures are insufficient, requiring prolonged hospitalization and even transfer to the pediatric intensive care unit (PICU) for intravenous (i.v.)

calcium administration. Alternate therapeutic options for these children should be considered.

Use of recombinant human (rh) PTH(1-34) (teriparatide) has been documented in adults, with successful control of serum calcium and phosphate levels [1]. However, due to occurrence of osteosarcoma in rat toxicology studies of rhPTH(1-34) there is concern about its long-term use in a pediatric population [2].

Recent studies have demonstrated the advantage of using rhPTH(1-34) to control hypocalcemia in children for periods up to 3 years [3–5]. The two cases presented here suggest a role for rhPTH(1-34) in the acute management of hypocalcemia and hyperphosphatemia. This treatment can accelerate

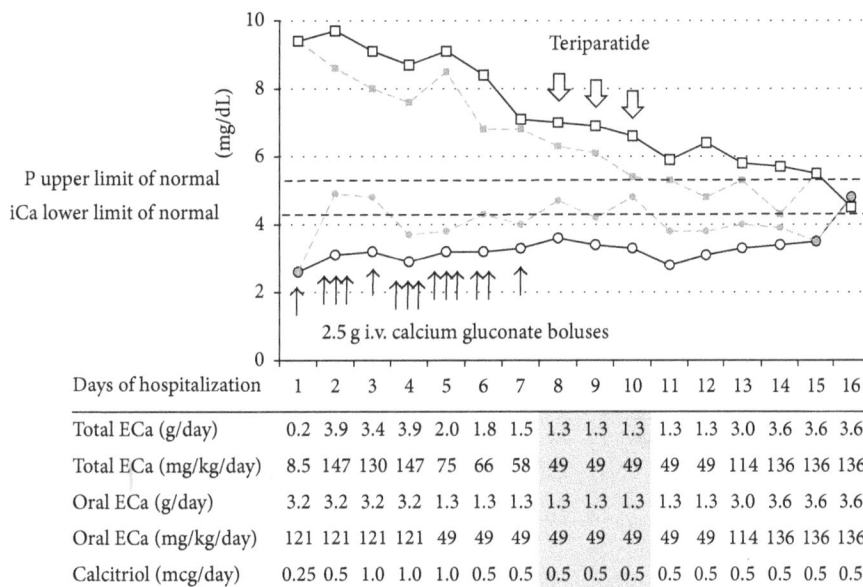

Days of hospitalization	1	2	3	4	5	6	7	8	9	10	11	12	13	14	15	16
Total ECa (g/day)	0.2	3.9	3.4	3.9	2.0	1.8	1.5	1.3	1.3	1.3	1.3	1.3	3.0	3.6	3.6	3.6
Total ECa (mg/kg/day)	8.5	147	130	147	75	66	58	49	49	49	49	49	114	136	136	136
Oral ECa (g/day)	3.2	3.2	3.2	3.2	1.3	1.3	1.3	1.3	1.3	1.3	1.3	1.3	3.0	3.6	3.6	3.6
Oral ECa (mg/kg/day)	121	121	121	121	49	49	49	49	49	49	49	49	114	136	136	136
Calcitriol (mcg/day)	0.25	0.5	1.0	1.0	1.0	0.5	0.5	0.5	0.5	0.5	0.5	0.5	0.5	0.5	0.5	0.5

FIGURE 1: Trends in serum ionized calcium and phosphorus levels in a 10-year-old girl with hypoparathyroidism over the course of hospitalization. Minimum and maximum daily levels of iCa (circles and solid and dashed lines, resp.) and P (squares and dashed and solid lines, resp.) are shown. Black arrows indicate individual calcium gluconate boluses (2.5 g each). Open arrows point to once daily subcutaneous administration of teriparatide. Oral supplementation consisted of calcium carbonate except for Days 5–12 when calcium glubionate was given. ECa, elemental calcium.

2. Case Presentations

2.1. Patient 1. A 10-year-old female presented to dermatology clinic with a 4-year history of alopecia universalis and nail dystrophy, hypocalcemic seizures at 4 years of age (seizure-free on calcium and vitamin D supplements), and frequent thrush during infancy. A clinical diagnosis of autoimmune polyglandular syndrome type 1 was made and confirmed with a pathogenic mutation in the autoimmune regulator (*AIRE*) gene. She had a normal ACTH level and adequate peak cortisol level of 17.8 μg/dL after 250 μg of cosyntropin i.v.

A week later, she presented to the Emergency Department with tetany and a 3-day history of cramping in the hands and legs. Her serum iCa level was 2.3 mg/dL (reference range 4.4–5.2 mg/dL) and phosphate level was 9.2 mg/dL (reference range 2.9–5.4 mg/dL). She was given an i.v. bolus of 2.5 g calcium gluconate and 0.25 μg of calcitriol before being transferred to PICU. Repeat testing showed persistent hypocalcemia and hyperphosphatemia and low PTH level (<3 pg/mL, reference range 12–72 pg/mL). She required multiple calcium gluconate boluses. Figure 1 shows trends in iCa and P levels along with calcium and calcitriol doses. She received ergocalciferol 50,000 IU daily by mouth on days 2–4. On Day 5, her 25-hydroxyvitamin D level was normal (43 μg/L, reference range 20–75 μg/L) and ergocalciferol was discontinued.

On Day 3, due to persistently high serum phosphate, she was started on phosphate binder aluminum hydroxide (600 mg three times daily), and then Renagel (up to 9.6 g per day). Despite high dose calcium supplementation (up to 8 g of calcium carbonate per day) and renal protective measures, she continued to have hypocalcemia and hyperphosphatemia. On Day 8, she was started on rhPTH(1-34) (20 μg once a day subcutaneously) and i.v. calcium boluses were discontinued. Within 48 hours, there was a significant rise in iCa and a drop in serum phosphate levels. rhPTH(1-34) was discontinued after 3 days of treatment. Hydrochlorothiazide (12.5 mg twice daily) was added on Day 13 to reduce renal calcium excretion because of nephrocalcinosis found on renal ultrasound. She was discharged on Day 15 with normal iCa (4.8 mg/dL) and P (4.5 mg/dL) levels a day later.

2.2. Patient 2. Patient 2 is a 12-year-old girl diagnosed with Graves' disease five weeks prior to admission, treated with methimazole. Two weeks later she was found to have a thyroid nodule and was diagnosed with papillary thyroid cancer. She underwent total thyroidectomy with central neck dissection without removal of the parathyroid glands. Following surgery she was started on 112 mcg of L-thyroxine daily, calcium carbonate 1000 mg four times a day, and calcitriol 0.25 μg daily. She presented to the Emergency Department five days later with muscle spasms, irritability, and difficulty in swallowing. Laboratory evaluation revealed severe hypocalcemia (iCa 2.8 mg/dL, Figure 2) and hyperphosphatemia (8.6 mg/dL). PTH level was <0.3 pg/mL. Free T4 level was normal (0.99 ng/dL, reference range 0.76–1.46 ng/dL), but TSH was still suppressed at <0.01 mU/L (reference range 0.4–4.0 mU/L).

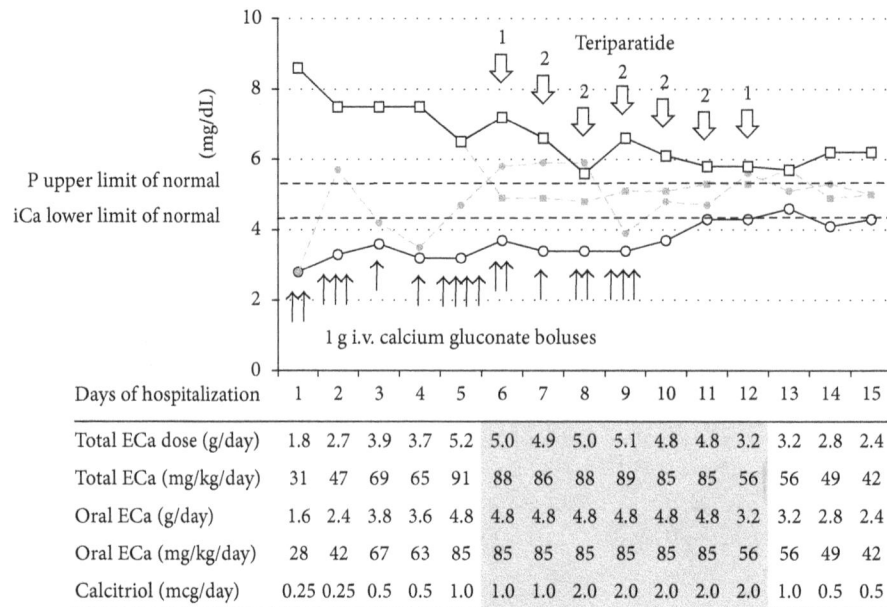

Days of hospitalization	1	2	3	4	5	6	7	8	9	10	11	12	13	14	15
Total ECa dose (g/day)	1.8	2.7	3.9	3.7	5.2	5.0	4.9	5.0	5.1	4.8	4.8	3.2	3.2	2.8	2.4
Total ECa (mg/kg/day)	31	47	69	65	91	88	86	88	89	85	85	56	56	49	42
Oral ECa (g/day)	1.6	2.4	3.8	3.6	4.8	4.8	4.8	4.8	4.8	4.8	4.8	3.2	3.2	2.8	2.4
Oral ECa (mg/kg/day)	28	42	67	63	85	85	85	85	85	85	85	56	56	49	42
Calcitriol (mcg/day)	0.25	0.25	0.5	0.5	1.0	1.0	1.0	2.0	2.0	2.0	2.0	2.0	1.0	0.5	0.5

FIGURE 2: Trends in serum ionized calcium and phosphorus levels in a 12-year-old girl with hypoparathyroidism over the course of hospitalization. Minimum and maximum daily levels of iCa (circles and solid and dashed lines, resp.) and P (squares and dashed and solid lines, resp.) are shown. Black arrows indicate individual calcium gluconate boluses (1 g each). Open arrows point to days of subcutaneous administration of teriparatide with the numbers above the arrows indicating once daily (1) or twice daily (2) injections. Oral supplementation consisted of calcium carbonate except for Days 2-3 when calcium citrate was also given. ECa, elemental calcium.

She was given two i.v. boluses of 1 g calcium gluconate and was transferred to PICU for further management. She required repeated i.v. calcium boluses in addition to oral supplementation with increasing doses of calcium carbonate (up to 12 g per day). The dose of calcitriol was gradually increased to 2 µg per day. Her 25-hydroxy-vitamin D level was 27 µg/L. She received 50,000 IU of ergocalciferol on Days 4 and 11, cholecalciferol 1,000 IU daily on Days 3–7, and then 4,000 IU daily starting on Day 8. Due to persistent signs and symptoms of hypocalcemia (prominent Chvostek sign, paresthesias, and QTc prolongation), rhPTH(1-34) treatment was started on Day 6 at a dose of 20 µg once a day subcutaneously. The same day, serum phosphate level decreased rapidly from 7.2 to 4.9 mg/dL, and serum iCa increased from 3.7 to 5.8 mg/dL. The dose of rhPTH(1-34) was temporarily increased to 20 µg twice daily on Days 7–11 because the effect diminished before the next scheduled dose. After 4 days of rhPTH(1-34) treatment, the patient no longer required i.v. calcium boluses. With near normalization of serum calcium and phosphate levels, rhPTH(1-34) was discontinued on Day 12. On discharge (Day 15), her iCa level was 4.8 mg/dL and phosphate level was 5.6 mg/dL.

3. Discussion

Standard therapeutic approaches in patients with hypoparathyroidism include calcium and vitamin D supplementation. Persistent severe hypocalcemia requires i.v. calcium gluconate administration in the form of i.v. boluses or as a continuous infusion. The latter may have to be continued for a week to ensure enterocyte recovery and adequate intestinal absorption of oral calcium and carries significant risks (cardiac arrhythmia, extravasation, and thrombophlebitis). Moreover, traditional therapy is not causative because it does not replace the deficient hormone.

While there is accumulating evidence for the benefits of rhPTH(1-34) replacement in children on a long-term basis [3], these two cases illustrate that a short-term treatment may also benefit children with refractory hypoparathyroidism by allowing faster normalization of calcium and phosphorus levels and shortening hospitalization, particularly when continuous i.v. calcium infusion is neither feasible nor effective. Similar benefits of short-term rhPTH(1-34) therapy have been demonstrated in adults with postsurgical hypoparathyroidism [6]. Certain patient populations are at a particularly high risk for severe hypocalcemia, for example, after thyroidectomy for thyroid cancer or Graves' disease, partly due to "hungry bone syndrome" in the latter [7], as illustrated by Patient 2.

Twice daily dosing of rhPTH was required in Patient 2 due to significant excursions in serum calcium levels, consistent with previous data showing less variation on a twice daily regimen compared to a once daily injections [8]. It remains to be determined if a longer acting rhPTH(1-84) molecule with favorable long-term safety and efficacy in adults [9] would benefit children as well.

References

[1] K. K. Winer, C. W. Ko, J. C. Reynolds et al., "Long-term treatment of hypoparathyroidism: a randomized controlled study comparing parathyroid hormone-(1–34) versus calcitriol and calcium," *Journal of Clinical Endocrinology and Metabolism*, vol. 88, no. 9, pp. 4214–4220, 2003.

[2] J. L. Vahle, M. Sato, G. G. Long et al., "Skeletal changes in rats given daily subcutaneous injections of recombinant human parathyroid hormone (1-34) for 2 years and relevance to human safety," *Toxicologic Pathology*, vol. 30, no. 3, pp. 312–321, 2002.

[3] K. K. Winer, N. Sinaii, J. Reynolds, D. Peterson, K. Dowdy, and G. B. Cutler Jr., "Long-term treatment of 12 children with chronic hypoparathyroidism: a randomized trial comparing synthetic human parathyroid hormone 1-34 versus calcitriol and calcium," *Journal of Clinical Endocrinology and Metabolism*, vol. 95, no. 6, pp. 2680–2688, 2010.

[4] P. Matarazzo, G. Tuli, L. Fiore et al., "Teriparatide (rhPTH) treatment in children with syndromic hypoparathyroidism," *Journal of Pediatric Endocrinology and Metabolism*, vol. 27, no. 1-2, pp. 53–59, 2014.

[5] R. I. Gafni, J. S. Brahim, P. Andreopoulou et al., "Daily parathyroid hormone 1–34 replacement therapy for hypoparathyroidism induces marked changes in bone turnover and structure," *Journal of Bone and Mineral Research*, vol. 27, no. 8, pp. 1811–1820, 2012.

[6] M. Shah, I. Bancos, G. B. Thompson et al., "Teriparatide therapy and reduced postoperative hospitalization for postsurgical hypoparathyroidism," *JAMA Otolaryngology—Head and Neck Surgery*, vol. 141, no. 9, pp. 822–827, 2015.

[7] C. E. Pesce, Z. Shiue, H.-L. Tsai et al., "Postoperative hypocalcemia after thyroidectomy for Graves' disease," *Thyroid*, vol. 20, no. 11, pp. 1279–1283, 2010.

[8] K. K. Winer, N. Sinaii, D. Peterson, B. Sainz Jr., and G. B. Cutler Jr., "Effects of once versus twice-daily parathyroid hormone 1–34 therapy in children with hypoparathyroidism," *Journal of Clinical Endocrinology and Metabolism*, vol. 93, no. 9, pp. 3389–3395, 2008.

[9] M. R. Rubin, N. E. Cusano, W. Fan et al., "Therapy of hypoparathyroidism with PTH(1–84): a prospective six year investigation of efficacy and safety," *The Journal of Clinical Endocrinology & Metabolism*, vol. 101, no. 7, pp. 2742–2750, 2016.

46

Megace Mystery: A Case of Central Adrenal Insufficiency

Kunal Mehta, Irene Weiss, and Michael D. Goldberg

Westchester Medical Center, Department of Medicine, Division of Endocrinology, Taylor Care Pavilion, Room D342, 100 Woods Road, Valhalla, NY 10595, USA

Correspondence should be addressed to Michael D. Goldberg; michael.goldberg@wmchealth.org

Academic Editor: Carlo Capella

Megestrol acetate (MA) is a synthetic progestin with both antineoplastic and orexigenic properties. In addition to its effects on the progesterone receptor, MA also binds the glucocorticoid receptor. Some patients receiving MA therapy have been reported to develop clinical features of glucocorticoid excess, while others have experienced the clinical syndrome of cortisol deficiency—either following withdrawal of MA therapy or during active treatment. We describe a patient who presented with clinical and biochemical features of central adrenal insufficiency. Pituitary function was otherwise essentially normal, and the etiology of the isolated ACTH suppression was initially unclear. The use of an exogenous glucocorticoid was suspected but was initially denied by the patient; ultimately, the culprit medication was uncovered when a synthetic steroid screen revealed the presence of MA. The patient's symptoms improved after she was switched to hydrocortisone. Clinicians should be aware of the potential effects of MA on the hypothalamic-pituitary-adrenal (HPA) axis.

1. Introduction

When evaluating a patient who presents with central adrenal insufficiency, it is important to assess recent exposure to exogenous glucocorticoids, as this is the most common etiology of a suppressed hypothalamic-pituitary-adrenal (HPA) axis. In addition to systemic oral glucocorticoids, one must screen for the use of injectable and topical agents and for antifungal therapies (e.g., ketoconazole), opiates, and other drugs that may impair HPA axis function [1]. Megestrol acetate (MA) is a synthetic progestin approved in the United States for the palliative treatment of advanced breast and endometrial cancers and for the treatment of anorexia or weight loss in patients with AIDS. In addition to being a potent activator of the progesterone receptor, MA activates the glucocorticoid receptor, with a binding affinity almost twice that of cortisol. Patients receiving MA therapy are therefore susceptible to developing clinical dysfunction of the hypothalamic-pituitary-adrenal axis, similar to that seen with exogenous glucocorticoids.

2. Case Presentation

A 60-year-old female of Haitian descent presented to the emergency department with chief complaints of progressive nausea and constipation for two months. Review of systems was positive for poor appetite, fatigue, weakness, episodes of dizziness, and a recent 20-pound weight loss. The patient's medical history was significant for hypertension, type 2 diabetes, and overactive bladder, and she had undergone a total hysterectomy. Her home medications included lisinopril, metformin, oxybutynin, aspirin, and omeprazole. She denied the use of alcohol, tobacco, or illicit drugs. There were no known drug allergies. The patient was afebrile, with a blood pressure of 118/58 mm Hg. She appeared cachectic, her mucous membranes were dry, and there was poor skin turgor. She was fully oriented and in no acute distress. Cardiac, pulmonary, abdominal, and musculoskeletal examinations were unremarkable, and there were no gross neurologic deficits. Abnormalities on the blood chemistry panel included a low sodium of 130 mEq/L (normal range, 136–145), low carbon dioxide content of 10 mEq/L (normal range, 22–30), elevated creatinine of 1.8 mg/dL (normal range, 0.6–1.1), and low phosphorus of 1.4 mg/dL (normal range, 2.3–4.7). Abdominal X-ray revealed a large amount of stool in the colon, without obstruction or free air. Initial management in the emergency department included intravenous hydration, antiemetics, laxatives, and stool softeners, and the patient was admitted to the hospital for further evaluation.

TABLE 1: Endocrine lab results.

	Hospital day 1, 7:00 am	Hospital day 1, 5:30 pm	Hospital day 5	Normal range
Cortisol	0.6 mcg/dL	1.0 mcg/dL		6.2–19.4
Adrenocorticotropic hormone (ACTH)		<5 pg/mL		10–60
Thyroid stimulating hormone (TSH)		1.05 mIU/L		0.35–4.70
Free thyroxine		0.8 ng/dL		0.7–1.9
Luteinizing hormone (LH)		12.0 mIU/mL		
Follicle stimulating hormone (FSH)		28.6 mIU/mL		
Prolactin		16.0 ng/mL		1.2–29.9
Insulin-like growth factor-1 (IGF-1)			178 ng/mL	45–173

Among the diagnoses considered by the admitting team was adrenal insufficiency, and a serum cortisol level was drawn at 7:00 am the next morning. When the result returned at 0.6 mcg/dL, the endocrinology service was consulted. On further questioning, the patient denied having been prescribed oral or injectable steroids or having used over-the-counter supplements of any kind. Fluticasone nasal spray had been prescribed, but it had been used only on rare occasions, and not since several months prior to admission. The patient's last menstrual period had been at age 53. She denied galactorrhea, headaches, vision changes, and frequent urination. There was no family history of pituitary or adrenal gland disease. The patient did not have phenotypic features of Cushing's syndrome or acromegaly, and there was no hyperpigmentation of the palmar creases or buccal mucosa. Blood was drawn for a repeat cortisol level, adrenocorticotropic hormone (ACTH) level, and additional pituitary hormones, after which oral hydrocortisone was started at a dose of 20 mg twice daily.

Within 24 hours, the patients' symptoms had improved and she appeared much more energetic; hydrocortisone was continued. The endocrine laboratory results are shown in Table 1. A magnetic resonance imaging (MRI) scan with and without gadolinium revealed a slightly asymmetric contour of the pituitary that was felt most likely to reflect a normal anatomic variant. On hospital day 10, a urine specimen was sent for a synthetic glucocorticoid screen. The patient was discharged home on hospital day 11 with a hydrocortisone regimen of 20 mg in the morning and 10 mg in the afternoon, potassium citrate to manage the newly diagnosed proximal renal tubular acidosis (RTA), stool softeners, and laxatives, in addition to her prior maintenance medications. Outpatient follow-up in the endocrinology clinic was planned.

The results of the urine synthetic glucocorticoid screen became available shortly after discharge. Megestrol acetate (MA) was detected, and the remainder of the screen was negative. The results were discussed with the patient over the telephone, and she denied ever having been prescribed MA. The patient's internist confirmed that this medication had not been prescribed in her office. Several days later, the patient revealed that she had HIV infection, a fact that she had previously withheld from her family, her internist, and the treating physicians in the hospital. She had been under the care of an infectious disease specialist, and in addition to being prescribed highly active antiretroviral therapy, she had been started within the past three months on MA 800 mg

daily as an appetite stimulant. MA was discontinued and she is being followed in the endocrinology clinic, with the plan to gradually taper her off the glucocorticoid replacement therapy. She is also being continued on potassium citrate; her proximal RTA was felt to be related to her antiretroviral therapy.

3. Discussion

This patient presented to the hospital with symptomatic central adrenal insufficiency, as manifested by fatigue, dizziness, and anorexia in the context of very low serum cortisol and plasma ACTH levels (see Table 1). Given the frank degree of suppression of these hormones, we did not feel it was necessary to perform a cosyntropin stimulation test to confirm the diagnosis. There was no biochemical evidence for additional anterior pituitary hormone deficiencies, nor was there hyperprolactinemia, though the gonadotropin levels were somewhat lower than expected for the postmenopausal state. The very slight elevation in IGF-1, in the absence of any clinical features of acromegaly, was felt most likely to be a nonsignificant result. Therefore, our clinical impression was that the patient had isolated ACTH suppression; the etiology, however, was not readily apparent.

The differential diagnosis of isolated ACTH deficiency includes genetic defects such as mutations in the proopiomelanocortin (POMC) gene [2] and in the gene for TPIT, a T-box transcription factor involved in the differentiation of corticotrophs [3]. However, these are rare conditions that typically present in infancy or childhood. Therefore, the use of exogenous glucocorticoids was strongly suspected to be the cause of our patient's central adrenal insufficiency. However, other than the infrequent use of nasal fluticasone several months prior to admission, she denied having taken any steroid preparations. Ultimately, the culprit drug, megestrol acetate, was detected using a urine synthetic glucocorticoid screen. Even after being confronted with this laboratory finding, it took some time for the patient to admit to having been prescribed megestrol acetate by an infectious disease specialist, as she had not yet revealed her HIV-positive status to her family or her primary care physician.

Megestrol acetate (MA) is an orally active, synthetic 17-hydroxyprogesterone derivative. It is approved by the United States Food and Drug Administration for the palliative treatment of advanced breast and endometrial cancers and for the treatment of anorexia, cachexia, or unexplained weight loss in patients with AIDS. Though the exact mechanism of its antineoplastic action remains unclear, it is postulated that progesterone receptor binding leads to feedback inhibition of gonadotropin releasing hormone and gonadotropins, which results in a reduction in circulating sex steroid hormones and downregulation of androgen and estrogen receptors [4]. Of note, this may explain the lower-than-expected gonadotropin levels that were seen in our patient. The mechanism by which MA stimulates appetite also has yet to be fully elucidated [5].

Many naturally occurring and synthetic steroid hormones bind to multiple steroid hormone receptors, and MA is no exception. In 1983, Kontula et al. demonstrated that MA displayed a considerable binding affinity to the glucocorticoid receptor (GR), almost twice that of the natural ligand cortisol [6]. Once MA was introduced into clinical practice, reports appeared in the literature describing biochemical evidence of endogenous HPA axis suppression in patients taking this medication [7–9]. In addition, reports emerged describing weight gain, new onset diabetes, worsening hyperglycemia in patients with preexisting diabetes, or the development of Cushingoid features, in patients receiving MA for advanced hormone-responsive cancers [10–12] and for AIDS cachexia [13–15]. These features of glucocorticoid excess typically resolved after discontinuation of the MA therapy. A survey of adverse drug event reports submitted to the US Food and Drug Administration between 1984 and 1996 revealed a total of 12 cases of new onset hyperglycemia, 12 cases of worsening hyperglycemia in patients with diabetes, and 5 cases of frank Cushing's syndrome in patients receiving MA [16].

In patients who have been treated chronically with exogenous glucocorticoids, abrupt withdrawal of these agents may result in the clinical syndrome of adrenal insufficiency. Given the ability of MA to bind the glucocorticoid receptor and produce symptoms and signs of glucocorticoid excess, while suppressing endogenous cortisol secretion, one expects that patients withdrawn from MA therapy may also be at risk for a steroid withdrawal syndrome. Case reports have described such an occurrence, with patients experiencing prompt clinical improvement after the initiation of oral hydrocortisone treatment [14, 17]. Our patient, however, developed clinically significant central adrenal insufficiency while *actively* receiving treatment with MA—not following its withdrawal. This has been reported to occur in patients receiving MA therapy for hormone-responsive cancers [18] and for cachexia syndromes [19, 20], as well as in a population of acutely ill hospitalized patients [21]. The aforementioned review of adverse events submitted to the FDA uncovered a total of 16 cases of clinically apparent adrenal insufficiency between 1984 and 1996, with some occurring during active treatment with MA and others developing after its discontinuation [16]. Daily doses of MA in these reports ranged from 60 to 1,600 mg, and durations of therapy ranged from days to months.

The mechanism by which the active use of an agent with glucocorticoid-like activity, not its withdrawal, may cause clinical adrenal insufficiency has yet to be fully elucidated. Mann et al. outlined a number of possible explanations, including unreported discontinuation of MA, the presence of intercurrent acute stress or illness in the context of

an already suppressed HPA axis, a dual agonist-antagonist action of MA (binding to the GR as a weak agonist, but also antagonistically blocking the binding of more potent endogenous glucocorticoids to the GR), and an inherently greater potential for MA to suppress the HPA axis than to induce glucocorticoid-like clinical effects [16]. Leinung et al. proposed several factors that may contribute to the clinical variability in individual responses to MA, including the apparent combined central agonism/peripheral antagonism observed clinically in the subset of patients with HPA axis suppression and symptomatic glucocorticoid deficiency. These included variations in pharmacokinetic properties of MA across individuals, the effects of progestational actions of MA on the mineralocorticoid receptor, and differences in the interactions of the MA-GR complex with DNA and transcription modulators across different tissues [22].

To our knowledge, this is the first report of MA-induced central adrenal insufficiency in which the patient's use of MA was unknown at the time of initial presentation. This case highlights, therefore, the clinical utility of the urine synthetic glucocorticoid screen when the etiology of isolated ACTH suppression is not readily apparent. This panel, which is performed at the Mayo Medical Laboratories, utilizes a high-performance liquid chromatography system and tandem mass spectrometry (LC-MS/MS) to detect the current or recent use of fourteen synthetic steroids [23]. While much of the literature on synthetic glucocorticoid analyses has focused on veterinary applications [24], or screening for "doping" in athletes [25], the value of such testing has also been demonstrated in the contexts of factitious Cushing's syndrome [26] and cases of clinical adrenal dysfunction due to intra-articular and epidural glucocorticoid administration [27].

In summary, clinicians are well advised to consider the potential for megestrol acetate therapy to cause adrenal dysfunction. Clinical manifestations of adrenal insufficiency may occur after abrupt withdrawal of MA, or even during active treatment, as was seen in our patient. Additionally, when the cause of central adrenal insufficiency is difficult to ascertain, the use of a synthetic glucocorticoid screen can be invaluable in uncovering the occult use of traditional oral, parenteral, or topical steroids, as well as megestrol acetate: a progestin with important glucocorticoid activity.

Disclosure

This case was presented as a poster at The Endocrine Society's 97th Annual Meeting and Expo, San Diego, CA, USA, March 5–8, 2015.

References

[1] S. R. Bornstein, "Predisposing factors for adrenal insufficiency," *The New England Journal of Medicine*, vol. 360, no. 22, pp. 2328–2339, 2009.

[2] H. Krude, H. Biebermann, W. Luck, R. Horn, G. Brabant, and A. Grüters, "Severe early-onset obesity, adrenal insufficiency and red hair pigmentation caused by POMC mutations in humans," *Nature Genetics*, vol. 19, no. 2, pp. 155–157, 1998.

[3] C. Couture, A. Saveanu, A. Barlier et al., "Phenotypic homogeneity and genotypic variability in a large series of congenital isolated ACTH-deficiency patients with TPIT gene mutations," *Journal of Clinical Endocrinology and Metabolism*, vol. 97, no. 3, pp. E486–E495, 2012.

[4] S. Lundgren, S. I. Helle, and P. E. Lønning, "Profound suppression of plasma estrogens by megestrol acetate in postmenopausal breast cancer patients," *Clinical Cancer Research*, vol. 2, no. 9, pp. 1515–1521, 1996.

[5] S.-S. Yeh and M. W. Schuster, "Megestrol acetate in cachexia and anorexia," *International Journal of Nanomedicine*, vol. 1, no. 4, pp. 411–416, 2006.

[6] K. Kontula, T. Paavonen, T. Luukkainen, and L. C. Andersson, "Binding of progestins to the glucocorticoid receptor," *Biochemical Pharmacology*, vol. 32, no. 9, pp. 1511–1518, 1983.

[7] J. Alexieva-Figusch, M. A. Blankenstein, W. C. J. Hop et al., "Treatment of metastatic breast cancer patients with different dosages of megestrol acetate; dose relations, metabolic and endocrine effects," *European Journal of Cancer and Clinical Oncology*, vol. 20, no. 1, pp. 33–40, 1984.

[8] C. L. Loprinzi, M. D. Jensen, N.-S. Jiang, and D. J. Schaid, "Effect of megestrol acetate on the human pituitary-adrenal axis," *Mayo Clinic Proceedings*, vol. 67, no. 12, pp. 1160–1162, 1992.

[9] K. K. Naing, J. A. Dewar, and G. P. Leese, "Megestrol acetate therapy and secondary adrenal suppression," *Cancer*, vol. 86, no. 6, pp. 1044–1049, 1999.

[10] P. H. B. Willemse, E. van der Ploeg, D. T. H. Sleijfer, T. Tjabbes, and H. van Veelen, "A randomized comparison of megestrol acetate (MA) and medroxyprogesterone acetate (MPA) in patients with advanced breast cancer," *European Journal of Cancer and Clinical Oncology*, vol. 26, no. 3, pp. 337–343, 1990.

[11] K. A. Steer, A. B. Kurtz, and J. W. Honour, "Megestrol-induced Cushing's syndrome," *Clinical Endocrinology*, vol. 42, no. 1, pp. 91–93, 1995.

[12] P. G. Rose, "Hyperglycemia secondary to megestrol acetate for endometrial neoplasia," *Gynecologic Oncology*, vol. 61, no. 1, pp. 139–141, 1996.

[13] K. Henry, S. Rathgaber, C. Sullivan, and K. McCabe, "Diabetes mellitus induced by megestrol acetate in a patient with AIDS and cachexia," *Annals of Internal Medicine*, vol. 116, no. 1, pp. 53–54, 1992.

[14] M. C. Leinung, R. Liporace, and C. H. Miller, "Induction of adrenal suppression by megestrol acetate in patients with AIDS," *Annals of Internal Medicine*, vol. 122, no. 11, pp. 843–845, 1995.

[15] S. Padmanabhan and A. S. Rosenberg, "Cushing's syndrome induced by megestrol acetate in a patient with AIDS," *Clinical Infectious Diseases*, vol. 27, no. 1, pp. 217–218, 1998.

[16] M. Mann, E. Koller, A. Murgo, S. Malozowski, J. Bacsanyi, and M. Leinung, "Glucocorticoidlike activity of megestrol: a summary of food and drug administration experience and a review of the literature," *Archives of Internal Medicine*, vol. 157, no. 15, pp. 1651–1656, 1997.

[17] G. Fried, M. Stein, and N. Haim, "A rare event of megestrol acetate (Megace)-induced adrenal suppression in a breast cancer patient," *American Journal of Clinical Oncology*, vol. 20, no. 6, pp. 628–629, 1997.

[18] A. P. Delitala, G. Fanciulli, M. Maioli, G. Piga, and G. Delitala, "Primary symptomatic adrenal insufficiency induced by megestrol acetate," *The Netherlands Journal of Medicine*, vol. 71, no. 1, pp. 17–21, 2013.

[19] M. Maurer, "Megestrol for AIDS-related anorexia," *Annals of Internal Medicine*, vol. 122, no. 11, p. 880, 1995.

[20] D. Bulchandani, J. Nachnani, A. Amin, and J. May, "Megestrol acetate-associated adrenal insufficiency," *The American Journal Geriatric Pharmacotherapy*, vol. 6, no. 3, pp. 167–172, 2008.

[21] A. R. Chidakel, S. B. Zweig, J. R. Schlosser, P. Homel, J. W. Schappert, and A. M. Fleckman, "High prevalence of adrenal suppression during acute illness in hospitalized patients receiving megestrol acetate," *Journal of Endocrinological Investigation*, vol. 29, no. 2, pp. 136–140, 2006.

[22] M. Leinung, E. A. Koller, and M. J. Fossler, "Corticosteroid effects of megestrol acetate," *The Endocrinologist*, vol. 8, no. 3, pp. 153–159, 1998.

[23] Mayo Clinic Laboratories Test Catalog, "Synthetic glucocorticoid screen, urine," 2015, http://www.mayomedicallaboratories.com/test-catalog/Overview/81035.

[24] E. Grippa, L. Santini, G. Castellano, M. T. Gatto, M. G. Leone, and L. Saso, "Simultaneous determination of hydrocortisone, dexamethasone, indomethacin, phenylbutazone and oxyphenbutazone in equine serum by high-performance liquid chromatography," *Journal of Chromatography B: Biomedical Sciences and Applications*, vol. 738, no. 1, pp. 17–25, 2000.

[25] M. Mazzarino, S. Turi, and F. Botrè, "A screening method for the detection of synthetic glucocorticosteroids in human urine by liquid chromatography-mass spectrometry based on class-characteristic fragmentation pathways," *Analytical and Bioanalytical Chemistry*, vol. 390, no. 5, pp. 1389–1402, 2008.

[26] G. Cizza, L. K. Nieman, J. L. Doppman et al., "Factitious Cushing syndrome," *Journal of Clinical Endocrinology and Metabolism*, vol. 81, no. 10, pp. 3573–3577, 1996.

[27] M. C. Lansang, T. Farmer, and L. Kennedy, "Diagnosing the unrecognized systemic absorption of intra-articular and epidural steroid injections," *Endocrine Practice*, vol. 15, no. 3, pp. 225–228, 2009.

47

A Novel Mutation of the *CYP11B2* in a Saudi Infant with Primary Hypoaldosteronism

Lama Alfaraidi,[1] Abrar Alfaifi,[1] Rawan Alquaiz,[1] Faten Almijmaj,[2] and Horia Mawlawi[2]

[1]*College of Medicine, King Saud University, Riyadh, Saudi Arabia*
[2]*Department of Pediatrics, Prince Sultan Military Medical City, Riyadh 11159, Saudi Arabia*

Correspondence should be addressed to Lama Alfaraidi; lama.al.faraidi@gmail.com

Academic Editor: Takeshi Usui

Isolated hypoaldosteronism is a rare autosomal recessive disease presenting with severe salt wasting and failure to thrive in infancy. A 6-month-old Saudi girl born to consanguineous parents was referred from primary health care for failure to thrive and developmental delay. Laboratory tests revealed hyponatremia, hyperkalemia, and metabolic acidosis with high renin and low aldosterone. Blood samples were collected for endocrine and genetic studies. Sequence analysis of the *CYP11B2* revealed a T to A transition at position 1398 + 2 in exon 8 of the gene in a homozygous state (c.1398+T>A). This result was confirmed by sequencing an independent PCR product. Given the position of the transition at a highly conserved nucleotide and the predictions of different bioinformatic algorithms, it is likely that the mutation is the pathogenic cause of this condition. This result was compared with the reference NM_000498.3. Here, we report a novel homozygous mutation resulting in aldosterone synthase deficiency. To the best of our knowledge, this mutation has not been described in the literature or in any database thus far. The mutation manifested as a rare inherited disease in an infant exhibiting critical salt loss. An adequate replacement treatment will give a good long-term prognosis.

1. Background

Aldosterone is a hormone exhibiting potent mineralocorticoid activity that is synthesized in the zona glomerulosa of the adrenal gland and is responsible for maintaining electrolyte balance and intravascular volume [1].

CYP11B1 (11b-hydroxylaze) and *CYP11B2* (aldosterone synthase), which share more than 90% of their amino acid sequences, encode the enzymes responsible for the three terminal steps in aldosterone formation [2]. *CYP11B2* is located on chromosome 8q24 and catalyzes three reactions: the 11-hydroxylation of deoxycorticosterone (DOC) to corticosterone, the 18-hydroxylation of corticosterone to 18-hydroxycorticosterone (18-OHB), and the 18-oxidation of 18-hydroxycorticosterone to aldosterone [3, 4].

Congenital isolated hypoaldosteronism, formerly known as corticosterone methyloxidase deficiency (CMO), is a rare autosomal recessive disorder caused by aldosterone synthase deficiency (ASD) [3]. Most cases have been attributed to approximately 80 different mutations within *CYP11B2*.

Patients with this deficiency experience recurrent dehydration, salt wasting, and failure to thrive [4]. ASD is subdivided into CMO types I and II, both of which are characterized by low aldosterone levels and elevated renin activity, accompanied by the accumulation of steroid precursors prior to a biosynthetic block. CMO I is characterized by low levels of 18-hydroxycorticosterone, whereas CMO II is characterized by high levels of 18-OHB and an increase of the urinary excretion of the major metabolite of 18-OHB [3].

ASD has been identified in Jews of European, North American, and Iranian descent [3]. In Asians, it has been reported among Thai [5], Indian [5], and Japanese [6] populations. In this paper, we present a case of isolated primary hypoaldosteronism in a 6-month-old Saudi female infant and the results of her *CYP11B2* analysis.

2. Case Report

A female infant born to consanguineous Saudi parents presented at 6 months of age to primary health care workers with

TABLE 1: Growth parameters progression.

Growth parameters	On admission at 6 months	After 6 months at 12 months	After 1 year at 18 months	Recently at 2 years
Weight	−5.20 SD (3.6 kg)	−2.80 SD (7.1 kg)	−0.64 SD (10.3 kg)	−0.67 SD (11.3 kg)
Height	−3.90 SD (55 cm)	−1.99 SD (68 cm)	−1.00 SD (77 cm)	−0.40 SD (84.7 cm)

TABLE 2: Laboratory investigations.

Test	Result	Normal reference level
Sodium	128 mmol/L	135–145 mmol/L
Potassium	7 mmol/L	3.6–5.2 mmol/L
Corrected calcium	2.6 mmol/L	2.1–2.6 mmol/L
Bicarbonate	15.5 mEq/L	22–28 mEq/L
Cortisol (prestimulation)	761 nmol/L	140–700 nmol/L
Cortisol (poststimulation)	1305 nmol/L	
ACTH	5.6 Pmol/L	1.6–13.9 Pmol/L
Dehydroepiandrosterone	0.118 nmol/L	0.090–3.350 nmol/L
17-Hydroxyprogesterone	2.3 mmol/L	0–5 nmol/L
Renin	3310 pmol/L	0.15–3.53 pmol/L
Aldosterone	68.4 pmol/L	139–3660 pmol/L

failure to thrive and developmental delay. Routine laboratory investigations revealed hyponatremia with hyperkalemia. The infant was delivered prematurely by C-section at 32 weeks with a birth weight 2.4 kg. The child was referred to the Prince Sultan Medical Military Hospital Emergency Center for treatment by an endocrinologist.

On admission, the patient was not dehydrated, and the vital signs were normal. Her weight and length were both below 3rd centile, weight was 3.6 kg (−5.2 SD), and length was 55 cm (−3.9 SD) (Table 1). The systemic examination results were normal; no hyperpigmentation was observed, and the external genitalia were normal. Regarding the patient's development, she was experiencing global developmental delay. She was not able to support her head or hold objects, was not cooing or laughing, had no social smile, and did not recognize her mother. The results of initial investigations were as follows: Na 128 mmol/L, K 7 mmol/L, corrected calcium (CC) 2.6 mmol/L, bicarbonate 15.5 mmol/L, and normal renal function. An adrenocorticotropic hormone (ACTH) stimulation test was performed: before test, the cortisol level was 761 nmol/L and the ACTH level was 5.6 nmol/L (normal), while after test, the cortisol level was 1305 nmol/L, the dehydroepiandrosterone level was 0.118 nmol/L (0.090–3.350), the renin level was 3310 pmol/L (0.15–3.53), and the aldosterone level was 68.4 (139–3660 pmol/L). A 17-hydroxyprogesterone test was normal (Table 2).

Based on the infant's clinical presentation and test results, she was diagnosed with primary hypoaldosteronism. The patient improved clinically, both growth and psychomotor development have matched her chronological age of 2 years, and biochemically when treated with 0.1 mg fludrocortisone twice daily and 1 ml NaCl delivered orally three times per day.

3. Methods

3.1. Genetic Study. Molecular genetic analysis of *CYP11B2* was performed. Written informed consent was obtained from the patient's parents. A blood sample was obtained from which DNA was extracted, and molecular genetic analysis of *CYP11B2* was performed. *CYP11B2* (OMIM 124080) exons 1–9 and their respective exon-intron boundaries were amplified by PCR and analyzed by direct sequencing. The resulting sequence data were compared with the reference sequence (NM_000498.3). The patient carried the homozygous mutation c.1398+2T>A(p.?) in *CYP11B2* (Figure 1). The result was confirmed by sequencing of an independent PCR product. Prediction of potential pathogenic effect of the detected mutation was performed utilizing ESE finder (http://krainer01.cshl.edu/cgi-bin/tools/ESE3/esefinder.cgi) [7] and Fruit Fly (http://www.fruitfly.org/) [8].

4. Discussion

We describe an infant girl who presented with failure to thrive, poor feeding, and developmental delay. Laboratory tests revealed hyponatremia and hyperkalemia, metabolic acidosis, normal cortisol levels, and high renin and low aldosterone levels. Genetic testing confirmed a diagnosis of primary hypoaldosteronism. The patient improved dramatically after treatment with fludrocortisone.

The ASD *(CYP11B2)* encodes the steroid 11/18 B hydroxylase and is expressed in the zona glomerulosa of the adrenal gland, where it synthesizes the mineralocorticoid aldosterone. ASD type I (CMO type I) is caused by a deficiency in the 18-hydroxylase enzyme, which results in low levels of

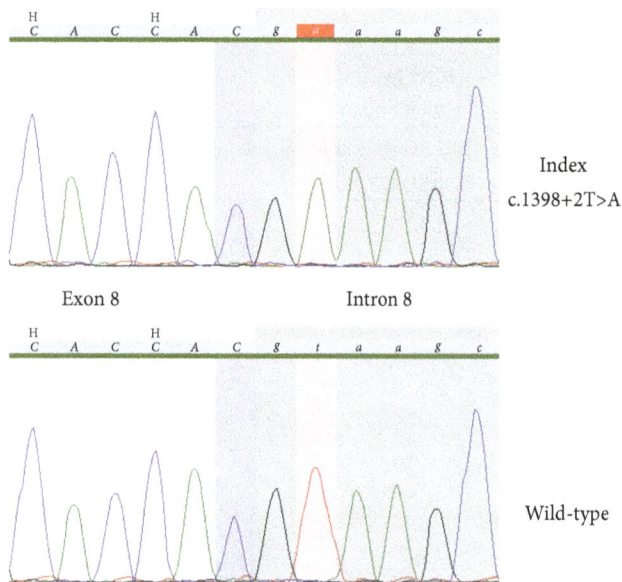

FIGURE 1: Chromatography.

OHB and aldosterone and low urinary metabolites; in ASD type II (CMO II), 18- OHB levels are markedly elevated, and the levels of aldosterone and its urinary metabolites are low [3]. The plasma renin activity levels are low in both disorders. The ratio of plasma 18- OHB/aldosterone can be differentiated between the two disorders, but this biochemical phenotype has overlapping features and is better considered a continuous spectrum of the same disease [5, 9].

Patients with ASD experience recurrent dehydration, salt wasting, and failure to thrive [4]. The clinical picture varies with age and is most severe during infancy. The severity of salt wasting decreases with age, but the abnormal steroid pattern persists throughout life, possibly due to increases in mineralocorticoid sensitivity and sodium intake with age [10]. However, the initial presentation of life-threating salt wasting that is a hallmark of ASD can be differentiated biochemically from defects in steroid biosynthesis, such as congenital adrenal hyperplasia with salt loss [11].

Primary hypoaldosteronism can be caused by different defects in CYP11B2, such as nonsense, missense, and frame shift mutations [10, 11]. However, in this case, we discovered a novel mutation in CYP11B2 that caused aldosterone deficiency. Genetic analysis revealed a T to A transition at position c.1398+2 in the homozygous state (c.1398+2T>A). Given the position of the transition at a highly evolutionarily conserved nucleotide and the predictions of different bioinformatic algorithms, it is likely that the mutation is pathogenic. The nucleotide exchange is located in intron 8 and affects the donor splice site of exon 8. A computer-based comparison of the modified donor splice site of exon 8 of CYP11B2 with the wild-type sequence was performed using different bioinformatic tools. This analysis revealed a loss of the constitutive donor splice site of exon 8 due to the alteration c.1398+2T>A. Although sequencing analysis cannot exclude a large heterozygous deletion in the CYP11B2 gene

in trans to c.1398+2T>A (i.e., hemizygosity), homozygosity of c.1398+2T>A is most likely.

Both homozygosity and hemizygosity of c.1398+2T>A in the CYP11B2 gene would be compatible with the clinical diagnosis of primary hypoaldosteronism in this patient. To distinguish between homozygosity and compound heterozygosity for c.1398+2T>A with a large deletion comprising this position on the other allele, we are in the process of sequencing the parents' DNA for the mutation.

5. Conclusion

To the best of our knowledge, this is the first reported case of a Saudi infant with aldosterone synthase deficiency due to a homozygous alteration (c.1398+2T>A) in CYP11B2 that has not been described in the literature or any databases thus far. Although it is a rare inherited disease, there is a high index of suspicion of cases with life-threating salt wasting in infancy because of dramatic clinical improvements and good long-term prognosis can be achieved with replacement treatment.

Additional Points

Limitations. We could not differentiate between biochemical types of ASD due to limited resources. The results of genetic testing of the parents are forthcoming.

References

[1] M. H. Bassett, P. C. White, and W. E. Rainey, "The regulation of aldosterone synthase expression," *Molecular and Cellular Endocrinology*, vol. 217, no. 1-2, pp. 67–74, 2004.

[2] E. Mornet, J. Dupont, A. Vitek, and P. C. White, "Characterization of two genes encoding human steroid 11β-hydroxylase (P-450(11β))," *The Journal of Biological Chemistry*, vol. 264, no. 35, pp. 20961–20967, 1989.

[3] P. C. White, "Aldesterone synthase deficiency and related disorder," *Molecular and Cellular Endocrinology*, 18187, 2004.

[4] S. Ulick, J. Z. Wang, and D. H. Morton, "The biochemical phenotypes of two inborn errors in the biosynthesis of aldosterone," *The Journal of Clinical Endocrinology & Metabolism*, vol. 74, no. 6, pp. 1415–1420, 1992.

[5] T. Klomchan, V. Supornsilchai, S. Wacharasindhu, V. Shotelersuk, and T. Sahakitrungruang, "Novel CYP11B2 mutation causing aldosterone synthase (P450c11AS) deficiency," *European Journal of Pediatrics*, vol. 171, no. 10, pp. 1559–1562, 2012.

[6] E. Kondo, A. Nakamura, K. Homma et al., "Two novel mutations of the CYP11B2 gene in a Japanese patient with aldosterone deficiency type 1," *Endocrine Journal*, vol. 60, no. 1, pp. 51–55, 2013.

[7] http://krainer01.cshl.edu/cgi-bin/tools/ESE3/esefinder.cgi.

[8] http://www.fruitfly.org/.

[9] G. Zhang, H. Rodriguez, C. E. Fardella, D. A. Harris, and W. L. Miller, "Mutation T318M in the CYP11B2 gene encoding P450c11AS (aldosterone synthase) causes corticosterone methyl

oxidase II deficiency," *American Journal of Human Genetics*, vol. 57, no. 5, pp. 1037–1043, 1995.

[10] L. Martinerie, S. Viengchareun, A.-L. Delezoide et al., "Low renal mineralocorticoid receptor expression at birth contributes to partial aldosterone resistance in neonates," *Endocrinology*, vol. 150, no. 9, pp. 4414–4424, 2009.

[11] M. Wasniewska, F. De Luca, M. Valenzise, F. Lombardo, and F. De Luca, "Aldosterone synthase deficiency type I with no documented homozygous mutations in the CYP11B2 gene," *European Journal of Endocrinology*, vol. 144, no. 1, pp. 59–62, 2001.

48

Seemingly Harmless Differentiated Thyroid Carcinoma Presenting as Bone Metastasis

D. Magalhães ⓘ,[1,2,3] C. Costa ⓘ,[4] I. Furtado ⓘ,[5] M. J. Matos,[4]
A. P. Santos,[4] H. Duarte,[6] M. Afonso,[7] J. Lobo ⓘ,[7,8,9] and I. Torres[4]

[1]Endocrinology, Diabetes and Metabolism Department, Centro Hospitalar São João, Porto, Portugal
[2]Faculty of Medicine of University of Porto, Porto, Portugal
[3]Instituto de Investigação e Inovação em Saúde, University of Porto, Porto, Portugal
[4]Endocrinology Department, Instituto Português de Oncologia, Porto, Portugal
[5]Internal Medicine Department, Centro Hospitalar do Porto, Porto, Portugal
[6]Nuclear Medicine Department, Instituto Português de Oncologia, Porto, Portugal
[7]Pathology Department, Instituto Português de Oncologia, Porto, Portugal
[8]Cancer Biology and Epigenetics Group, Research Center, Instituto Português de Oncologia, Porto, Portugal
[9]Pathology and Molecular Immunology Department, Institute of Biomedical Sciences Abel Salazar (ICBAS),
  University of Porto, Porto, Portugal

Correspondence should be addressed to D. Magalhães; danielascmagalhaes@gmail.com

Academic Editor: Osamu Isozaki

Thyroid carcinoma is the most common endocrine neoplasia. Differentiated thyroid carcinomas (DTCs) represent the majority of cases, which usually follow an indolent clinical course with low mortality rates. The authors describe two cases of well DTC without classic histological poor prognosis features, presenting as extensive and unresectable osteolytic bone metastases. DTCs are considered harmless tumours, due to their benign and silent behaviour. The authors want to underline the importance of clinical awareness during follow-up in cases of DTC, which can be aggressive in presentation and behaviour. Timely identification and diagnosis of these tumours are essential for prompt treatment initiation and improvement of overall survival.

1. Introduction

The most common endocrine neoplasia is the thyroid carcinoma, with a rapidly increasing incidence worldwide [1–3]. The majority (>90%) of thyroid cancers are differentiated thyroid carcinomas (DTC)—papillary or follicular—which follow, in most cases, an indolent clinical course with low mortality rates [4, 5].

When distant metastases occur, the bone is the second most frequently affected site [6]. The incidence of bone metastases is about 1 to 7% in papillary carcinoma and 7 to 20% in follicular carcinoma. When present, the lesions are mostly osteolytic in nature [2, 7]. Bone metastases can result in clinically significant morbidity, coursing with

important pain, pathological fractures, and neurological dysfunction [2, 6]. However, clinically silent presentation of bone metastases can also occur [2]. The presence of bone metastases is associated with a worse prognosis, lower survival rates, and significant deterioration of quality of life [2].

The authors report two cases of DTC without significant microscopic adverse features presenting as lytic bone metastases.

2. Case 1

A 62-year-old male presented with refractory sacral coccygeal pain. The patient had past medical history of type 2

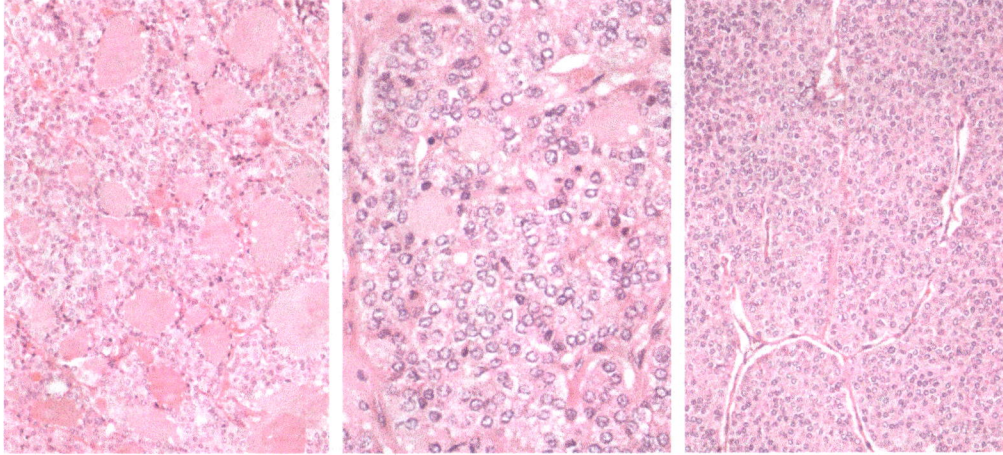

FIGURE 1: Fragments of bone tissue involved by epithelial neoplasia of follicular architecture, with foci of nondifferentiated (insular) carcinoma [Case 1].

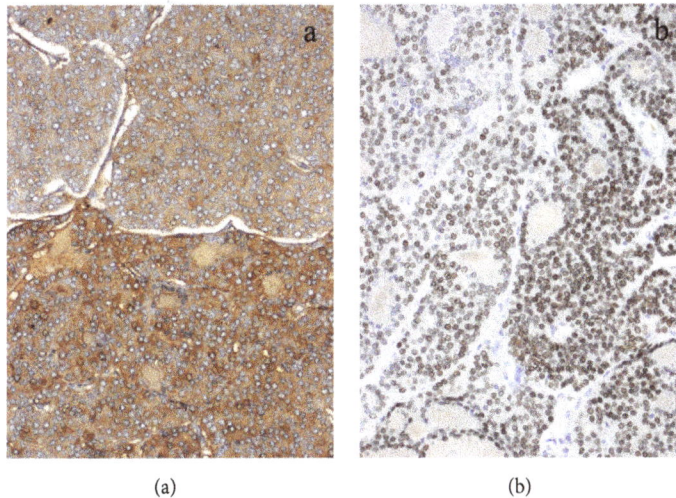

(a)   (b)

FIGURE 2: Malignant cells revealing intense and diffuse immunoexpression of thyroglobulin (cytoplasmic) (a) and TTF-1 (nuclear) (b) [Case 1].

diabetes mellitus (treated with linagliptin/metformin), non-treated high blood pressure, right-sided hemiparesis following meningitis in childhood, nephrolithiasis, and smoking history. The pelvic computed tomography (CT) revealed a 9x7.5x9 cm bulky mass in the sacrum with locally increased soft tissue density, causing extensive lytic lesions of the sacred vertebrae and extending to the left iliac bone, suggestive of chordoma. The patient underwent total sacrectomy with partial excision and reconstruction of the left iliac bone. The anatomopathological examination revealed sacrococcygeal involvement by a thyroid carcinoma, as verified by immunohistochemical staining for thyroglobulin and TTF-1, predominantly papillary (follicular variant), however with foci of nondifferentiated (insular) carcinoma (Figures 1 and 2). Thyroid ultrasonography showed a solid nodule of 20 mm in the right lobe and two solid hypoechogenic nodules of 11 and 9 mm in the left lobe, the smallest with coarse calcifications. No lymphadenopathies were found. 18F-fluorodeoxyglucose positron-emission tomography (18F-FDG-PET) revealed a hypermetabolic focus in the left lobe of the thyroid, consistent with the suspected malignant neoplasia, and uptake of the radiopharmaceutical drug in the fifth lumbar vertebra and pelvic bones, consistent with secondary involvement (Figure 3). Consequently, the patient underwent total thyroidectomy. Histological examination revealed only follicular and oxyphilic variants of multifocal papillary carcinoma (at least six foci) and none of insular carcinoma, with dimensions ranging from 2 to 15 mm, without signs of hematogenic, lymphatic, or perineural permeation, as well as no signs of invasion of the capsule or extrathyroidal extension, with resection margins uninvolved by tumour (pT1b[m]NxM1R0) (Figure 4). Radioactive iodine therapy (RAI) was then performed. Posttherapy scintigraphy showed hyperfixation in the remnants of the sacrum and lower lumbar spine, bilateral iliac bone, and anterior cervical region (Figure 5). TSH-stimulated thyroglobulin was 24490 ng/mL. Follow-up

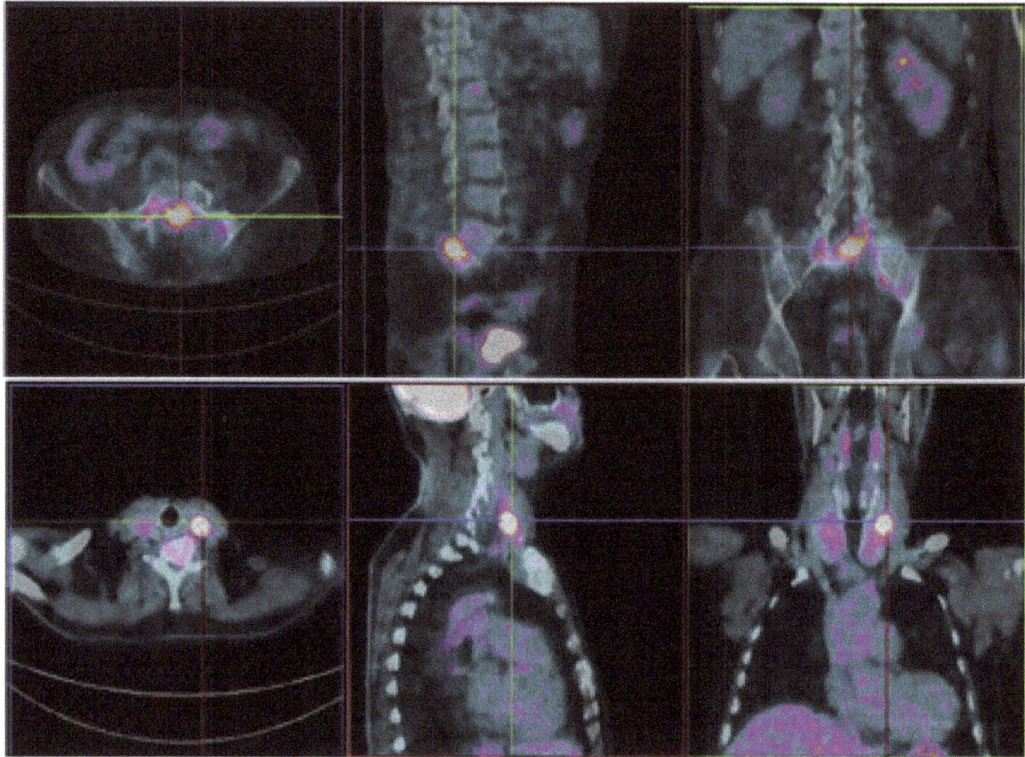

FIGURE 3: 18F-FDG-PET showing uptake of the radiopharmaceutical drug in thyroid left lobe, L5 vertebrae, and pelvic bones [Case 1].

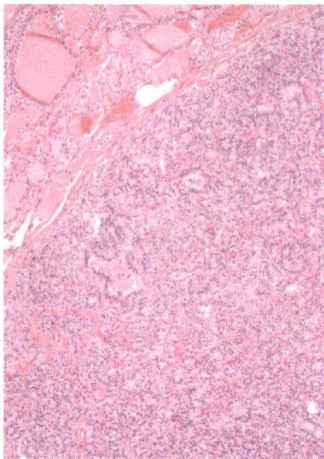

FIGURE 4: Fragments of thyroid involved by papillary thyroid carcinoma of follicular and oxyphilic variants [Case 1].

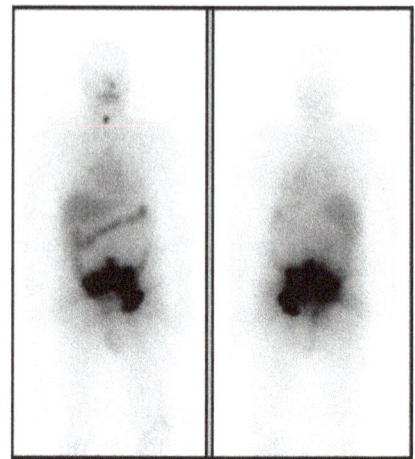

FIGURE 5: Posttherapy scintigraphy showing hyperfixation in the remnants of the sacrum and lower lumbar spine, bilateral iliac bone, and anterior cervical region [Case 1].

magnetic resonance imaging (MRI) revealed persistence and progression of the pelvic lesion. At this time the patient was unable to walk, had a chronic indwelling bladder catheter, suffered from fecal incontinence, and presented with uncontrolled refractory chronic pain.

3. Case 2

A 64-year-old male presented with pain in the left iliac region for 6 months. His past medical history was significant for gastric peptic ulcer disease (submitted to partial gastrectomy and

chronically treated with lansoprazole), nephrolithiasis, and hyperuricemia. At admission a poorly defined mass on the left posterior iliac crest was palpable. The patient underwent a pelvic CT, which revealed a 9 cm lytic lesion of left iliac bone with soft tissue involvement (Figure 6). A biopsy was performed and the histological examination and immuno-histochemical staining for thyroglobulin and TTF-1 showed iliac involvement of a well-differentiated thyroid carcinoma (Figures 7 and 8). Thyroid ultrasonography disclosed a poorly

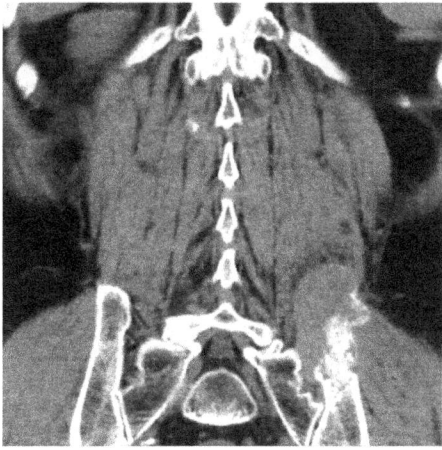

FIGURE 6: Pelvic CT revealing a 9 cm lytic lesion of left iliac bone [Case 2].

defined 8 mm nodule in the left inferior lobe, heterogeneous and partially calcified, and a 4 mm hypoechoic nodule in the right lobe, without associated lymphadenopathies. The patient was submitted to total thyroidectomy and anatomopathological examination revealed a 1.1 cm papillary carcinoma, of follicular variant, with capsular invasion and limited extrathyroidal extension (ETE). Consequently, RAI therapy was performed. Postablative 131 iodine scintigraphy and 18F-FDG-PET (Figure 9) did not reveal further lesions. TSH-stimulated thyroglobulin was 185051 ng/mL. The patient is currently waiting for a hemipelvectomy.

4. Discussion

The authors present two rare cases of well DTC without significant histological poor prognosis features presenting as osteolytic bone metastases. DTCs, in particular those that are small and organ confined as in the above-mentioned cases, are often characterized by a slowly progressive course with a 5-year survival rate of 98.2% [8]. Of the several histological subtypes of papillary carcinoma, the follicular variants are probably the most common. At the time of diagnosis, distant metastases are seen in 2 to 10% of patients: two-thirds are pulmonary and one-fourth is represented by skeletal metastases [9]. Metastization at the time of the diagnosis of well DTC is an unusual combination, with poor prognosis. Moreover, according to the most recent data from Cancer Care Ontario, distant metastases occur in less than 1% of all thyroid cancer patients [10].

However, the bone is the third most common site of metastatic cancer of unknown origin, particularly of the spine, followed by the pelvis and long bones [11]. In such cases, bone biopsy is mandatory, since histological findings often provide important diagnostic clues, as well as important information regarding the prognosis and treatment of these patients [11]. This is particularly true in bone metastases from DTC [11]. In the first described case the radiological features were highly suggestive of a chordoma, dictating the choice of immediate resection, and pathological examination established the diagnosis of a thyroid carcinoma. In the second case, bone biopsy was diagnostic.

The described cases are unusual due to the aggressive presentation in the absence of previous poor prognosis anatomopathological features of the primitive tumours. In the first case report, beyond multifocality no other unfavourable features were present, predicting a low risk DTC [4]. However, the histological examination of the excised bone metastasis revealed insular carcinoma foci, suggesting primary tumour dedifferentiation during the process of distant metastization. In fact, DTCs can undergo dedifferentiation through a process of multiple genetic and epigenetic alterations, evolving into poor differentiated or even undifferentiated/anaplastic carcinomas [12]. The histological findings of bone metastasis in the first case, according to the Turin criteria, are compatible with a poorly differentiated thyroid carcinoma (PDTC), defined as a follicular-cell neoplasm with insular, solid, or trabecular growth [12, 13]. This type of tumour constitutes an entity that, in terms of morphology and behaviour, is considered of intermediate risk between papillary and follicular well DTCs and anaplastic carcinomas [12]. Significant regional differences in the incidence of this type of tumour are found, suggesting that their etiology is multifactorial and results from the interaction of genetic, environmental, and diet related factors [12, 14]. Furthermore, there are reports of tumours, which, even in the absence of any identifiable dedifferentiation marker, behave aggressively. In the second case report, capsular and microscopically immediate perithyroidal soft tissue invasion was present, estimating an intermediate risk DTC following 2015 ATA guidelines [4]. Nevertheless, the definition of limited/microscopic ETE is subjective, as the thyroid lacks a well-defined capsule and is often intermingled with adipose tissue or even peripheral skeletal muscle. Even so, recent studies have shown that gross ETE constitutes a strong predictor for recurrence and disease-related death, and that limited ETE alone does not have a significant impact on survival. Consequently, some authors questioned whether microscopic ETE should be sufficient to increase the risk of persistent/recurrent disease from low to intermediate or to upstage a DTC as T3 [1]. Furthermore, none of the cases presented with vascular or lymphoid invasion, which could predict a more aggressive conduct and the presence of extensive bone metastases.

Nevertheless, the factors predicting a worse outcome in DTCs also include demographic features. There is established evidence that male sex and increasing age are important risk modifiers [12]. The latest study from The Cancer Genome Atlas (TCGA) Research Network has shown that mutation density correlates with age and therefore age should always be considered as a continuous variable in risk stratification, rather than a static threshold from which patients are classified as having low or high risk [15]. The patients abovementioned were both men and over 60 years old.

Although DTC has often an indolent course and usually poses minimal risk to human health, without apparent symptoms or adverse impact from their disease burden for many years, the cases mentioned above mean to underline the notion that patients can have an aggressive presentation and behaviour despite relatively "benign" histological features. In order to complement the histological study, it would be interesting to design a molecular study of the described

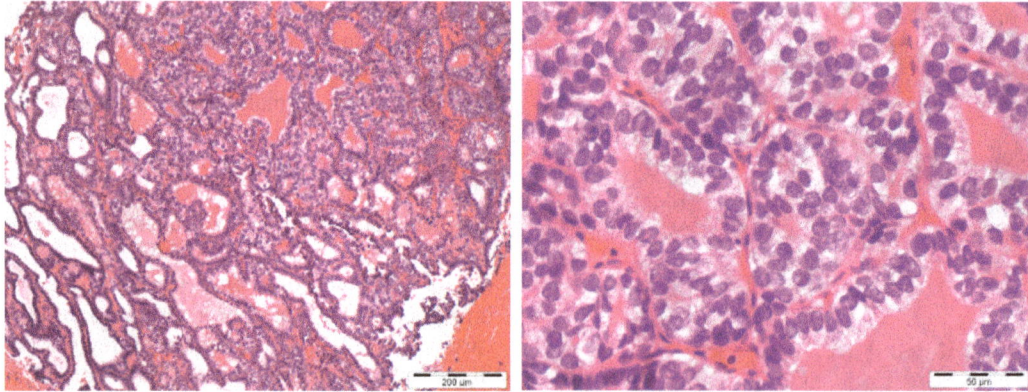

FIGURE 7: Fragments of bone tissue involved by epithelial neoplasia of follicular architecture [Case 2].

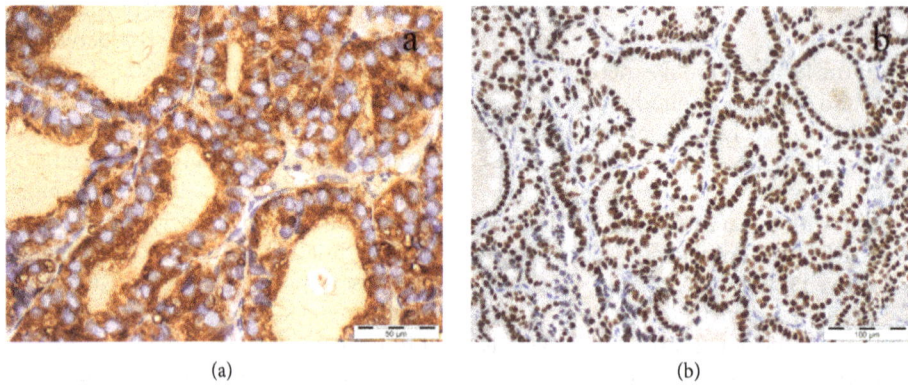

(a)

(b)

FIGURE 8: Malignant cells revealing intense and diffuse immunoexpression of thyroglobulin (cytoplasmic) (a) and TTF-1 (nuclear) (b) [Case 2].

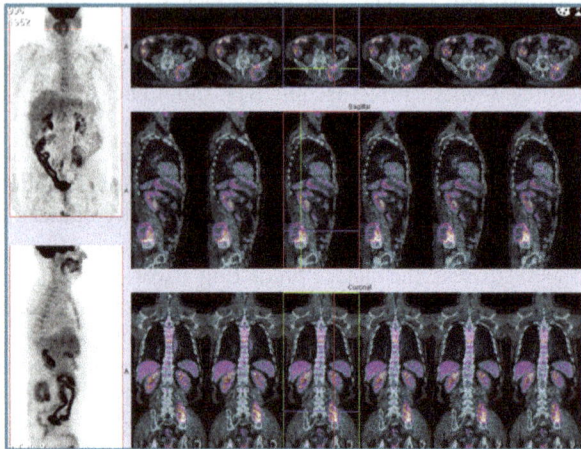

FIGURE 9: 18F-FDG-PET revealing the pelvic lesion found on CT, without no other metabolically active lesions [Case 2].

angiogenesis mediators, cellular regulators, and adhesion molecules. Because overall survival is improved by complete resection of the primary tumour and its metastases, early diagnosis and treatment are crucial.

5. Conclusions

DTC are commonly tumours with a benign clinical course. However, patients presenting with seemingly innocent features may have aggressive tumours with bone metastization upon diagnosis. Prompt treatment initiation is crucial for patient survival. The authors want to underline the necessity of high clinical awareness and close follow-up to decrease morbidity and mortality in these patients. Further studies are needed to disclose clinical and histological patterns of poor prognosis.

Abbreviations

DTC: Differentiated thyroid carcinoma
RAI: Radioactive iodine therapy
ETE: Extrathyroidal extension.

tumours in an attempt to identify mutations that could serve as predictors for a more aggressive behaviour. DTCs are heterogeneous with different molecular signatures and variable presentation. A variety of molecular markers is involved in the processes of tumorigenesis, tumour progression, and development, including focal mutations, rearrangements, epigenetic changes of growth factors and their receptors,

Ethical Approval

All procedures performed in this study involving human participants were in accordance with the ethical standards of the institutional and/or national research committee and with the 1964 Helsinki Declaration and its later amendments or comparable ethical standards.

Disclosure

This research did not receive any specific grant from any funding agency in the public, commercial, or not-for-profit sector.

Authors' Contributions

D. Magalhães collected and interpreted the data and wrote the manuscript. I. Furtado revised the manuscript. C. Costa, M. J. Matos, A. P. Santos, and I. Torres participated in the medical treatment. All authors read and approved the final manuscript.

References

[1] B. Xu and R. Ghossein, "Evolution of the histologic classification of thyroid neoplasms and its impact on clinical management," *European Journal of Surgical Oncology*, vol. 44, no. 3, pp. 338–347, 2018.

[2] J.-D. Lin, S.-F. Lin, S.-T. Chen, C. Hsueh, C.-L. Li, and T.-C. Chao, "Long-term follow-up of papillary and follicular thyroid carcinomas with bone metastasis," *PLoS ONE*, vol. 12, no. 3, Article ID e0173354, 2017.

[3] R. Siegel, J. Ma, Z. Zou, and A. Jemal, "Cancer statistics, 2014," *CA: A Cancer Journal for Clinicians*, vol. 64, no. 1, pp. 9–29, 2014.

[4] B. R. Haugen, E. K. Alexander, K. C. Bible, G. M. Doherty, S. J. Mandel, Y. E. Nikiforov et al., "2015 American association management guidelines for adult patients with nodules and differentiated cancer—the american association guidelines task force on nodules and differentiated cancer," *Thyroid*, vol. 26, no. 2, pp. 319–321, 2016.

[5] N. Mizoshiri, T. Shirai, R. Terauchi et al., "Metastasis of differentiated thyroid cancer in the subchondral bone of the femoral head: a case report," *BMC Musculoskeletal Disorders*, vol. 9, no. 16, article 286, 2015.

[6] Y. M. Choi, W. G. Kim, H. Kwon et al., "Early prognostic factors at the time of diagnosis of bone metastasis in patients with bone metastases of differentiated thyroid carcinoma," *European Journal of Endocrinology*, vol. 175, no. 3, pp. 165–172, 2016.

[7] J. A. Wexler, "Approach to the thyroid cancer patient with bone metastases," *The Journal of Clinical Endocrinology & Metabolism*, vol. 96, no. 8, pp. 2296–2307, 2011.

[8] http://seer.cancer.gov/statfacts/html/thyro.html accessed on June 5, 2017.

[9] https://www.uptodate.com/contents/papillary-thyroid-cancer?source=search_result&search=differentiated%20thyroid%20carcinoma&selecselected=10~150 accessed on June 5, 2017.

[10] O. Mete and S. L. Asa, "Pathological definition and clinical significance of vascular invasion in thyroid carcinomas of follicular epithelial derivation," *Modern Pathology*, vol. 24, no. 12, pp. 1545–1552, 2011.

[11] A. Piccioli, G. Maccauro, M. S. Spinelli, R. Biagini, and B. Rossi, "Bone metastases of unknown origin: epidemiology and principles of management," *Journal of Orthopaedics and Traumatology*, vol. 16, no. 2, article 344, pp. 81–86, 2015.

[12] S. Papp and S. L. Asa, "When thyroid carcinoma goes bad: a morphological and molecular analysis," *Head & Neck Pathology*, vol. 9, no. 1, pp. 16–23, 2015.

[13] M. Volante, P. Collini, Y. E. Nikiforov et al., "Poorly differentiated thyroid carcinoma: the Turin proposal for the use of uniform diagnostic criteria and an algorithmic diagnostic approach," *The American Journal of Surgical Pathology*, vol. 31, no. 8, pp. 1256–1264, 2007.

[14] J. Hannallah, J. Rose, and M. A. Guerrero, "Comprehensive literature review: recent advances in diagnosing and managing patients with poorly differentiated thyroid carcinoma," *International Journal of Endocrinology*, vol. 2013, Article ID 317487, 7 pages, 2013.

[15] The Cancer Genome Atlas Research Network, "Integrated genomic characterization of papillary thyroid carcinoma," *Cell*, vol. 159, pp. 676–690, 2014.

49

Ectopic Papillary Thyroid Cancer with Distant Metastasis

Oscar R. Vázquez ⓘ,[1] **Frieda Silva,**[1] **Eduardo Acosta-Pumarejo,**[2] **and Maria L. Marín**[3]

[1]*Nuclear Medicine Section, Radiological Sciences Department, University of Puerto Rico, San Juan, Puerto Rico, USA*
[2]*Radiology Department, VA Caribbean Healthcare System, San Juan, Puerto Rico, USA*
[3]*Pathology Department, Isaac Gonzalez Oncologic Hospital, San Juan, Puerto Rico, USA*

Correspondence should be addressed to Oscar R. Vázquez; oscar.vazquez2@upr.edu

Academic Editor: Eli Hershkovitz

Ectopic thyroid tissue is a rare clinical entity wherein malignant lesions may arise, the most common one being papillary carcinoma. We present a case of a 68-year-old female who presented with a growing mass in the right clavicle. An MR of the shoulder showed a soft tissue mass arising from the anterior margin of the right distal clavicle. A fine needle aspiration of the mass showed papillary thyroid carcinoma. PET/CT confirmed the clavicular and mediastinal mass. Excision of the clavicular mass and total thyroidectomy with modified right neck dissection were performed. Pathology revealed no evidence of malignancy in the thyroid; lymph nodes were positive for metastatic thyroid carcinoma. Postsurgery CT showed the superior mediastinal mass with surrounding adenopathy; radioiodine (RAI) treatment with dose of 142.1 mCi [5257.7 MBq] was recommended. Posttherapy whole-body scan (WBS) showed RAI avid tissue in the neck and superior mediastinum. Follow-up chest CT revealed pulmonary nodules that increased in number and size; a second RAI therapeutic dose was given. The posttherapy RAI WBS was negative. Repeat PET/CT showed multiple hypermetabolic lesions in the mediastinum, neck, lymph nodes, pulmonary nodes, and right shoulder. The FDG avid lesions with no RAI uptake suggested tumor dedifferentiation.

1. Introduction

Ectopic thyroid tissue is a rare clinical entity, with a prevalence of 1: 300,000 in the general population. The ectopic tissue may be located anywhere from the base of the tongue to the diaphragm, the most frequent sites being lingual, thyroglossal, laryngotracheal, and lateral cervical regions. It may also occur in less frequent sites such as the esophagus, mediastinum, heart, adrenal glands, and pancreas [1]. The mediastinum is the most frequent location after the neck [2].

Ectopic thyroid tissue can undergo the same pathologic processes of a normal thyroid gland. Even when the probability of cancer on ectopic tissue is less than 1%, malignant lesions may arise. Differentiated carcinoma accounts for the majority of these tumors, papillary carcinoma being the most common. As in the native thyroid, papillary tumors are the more frequent malignant lesions in ectopic tissue. Lymph node metastasis is common; distant metastases can occur in 10 % of cases. Most of papillary tumors are radioiodine avid

and have an excellent prognosis [3]. Lymph node metastases in malignant ectopic lesions are present in 30% of cases.

We present a case of ectopic thyroid tissue in the mediastinum with papillary carcinoma that presented with an unusual aggressive behavior.

2. Case Summary

A 68-year-old female patient with history of hypothyroidism came to the clinic for evaluation because of a growing mass in the right distal clavicular lesion. An MR of the shoulder region was performed revealing a 5.5 cm soft tissue mass arising from the anterior margin of the right distal clavicle. A fine needle aspiration of the mass was performed; histology showed papillary thyroid carcinoma [Figure 1]. Immuno-histochemistry was positive for TTF-1, thyroglobulin, CK19, CK7, and EMA. A whole-body 18F-FDG PET-CT study was ordered. The study was done with 15.5 mCi [576 MBq] of 18F-FDG and it showed a hypermetabolic lesion in the

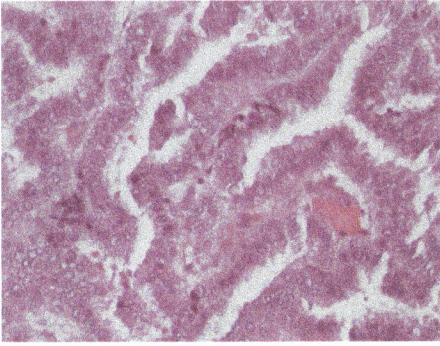

FIGURE 1: Surgical pathology of the right clavicular mass revealing metastatic papillary adenocarcinoma.

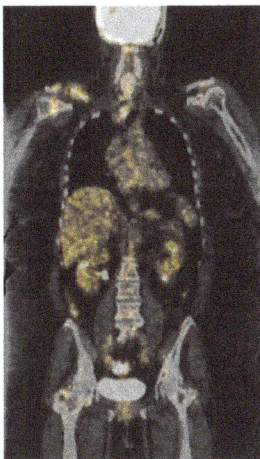

FIGURE 2: Coronal-fused 18F-FDG PET/CT shows FDG avid lesion in the distal right clavicle with osseous destruction and an FDG avid mediastinal mass displacing the trachea to the left.

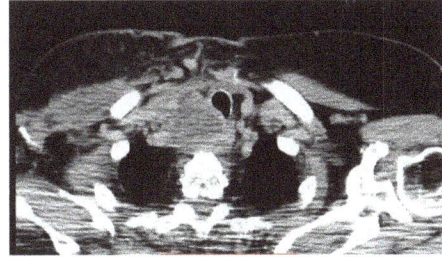

FIGURE 3: Axial chest CT showing a hypodense, solid, infrahyoid mass extending to the superior mediastinum.

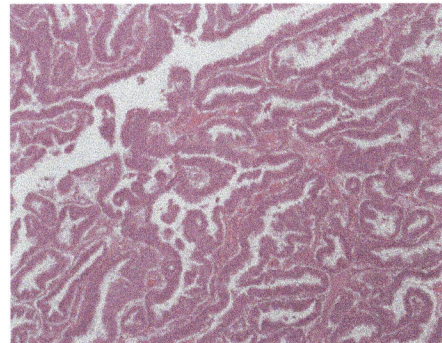

FIGURE 4: Pathology report of central neck biopsy of superior mediastinal mass revealing papillary thyroid carcinoma.

distal right clavicle with evidence of osseous destruction and enlarged retro- and infraclavicular lymph nodes [SUV max: 12.5 g/mL]. There was also an FDG avid mediastinal mass displacing the trachea and esophagus [SUV max: 7.9 g/mL]. The thyroid gland was small and atrophic [Figure 2].

Complete excision of the right clavicular mass and the distal clavicle was performed. This was followed by a total thyroidectomy, with modified right neck dissection of levels 3, 4, and 5. The pathology report of the thyroid gland was negative for malignancy; however, the neck dissection procedure was positive for metastatic papillary thyroid carcinoma in level III cervical lymph nodes. Postsurgery CT scan showed a hypodense, solid, infrahyoid mass extending to the superior mediastinum with surrounding adenopathy [Figure 3].

The patient was subsequently treated with external beam radiation therapy to the distal clavicular region. Central neck biopsy of the superior mediastinal mass was performed. The biopsy reported papillary carcinoma, with similar cellular characteristics as that reported in the clavicular mass; surgical pathology report revealed papillary thyroid carcinoma with tumor cells positive for TTF-1 and focally positive for thyroglobulin [Figure 4]. Due to the morbidity of the procedure,

surgical excision of the mediastinal mass was not recommended at the moment. Instead, the patient was referred to the nuclear medicine service for evaluation with a 131-iodine whole-body scan (WBS) and possible treatment with radioiodine (RAI). The study was performed with 3 mCi [111 MBq] of 131-iodine [TSH level: 42.6 uU/mL; stimulated Tg: 66.4 ng/mL; TgAb: 3.8]. It revealed abnormal tracer uptake in the region of the thyroid bed and upper mediastinum. The patient was then prepared for RAI adjuvant therapy for residual thyroid tissue. A dose of 142.1 mCi [5257.7 MBq] of 131-iodine was administered and the posttherapy WBS revealed focal tracer uptake in the lower anterior neck extending to the thoracic inlet and superior mediastinum, consistent with persistent functional thyroid tissue; no focal RAI uptake was observed in the region of the right clavicle. Neck sonogram and CT scan of the neck and superior mediastinum with IV contrast performed afterwards showed multiple abnormal lymph nodes in the thyroid bed and neck arguing in favor of recurrent or metastatic disease. The CT also showed additional pulmonary nodules and interval size decrease of the superior mediastinal mass. The patient was reevaluated and a second dose of RAI was recommended to be given three [3] months after the contrast enhanced CT. A dose of 172.1 mCi [6367.7 MBq] of 131-iodine was administered [TSH level 74.3 uIU/mL]; at this time, the stimulated Tg was 1,216.6 ng/mL and the TgAb < 1 IU/mL. The posttherapy WBS showed no evidence of radioiodine concentration in the thyroid bed, mediastinum, supraclavicular area, or neck. Follow-up PET/CT performed with 15

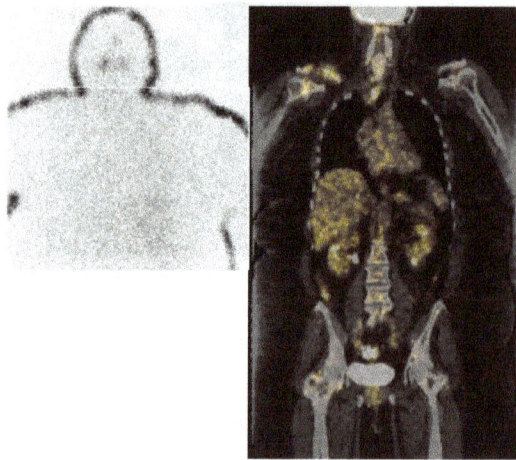

FIGURE 5: Left: posttherapy 131-iodine WBS shows no evidence of functional thyroid tissue. Right: coronal-fused images of 18F-FDG PET/CT study performed after posttherapy WBS show the FDG avid mediastinal and right shoulder masses.

mCi [555 MBq] of 18F-FDG showed the previously described mediastinal FDG avid mass, with a cystic or necrotic area, development of hypermetabolic neck lymph nodes, axillary nodes, and pulmonary nodes and a large mass in the right shoulder area [SUV max: 5.5] [Figure 5]. At this time the tumor was considered to be dedifferentiated and patient was started on tyrosine kinase inhibitor therapy with good short term therapeutic response.

3. Discussion

The thyroid gland develops around the 4th week of embryonal development and originates from a diverticulum located in the median ventral wall of the pharynx, between the first and second pharyngeal pouches dorsal to the aortic sac [4]. The primitive thyroid tissue penetrates the underlying mesenchymal tissue and descends anterior to the hyoid bone and laryngeal cartilages until it reaches the lower neck. This process takes three weeks and is usually complete by the seventh week of gestation. Abnormal descent of the thyroid tissue may occur and gives rise to ectopic thyroid tissue, which can be found anywhere from the base of the tongue to the diaphragm. The probability of cancer on ectopic thyroid tissue is less than 1% and when it occurs papillary carcinoma is the most common histology [5–7].

Several criteria have been described to establish the presence of ectopic thyroid tissue in the mediastinum versus a substernal or a retrosternal extension of the thyroid gland. These are as follows: the tissue has blood supply from intrathoracic vessels rather than from cervical arteries, there is a normal or absent [without history of surgery] cervical thyroid gland, and the cervical thyroid gland does not have a similar pathologic process as the ectopic tissue and has no history or evidence of documented malignancy [5, 8].

This case presented meets the above-mentioned criteria of an ectopic tissue. The native thyroid was negative for malignancy and the thyroid gland had no intrathoracic extension

as demonstrated in the CT. Unfortunately, the mediastinal mass was not excised, and we could not demonstrate the intrathoracic source of the blood supply. However, the patient had no bleeding complications during the excision of the thyroid gland. Furthermore, the tumor had an aggressive evolution, initially presenting with a clavicular mass and bone involvement. This makes the case a very unusual one, since as stated before most malignant ectopic thyroid tissue presents a papillary histology, usually not aggressive in nature.

The whole-body scan performed after the first radioiodine therapy failed to reveal radioiodine uptake in the clavicular region, the mediastinal masses, or the lung lesions. Tumors with high thyroglobulin levels, negative radioiodine scan, and FDG avidity tend to be more aggressive and dedifferentiated. PET studies have been used for several years in such cases for diagnostic and prognostic purposes. PET/CT may change patient management in up to 40% of cases. The volume of the FDG avid lesions and the SUV were considered strong predictors of survival. Overall survival and cancer specific survival have been reported to be 8.9 and 9.6 years, respectively, in radioiodine refractory thyroid cancer. The time of tumor dedifferentiation was found to be the second most important prognostic factor for the survival. Patients with less than 3 years of tumor dedifferentiation had a worse prognosis [3, 9, 10].

In our case, the elapsed time for dedifferentiation was 6 months. There was no uptake in the mediastinal and clavicular masses in the posttherapy radioiodine study, suggesting the tumor had dedifferentiated and furthermore became more aggressive in nature. The whole-body scan performed after the second therapeutic dose of radioiodine did not reveal any foci of abnormal RAI uptake, further confirming the loss of the sodium iodine symporter to concentrate iodine, as a sign of dedifferentiation.

To our knowledge, this is the first report of an unusually aggressive ectopic thyroid tumor. There are several important facts in the presentation and evolution of the case that should raise the suspicion of a possible dedifferentiated aggressive ectopic tumor. The presence of early distant metastasis, the rapidly rising thyroglobulin levels, and the poor radioiodine uptake are ominous signs in thyroid malignancies. The early identification of bad prognostic signs is important in the therapy planning and follow-up.

4. Conclusion

Ectopic thyroid tissue is a rare entity. The chances of harboring malignant cells are low. When malignant lesions occur, they are usually papillary carcinomas. Even when the incidence of thyroid carcinoma has been increasing in the last years, the mortality has not changed, except in radioiodine refractory tumors.

Tumoral lesions in ectopic mediastinal lesions are a rare entity; an aggressive papillary carcinoma is even less common. To our knowledge, this is the first report of a widely metastatic tumor in ectopic thyroid tissue. It is important to keep in mind that tumor dedifferentiation may occur in ectopic tumors in order to provide patients with early therapeutic options.

References

[1] G. Lianos, C. Bali, V. Tatsis et al., "Ectopic thyroid carcinoma. Case report," *Giornale di Chirurgia*, vol. 34, no. 4, pp. 114–116, 2013.

[2] A. D. Mace, A. Taghi, S. Khalil, and A. Sandison, "Ectopic sequestered thyroid tissue: an unusual cause of a mediastinal mass," *ISRN Surgery*, 2011.

[3] T. Abraham and H. Schöder, "Thyroid cancer—indications and opportunities for positron emission tomography/computed tomography imaging," in *Seminars in Nuclear Medicine*, vol. 41, no. 2, pp. 121–138, Elsevier, 2011.

[4] A. R. Mansberger Jr. and J. P. Wei, "Surgical embryology and anatomy of the thyroid and parathyroid glands," *Surgical Clinics of North America*, vol. 73, no. 4, pp. 727–746, 1993.

[5] A. Sahbaz, N. Aksakal, B. Ozcinar, F. Onuray, K. Caglayan, and Y. Erbil, "The "forgotten" goiter after total thyroidectomy," *International Journal of Surgery Case Reports*, vol. 4, no. 3, pp. 269–271, 2013.

[6] Y. Agosto-Vargas, M. Gutiérrez, J. H. Martínez et al., "Papillary Thyroid Carcinoma: Ectopic Malignancy versus Metastatic Disease," *Case Reports in Endocrinology*, vol. 2017, Article ID 9707031, 3 pages, 2017.

[7] B. C. Shah, C. S. Ravichand, S. Juluri, A. Agarwal, C. S. Pramesh, and R. C. Mistry, "Ectopic thyroid cancer," *Annals of Thoracic and Cardiovascular Surgery*, vol. 13, no. 2, pp. 122–124, 2007.

[8] U. Kesici, Ö. Koral, S. Karyağar et al., "Missed retrosternal ectopic thyroid tissue in a patient operated for multinodular goiter," *Turkish Journal of Surgery/Ulusal Cerrahi Dergisi*, vol. 32, no. 1, article 67, 2016.

[9] S. Shafiee, A. Sadrizade, A. Jafarian, S. R. Zakavi, and N. Ayati, "Ectopic papillary thyroid carcinoma in the mediastinum without any tumoral involvement in the thyroid gland. A Case Report," *Journal of Nuclear Medicine and Biology*, vol. 1, no. 1, article 44, 2013.

[10] J. Wassermann, M. Bernier, J. Spano et al., "Outcomes and Prognostic Factors in Radioiodine Refractory Differentiated Thyroid Carcinomas," *The Oncologist*, vol. 21, no. 1, pp. 50–58, 2016.

50

Bilateral Pheochromocytomas in a Patient with Y175C Von Hippel-Lindau Mutation

Olga Astapova ⓘⒹ, **Anindita Biswas, Alessandra DiMauro, Jacob Moalem,** and **Stephen R. Hammes**

Division of Endocrinology and Metabolism, Department of Medicine, University of Rochester School of Medicine and Dentistry, Rochester, New York 14642, USA

Correspondence should be addressed to Olga Astapova; olga_astapova@urmc.rochester.edu

Academic Editor: Carlo Capella

Von Hippel-Lindau (VHL) disease, caused by germline mutations in the *VHL* gene, is characterized by metachronously occurring tumors including pheochromocytoma, renal cell carcinoma (RCC), and hemangioblastoma. Although VHL disease leads to reduced life expectancy, its diagnosis is often missed and tumor screening guidelines are sparse. VHL protein acts as a tumor suppressor by targeting hypoxia-inducible factors (HIFs) for degradation through an oxygen-dependent mechanism. *VHL* mutants with more severely reduced HIF degrading function carry a high risk of RCC, while mutants with preserved HIF degrading capacity do not cause RCC but still lead to other tumors. VHL disease is classified into clinical types (1 and 2A-2C) based on this genotype-phenotype relationship. We report a case of bilateral pheochromocytomas and no other VHL-related tumors in a patient with Y175C VHL and show that this mutant preserves the ability to degrade HIF in normal oxygen conditions but, similar to the wild-type VHL protein, loses its ability to degrade HIF under hypoxic conditions. This study adds to the current understanding of the structure-function relationship of *VHL* mutations, which is important for risk stratification of future tumor development in the patients.

1. Introduction

Von Hippel-Lindau (*VHL*) is a tumor suppressor gene associated with inhibition of angiogenesis, apoptosis, cell cycle exit, fibronectin matrix assembly, and proteolysis. Germline mutations in *VHL* occur with a frequency of 1:36,000 in Europe [1] and a 20% de novo rate. Mutations are passed down in an autosomal dominant pattern with almost complete penetrance by the age of 60 [2]. People with *VHL* mutations metachronously develop various benign and malignant tumors. More than half of the patients develop CNS and retinal hemangioblastomas (most commonly in the cerebellum or spinal cord). Other common life-threatening tumors are pheochromocytoma and clear cell renal cell carcinoma (RCC). An increased frequency of pancreatic neuroendocrine tumors, endolymphatic sac tumors, epididymal tumors, and benign cysts in the pancreas and the kidneys is also reported. Because of time lag between occurrences of different tumors, the diagnosis of VHL disease is often delayed, resulting in increased mortality [3].

VHL regulates the cellular response to low oxygen conditions by interacting with hypoxia-inducible factors (HIFα: HIF1α and HIF2α). In normoxic conditions, HIFα is hydroxylated on conserved proline residues by prolyl hydroxylases, which require oxygen as a cofactor. Hydroxylated HIFα is recognized by VHL which acts in complex with its cofactors elongin B and elongin C to ultimately target HIFα for ubiquitination and proteasomal degradation [4]. In hypoxic conditions, prolyl hydroxylases become inactive, and unhydroxylated HIFα is not recognized by VHL. This leads to accumulation of HIFα, which forms heterodimers that translocate to the nucleus, bind to hypoxia-response elements, and induce the transcription of genes involved in adaptations to hypoxia, including angiogenesis. The same process occurs in the absence of functional VHL and leads to tumorigenesis in patients with VHL disease, most likely through the two-hit model [2, 5].

Studies of over a dozen different *VHL* mutations have identified several phenotypic subtypes revealing a structure-function relationship in which the severity of the mutation

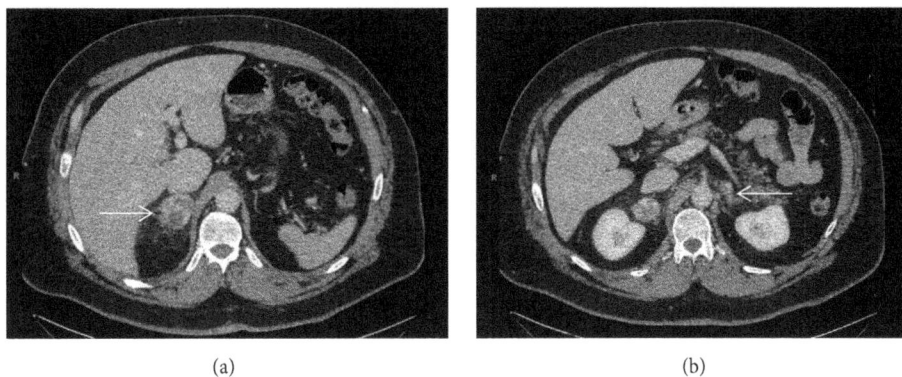

FIGURE 1: CT scan of the abdomen showing the right adrenal tumor ((a), arrow) and the left adrenal tumor ((b), arrow) prior to adrenalectomy.

predicts the likelihood of RCC [6]. *VHL* mutants that retain the ability to downregulate HIFα are less likely to be associated with RCC than those that lose that ability [4, 7, 8]. Patients with type 1 VHL have deletion or truncation mutations that completely abolish any functional protein expression. They have a high risk of RCC and also present with both retinal and CNS hemangioblastomas; however, pheochromocytomas are uncommon [9]. Type 2 VHL is characterized by pheochromocytomas and is caused by point mutations with variable degrees of limitation of VHL activity. It is further subdivided into 2A, 2B, and 2C based on the frequency of RCC and hemangioblastomas. RCC appears more frequently in patients with the more severely dysfunctional VHL resulting in higher expression of HIFα, such as types 1 and 2B. By contrast, type 2C mutations retain their ability to fully downregulate HIFα and present with only pheochromocytomas, indicating that HIFα-independent mechanisms are at play in the pathogenesis of VHL-related pheochromocytomas. Some *in vitro* studies suggest that type 2C VHL mutants cause defective fibronectin matrix assembly, while retaining the ability to suppress HIFα and stop the growth of RCC cells in culture [10, 11].

2. Case Presentation

A 53-year-old man of Puerto-Rican origin presented to the endocrinology clinic after undergoing bilateral adrenalectomy for multifocal pheochromocytomas. He had a prior history of morbid obesity, obstructive sleep apnea, diabetes, and hypertension. He was followed by his primary care physician for persistent hematuria ranging from 3 to 35 red blood cells per high power field on urinalysis, as well as urinary frequency, weak stream, and nocturia three times per night for the previous three years. He had been unable to tolerate an empiric trial of tamsulosin for benign prostate hypertrophy due to orthostatic dizziness. Negative symptoms pertinent to this case include flushing, headaches, sweating, palpitations, anxiety, blurry vision, or dizziness. His family history was notable for death from a myocardial infarction in his father at the age of 57 and an unknown genitourinary cancer in his sister. There was no family history of adrenal tumors, hyperparathyroidism, medullary thyroid cancer, renal cancer,

or pituitary tumors. The patient was a smoker with several past attempts at quitting.

Due to the persistent hematuria, smoking, and the family history of cancer, a CT urogram was performed to screen for bladder cancer. While no abnormalities were seen within the urogenital tract, bilateral, irregular, heterogeneous large adrenal masses (Figure 1) measuring 4.7 cm (R) and 1.6 cm (L) were noted. In addition, a prominent and suspicious lymph node was identified. Biochemical characterization of the adrenal masses revealed significantly elevated 24-hour urine normetanephrine (1090 micrograms/gram of creatinine; normal range, 0–400 micrograms/gram of creatinine), leading to the diagnosis of pheochromocytoma. Urine metanephrine level was within normal range. Cushing's syndrome was ruled out with an undetectable late-night salivary cortisol level. Electrolyte levels, kidney function, and complete blood count were within normal limits. In search for additional, extra-adrenal foci, a metaiodobenzylguanidine (MIBG) scan was performed but was nondiagnostic due to lack of cardiac activity. Nevertheless, given the available imaging and biochemical findings, there was concern for malignant pheochromocytoma, and the patient ultimately underwent an open bilateral adrenalectomy and paracaval lymph node excision. Intraoperatively, the patient required vasopressor support and a large amount of crystalloid resuscitation (13 liters) to maintain hemodynamic stability. Intraoperative ultrasound was used to identify one mesenteric lymph node of mildly suspicious appearance which was resected, in addition to a large retroperitoneal paracaval lymph node.

Surgical pathology confirmed pheochromocytomas in the bilateral adrenal glands (right, 5.0 x 3.5 x 2.5 cm, and left, 1.5 x 1.3 x 1.0 cm) which were both confined to the adrenal glands. The paracaval lymph node was described as paraganglioma versus metastatic pheochromocytoma measuring 1.6 cm in the greatest dimension with no lymphoid tissue identified. The immediate postoperative course was unremarkable. The patient was started on life-long glucocorticoid and mineralocorticoid replacement. His diabetes and hypertension resolved.

Due to the multifocal nature of the pheochromocytomas and the presence of first-degree relatives likely to be affected, the patient was offered genetic screening for familial

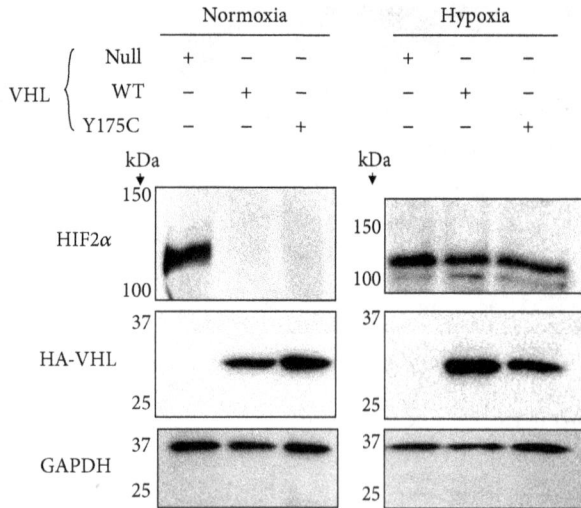

FIGURE 2: Western blot of HIF2α, HA-VHL, and GAPDH expression in normal oxygen (left) and hypoxic (right) conditions. VHL-null 786-O cells were transfected and clonally selected for stable expression of either WT or Y175C VHL or GFP (null), as indicated.

paraganglioma syndromes. With the patient's informed written consent, genomic DNA was isolated from a peripheral blood sample and targeted gene sequencing was performed using PGLNext. Coding exons and adjacent intron nucleotides of the 12 targeted genes associated with hereditary pheochromocytoma syndromes were amplified and then sequenced using PCR and next-generation sequencing. Gross deletion and duplication analysis was also performed. The patient was found to have a heterozygous germline mutation, c.524A>G in the *VHL* gene, corresponding to the Y175C substitution in the protein. This was identified as a likely pathogenic variant and confirmed by Sanger sequencing. In one study, this alteration was described in a patient with a personal and family history of pheochromocytoma and no other VHL-associated tumors and segregated with disease in this family [12].

In order to better define the risk of RCC in this patient and others with this mutation, we assessed the ability of Y175C VHL to degrade HIFα *in vitro*. Stable wild-type (WT) or Y175C VHL-expressing cells lines were generated by transfection and clonal selection of *VHL*-null 786-O cells derived from a human RCC as previously described [10, 13]. Control cells were transfected with GFP. We detected HIF2α expression in the control *VHL*-null cell line, while stable overexpression of either WT or Y175C VHL resulted in the disappearance of HIF2α (Figure 2, left panel). To further characterize the function of Y175C VHL under hypoxic conditions, the cells were placed into a hypoxia incubator at 1% O_2 for 24 hours. As expected, the WT VHL lost the ability to induce HIF2α degradation in hypoxia (Figure 2, right panel). The Y175C VHL similarly did not reduce HIF2α abundance in hypoxia. HIF2α abundance was also similar in WT and Y175C VHL-expressing cells after 6 hours and 12 hours of hypoxia (data not shown). Thus, under both

normoxic and hypoxic conditions, Y175C VHL functions similarly to the WT with regard to HIFα degradation.

3. Discussion

Differential diagnoses of VHL include other hereditary syndromes such as multiple endocrine neoplasia type 2, polycystic kidney disease, type 1 neurofibromatosis, and hereditary pheochromocytoma-paraganglioma syndrome. Germline mutations in known susceptibility genes including *SDHB* (succinate dehydrogenase complex B) and others are identified in 11-13% of patients with sporadic pheochromocytomas [14]. While screening should not be offered to every patient with a pheochromocytoma, guidelines including those from the Massachusetts General Hospital [1] suggest consideration of genetic screening for syndromes of pheochromocytoma in patients with other factors such as certain other tumors, pancreatic cysts, and multiple pheochromocytomas or those under 40 years of age. In general, genetic screening is likely underutilized according to these guidelines. Genetic screening was recommended for this patient due to the presence of bilateral pheochromocytomas.

Although Y175C VHL has been reported in another family with a similar phenotype, its molecular function has not been studied to date. We have shown that the Y175C mutation preserves the ability of VHL to degrade HIFα under normal oxygen conditions. The mutant also functions similarly to the wild-type protein in hypoxia, which abrogates VHL-mediated HIFα degradation. This is the first reported molecular study of Y175C VHL and it adds to the growing body of knowledge about various *VHL* mutants. Based on our findings, this patient has type 2C VHL, the subtype with preserved HIFα degradation ability and with pheochromocytomas as the sole presenting feature. Previously reported type 2C VHL mutants with pheochromocytoma as the only notable disease manifestation include L188V and V84L. These mutants also demonstrated preserved ability to ubiquitinate HIFα [10].

Our case is similar to a previously described Spanish cohort with the same mutation [12] that presented with pheochromocytomas in mutation carriers and no other VHL-associated tumors. The authors of that study calculated the folding energy of Y175C VHL and found that it was only slightly higher than that of the wild-type, indicating that Y175C VHL is predicted to be fairly stable. In contrast, the folding energies of mutants with more severe disease phenotypes are dramatically higher than the wild-type, resulting in unstable proteins and predicted loss of function. Our *in vitro* findings are in line with this *in silico* prediction which supports a low risk of RCC in this patient.

Although HIFα degradation is better characterized, many studies have shown that VHL is also important in extracellular matrix assembly and cell membrane structure through regulating fibronectin and integrins, and loss of this function leads to tumor development as well. Fibronectin is upregulated by VHL at the mRNA level and independently of hypoxia [15] or the HIFα pathway [16] and requires covalent modification of VHL by NEDD8, a ubiquitin-like molecule [16]. Mutants that escape this modification are involved in tumorigenesis despite adequate HIFα suppression. VHL also reduces the protein abundance of several subtypes of integrins in an oxygen-independent manner, via proteasomal degradation, suggesting that VHL is important in cell adhesion and maintenance of tight junctions [17]. Further, depletion of HIF-2α alone does not fully recapitulate the effects of VHL replacement in a *VHL*-null cell line [18], particularly the downregulation of integrins and resulting morphological changes. These mechanisms are likely involved in VHL-associated tumorigenesis, particularly in pheochromocytoma, where the HIFα pathway does not play a significant role.

Acknowledgments

The authors thank Dr. Keith Nehrke and Dr. Teresa Sherman for providing the hypoxia chamber used in this experiment.

References

[1] S. Schmid, S. Gillessen, I. Binet et al., "Management of von Hippel-Lindau disease: An interdisciplinary review," *Oncology Research and Treatment*, vol. 37, no. 12, pp. 761–771, 2014.

[2] C. Cassol and O. Mete, "Endocrine manifestations of von Hippel-Lindau disease," *Archives of Pathology & Laboratory Medicine*, vol. 139, no. 2, pp. 263–268, 2015.

[3] M. L. M. Binderup, A. M. Jensen, E. Budtz-Jørgensen, and M. L. Bisgaard, "Survival and causes of death in patients with von Hippel-Lindau disease," *Journal of Medical Genetics*, vol. 54, no. 1, pp. 11–18, 2017.

[4] S. C. Clifford and E. R. Maher, "Von hippel-lindau disease: Clinical and molecular perspectives," *Advances in Cancer Research*, vol. 82, pp. 85–105, 2001.

[5] L. Gossage, T. Eisen, and E. R. Maher, "VHL, the story of a tumour suppressor gene," *Nature Reviews Cancer*, vol. 15, no. 1, pp. 55–64, 2015.

[6] M. Barontini and P. L. M. Dahia, "VHL Disease," *Best Practice & Research Clinical Endocrinology & Metabolism*, vol. 24, no. 3, pp. 401–413, 2010.

[7] L. Li, L. Zhang, X. Zhang et al., "Hypoxia-inducible factor linked to differential kidney cancer risk seen with type 2A and type 2B VHL mutations," *Molecular and Cellular Biology*, vol. 27, no. 15, pp. 5381–5392, 2007.

[8] M. P. Rechsteiner, A. Von Teichman, A. Nowicka, T. Sulser, P. Schraml, and H. Moch, "VHL gene mutations and their effects on hypoxia inducible factor HIFα: identification of potential driver and passenger mutations," *Cancer Research*, vol. 71, no. 16, pp. 5500–5511, 2011.

[9] R. R. Lonser, G. M. Glenn, M. Walther et al., "Von Hippel-Lindau disease," *The Lancet*, vol. 361, no. 9374, pp. 2059–2067, 2003.

[10] M. A. Hoffman, M. Ohh, H. Yang, J. M. Klco, M. Ivan, and W. G. Kaelin Jr., "Von Hippel-Lindau protein mutants linked to type 2C VHL disease preserve the ability to downregulate HIF," *Human Molecular Genetics*, vol. 10, no. 10, pp. 1019–1027, 2001.

[11] S. C. Clifford, M. E. Cockman, A. C. Smallwood et al., "Contrasting effects on HIF-1alpha regulation by disease-causing pVHL mutations correlate with patterns of tumourigenesis in von Hippel-Lindau disease," *Human Molecular Genetics*, vol. 10, no. 10, pp. 1029–1038, 2001.

[12] S. Ruiz-Llorente, J. Bravo, A. Cebrián et al., "Genetic characterization and structural analysis of VHL spanish families to define genotype-phenotype correlations," *Human Mutation*, vol. 23, no. 2, pp. 160–169, 2004.

[13] Z. Ding, P. German, S. Bai et al., "Genetic and pharmacological strategies to refunctionalize the von hippel lindau R167Q mutant protein," *Cancer Research*, vol. 74, no. 11, pp. 3127–3136, 2014.

[14] J. P. Brito, N. Asi, I. Bancos et al., "Testing for germline mutations in sporadic pheochromocytoma/paraganglioma: A systematic review," *Clinical Endocrinology*, vol. 82, no. 3, pp. 338–345, 2015.

[15] H. A. R. Bluyssen, M. P. J. K. Lolkema, M. Van Beest et al., "Fibronectin is a hypoxia-independent target of the tumor suppressor VHL," *FEBS Letters*, vol. 556, no. 1-3, pp. 137–142, 2004.

[16] N. H. Stickle, J. Chung, J. M. Klco, R. P. Hill, W. G. Kaelin Jr., and M. Ohh, "pVHL modification by NEDD8 is required for fibronectin matrix assembly and suppression of tumor development," *Molecular and Cellular Biology*, vol. 24, no. 8, pp. 3251–3261, 2004.

[17] Q. Ji and R. D. Burk, "Downregulation of integrins by von Hippel-Lindau (VHL) tumor suppressor protein is independent of VHL-directed hypoxia-inducible factor alpha degradation," *The International Journal of Biochemistry & Cell Biology*, vol. 86, no. 3, pp. 227–234, 2008.

[18] M. D. Hughes, E. Kapllani, A. E. Alexander, R. D. Burk, and A. R. Schoenfeld, "HIF-2alpha downregulation in the absence of functional VHL is not sufficient for renal cell differentiation," *Cancer Cell International*, vol. 7, p. 13, 2007.

51

Diagnostic Dilemma in Two Cases of Hyperandrogenism

Ibrahim Alali ⓘ,[1] Lilianne Haj Hassan ⓘ,[2] Ghadeer Mardini,[1] Nermeen Hijazi,[1] Lama Hadid,[1] and Younes Kabalan[1]

[1]*Endocrinology Department, Al-Assad University Hospital, Damascus University, Syria*
[2]*Endocrinology Department, Al-Mouwassat University Hospital, Damascus University, Syria*

Correspondence should be addressed to Ibrahim Alali; ibali2012@gmail.com

Academic Editor: Carlo Capella

Hirsutism is a common endocrine complaint affecting about 10 percent of women. It may be caused by multiple etiologies including adrenal and ovarian disorders. Usually, it is a result of a benign entity such as PCOs and idiopathic hirsutism. However, sometimes especially when it is severe and rapid in progression an androgen-secreting tumor should be excluded. Sertoli-Leydig cell tumors constitute fewer than 0.5 percent of ovarian tumors and it may be benign or malignant. In this article, we present two cases of hyperandrogenism caused by occult ovarian Leydig cell tumors. one of them was confounded by the presence of coincidental bilateral adrenal nodules that complicated the diagnostic process. Tumor dissection was curative in both cases and the diagnosis was confirmed by pathological and hormonal testing after surgery.

1. Introduction

Hirsutism is known as excess male-pattern hair growth in women; it produces a significant emotional stress regardless of its etiology [1].

Endogenous androgens are made by the adrenal glands and the ovaries in both post- and premenopausal women [2].

Hirsutism is usually caused by benign etiologies such as polycystic ovary syndrome PCOs and idiopathic hirsutism. However, when it is severe and/or associated with virilization, an androgen-secreting tumor should be excluded [3].

These tumors may originate from adrenals or ovaries, where they arise from sex cord such as Sertoli-Leydig cell tumors [4].

They may be so small in contrast to adrenal tumors which are often large in size and aggressive in behavior.

Due to the high incidence of adrenal incidentalomas, the incidence of an adrenal mass does not exclude the ovarian origin of androgen secretion and then the differential diagnosis is sometimes so complex [5].

Here we describe two cases of hyperandrogenism in post- and premenopausal women caused by androgen-secreting ovarian tumors.

2. Case 1 Presentation

A 60-year-old woman came to the endocrinology clinic with a complaint of rapidly progressive signs and symptoms of hyperandrogenism over 6 months. She mentioned hirsutism noticed especially in the face and chin, hair loss that took a male-pattern baldness in all over the head, deepening voice, and increased libido.

She had no galactorrhea, muscle weakness, hyperpigmentation, bruising, weight loss, or anorexia.

She was married, housewife, and smoker (5 pack-years), got 6 children, did not consume alcohol; she had regular menses since puberty until she had amenorrhea 22 years ago after hysterectomy (because of leiomyoma). She was diagnosed with hypothyroidism 15 years ago treated with L-Thyroxine (700 μg\weekly) and osteoporosis 7 years ago treated with Calcium supplements + alendronate 70 mg weekly. She denied the use of any drugs that may cause hyperandrogenism.

On examination, the patient seemed well. The blood pressure was 120/80 mm Hg, the pulse 83 beats per minute, the height 154 cm, the weight 72 kg, and the body mass index (BMI; the weight in kilograms divided by the square of the

TABLE 1: Hormonal study at initial assessment and normalization of androgens one-month postsurgery.

Test (Normal range) unit	Initial evaluation		1 month after surgery	
	Case 1	Case 2	Case 1	Case 2
Testosterone (0.23-0.73) ng/mL	7.05	15	0.03	0.2
DHEAS(60-338)μg/dL	113.4	62.9		
17OHP(0.2-0.9) ng/mL	3.83	-	0.197	-
TSH(0.5-4.5) mIU/L	0.99	1.96		
PRL(up to 25) ng/mL	13.34	16		

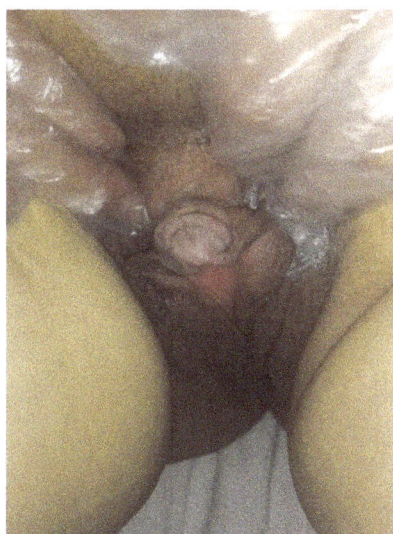

FIGURE 1: Clitoromegaly.

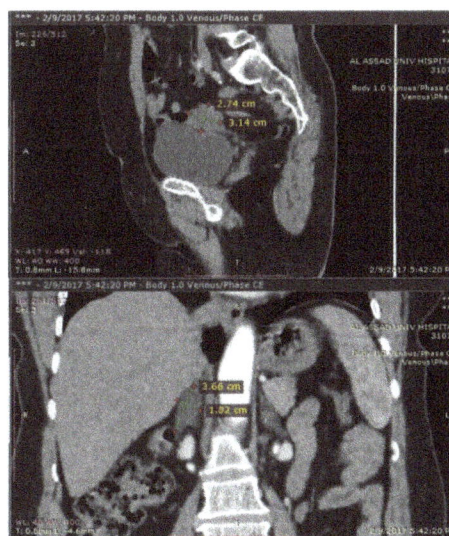

FIGURE 2: On the top, the figure shows sagittal CT section of the left ovary measures 2.74 cm by 3.14 cm. On the bottom, it shows coronal section adrenals with the largest nodule in right adrenal gland measures 3.66 cm by 1.82 cm with a left adrenal nodule.

height in meters) 30.2 (obesity class I). The Ferriman-Gallwey score for hirsutism estimation was 6 (4 in the chin, 2 in upper lip); she had acanthosis nigricans, frontal baldness, and clitoromegaly (2 cm by 3 cm) as shown in (Figure 1). Except for a cesarean scar in the abdomen, the rest of examination was unremarkable.

Laboratory studies revealed a hemoglobin concentration of 15 g/dL, serum sodium level of 141 mEq/L, and potassium level of 4.5 mEq/L. An automated chemistry panel showed normal findings. Hormonal studies were as in Table 1.

Transvaginal ultrasonography showed that uterine and left ovary was removed, right ovary measured 2.1 cm by 2 cm by 4.5 cm with a volume of 7.8 cm^3. Abdominal computed tomography (CT) showed bilateral adrenal nodular hyperplasia as in (Figure 2). All adrenal function tests (hypo- and hypersecretion) were proved to be normal: 24-hour urine normetanephrine 47.3 μ/24hours (up to 600), metanephrine 107 μ/24hours (up to 350), 8 A.M cortisol 13.02 μg/dL, adrenocorticotrophic hormone ACTH 19.69 pg/mL (7-63), and 11 P.M cortisol 1.66 μg/dL

In order to distinguish ACTH-dependent hyperandrogenism from other causes of hyperandrogenism, a 48-h low-dose (2mg) dexamethasone-suppression test was carried out [6], without a decrease in testosterone value (10.94 ng/mL) though enough cortisol suppression at the end of the test 0.58 μg/dL.

In such cases the catheterization of the adrenal and ovarian veins may be useful in identifying the source of hyperandrogenism but it was not available at our center. Since the lack of dexamethasone-induced inhibition of testosterone was suggestive of an ACTH-independent etiology mainly ovarian, and the patient was postmenopausal, the decision of laparoscopic oophorectomy was made. The pathology report confirmed the diagnosis of 2.8 cm Leydig cell tumor (Figure 3). Testosterone was performed 72-hour postsurgery and it was 0.03 ng/mL. 17 hydroxy-progesterone and testosterone were performed 1 month later and they were in normal limits.

3. Case 2 Presentation

A 39-year-old woman came to endocrinology clinic with a complaint of hirsutism started 4 years ago, alongside with oligomenorrhea followed by amenorrhea two years ago. There was no temporal baldness or deepening voice.

The patient was treated for a period of 3 months with combined oral contraceptive pills COCP and cyproterone acetate without improvement in symptoms, 6 months earlier to admission.

She was married, got 3 children and was nonsmoking or alcohol consuming. She was diagnosed 5 years ago with

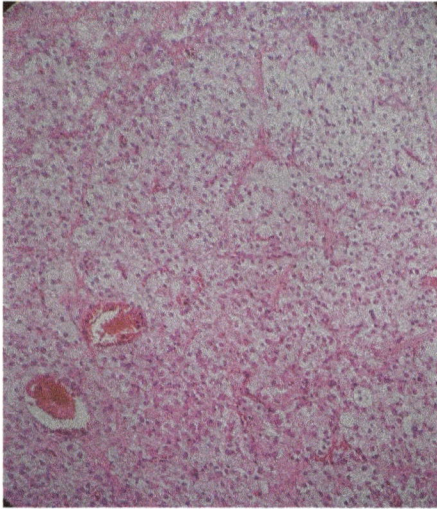

FIGURE 3: Leydig cell tumor composed by granular cells with eosinophilic cytoplasm and round nuclei (hematoxylin and eosin stain).

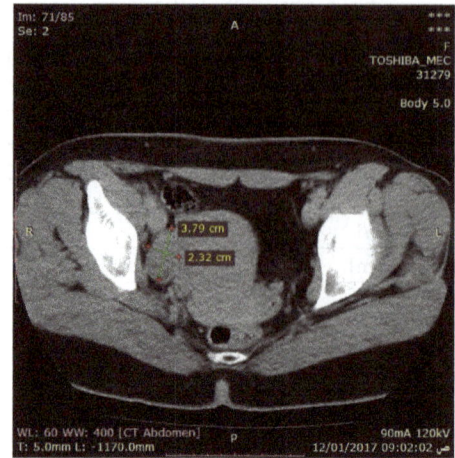

FIGURE 4: Right ovary measures 3.8 by 2.3 cm.

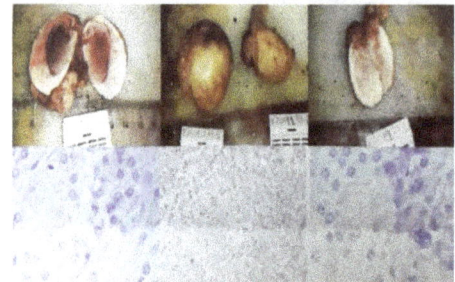

FIGURE 5: Upper left shows Leydig cell tumor of the right ovary. Upper right shows normal left ovary; microscopic examination shows cells abundant eosinophilic cytoplasm. Reinke crystals are noted.

rheumatoid arthritis and treated for only one month with prednisolone and methotrexate.

On examination, she seemed well. The blood pressure was 120/80 mm Hg, the height 155 cm, the weight 65 kg, and the body mass index BMI 27.1 (overweight). The Ferriman-Gallwey score for hirsutism estimation was 16 (4 points for each chin, upper lip, low abdomen, and medial thigh), clitoromegaly (1 cm by 0.5 cm); she had no acanthosis nigricans or frontal baldness. Otherwise, she had normal findings.

Laboratory studies revealed a hemoglobin concentration of 10.3 g/dL, ferritin 10 ng/mL, serum sodium level of 138 mEq/L, and potassium level of 4.15 mEq/L. An automated chemistry panel showed normal findings except for fasting glucose 119 mg/dL. She started metformin therapy and ferrous replacement. Hormonal studies were as in Table 1.

Transvaginal ultrasonography showed that ovaries measured 3.3 by 2 cm and 3.2 by 2 cm for right and left ovary, respectively, without masses. CT scan for adrenals was within normal also and right ovary measured 3.8 by 2.3cm as shown in Figure 4.

Since catheterization of the adrenal and ovarian veins was not available, the diagnostic and therapeutic options were explained to the patient and giving that she was not interested in future fertility, she underwent laparoscopic exploration for oophorectomy.

Pathologic report sowed 2.5 cm of Leydig cell tumor in the right ovary, while the left ovary was within normal as shown in (Figure 5). Testosterone was normalized after surgery.

4. Discussion

Androgen-secreting tumors typically come with quickly progressive hyperandrogenism resulting in virilization. These tumors may ascend from adrenal glands or ovaries representing the least common cause of the hyperandrogenism in women with a prevalence of 0.2% [7].

Androgen-secreting adrenal tumors are very infrequent, large, and aggressive and usually associated with high cortisol levels, while purely androgen-secreting adrenal tumors are very rare [8, 9].

Virilizing ovarian tumors are rare medical condition representing less than 0.2% of all causes of hyperandrogenism and fewer than 1% of all ovarian tumors [10].

Although DHEAs level might help to differentiate ovarian from the adrenal source of hyperandrogenism, adrenocortical tumors might sometimes present with normal DHEAs level [11]. Furthermore, ovarian tumors have been rarely reported to be associated with a high DHEAs level which makes final diagnosis very challenging [12].

Leydig cell tumors are a very uncommon type of virilizing ovarian tumors (less than 0.1 % of ovarian tumors) and might occasionally be small enough to pass detection even with careful radiological studies [10] leading to bilateral oophorectomy as both a diagnostic and therapeutic approach [13].

Here we represented two cases of occult Leydig ovarian tumors. One of these cases was associated with bilateral nodular adrenal hyperplasia; these cases highlight the challenges in the diagnosis of Leydig cell tumors.

In the first case, the patient denied the use of any drugs that may lead to hyperandrogenism and because of her severe symptoms, other etiologies should be excluded [14].

In women with PCOS symptoms generally begin in puberty and gradually develop through reproductive years [14] so new onset virilization symptoms and very high testosterone levels proposed to rule out PCOS. Patient's age and absence of adrenal insufficiency excluded classical congenital adrenal hyperplasia CAH, but not the nonclassic form of CAH, although it was theoretically excluded because of the recent onset and severity of symptoms, very high values of testosterone, and the absence of testosterone suppression after dexamethasone. However, we depended on 17 OH progesterone monitoring after surgery to make a definite diagnosis.

A suppression test with dexamethasone was performed [6], and plasma cortisol levels decreased, but total testosterone inhibition did not occur discarding the functional adrenal hyperandrogenism and indicated tumorous origin, with the absence of cortisol cosecretion and normal DHEAS values suggested the presence of an occult ovarian tumor.

Catheterization of both the adrenal and ovarian veins was not suggested because it is unavailable at Al-Assad Center so the patient went to oophorectomy and the diagnosis was made.

The 17OH progesterone returned to normal one month after surgery confirming the ovarian source and excluding nonclassic CAH.

Some cases of unilateral adrenal nodule correlation with Leydig cell tumor were reported [5, 15], but according to our knowledge, this is the first reported case of coincidence bilateral adrenal incidentalomas with Leydig cell tumor in a postmenopausal woman.

In the second case, the absence of adrenal or ovarian mass suggested the use of catheterization of both the adrenal and ovarian veins, but this procedure was not available at Al-Mouwassat Center and the patient was not interested in another pregnancy so after discussing the possibility of an occult ovarian tumor as a cause of her complaint she decided to have bilateral oophorectomy to make a final diagnosis.

The establishment of the precise cause of androgen excess may not always be apparent, necessitating engagement of a combination of clinical talents complemented with appropriate laboratory and imaging techniques [16].

References

[1] J. Mihailidis, R. Dermesropian, P. Taxel, P. Luthra, and J. M. Grant-Kels, "Endocrine evaluation of hirsutism," *International Journal of Women's Dermatology*, vol. 3, no. 1, pp. S6–S10, 2017.

[2] H. G. Burger, "Androgen production in women," *Fertility and Sterility*, vol. 77, supplement 4, pp. S3–S5, 2002.

[3] D. Bode, D. A. Seehusen, and D. Baird, "Hirsutism in women," *American Family Physician*, vol. 85, no. 4, pp. 373–380, 2012.

[4] F. A. Tavassoli, P. Devilee, and World Health Organization, *Classification of Tumours. Pathology and Genetics of the Breast and Female Genital Organs*, IARC Press, Lyon, 2003.

[5] M. Tutzer, I. Winnykamien, J. Davila Guardia, and C. Castelo-Branco, "Hyperandrogenism in post-menopausal women: A diagnosis challenge," *Gynecological Endocrinology*, vol. 30, no. 1, pp. 23–25, 2014.

[6] G. A. Kaltsas, A. M. Isidori, B. P. Kola et al., "The value of the low-dose dexamethasone suppression test in the differential diagnosis of hyperandrogenism in women," *The Journal of Clinical Endocrinology & Metabolism*, vol. 88, no. 6, pp. 2634–2643, 2003.

[7] E. Carmina, F. Rosato, A. Jannì, M. Rizzo, and R. A. Longo, "Relative prevalence of different androgen excess disorders in 950 women referred because of clinical hyperandrogenism," *The Journal of Clinical Endocrinology & Metabolism*, vol. 91, no. 1, pp. 2–6, 2006.

[8] D. Cavlan, N. Bharwani, and A. Grossman, "Androgen- and estrogen-secreting adrenal cancers," *Seminars in Oncology*, vol. 37, no. 6, pp. 638–648, 2010.

[9] F. Cordera, C. Grant, J. Van Heerden et al., "Androgen-secreting adrenal tumors," *Surgery*, vol. 134, no. 6, pp. 874–880, 2003.

[10] R. H. Young, "Ovarian sex cord-stromal tumours and their mimics," *Pathology*, vol. 50, no. 1, pp. 5–15, 2018.

[11] W. Waggoner, L. R. Boots, and R. Azziz, "Total testosterone and DHEAS levels as predictors of androgen-secreting neoplasms: A populational study," *Gynecological Endocrinology*, vol. 13, no. 6, pp. 394–400, 1999.

[12] R. Azziz, J. E. Nestler, and D. Dewailly, *Androgen Excess Disorders in Women - Polycystic Ovary Syndrome and Other Disorders*, Humana Press, Totowa, NJ, 2007.

[13] M. C. Markopoulos, E. Kassi, K. I. Alexandraki, G. Mastorakos, and G. Kaltsas, "Hyperandrogenism after menopause," *European Journal of Endocrinology*, vol. 172, no. 2, pp. R79–R91, 2015.

[14] G. Conway, D. Dewailly, E. Diamanti-Kandarakis et al., "The polycystic ovary syndrome: A position statement from the European Society of Endocrinology," *European Journal of Endocrinology*, vol. 171, no. 4, pp. P1–P29, 2014.

[15] M. L. C. Rivera-Arkoncel, D. Pacquing-Songco, and F. L. Lantion-Ang, "Virilising ovarian tumour in a woman with an adrenal nodule," *BMJ Case Reports*, vol. 2010, 2010.

[16] M. Alpañés, J. M. González-Casbas, J. Sánchez, H. Pián, and H. F. Escobar-Morreale, "Management of postmenopausal virilization," *The Journal of Clinical Endocrinology and Metabolism*, vol. 97, no. 8, pp. 2584–2588, 2012.

52

Panhypopituitarism due to Absence of the Pituitary Stalk: A Rare Aetiology of Liver Cirrhosis

Marta Gonzalez Rozas,[1] **Lidia Hernanz Roman,**[2] **Diego Gonzalez Gonzalez,**[3] **and José Luis Pérez-Castrillón**[2]

[1]*Internal Department, Hospital de Segovia, Segovia, Spain*
[2]*Internal Department, Hospital Universitario Río Hortega, Valladolid, Spain*
[3]*Pathology Department, Hospital Universitario Río Hortega, Valladolid, Spain*

Correspondence should be addressed to José Luis Pérez-Castrillón; castrv@terra.com

Academic Editor: Osamu Isozaki

Studies have established a relationship between hypothalamic-pituitary dysfunction and the onset of liver damage, which may occasionally progress to cirrhosis. Patients with hypopituitarism can develop a metabolic syndrome-like phenotype. Insulin resistance is the main pathophysiological axis of metabolic syndrome and is the causal factor in the development of nonalcoholic fatty liver disease (NAFLD). We present the case of a young patient with liver cirrhosis of unknown aetiology that was finally attributed to panhypopituitarism.

1. Introduction

Studies have established a relationship between hypothalamic-pituitary dysfunction and the onset of liver damage, which may occasionally progress to cirrhosis. Patients with hypopituitarism develop a metabolic syndrome-like phenotype, including secondary hormonal alterations, central obesity, insulin resistance, diabetes mellitus, dyslipidaemia, and, occasionally, hyperphagia [1, 2]. Insulin resistance is the main pathophysiological axis of metabolic syndrome and is the causal factor in the development of nonalcoholic fatty liver disease (NAFLD), which may evolve independently from liver cirrhosis.

We present the case of a young patient with liver cirrhosis of unknown aetiology that was finally attributed to panhypopituitarism.

2. Case Study

A 24-year-old man attended our hospital with fever of two days of evolution accompanied by chills and periumbilical abdominal pain, with no other associated clinical features, except for occasional episodes of epistaxis and gingival bleeding. The medical history was remarkable only for hepatitis in childhood.

At admission, the patient was conscious and oriented. Physical examination revealed obesity (body mass index [BMI] = 30), height 174 cm, waist circumference 117 cm, blood pressure systolic 127 mmHg, blood pressure diastolic 75 mmHg, cutaneous-mucous paleness, hepatomegaly (3 cm), hypermobility in the lower limbs, and macrodactylia, without other remarkable features.

Laboratory tests showed leukocytes $7.2 \times 1000/\mu L$, haemoglobin 12.9 g/dL, mean corpuscular volume 88.5 fl, and platelets $98 \times 1000/\mu L$. Clotting and blood smears were normal. Biochemical tests showed glucose 97 mg/dL, HbA1c 4.3%, urea 43 mg/dL, total cholesterol 201 mg/dL, triglycerides 125 mg/dL, uric acid 7.91 mg/dL, creatinine 1.6 mg/dL, total bilirubin 1.29 mg/dL, calcium 9.9 mg/dL, glutamic-oxaloacetic transaminase (GOT) 30 U/L, glutamic-pyruvic transaminase (GPT) 58 U/L, alkaline phosphatase 139 U/L, sodium 141 mEq/L, and potassium 4 mEq/L.

Serology for hepatitis B and C, cytomegalovirus, and toxoplasma was negative. Autoimmune tests were negative for

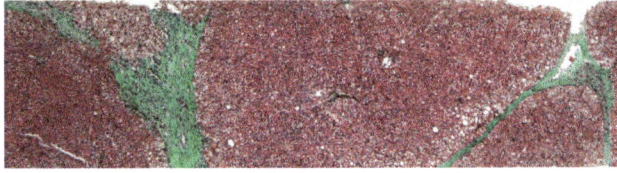

FIGURE 1: Liver biopsy. Architectural distortion with nodular areas bounded by fibrous tract (Masson).

antinuclear antibodies, anti-smooth muscle antibodies, and antimitochondrial antibodies. Other causes of chronic liver disease such as drug-induced and cholestatic liver disease and metabolic disease were ruled out (alpha-antitrypsin (199 mg/dL), ceruloplasmin (38 mg/dL), and copper (127 mg/dL) were normal).

Hormone testing showed ACTH 14.5 pg/mL, GH < 0.11 ng/mL, somatomedin C 3.56 ng/mL, TSH 0 mUI/L, FT4 0.6 ng/dL, cortisol 1.4 μg/dL, FSH 0.2 U/L, prolactin < 0.6 ng/mL, testosterone < 0.1 ng/dL, and insulin 19.8 μUI/mL. A TRH and LH-FH test was performed with no response. The patient had a normal karyotype (46XY).

Chest X-ray, abdominal CT scan, electrocardiogram, and echocardiogram were normal. Abdominal ultrasound confirmed dilation of the portal vein (14 mm) and hepatosplenomegaly. Hip radiography showed bilateral hip dysplasia without closing of growth plates, and cerebral MRI showed absence of the pituitary stalk.

Finally, liver biopsy showed architectural distortion with nodular areas bounded by fibrous tracts, with ductal proliferation without iron deposits, suggestive of liver cirrhosis with mild steatosis and minimal inflammatory activity (Figure 1).

The patient received hormone replacement therapy with cortisol, thyroid hormones, and testosterone.

3. Relationship between Cirrhosis and Panhypopituitarism

The first cases establishing an association between hypothalamic-pituitary dysfunction and liver damage were reported in 2004. Most cases occur in children or adolescents who present hypothalamic dysfunction secondary to structural lesions such as perinatal asphyxia and craniopharyngiomas or genetic disorders such as Prader-Willi disease [1–3].

NAFLD affects 20–50% of adults in developed countries and includes histological alterations that range from simple steatosis to nonalcoholic steatohepatitis (NASH) and cirrhosis. Simple steatosis is often associated with obesity and is characterized by fat accumulation in the liver, without inflammation, and is considered benign [4].

NASH occurs in 2-3% of cases and is characterized by steatosis, inflammation, and pericellular fibrosis that may progress to cirrhosis and hepatocellular carcinoma. The definitive diagnosis of NAFLD requires a liver biopsy [4]. NAFLD is characterized by insulin resistance, central obesity, and impaired glucose tolerance and is considered a hepatic manifestation of metabolic syndrome. The increased prevalence of obesity and diabetes has increased the incidence of NAFLD, which is now the leading cause of chronic liver disease in North America [5].

Furthermore, patients with hypopituitarism that have a growth hormone deficiency (GHD) and other hypothalamic dysfunctions show a similar phenotype. Due to the similarity of the two phenotypes, it is hypothesized that patients with hypothalamic-pituitary dysfunction might develop liver disease.

4. Pathogenesis of NAFLD

The pathogenesis of NAFLD is very complex and involves different mechanisms that suggest an association between adipose tissue and the liver. Three possible underlying mechanisms have been proposed: first, the excessive accumulation of lipids; second, an inflammatory response that causes cell apoptosis; and, third, a probable defect in the reparative response to the damage suffered. Hormonal deficiencies may contribute to the occurrence of any of these mechanisms.

Altered lipid homeostasis in the liver is a key point in the pathogenesis of NAFLD. Initially, it was thought that elevated levels of free fatty acids (FFA) were the main cause of cell damage, due to their ability to induce apoptosis, which promotes hepatocyte death [6].

Circulating FFA constitute 60% of body fat and correlate with the severity of NAFLD. A lipidomic analysis by Puri et al. showed that despite the increased hepatic lipid content, FFA levels were not altered and found high concentrations of triacylglycerol and diacylglycerol with an increase in saturated FFA, which are more hepatotoxic [7]. Other lipid abnormalities such as increased free cholesterol and reduced phosphatidylcholine are also involved [7].

The oxidation of FFA within hepatocytes is the main source of reactive oxygen species (ROS). When ROS production exceeds the antioxidant capacity of the cell this causes mitochondrial and nuclear DNA damage, disruption of the phospholipid membrane and the release of proinflammatory cytokines and toxic products that perpetuate the damage, causing cell death. Some of these products activate fibrogenic hepatic stellate cells and this continues the inflammatory process [8].

Different cytokines and adipokines, in addition to genetic factors, participate in the pathogenesis of NAFLD. Tumour necrosis factor (TNF-α) is a proinflammatory cytokine that is induced, in part by FFA, and, experimentally, seems to promote hepatic lipotoxicity [9]. Patients with NASH have higher levels of TNF-α than those with isolated steatosis, possibly caused by increased intestinal permeability that allows a high level of endotoxins in the systemic and portal circulation [10]. The imbalance in the inflammatory pathway mediated by TNF-α is important in the transition from NASH to hepatocellular carcinoma.

Adiponectin, an adipokine with anti-inflammatory, insulin-sensitizing, and antifibrotic properties, is reduced in patients with NASH and those with visceral obesity and insulin resistance. It exercises a hepatoprotective effect through inactivation of TNF-α synthesis.

Leptin, a hormone that regulates appetite and fat metabolism through the CNS, has a proinflammatory effect and stimulates adipocyte production of TNF-α. In animal models of fibrotic or fatty liver, it behaves as a profibrotic cytokine, while in humans with NAFLD it correlates with the severity of liver fibrosis, regardless of the degree of insulin resistance and the BMI [2, 11]. In patients with hypopituitarism and GHD, leptin levels are higher than those corresponding to their obesity [12].

5. Insulin Resistance and Hormone Deficiencies

Insulin resistance is closely linked to visceral obesity and metabolic syndrome and is clearly accepted as the central axis of the pathogenesis of NAFLD in the context of type 2 DM [13, 14]. The main metabolic changes that establish a relationship between hypopituitarism and cirrhosis are insulin resistance, the accumulation of hepatic triglycerides, and increased oxidative stress. In addition, GHD, insulin-like growth factor 1 (IGF-1) and other factors such as gonadotropins or cortisol are also involved [15].

In physiological conditions, insulin suppresses lipolysis and glucose production and promotes lipogenesis and the uptake, utilization, and storage of glucose [16]. Insulin resistance favours the mobilization and deposition of fatty acids outside the adipose tissue, reduces the inhibition of lipolysis, and increases de novo hepatic lipogenesis [17]. It increases the hepatic expression of fatty acid transport proteins and their reesterification [18] and produces alterations in the insulin receptor and the GLUT 4 transporter and in the phosphorylation of both substrates and insulin receptors. This increases oxidative stress, mitochondrial toxicity, and the dysregulation of adipokines with subsequent inflammation and, finally, fibrosis [19].

GH and insulin-like growth factor 1 (IGF-1) appear to play an important role in the regulation of hepatic lipid metabolism [20]. The mechanism by which their deficiency contributes to hepatic steatosis and fibrosis is not fully known. Reductions in or an absence of GH secretion in the anterior pituitary gland may cause a reduction in the hepatic secretion of IGF-1, which is secreted by the hepatocytes after stimulation by GH. IGF-1 is a catabolic hormone that plays an important role in protein synthesis and also stimulates IGFBP-3 secretion by the Kupffer cells. It has antifibrotic, cell-protective, insulin-like effects. Therefore, absence of or reduction in IGF-1 secretion would lead to increased hepatic glucose production and favour peripheral insulin resistance [21]. GH promotes lipolysis in adipose tissue and the secretion of very low density lipoproteins by the liver, and therefore low levels of GH promote severe hypertriglyceridemia in the liver [21].

Patients with GHD have greater fat infiltration than those without this deficiency and NAFLD patients have lower levels of GH, although this might reflect a decrease in GH due to obesity. Furthermore, it appears that the level of insulin resistance is higher in patients with GH deficiency than in healthy persons with the same BMI. Studies have found that NAFLD patients have lower serum GH [22] and IFG-1 [23].

Although GH is the major stimulant of IGF-1 synthesis in hepatocytes, other cytokines, such as interleukin 1 beta (IL-1β), TNF-α, and interleukin 6 (IL-6), inhibit IGF-1 secretion [21]. IGF-1 bioactivity is also reduced by high levels of IGFBP1-2, which act primarily by blocking the actions of IGF-1 [24].

The chronic liver disease was due, therefore, to IGF-1 deficiency and GH resistance, because the hepatic response to GH is diminished in the presence of liver disease [25]. Hepatic fibrosis is caused by activation of hepatic stellate cells which are activated by inflammatory cytokines.

Associations have been established between different hormones and NAFLD, although clinical data is scarce and less validated. There is an association between liver steatosis and low testosterone levels, probably due to increased BMI and waist circumference [26]. Testosterone therapy decreases the accumulation of liver fat measured by CT scan [27], while oestrogen appears to protect against the development of NAFLD [28]. Glucocorticoids appear to increase FFA levels and hypothyroidism [29], while low vitamin D levels [30] are associated with the development of NAFLD. Glucagon-like peptide (GLP-1) is secreted by L cells in the small intestine and reduces intrahepatic lipid accumulation via its incretin effect, increasing the secretion of insulin-dependent glucose and a reduction in pancreatic beta cells and the appetite [31].

In patients with hypothalamic and pituitary dysfunction, NAFLD develops relatively rapidly, with a high prevalence of cirrhosis, and is a serious complication in patients with GH, IGF-1, and IGFBP3 deficiencies.

6. Treatment

GH replacement therapy improves the hepatic process and dyslipidaemia and has a protective endothelial effect in patients with GH deficiency, although the effects are minor, probably due to the persistence of GH resistance. It also seems to have a direct or indirect effect on the reduction of hepatic oxidative stress. Furthermore, it reduces levels of C-reactive protein (CRP) and TNF-α, which play an important role in inflammation and insulin resistance [20, 21].

IGF1 overexpression or supplementation attenuates fibrogenesis in mouse models. It improves hepatocellular function, promotes liver regeneration, reduces oxidative damage increases albumin, and has protective effects on the endothelium and vascular cells. It also has extrahepatic effects such as increased food intake, muscle mass, bone density, and gonadal function. Treatment with recombinant human IGF-1, which seems to reverse fibrotic effects, is beginning to be used in patients with cirrhosis, although further studies on its use are required [24, 32].

Other treatments aimed at treating NASH are those used in the treatment of the components of the metabolic syndrome: hypertension, obesity, dyslipidaemia, and insulin resistance. Novel treatments such as caspase inhibition, agonism/antagonism of the adenosine system, PPAR alpha and delta, peripheral cannabinoid 1 receptor agonism, farnesoid x receptor agonism, monoclonal antibodies to TNF-α, thyroid hormones analogues, and enzymatic modulation are under investigation [33].

Our patient had a GH deficiency, among others, in the context of hypopituitarism with abdominal obesity. Insulin resistance and hormonal deficiencies contributed to the rapid development of cirrhosis, which improved with replacement therapy.

References

[1] K. Nakajima, E. Hashimoto, H. Kaneda et al., "Pediatric nonalcoholic steatohepatitis associated with hypopituitarism," *Journal of Gastroenterology*, vol. 40, no. 3, pp. 312–315, 2005.

[2] L. A. Adams, A. Feldstein, K. D. Lindor, and P. Angulo, "Nonalcoholic fatty liver disease among patients with hypothalamic and pituitary dysfunction," *Hepatology*, vol. 39, no. 4, pp. 909–914, 2004.

[3] A. Nyunt, N. Kochar, D. T. Pilz, J. G. C. Kingham, and M. K. Jones, "Adult cirrhosis due to untreated congenital hypopituitarism," *Journal of the Royal Society of Medicine*, vol. 98, no. 7, pp. 316–317, 2005.

[4] R. S. Ahima, "The natural history of nonalcoholic fatty liver disease: insights from children and mice," *Gastroenterology*, vol. 135, no. 6, pp. 1860–1862, 2008.

[5] P. M. Gholam, L. Flancbaum, J. T. Machan, D. A. Charney, and D. P. Kotler, "Nonalcoholic fatty liver disease in severely obese subjects," *The American Journal of Gastroenterology*, vol. 102, no. 2, pp. 399–408, 2007.

[6] A. E. Feldstein, A. Canbay, M. E. Guicciardi, H. Higuchi, S. F. Bronk, and G. J. Gores, "Diet associated hepatic steatosis sensitizes to Fas mediated liver injury in mice," *Journal of Hepatology*, vol. 39, no. 6, pp. 978–983, 2003.

[7] P. Puri, R. A. Baillie, M. M. Wiest et al., "A lipidomic analysis of nonalcoholic fatty liver disease," *Hepatology*, vol. 46, no. 4, pp. 1081–1090, 2007.

[8] J. D. Browning and J. D. Horton, "Molecular mediators of hepatic steatosis and liver injury," *The Journal of Clinical Investigation*, vol. 114, no. 2, pp. 147–152, 2004.

[9] A. E. Feldstein, N. W. Werneburg, A. Canbay et al., "Free fatty acids promote hepatic lipotoxicity by stimulating TNF-α expression via a lysosomal pathway," *Hepatology*, vol. 40, no. 1, pp. 185–194, 2004.

[10] J. Crespo, A. Cayón, P. Fernández-Gil et al., "Gene expression of tumor necrosis factor α and TNF-receptors, p55 and p75, in nonalcoholic steatohepatitis patients," *Hepatology*, vol. 34, no. 6, pp. 1158–1163, 2001.

[11] K. Ikejima, Y. Takei, H. Honda et al., "Leptin receptor-mediated signaling regulates hepatic fibrogenesis and remodeling of extracellular matrix in the rat," *Gastroenterology*, vol. 122, no. 5, pp. 1399–1410, 2002.

[12] K. A. S. Al-Shoumer, V. Anyaoku, W. Richmond, and D. G. Johnston, "Elevated leptin concentrations in growth hormone-deficient hypopituitary adults," *Clinical Endocrinology*, vol. 47, no. 2, pp. 153–159, 1997.

[13] H. C. Masuoka and N. Chalasani, "Nonalcoholic fatty liver disease: an emerging threat to obese and diabetic individuals," *Annals of the New York Academy of Sciences*, vol. 1281, no. 1, pp. 106–122, 2013.

[14] I. Doycheva, N. Patel, M. Peterson, and R. Loomba, "Prognostic implication of liver histology in patients with nonalcoholic fatty liver disease in diabetes," *Journal of Diabetes and Its Complications*, vol. 27, no. 3, pp. 293–300, 2013.

[15] Y. Takahashi, K. Iida, K. Takahashi et al., "Growth hormone reverses nonalcoholic steatohepatitis in a patient with adult growth hormone deficiency," *Gastroenterology*, vol. 132, no. 3, pp. 938–943, 2007.

[16] A. R. Saltiel and C. R. Kahn, "Insulin signalling and the regulation of glucose and lipid metabolism," *Nature*, vol. 414, no. 6865, pp. 799–806, 2001.

[17] K. M. Utzschneider and S. E. Kahn, "The role of insulin resistance in nonalcoholic fatty liver disease," *The Journal of Clinical Endocrinology & Metabolism*, vol. 91, pp. 4753–4761, 2006.

[18] M. E. Miquilena-Colina, E. Lima-Cabello, S. Sánchez-Campos et al., "Hepatic fatty acid translocase CD36 upregulation is associated with insulin resistance, hyperinsulinaemia and increased steatosis in non-alcoholic steatohepatitis and chronic hepatitis C," *Gut*, vol. 60, no. 10, pp. 1394–1402, 2011.

[19] A. J. Sanyal, C. Campbell-Sargent, F. Mirshahi et al., "Nonalcoholic steatohepatitis: association of insulin resistance and mitochondrial abnormalities," *Gastroenterology*, vol. 120, no. 5, pp. 1183–1192, 2001.

[20] Y. Takahashi, "Essential roles of growth hormone (GH) and insulin-like growth factor-I (IGF-I) in the liver," *Endocrine Journal*, vol. 59, no. 11, pp. 955–962, 2012.

[21] T. Ichikawa, K. Nakao, K. Hamasaki et al., "Role of growth hormone, insulin-like growth factor 1 and insulin-like growth factor-binding protein 3 in development of non-alcoholic fatty liver disease," *Hepatology International*, vol. 1, no. 2, pp. 287–294, 2007.

[22] L. Xu, C. Xu, C. Yu et al., "Association between serum growth hormone levels and nonalcoholic fatty liver disease: a cross-sectional Study," *PLoS ONE*, vol. 7, no. 8, Article ID e44136, 2012.

[23] A. Fusco, L. Miele, A. D'Uonnolo et al., "Nonalcoholic fatty liver disease is associated with increased GHBP and reduced GH/IGF-I levels," *Clinical Endocrinology*, vol. 77, no. 4, pp. 531–536, 2012.

[24] K. Bonefeld and S. Møller, "Insulin-like growth factor-I and the liver," *Liver International*, vol. 31, no. 7, pp. 911–919, 2011.

[25] A. Lonardo, P. Loria, F. Leonardi, D. Ganazzi, and N. Carulli, "Growth hormone plasma levels in nonalcoholic fatty liver disease," *American Journal of Gastroenterology*, vol. 97, no. 4, pp. 1071–1072, 2002.

[26] S. Kim, H. Kwon, J.-H. Park et al., "A low level of serum total testosterone is independently associated with nonalcoholic fatty liver disease," *BMC Gastroenterology*, vol. 12, article 69, 2012.

[27] C. M. Hoyos, B. J. Yee, C. L. Phillips, E. A. Machan, R. R. Grunstein, and P. Y. Liu, "Body compositional and cardiometabolic effects of testosterone therapy in obese men with severe obstructive sleep apnoea: a randomised placebo-controlled trial," *European Journal of Endocrinology*, vol. 167, no. 4, pp. 531–541, 2012.

[28] G.-X. Tian, Y. Sun, C.-J. Pang et al., "Oestradiol is a protective factor for non-alcoholic fatty liver disease in healthy men," *Obesity Reviews*, vol. 13, no. 4, pp. 381–387, 2012.

[29] T. Ittermann, R. Haring, H. Wallaschofski et al., "Inverse association between serum free thyroxine levels and hepatic steatosis: results from the study of health in pomerania," *Thyroid*, vol. 22, no. 6, pp. 568–574, 2012.

[30] E.-J. Rhee, M. K. Kim, S. E. Park et al., "High serum vitamin D levels reduce the risk for nonalcoholic fatty liver disease in healthy men independent of metabolic syndrome," *Endocrine Journal*, vol. 60, no. 6, pp. 743–752, 2013.

[31] J. E. Mells, P. P. Fu, S. Sharma et al., "Glp-1 analog, liraglu-
tide, ameliorates hepatic steatosis and cardiac hypertrophy
in C57BL/6J mice fed a western diet," *American Journal of
Physiology—Gastrointestinal and Liver Physiology*, vol. 302, no.
2, pp. G225–G235, 2012.

[32] M. Conchillo, R. J. de Knegt, M. Payeras et al., "Insulin-like
growth factor I (IGF-I) replacement therapy increases albumin
concentration in liver cirrhosis: results of a pilot randomized
controlled clinical trial," *Journal of Hepatology*, vol. 43, no. 4,
pp. 630–636, 2005.

[33] A. Federico, C. Zulli, I. de Sio et al., "Focus on emerging
drugs for the treatment of patients with non-alcoholic fatty liver
disease," *World Journal of Gastroenterology*, vol. 20, no. 45, pp.
16841–16857, 2014.

53

A Large Isolated Hydatid Cyst of the Adrenal Gland: A Case Report and Review of the Literature

Fatehi Elnour Elzein,[1] Abdullah Aljaberi,[1] Abdullah AlFiaar,[2] and Abdullah Alghamdi[3]

[1]Division of Infectious Diseases, Department of Medicine, Prince Sultan Military Medical City, Riyadh 11159, Saudi Arabia
[2]Histopathology Department, Prince Sultan Military Medical City, Riyadh 11159, Saudi Arabia
[3]Urology Department, Prince Sultan Military Medical City, Riyadh 11159, Saudi Arabia

Correspondence should be addressed to Fatehi Elnour Elzein; fatehielzein@yahoo.com

Academic Editor: John Broom

A 44-year-old patient presented with two-year history of (R) lumbar pain. There was a strong history of childhood animals' contact, including dogs. A brother had multiple hydatid cysts requiring surgery. Initial ultrasound showed a large (R) adrenal mass measuring $10 \times 9 \times 8$ cm. Subsequent CT scan confirmed a heavily calcified cyst in the (R) adrenal gland. Hormonal studies were normal. He had an uneventful course following a total adrenalectomy. Isolated adrenal hydatid is extremely rare with an incidence of less than 0.5%; however, the diagnosis should always be suspected in all patients from an endemic area presenting with an adrenal cystic mass.

1. Introduction

Hydatid disease is a zoonotic infection caused by the parasite *Echinococcus granulosus*. Dogs are the principal definitive host while sheep are the most common intermediate one. Individuals get accidentally infected by ingesting the worm's eggs in contaminated food and water, or through close association with domestic dogs. Larvae producing cysts commonly involve the liver, the lungs, and the kidneys. The liver is involved in almost 70% of the cases. Larvae that escape filtration by the liver involve the lungs in 25% of the patients [1]. The disease is distributed throughout the world; it is endemic in the Mediterranean, Eastern Europe, the Middle East, South America, Australia, and South Africa region. Hence, echinococcal infestation should be suspected in any patients from these areas especially in the farming and pastoral locations. Overall adrenal cysts are rare, with a reported autopsy incidence of 0.073% [2], often presenting with broad clinical and radiologic findings, and are thus underrecognized. Occasionally malignant neoplasms greatly mimic benign cysts. As an illustration, only 2 cases (6%) of malignant neoplasms were detected among 31 cystic adrenal lesions diagnosed over a 20-year period (1 epithelioid angiosarcoma and 1 adrenocortical carcinoma) [3]. For this reason, differentiation of cystic adrenal hydatid from other adrenal cysts and adrenal solid tumors with cystic change presents a diagnostic challenge on imaging alone. This is particularly difficult in large sized cysts. One study showed that 1.2% of lesions are malignant, and all exceeded 5 cm [4]. Hydatid cysts account for only 6%-7% of all adrenal cysts. On the other hand, isolated adrenal hydatid cyst constitutes less than 1% of overall hydatid cases [5].

2. Case Report

A 44-years-old man was seen in the clinic for recurrent (R) flank pain of 2-year duration. Ultrasound and subsequent CT scan performed 2 years ago showed a (R) suprarenal mass. He denied a history of hypertension, palpitations, or syncopal attacks. Serum cortisol, ACTH, metanephrine, and normetanephrine were normal at 201 nmol/L, 2.8 pmol/L (NR 1.6–13.90), 29 ng/L (NR < 90), and 92.0 ng/L (NR < 129), sequentially. Similarly, aldosterone and renin levels were normal with aldosterone/renin ratio of 3.6. Serum

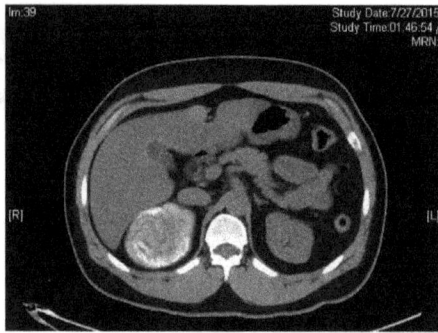

FIGURE 1: CT scan abdomen showing (R) adrenal mass.

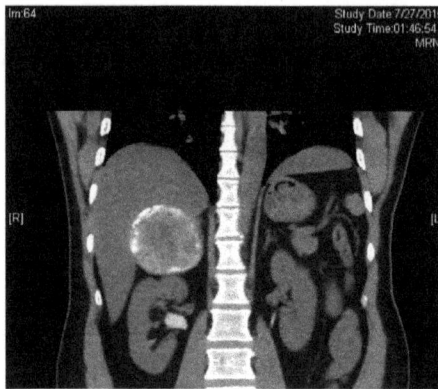

FIGURE 2: CT scan showing (R) adrenal mass with calcification.

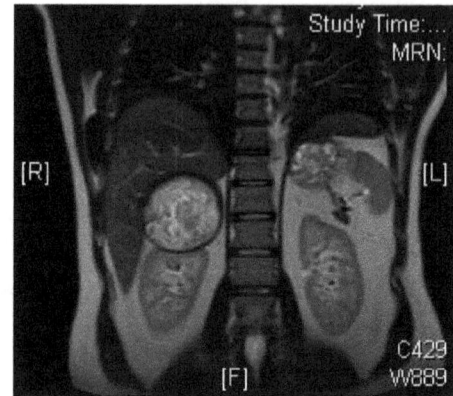

FIGURE 3: MRI with R adrenal mass.

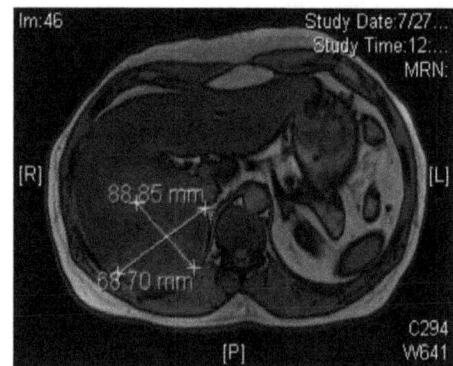

FIGURE 4: MRI (R) adrenal mass 88 × 68 mm.

testosterone and dehydroepiandrosterone sulphate were also normal, at 5.94 nmol/L and 3.61 μmol/L successively. He was labeled as a nonfunctioning (R) adrenal mass. He later admitted to a strong history of childhood contact with animals including dogs. His elder brother was operated for multiple hydatid cysts in the abdomen. There were no urinary or other systemic symptoms. General examination including the blood pressure was normal apart from mild tenderness in the (R) renal angle. CT scan abdomen in July 2015 showed a large well-defined oval shaped heavily calcified cystic mass at the right adrenal gland, measuring 8.5 × 6.6 cm on transverse and AP diameter, respectively (Figures 1 and 2). MRI confirmed the CT finding. The mass depicts low T1 and heterogeneous high T2 signal intensity with internal stripes in T2 resembling water lily sign but showed no enhancement. It is surrounded with thin rim of dark T2 signal likely representing calcification (Figures 3 and 4). There was a mass effect on the upper pole of the right kidney and in some areas it appears inseparable from segment VI of the liver. The radiological features were consistent with hydatid cyst. IHA for hydatid was negative at 1 : 80. He was started on albendazole (400 mg twice daily) and praziquantel 600 mg weekly, for four weeks prior to surgery. In view of the persistent loin pain and the large cysts (≥5 cm diameter), he underwent (R) adrenalectomy through a right subcostal incision without spillage of the cyst content. The patient tolerated the procedure well with uneventful postoperative course. Macroscopic appearance showed well circumscribed

cystic lesion measuring 10 × 8 × 4.5 cm (Figure 5) with focal multiloculated appearance. Histopathology revealed dense fibrous capsule with three layers showing a middle layer with characteristic lamination pattern and focal calcification. The cyst content is a lightly dense proteinaceous, with a jelly-like matrix material (Figures 6, 7, and 8). No scolices or hooks were seen and no associated granulomas or neoplasia. The histological features were consistent with hydatid cyst. He was finally discharged on albendazole 400 mg BD for another four weeks.

3. Discussion

Hydatid cyst involving the adrenals is rare and is usually a part of a generalized Echinococcosis. It is frequently discovered incidentally. Furthermore and similar to our patient, abdominal pain resulting from organ compression can be a presenting feature [6]. In very rare cases hypertension that subsides with resection of the cyst had mimicked a phaeochromocytoma [7]. The radiological findings in our patient are highly suggestive of hydatid disease despite a negative serology. The presence of solid mass and dense calcification is similar to a type 5 hepatic cyst. WHO classifies hydatid cyst into type 1 with a well-defined, anechoic lesion; type 2 demonstrates the separation of the membrane (the "water lily" sign formed by the undulating membrane); type

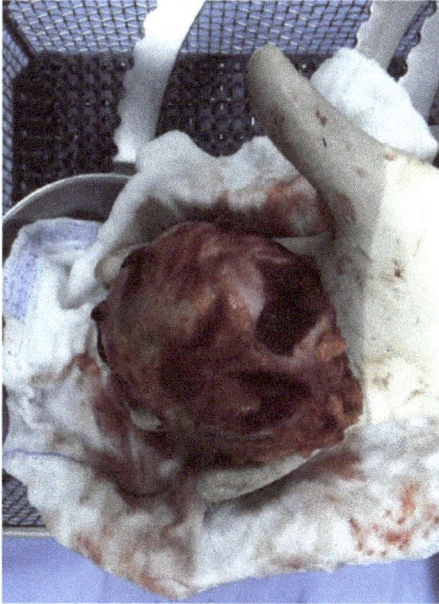

FIGURE 5: Gross pathology of the resected adrenal gland.

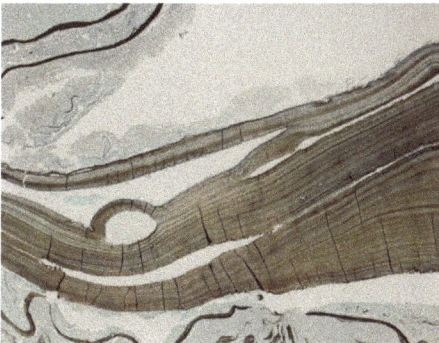

FIGURE 6: Microscopic image showing characteristic laminated pattern of cyst membrane (GMC stain magnification ×40).

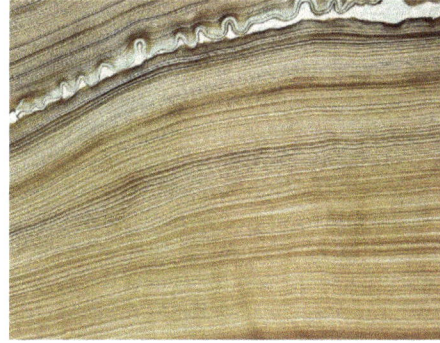

FIGURE 7: Microscopic image showing characteristic laminated pattern of the cyst membrane (GMC stain magnification ×200).

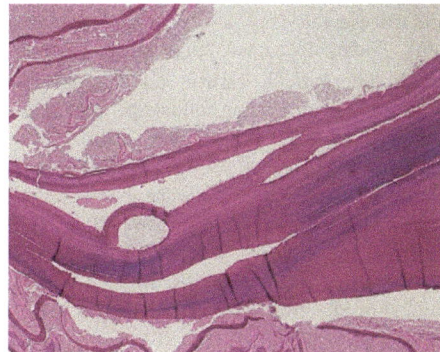

FIGURE 8: Laminated middle layer of the capsule (PAS stain).

3 is characterized by the presence of septa and intraluminal daughter cysts. Type 4 is a nonspecific solid mass while type 5 is characterized by a solid cyst with a calcified wall [8].

Although serology is useful in the diagnosis of hydatid disease, a number of patients may have a negative test. In some series 30–40% of patients with hepatic cystic echinococcosis are antibody negative. This could be due to the capacity of E. granulosus antigens to inhibit B cell activity and proliferation [9]. In general, the sensitivity of the serological tests is determined by the location and state of the cysts [10]. The indirect hemagglutination (IHA) test and ELISA have a sensitivity of 80% overall, (90% in hepatic echinococcosis, 40% in pulmonary echinococcosis). Our patient cyst's calcification adds further to the difficulty in the diagnosis. It has been previously reported that false negative serology ensues when the cyst is senescent, dead, or calcified [11]. Consequently, a negative serology does not exclude the diagnosis.

Hydatid cyst can be asymptomatic and need not any intervention except for doubt in the diagnosis and in large cyst causing mass effect. Treatment of adrenal hydatid, when indicated, is mainly surgical and by total cyst excision. Small asymptomatic nonfunctioning cts are treated conservatively. Total adrenalectomy may be considered when the cyst has completely destroyed the gland. Both laparoscopic resection of an adrenal hydatid and laparotomy are accepted surgical intervention [12]. Laparotomy nonetheless allows a better exploration of the peritoneal cavity. Adjuvant albendazole pre- and postoperatively reduced recurrences in hepatic hydatidosis. Of patients who received albendazole therapy for hydatid disease of the liver, no patient had viable cysts at the time of surgery, as compared to 94.45% of the patients who did not receive any preoperative albendazole ($P <$ 0.01). The recurrence rate without adjuvant albendazole was 16.66% while no recurrence was seen in patients who received albendazole [13]. It may be argued that our patient calcified hydatid cyst might have indicated dead parasites and hence does not require albendazole therapy. However, peripheral calcification has been described previously in both viable and nonviable cysts [14].

This patient's history of childhood contact with animals and the slowly progressive nature of his adrenal mass together with a history of hydatid in his brother are highly suggestive of hydatid disease. The radiological findings are characteristic though not pathognomonic. Both macroscopic and microscopic features are consistent with adrenal hydatid cyst. A caveat to the diagnosis is the absence of the scolices and/or hooks in the histopathology sections, albeit could be focally present within the specimen but not sampled in the tissue sections or on the glass slides.

Overall, isolated hydatid disease of the adrenals is rare. The diagnosis should be suspected in all patients from or who lived in endemic areas. Surgical excision with either laparotomy or laparoscopic approach remains the intervention of choice in such cases. Adjunctive medical treatment improves the outcome and decreases the recurrence rate.

References

[1] I. Pedrosa, A. Saíz, J. Arrazola, J. Ferreirós, and C. S. Pedrosa, "Hydatid disease: radiologic and pathologic features and complications," *Radiographics*, vol. 20, no. 3, pp. 795–817, 2000.

[2] Z. Ricci, V. Chernyak, K. Hsu et al., "Adrenal cysts: natural history by long-term imaging follow-up," *American Journal of Roentgenology*, vol. 201, no. 5, pp. 1009–1016, 2013.

[3] C. Sebastiano, X. Zhao, F.-M. Deng, and K. Das, "Cystic lesions of the adrenal gland: our experience over the last 20 years," *Human Pathology*, vol. 44, no. 9, pp. 1797–1803, 2013.

[4] M. F. Herrera, C. S. Grant, J. A. van Heerden, P. F. Sheedy, and D. M. Ilstrup, "Incidentally discovered adrenal tumors: an institutional perspective," *Surgery*, vol. 110, no. 6, pp. 1014–1021, 1991.

[5] G. Dionigi, G. Carrafiello, C. Recaldini et al., "Laparoscopic resection of a primary hydatid cyst of the adrenal gland: a case report," *Journal of Medical Case Reports*, vol. 1, article 61, 2007.

[6] M. N. Akçay, G. Akçay, A. A. Balik, and A. Böyük, "Hydatid cysts of the adrenal gland: review of nine patients," *World Journal of Surgery*, vol. 28, no. 1, pp. 97–99, 2004.

[7] M. D. Escudero, L. Sabater, J. Calvete, B. Camps, M. Labiós, and S. Liedó, "Arterial hypertension due to primary adrenal hydatid cyst," *Surgery*, vol. 132, no. 5, pp. 894–895, 2002.

[8] WHO Informal Working Group, "International classification of ultrasound images in cystic echinococcosis for application in clinical and field epidemiological settings," *Acta Tropica*, vol. 85, no. 2, pp. 253–261, 2003.

[9] D. O. Griffin, H. J. Donaghy, and B. Edwards, "Management of serology negative human hepatic hydatidosis (caused by echinococcus granulosus) in a young woman from bangladesh in a resource-rich setting: a case report," *IDCases*, vol. 1, no. 2, pp. 17–21, 2014.

[10] S. Kumar, B. Nanjappa, and K. K. Gowda, "Laparoscopic management of a hydatid cyst of the adrenal gland," *Korean Journal of Urology*, vol. 55, no. 7, pp. 493–495, 2014.

[11] A. Christopher and E. C. J. Sanford, *The Travel and Tropical Medicine Manual*, Elsevier Health Sciences: Elsevier Health Sciences, 4th edition, 2008.

[12] T. Defechereux, J. Sauvant, L. Gramatica, M. Puccini, C. De Micco, and J. F. Henry, "Laparoscopic resection of an adrenal hydatid cyst," *European Journal of Surgery*, vol. 166, no. 11, pp. 900–902, 2000.

[13] S. Ul-Bari, S. H. Arif, A. A. Malik, A. R. Khaja, T. A. Dass, and Z. A. Naikoo, "Role of albendazole in the management of hydatid cyst liver," *Saudi Journal of Gastroenterology*, vol. 17, no. 5, pp. 343–347, 2011.

[14] K. J. Mortelé, E. Segatto, and P. R. Ros, "The infected liver: radiologic-pathologic correlation," *Radiographics*, vol. 24, no. 4, pp. 937–955, 2004.

54

Thyroseq V3 Molecular Profiling for Tailoring the Surgical Management of Hürthle Cell Neoplasms

Sarah Pearlstein,[1] **Arash H. Lahouti,**[2] **Elana Opher,**[2]
Yuri E. Nikiforov,[3] **and Daniel B. Kuriloff** ⓘ [4,5]

[1]*Department of Surgery, Lenox Hill Hospital, New York, NY, USA*
[2]*Department of Pathology, Lenox Hill Hospital, New York, NY, USA*
[3]*Department of Pathology, University of Pittsburgh Medical Center, Pittsburgh, PA, USA*
[4]*New York Head & Neck Institute, Lenox Hill Hospital, New York, NY, USA*
[5]*Zucker School of Medicine at Hofstra/Northwell, New York, NY, USA*

Correspondence should be addressed to Daniel B. Kuriloff; dkuriloff@northwell.edu

Academic Editor: Osamu Isozaki

Hürthle cell predominant thyroid nodules often confound the diagnostic utility of fine needle aspiration biopsy (FNAB) with cytology often interpreted as a Hürthle cell lesion with an indeterminate risk of malignancy, Bethesda category (BC) III or IV. Molecular diagnostics for Hürthle cell predominant nodules has also been disappointing in further defining the risk of malignancy. We present a case of a slowly enlarging nodule within a goiter initially reported as benign on FNAB, BC II but on subsequent FNAB suspicious for a Hürthle cell neoplasm, BC IV. The patient had initially requested a diagnostic lobectomy for a definitive diagnosis despite a higher risk of malignancy based on the size of the nodule > 4 cm alone. To better tailor this patient's treatment plan, a newer expanded gene mutation panel, ThyroSeq® v3 that includes copy number alterations (CNAs) and was recently found to have greater positive predictive value (PPV) for identifying Hürthle cell carcinoma (HCC), was performed on the FNAB material. Molecular profiling with ThyroSeq® v3 was able to predict a greater risk of carcinoma, making a more convincing argument in favor of total thyroidectomy. Surgical pathology confirmed a Hürthle cell carcinoma with 5 foci of angioinvasion and foci of capsular invasion.

1. Introduction

Thyroid nodules with a predominance of Hürthle cells often confound the diagnostic utility of fine needle aspiration biopsy with cytology often interpreted as a Hürthle cell lesion with an indeterminate risk of malignancy, Bethesda category III or IV. Molecular diagnostics for Hürthle cell predominant thyroid nodules, with the exception of medullary thyroid carcinoma, has also been disappointing in further defining the risk of malignancy. This diagnostic challenge occurs because Hürthle cells or oncocytic metaplasia is associated with benign nodules (cell-mediated autoimmune thyroiditis, humoral-mediated Graves' disease, and hyperplastic nodules in multinodular goiters (MNG)). Hürthle cells also occur in neoplastic conditions such as Hürthle cell adenoma, Hürthle cell carcinoma, and the oncocytic variant of papillary thyroid carcinoma. Medullary carcinoma, a C-cell derived neoplasm, can also exhibit an oncocytic appearance and is included in the differential diagnosis of Hürthle cell lesions.

Furthermore, different areas within the same nodule may yield very different degrees of Hürthle cell differentiation further confusing the cytologic interpretation. There are additional challenges; a benign Hürthle cell adenoma cannot be distinguished from a HCC without demonstrating either capsular or vascular invasion found after surgical removal on careful histopathologic assessment at multiple levels. The biological behavior of HCC varies and can present either as a minimally invasive or as a widely invasive tumor. Hürthle cell carcinoma may have a more aggressive biological behavior compared with the other well-differentiated thyroid cancers and is associated with a higher rate of distant metastases. Hürthle cell carcinoma often has less radioiodine avidity compared with other well-differentiated thyroid cancers, mandating a more complete thyroidectomy, especially for optimal adjuvant therapy for a subset of tumors with some RAI avidity in the setting of locally aggressive HCC, regional lymph node involvement, or distant metastases [1].

We present a case of a slowly enlarging nodule within a MNG initially reported as benign on FNA cytology BC II but on subsequent FNA cytology interpreted as a Hürthle cell neoplasm or suspicious for a Hürthle cell neoplasm, BC IV. Molecular profiling using ThyroSeq® v2 next-generation gene sequencing [2] revealed an absence of gene mutations or fusions but strong overexpression of the MET gene. Since this finding alone could not reliably predict a HCC, the patient had initially requested a diagnostic lobectomy for a definitive pathologic diagnosis despite a higher risk of malignancy based on the size of the nodule > 4 cm alone. To better tailor this patient's treatment plan, the ThyroSeq® v3 panel, recently found to have greater positive predictive value (PPV) for identifying Hürthle cell malignancies, was performed on the FNA material. Molecular profiling with ThyroSeq® v3 was able to predict a greater risk of HCC, making a more convincing argument in favor of total thyroidectomy. This case report illustrates the important role of molecular diagnostics, specifically, ThyroSeq® v3 in tailoring the often difficult clinical management of Hürthle cell thyroid nodules for optimal surgical treatment.

2. Case Presentation

This patient was a generally healthy 62-year-old male with a left lobe complex nodule within a nontoxic multinodular goiter that had been enlarging for approximately 3 years. In 2015, the patient had a FNAB reported as benign, BC II. Because of continued growth, he had a second FNA biopsy approximately six months later reported as a Hürthle cell neoplasm or suspicious for a Hürthle cell neoplasm, BC IV with Oncocytic / Hürthle cells dispersed mostly singly and in small fragments in a background of lysed blood. CKAE1/AE3, TTF-1, and thyroglobulin immunostains were positive (Figure 1(a)). Molecular testing with ThyroSeq® v2 revealed an absence of gene mutations or fusions but overexpression of the MET gene with an uncertain increased risk of malignancy. After repeat ultrasound imaging, the nodule had grown from 4.9 to 6.0 cm over the course of 1 year. He was euthyroid with negative anti-thyroid antibodies. There was no family history of thyroid cancer or known radiation exposures in his youth. He had no obstructive symptoms despite the size of the mass and denied shortness of breath, dysphagia, neck pain, neck pressure, or recent voice changes. His weight had been stable and appetite good. His past medical history was significant for a retinal detachment, hypertension, and inguinal hernia with a surgical history limited to eye surgery and hernia repair. He denied tobacco or alcohol use. On exam, the patient had an enlarged, firm thyroid gland with the left thyroid lobe causing significant tracheal deviation to the right. A neck CT scan demonstrated a markedly enlarged left thyroid lobe (7.2 cm in sagittal height) causing significant rightward tracheal deviation, minimal tracheal compression, and slight early substernal extension (Figure 2). He had

multiple opinions from both endocrinologists and surgeons with various recommendations from left thyroid lobectomy to total thyroidectomy. The patient had initially contemplated a hemithyroidectomy due to concerns for voice impairment that could impact his occupation as an attorney.

After a second surgical consultation, he elected to have another, more advanced molecular test performed on the same FNAB specimen. The ThyroSeq® v3 test has been designed to improve the performance of its previous version, ThyroSeq v2, specifically with respect to Hürthle cell tumors. This has been achieved by expanding the number of gene markers analyzed for mutations and gene fusions and particularly by incorporating the analysis of copy number alterations (CNAs), which are common in Hürthle cell cancers. ThyroSeq® v3 test results in this case showed CNAs involving multiple chromosomes with the pattern of genome haploidization which predicted a much greater probability that the left lobe nodule represented a Hürthle cell malignancy rather than Hürthle cell metaplasia or an adenoma. Based on the additional information provided by ThyroSeq® v3, in July, 2017, the patient elected a total thyroidectomy. At surgery, the overlying strap muscles were superficially adherent to the thyroid capsule on the left with a suspicion of minimal extrathyroidal extension of the tumor and a layer of muscle was left attached to the specimen. There were no paratracheal lymph nodes. He did require single gland parathyroid autotransplantation. Postoperatively, his parathyroid hormone and calcium levels were within normal limits. On final surgical pathology, an encapsulated 7 cm Hürthle cell carcinoma with 5 foci of angioinvasion was found along with foci of capsular invasion, without extrathyroidal extension (Figure 1(b)). A second opinion was sought and the reviewing pathologist reported 4 foci of capsular invasion and 3 foci of vascular invasion. The number of foci of vascular invasion was prognostically important and prompted more aggressive treatment and follow-up.

One month postoperatively, thyroglobulin was 308 ng/mL. A small thyroid remnant with 2.4% uptake in the surgical bed was found on I-131 whole body scan. An FDG-PET scan was negative for any activity in the thyroidectomy bed or for distant metastatic disease; therefore he was given 30 mCi of radioactive iodine to ablate the remnant. At this time, his thyroglobulin had decreased from 308 to 8.71 ng/mL. His postablation, I-131 whole body scan showed ablation of the thyroid remnant and no evidence of metastatic disease. By 10/27/2017, the thyroglobulin had decreased further to 0.2 ng/mL with no detectable thyroglobulin antibodies and a TSH of 0.09 uIU/ml indicating a favorable early response to initial treatment.

3. Discussion

In the past, cytologic assessment, with or without molecular profiling, of Hürthle cell nodules failed to accurately predict the risk of HCC. The presence of Hürthle or oncocytic cells in cytologic specimens from FNA samples is often seen in a wide range of thyroid pathologies, the majority of which are benign. The finding of predominance of Hürthle cells is usually interpreted as suspicious for a follicular neoplasm,

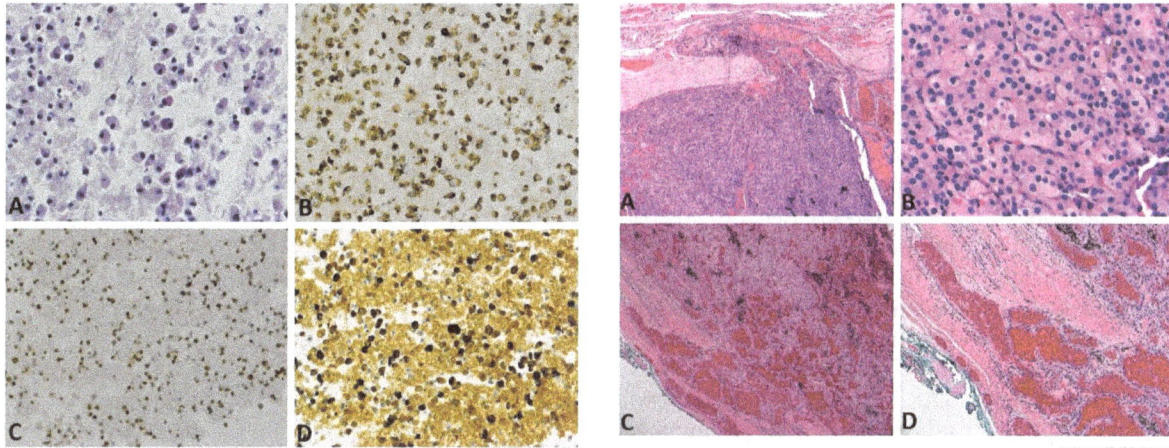

(a) FNA diagnosis: Hürthle cell neoplasm or suspicious for a Hürthle cell neoplasm, Bethesda Category IV. The aspirate shows predominantly single cells, many with degenerated friable cytoplasm, imparting a pseudo-necrotic background (A). The cells have abundant granular eosinophilic cytoplasm with eccentric and slightly enlarged nuclei, giving a plasmacytoid appearance (ThinPrep, Papanicolaou x 40). The neoplastic cells stain with pankeratin AE1/AE3 (B), TTF-1 (C), and thyroglobulin (D), confirming their thyroid follicular origin and excluding medullary carcinoma or histiocytes

(b) Invasive, follicular carcinoma, oncocytic (Hürthle cell) variant. The tumor shows a trabecular/solid architecture (A), composed of large, polygonal cells with abundant granular eosinophilic cytoplasm. The cells have round to slightly irregular nuclei with prominent centrally placed nucleoli (B). Foci of capsular (A) and vascular invasion are identified (C, D)

FIGURE 1

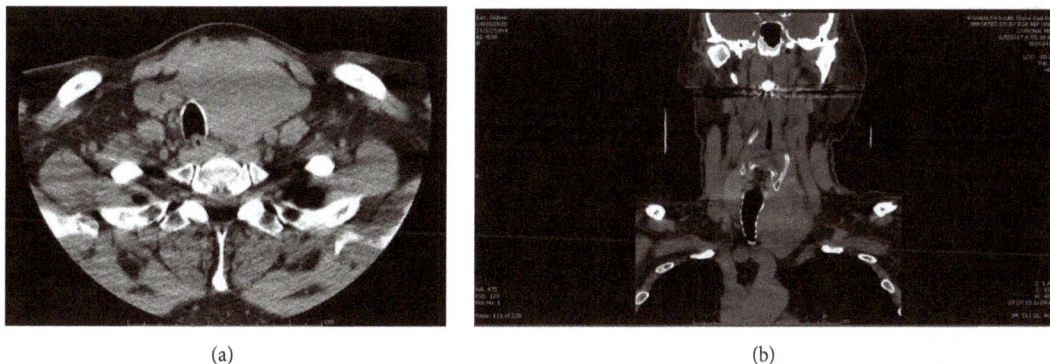

(a)   (b)

FIGURE 2: Preoperative neck CT without contrast, demonstrating a large left thyroid lobe mass with displacement of the trachea, mild compression, and early substernal extension; representative axial (a) and coronal views (b).

Hürthle cell type, BC IV, conferring a positive predictive value (PPV) for malignancy of approximately 15-30%. The high frequency of nonneoplastic Hürthle cell proliferation in patients with Hashimoto's thyroiditis can be a diagnostic dilemma for the cytopathologist [3]. With the advent of molecular profiling, the hope was to minimize the need for diagnostic thyroid lobectomy for benign nodules, for tumor prognostication to tailor the extent of thyroid surgery for optimal cure and to prevent tumor recurrence. The Afirma® Gene Expression Classifier developed by Veracyte, Inc. (South San Francisco, CA) has been shown to have a high negative predictive value (NPV) for most benign thyroid nodules but with a poor PPV for malignancy and renders a large number of FNA samples with various proportions of nonneoplastic Hürthle cells as suspicious for malignancy, thus triaging most of these patients to thyroid surgery [4].

ThyroSeq is a multigene next-generation sequencing-based test for thyroid nodules. The early version, ThyroSeq v2, utilized the analysis of 56 genes predominantly for point mutations and gene fusions, as well as for limited gene expression alterations [2]. The expanded version of the test, ThyroSeq v3, interrogated 112 genes and is based not only on the analysis of point mutations, gene fusions, and gene expression alterations, but also on copy number alterations (CNAs) [5]. The latter is particularly important for predicting Hürthle cell carcinomas, which are known to have a characteristic pattern of CNAs with almost complete genome haploidization [6]. Taking advantage of the analysis of CNAs, in the validation study, ThyroSeq v3 showed reliable performance in Hürthle cell cancers, offering 93% sensitivity and 69% specificity [5]. In a preliminary report from a recent multicenter study which included 10 Hürthle cell carcinomas,

34 Hürthle cell adenomas, and 5 hyperplastic nodules with Hürthle cell predominance, the performance of ThyroSeq® v3 allowed for the detection of all HCCs (sensitivity, 100%; 95%CI: 69.2- 100%), with all 5 hyperplastic nodules with Hürthle cell predominance classified as negative and overall test specificity of 66.7% (95%CI: 49.8-80.9%) [7].

In an era of patient-guided decision-making and the ability to tailor the extent of surgery based on preoperative FNA biopsy prognostication, molecular profiling of thyroid nodules has become increasingly utilized. Despite the limitations of molecular testing and the variance in both PPV and NPV with a varying prevalence of malignancy in different populations, its utility in selecting patients for active surveillance, thyroid lobectomy, and total thyroidectomy will likely increase, especially as their overall accuracy improves over time. The particular advantages of ThyroSeq® v3 over ThyroSeq® v2 in guiding the extent of thyroid surgery for indeterminate Hürthle cell cytopathology are illustrated by this case report and helped tailor the best treatment for this patient with a Hürthle cell carcinoma who would otherwise have likely needed a completion thyroidectomy.

References

[1] S. Ahmadi, M. Stang, X. S. Jiang, and J. A. Sosa, "Hürthle cell carcinoma: Current perspectives," *OncoTargets and Therapy*, vol. 9, pp. 6873–6884, 2016.

[2] Y. E. Nikiforov, S. E. Carty, S. I. Chiosea et al., "Highly accurate diagnosis of cancer in thyroid nodules with follicular neoplasm/suspicious for a follicular neoplasm cytology by thyroseq V2 next-generation sequencing assay," *Cancer*, vol. 120, no. 23, pp. 3627–3634, 2014.

[3] M. H. Roh, V. Y. Jo, E. B. Stelow et al., "The predictive value of the fine-needle aspiration diagnosis "Suspicious for a follicular neoplasm, Hürthle cell type" in patients with Hashimoto thyroiditis," *American Journal of Clinical Pathology*, vol. 135, no. 1, pp. 139–145, 2011.

[4] E. Brauner, B. J. Holmes, J. F. Krane et al., "Performance of the Afirma Gene Expression Classifier in Hürthle Cell Thyroid Nodules Differs from Other Indeterminate Thyroid Nodules," *Thyroid*, vol. 25, no. 7, pp. 789–796, 2015.

[5] M. N. Nikiforova, S. Mercurio, A. I. Wald et al., "Analytical performance of the ThyroSeq v3 genomic classifier for cancer diagnosis in thyroid nodules," *Cancer*, vol. 124, no. 8, pp. 1682–1690, 2018.

[6] W. E. Corver, D. Ruano, K. Weijers et al., "Genome haploidisation with chromosome 7 retention in oncocytic follicular thyroid carcinoma," *PLoS ONE*, vol. 7, no. 6, Article ID e38287, 2012.

[7] L. David, E. Steward Sally, S. Rebecca et al., *Clinical Validation of ThyroSeq v3® Performance in Thyroid Nodules with Indeterminate Cytology: A Prospective Blinded Multi-Institutional Validation Study. Presented at the 87th Annual American Thyroid Association Meeting*, 2017.

55

Effect of Intranasal Calcitonin in a Patient with McCune-Albright Syndrome, Fibrous Dysplasia, and Refractory Bone Pain

Tayane Muniz Fighera[1] and Poli Mara Spritzer[1,2]

[1]Gynecological Endocrinology Unit, Division of Endocrinology, Hospital de Clinicas de Porto Alegre,
 Rua Ramiro Barcelos 2350, 90035-003 Porto Alegre, RS, Brazil
[2]Laboratory of Molecular Endocrinology, Department of Physiology, Federal University of Rio Grande do Sul,
 Rua Ramiro Barcelos 2350, 90035-003 Porto Alegre, RS, Brazil

Correspondence should be addressed to Poli Mara Spritzer; spritzer@ufrgs.br

Academic Editor: Mihail A. Boyanov

McCune-Albright syndrome (MAS) is a rare disease defined by the triad of polyostotic fibrous dysplasia of bone, café-au-lait skin spots, and precocious puberty. No available treatment is effective in changing the course of fibrous dysplasia of bone, but symptomatic patients require therapeutic support to reduce bone pain and prevent fractures and deformities. We report the case of a 27-year-old woman with MAS and severe fibrous dysplasia. She was diagnosed with MAS at 4 years of age and, during follow-up, she had multiple pathological fractures and bone pain refractory to treatment with bisphosphonates, tricyclic antidepressants, and opioids. The pain was incapacitating and the patient required a wheelchair. Intranasal calcitonin was then started, and, 30 days later, the patient already showed significant improvement in pain severity at the affected sites. After 3 months, she was able to walk without assistance. No adverse effects were observed, nor were any significant changes in serum levels of calcium, phosphorus, and alkaline phosphatase. Calcitonin has a well-recognized analgesic effect on bone tissue. Despite the small number of studies involving patients with MAS, calcitonin may be considered a short-term therapeutic option in cases of severe and refractory bone pain.

1. Introduction

McCune-Albright syndrome (MAS) is classically defined by the presence of fibrous dysplasia (FD), *café-au-lait* skin pigmentation, and precocious puberty. Other hyperfunctioning endocrinopathies may be involved, including hyperthyroidism, growth hormone excess, Cushing syndrome, and renal phosphate wasting. MAS has an estimated prevalence ranging from 1/100.000 to 1/1000.000, affects both sexes equally, and is generally diagnosed in children and young adults [1].

Patients with MAS have involvement of multiple bone sites (polyostotic FD) that is usually established early in life [2]. FD occurs when bone marrow cells are affected by somatic activating mutations of the gene encoding the α-subunit of the stimulatory G protein (Gs α). The mutation results in locally increased stimulation of adenylyl cyclase and cAMP overproduction, leading to autonomic secretion in endocrine tissues. At the bone tissue level, FD is characterized by dysplastic lesions consisting of abnormal and poorly organized fibrous tissue, with a lytic or cystic appearance [3]. The natural course of bone disease is highly variable. Lesions can remain stable for decades, but they can also progress to multiple fractures and severe bone pain and deformities, which can be extremely debilitating [1, 2].

Clinical studies on FD are difficult because this condition is rare and clinically heterogeneous. There are no available medical therapies capable of altering the disease course. Recently, a multidisciplinary workshop, including patients, clinicians, and researchers, discussed the priorities of diagnosis and treatment of patients with FD and MAS. Among these priorities is the management of chronic pain with typical and atypical analgesics as well as adjuvant interventions when necessary [4]. The primary target of treatment may be the relief of bone pain and reduction of fracture risk and deformity. Intravenous bisphosphonates, such as zoledronic acid and pamidronate, may be effective in reducing bone pain and bone resorption as well as in improving the radiographic appearance of lytic lesions. Calcium and vitamin D supplementation may also be considered [5]. However, some patients have poor response to available therapies.

We report here a case of MAS presenting severe FD and refractory bone pain and the effect of short-term treatment with intranasal calcitonin, highlighting the challenges of the management of this uncommon clinical presentation.

2. Case Presentation

A 4-year-and-8-month-old girl was referred to the endocrinology outpatient clinic in 1993 for evaluation of bilateral development of breast tissue followed by vaginal bleeding lasting 5 days. After 2 months, she had another episode of vaginal bleeding, with duration similar to that of the first episode. She was born from vaginal delivery at term, weighed 2,350 kg, and had adequate motor and cognitive development. She used no continuous medication. On physical examination, the patient had a weight of 15,5 kg (p25), height of 1,02 m (p25), Tanner stage M1P1, and absence of café-au-lait skin pigmentation. Bone age was compatible with chronological age. Pelvic ultrasound showed uterus with 3.2 cc, endometrium of 0.2 cm, right ovary with a volume of 0.5 cc, and left ovary with a cyst measuring 1.5×2.3 cm. Laboratory tests showed estradiol 18.3 pmol/L, LH 1.70 IU/L, FSH 2.10 IU/L, prolactin 15 μg/L, cortisol 400 nmol/L, TSH 1.3 mIU/L, and a prepubertal response to GnRH test. An initial diagnosis of autonomous ovarian follicular cyst was then made and the patient was kept on regular clinical follow-up with expectant management. After 7 months of follow-up, progression of premature thelarche (M2P1) was observed, with serum estradiol levels 38.2 pmol/L and normal prepubertal gonadotropin levels. Bone scintigraphy showed increased radioisotope concentration in the humerus, femur, tibia, and maxilla on the right side. Bone densitometry showed adequate bone mineral density (BMD) for age. The 24 h urine analysis showed a tubular phosphorus reabsorption rate of 88%, with phosphaturia of 16.9 mmol/24 h. Due to the presence of precocious puberty and FD, the patient was diagnosed with MAS.

At that time, letrozole was not yet available in the country and suppressive therapy was started with 200 mg of intramuscular medroxyprogesterone every 3 weeks, with regression of breast tissue. A bone age X-ray performed at follow-up was compatible with chronological age. No increase in ovarian volume was detected on pelvic ultrasound. She had menarche at age 11, with irregular cycles and facial acne that improved with oral contraceptives. At age 14, due to bone pain in the right thigh and radiographic evidence of

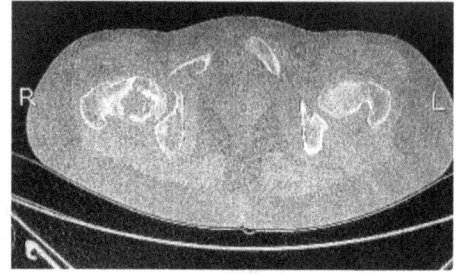

FIGURE 1: Computed tomography at age 17. Osteolytic lesions and areas of "ground-glass" opacity in the right femur.

cysts, the patient started receiving a treatment protocol with intravenous pamidronate every 6 months, 40 mg/day for 3 consecutive days, for five cycles. The dose was not increased because of patient intolerance to medication. Over the follow-up period, vitamin D levels were monitored and supplementation provided if necessary. Treatment response was assessed by subjective pain intensity, alkaline phosphatase levels, and serial bone scintigraphy. At age 17, the patient had severe spontaneous pain in the hip, and a computed tomography scan showed interruption of the cortex in the right femoral neck related to fracture (Figure 1). The patient then underwent local curettage followed by a lyophilized bovine bone grafting in the right proximal femur. Bone tissue biopsy showed areas of fibrosis and hyalinization, associated with immature trabecular bone, compatible with the diagnosis of FD. Two years after this procedure, the patient had a costal arch fracture after minimal trauma. During the past year, there was progressive worsening of pain, especially in the hip region, refractory to different analgesic regimens that included tricyclic antidepressants and opioids. Bone scintigraphy revealed diffusely increased osteoblastic activity in the right hemibody (Figure 2). Bone densitometry showed Z-score −0.7 in lumbar spine (BMD 1.091 g/cm^2), −1.3 in left total femur (BMD 0.840 g/cm^2), and −2.8 in forearm 33% (BMD 0.629 g/cm^2). The patient had severe pain, according to a visual scale of pain [6], and had great difficulty in walking and required a wheelchair, even at home. An Rx showed lesions compatible with fibrous dysplasia (Figure 3). She was seen by an orthopedist, who suggested conservative treatment, with no indication for further surgery. A new cycle of pamidronate, with 160 mg divided into 3 days (40 mg on the first day and 60 mg on the second and third days), produced no improvement. After obtaining written informed consent, we then started calcitonin administered as a nasal spray 200 UI once daily. The patient returned 2 weeks later reporting good tolerance and significant improvement in pain severity. The dose was increased to 200 UI twice daily and the patient returned after 30 days of treatment walking with the aid of crutches but without a wheelchair. She no longer needed opioids every day, which had a significant impact on quality of life, since the patient was intolerant of this class of medications. Three months after the start of nasal calcitonin, the patient is able to walk without assistance, with mild pain, estimated by the visual scale in the hip and sporadic opioid use. While

TABLE 1: Bone metabolism evaluation.

	Before calcitonin treatment	During calcitonin treatment	Reference values
Age (years)	27.3	27.6	
Total calcium (mmol/L)	2.2	2.3	2.1–2.5
Phosphorus (mmol/L)	1.1	1.2	0.8–1.4
Parathyroid hormone (ng/L)		53.3	15–68
Alkaline phosphatase (U/L)	454	341	35–104
25 (OH) vitamin D3 (nmol/L)	64.8	45.6	75–250
Creatinine (μmol/L)	70.7	61.8	44–80

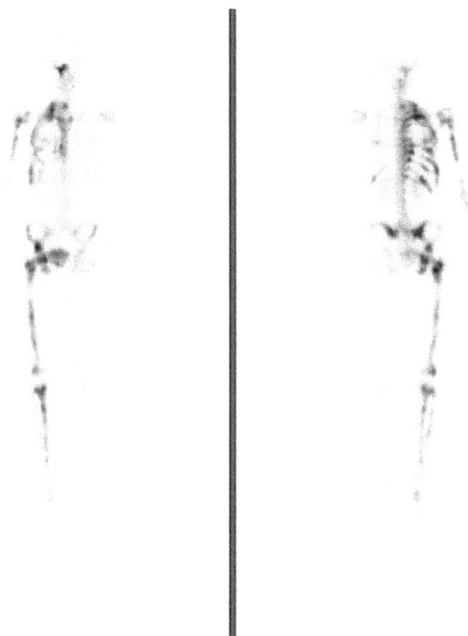

FIGURE 2: Bone scintigraphy at age 26. Diffusely increased osteoblastic activity on the right side of the body and tenth left costal arch.

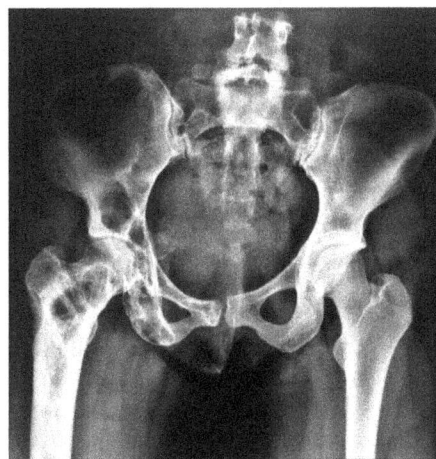

FIGURE 3: Hip Rx at age 27. Lesions in the iliac bone and right femur compatible with fibrous dysplasia.

no specific biochemical markers of bone turnover, such as amino-terminal propeptide (PINP) of type I collagen and carboxy-terminal collagen crosslinks (CTX), were available for this patient, serum alkaline phosphatase, an unspecific bone turnover marker, and calcium and phosphorus levels were assessed and did not change during treatment (Table 1).

3. Discussion

The present report shows the favorable outcome of a patient with MAS and severe bone pain after short-term treatment with nasal calcitonin. Calcitonin is a 32-amino acid polypeptide hormone produced by the parafollicular cells of the thyroid gland whose secretion is mainly regulated by serum calcium levels. Its main role is to inhibit bone resorption by reducing osteoclast activity [3].

FD is characterized by the development of fibrous bone lesions that replace normal skeletal structures. Abnormal fibroblast proliferation and defective osteoblast differentiation result in the replacement of cancellous bone and marrow with fibrous connective tissue. There is no cure or spontaneous resolution of FD, but, since bone pain, deformities, and pathological fractures are the main symptoms, the condition often requires treatment [7]. However, because it is a rare disease, few data are available in the literature addressing these concerns.

Benhamou et al. [8] recently conducted an analysis of 372 patients with FD, 42% of whom were diagnosed with a polyostotic form and 12% with MAS. The main symptom at diagnosis was bone pain, which occurred in 44% of patients, followed by fracture in 9%. In univariate analysis, younger age at diagnosis, renal phosphate wasting, a polyostotic form of FD, fracture, and bisphosphonate use were significant predictors. In the multivariate model, the polyostotic form and bisphosphonate use remained significant predictors. However, those who were treated were likely to have more severe disease.

Bisphosphonates are often used as a medical treatment to reduce the increased bone turnover in the affected bone tissue. Thomsen and Rejnmark [7] published a review on the treatment of 26 cases of FD, 4 of which were diagnosed with MAS. Most patients received bisphosphonate treatment (89%), but it did not result in significant relief of symptoms or radiological improvement of the lesions. The mean duration of treatment was 4 years (3–276 months), and the types of bisphosphonates prescribed changed during follow-up. Only

3 patients reported pain relief with treatment. Boyce et al. (2014) also evaluated 35 patients with FD with at least 2 skeletal lesions. Alendronate was administered over a 24-month period in 6-month cycles, with stratified doses by weight. There was no difference in mean pain score and functional tests between alendronate and placebo groups at any point during the treatment period [9].

The use of calcitonin in patients with FD is not new. The first study published by Bell et al. [10] in 1970 investigated the effects of calcitonin in 5 patients, 4 with a diagnosis of Paget's disease and 1 with polyostotic FD. Calcitonin was given intramuscularly every 12 hours for 16 days, with the patients hospitalized under medical care. No significant changes were observed in serum levels of calcium, phosphorus, and alkaline phosphatase. Calcitonin reduced calciuria in 3 patients and fecal calcium in all patients, but these changes occurred only during treatment. Urinary hydroxyproline levels decreased significantly in 2 patients and did not increase again even 30 days after the end of treatment. Similar findings were described by Yamamoto et al. [11] in a 12-year-old girl with a diagnosis of MAS. In this case, treatment with a synthetic analog of calcitonin administered twice weekly for 20 weeks led to a progressive reduction in urinary proline and hydroxyproline levels. Other study has not confirmed this effect of calcitonin on bone turnover markers [12].

The analgesic activity of calcitonin has been demonstrated in several trials in patients suffering from different painful skeletal conditions [13–15]. The mechanism of the analgesic effect of calcitonin remains unclear, but some evidence for its role in decreasing pain has already been described [16]. Indeed, calcitonin-binding sites have been detected in the hypothalamus and other areas of the central nervous system and seems to depend on the integrity of the serotonergic pathway [17]. In addition, calcitonin possibly inhibits the production of prostaglandins and other proinflammatory cytokines, through a reduction in cyclogenase activity [18]. It also induces a reduction of calcium influx in the neural membrane, which makes the target cells less reactive and decreases the stimulation of nociceptors located in the synovia and periosteum [18, 19]. Other putative mechanisms include elevated plasma β endorphin levels and effects on central serotonergic or monoaminergic pathways [13]. Although antibody formation against human calcitonin is rare, approximately 40 to 70% of patients receiving long-term therapy with salmon calcitonin produce specific antibodies. The clinical significance of these antibodies is unclear; however, clinical trials in postmenopausal osteoporosis have shown that these antibodies do not reduce the efficacy of long-term treatment [3].

Concerning potential adverse effects of calcitonin, the European Medicines Agency (EMA) recently published a press release stating that the increase in cancer rates with calcitonin varied between 0.7% in studies with the oral formulation and 2.4% in the studies with the nasal formulation [20]. However, the EMA did not advise against short-term use (less than 3 months), especially in patients with Paget's disease, bone loss associated with immobilization, and cancer related hypercalcemia. In addition, studies with

fracture-related bone pain have shown benefit of the analgesic properties of calcitonin when used for short term, but not for long periods [21, 22]. In a meta-analysis of 13 studies in patients with osteoporotic vertebral compression fractures, there was a significant reduction of bone pain with onset in less than 10 days, with continued improvement through 4 weeks. For patients with pain for more than 3 months, there was no significant improvement [22]. Another study evaluated 91 patients with breast cancer and anastrozole-induced bone pain. The results showed a significant reduction of pain in women receiving calcitonin for three months when compared to the control group [23].

We reported the case of a patient with a diagnosis of MAS and incapacitating bone pain refractory to treatment with intravenous bisphosphonate associated with opioids and tricyclic antidepressants. There are only a few references in the literature to the use of calcitonin in MAS, but, in the present case, there was a significant improvement in both bone pain severity and quality of life. The treatment was very well tolerated and no adverse effects were noted. Based on this experience, short-term use of calcitonin may be considered an effective alternative in selected patients with polyostotic FD and severe and refractory bone pain.

Disclosure

The funder had no role in the design, analysis, or writing of this article.

Acknowledgments

This work was supported by Conselho Nacional de Desenvolvimento Científico e Tecnológico (CNPq INCT 465482/2014-7), Brazil.

References

[1] C. E. Dumitrescu and M. T. Collins, "McCune-Albright syndrome," Orphanet Journal of Rare Diseases, vol. 3, no. 1, article no. 12, 2008.

[2] E. S. Hart, M. H. Kelly, B. Brillante et al., "Onset, progression, and plateau of skeletal lesions in fibrous dysplasia and the relationship to functional outcome," Journal of Bone and Mineral Research, vol. 22, no. 9, pp. 1468–1474, 2007.

[3] G. L. Plosker and D. McTavish, "A review of its pharmacological properties and role in the management of postmenopausal osteoporosis, Drugs aging," Intranasal Salcatonin (Salmon Calcitonin), vol. 8, no. 5, pp. 378–400, 1996.

[4] A. M. Boyce, A. Turner, L. Watts et al., "Improving patient outcomes in fibrous dysplasia/McCune-Albright syndrome: an international multidisciplinary workshop to inform an international partnership," Archives of Osteoporosis, vol. 12, no. 1, 6 pages, 2017.

[5] R. D. Chapurlat, "Medical therapy in adults with fibrous dysplasia of bone," Journal of Bone and Mineral Research, vol. 21, no. 2, pp. 114–119, 2006.

[6] H. M. McCormack, D. J. Horne, and S. Sheather, "Clinical applications of visual analogue scales: a critical review," *Psychological Medicine*, vol. 18, no. 4, pp. 1007–1019, 1988.

[7] M. D. Thomsen and L. Rejnmark, "Clinical and radiological observations in a case series of 26 patients with fibrous dysplasia," *Calcified Tissue International*, vol. 94, no. 4, pp. 384–395, 2014.

[8] J. Benhamou, D. Gensburger, C. Messiaen, and R. Chapurlat, "Prognostic Factors From an Epidemiologic Evaluation of Fibrous Dysplasia of Bone in a Modern Cohort: The FRANCEDYS Study," *Journal of Bone and Mineral Research*, vol. 31, no. 12, pp. 2167–2172, 2016.

[9] A. M. Boyce, M. H. Kelly, and B. A. Brillante, "A randomized, double blind, placebo-controlled trial of alendronate treatment for fibrous dysplasia of bone," *The Journal of Clinical Endocrinology & Metabolism*, vol. 99, no. 11, pp. 4133–4140, 2014.

[10] N. H. Bell, S. Avery, and C. Conrad Johnston, "Effects of calcitonin in Pagets disease and polyostotic fibrous dysplasia," *J Clin Endocrinol*, vol. 31, no. 3, pp. 283–290, 1970.

[11] K. Yamamoto, I. Maeyama, H. Kishimoto et al., "Suppressive Effect of Elcatonin, an Eel Calcitonin Analogue, on Excessive Urinary Hydroxyproline Excretion in Polyostotic Fibrous Dysplasia (McCune-Albright's Syndrome)," *Endocrinologia Japonica*, vol. 30, no. 5, pp. 651–656, 1983.

[12] Å. Hjelmstedt and S. Ljunghall, "A case of albright's syndrome treated with calcitonin," *Acta Orthopaedica*, vol. 50, no. 3, pp. 251–253, 1979.

[13] K. Mystakidou, S. Befon, K. Hondros, E. Kouskouni, and L. Vlahos, "Continuous subcutaneous administration of high-dose salmon calcitonin in bone metastasis: Pain control and beta-endorphin plasma levels," *Journal of Pain and Symptom Management*, vol. 18, no. 5, pp. 323–330, 1999.

[14] S. Tanaka, A. Yoshida, S. Kono, and M. Ito, "Effectiveness of monotherapy and combined therapy with calcitonin and minodronic acid hydrate, a bisphosphonate, for early treatment," *Journal of Orthopaedic Science*, vol. 22, no. 3, pp. 536–541, 2017.

[15] M. Esenyel, A. Içağasioğlu, and C. Z. Esenyel, "Effects of calcitonin on knee osteoarthritis and quality of life," *Rheumatology International*, vol. 33, no. 2, pp. 423–427, 2013.

[16] G. P. Lyritis and G. Trovas, "Analgesic effects of calcitonin," *Bone*, vol. 30, 5, pp. 71S–74S, 2002.

[17] C. H. Chesnut III, M. Azria, S. Silverman, M. Engelhardt, M. Olson, and L. Mindeholm, "Salmon calcitonin: A review of current and future therapeutic indications," *Osteoporosis International*, vol. 19, no. 4, pp. 479–491, 2008.

[18] R. Viana and M. W. C. Payne, "Use of calcitonin in recalcitrant phantom limb pain complicated by heterotopic ossification," *Pain Research and Management*, vol. 20, no. 5, pp. 229–233, 2015.

[19] C. Gennari, "Analgesic effect of calcitonin in osteoporosis," *Bone*, vol. 30, no. 5, pp. 67S–70S, 2002.

[20] *European Medicines Agency. European Medicines Agency recommends limiting long-term use of calcitonin medicines*, Press release, 2012.

[21] P. M. Foye, P. Shupper, and I. Wendel, "Coccyx fractures treated with intranasal calcitonin," *Pain Physician*, vol. 17, no. 2, pp. 233-229, 2014.

[22] J. A. Knopp-Sihota, C. V. Newburn-Cook, J. Homik, G. G. Cummings, and D. Voaklander, "Calcitonin for treating acute and chronic pain of recent and remote osteoporotic vertebral compression fractures: A systematic review and meta-analysis," *Osteoporosis International*, vol. 23, no. 1, pp. 17–38, 2012.

[23] P. Liu, D. Q. Yang, F. Xie, B. Zhou, and M. Liu, "Effect of calcitonin on anastrozole-induced bone pain during aromatase inhibitor therapy for breast cancer," *Genetics and Molecular Research*, vol. 13, no. 3, pp. 5285–5291, 2014.

56

Management of Refractory Noninsulinoma Pancreatogenous Hypoglycemia Syndrome with Gastric Bypass Reversal: A Case Report and Review of the Literature

Bhavana B. Rao,[1] Benjamin Click,[1] George Eid,[2] and Ronald A. Codario[3]

[1]*Department of Internal Medicine, University of Pittsburgh Medical Center, Pittsburgh, PA 15213, USA*
[2]*Division of Bariatric Surgery, Allegheny Health Network, Pittsburgh, PA 15212, USA*
[3]*Division of Endocrinology, Department of Internal Medicine, VA Pittsburgh Healthcare System, Pittsburgh, PA 15240, USA*

Correspondence should be addressed to Ronald A. Codario; ronald.codario@va.gov

Academic Editor: Yuji Moriwaki

Background. Roux-en-Y gastric bypass (RYGB) is a commonly performed, effective bariatric procedure; however, rarely, complications such as postprandial hypoglycemia due to noninsulinoma pancreatogenous hypoglycemia syndrome (NIPHS) may ensue. Management of refractory NIPHS is challenging. We report a case that was successfully treated with RYGB reversal. *Case Report.* A 58-year-old male with history of RYGB nine months earlier for morbid obesity presented for evaluation of postprandial, hypoglycemic seizures. Testing for insulin level, insulin antibodies, oral hypoglycemic agents, pituitary axis hormone levels, and cortisol stimulation was unrevealing. Computed tomography (CT) scan of the abdomen was unremarkable. A 72-hour fast was completed without hypoglycemia. Mixed meal testing demonstrated endogenous hyperinsulinemic hypoglycemia (EHH) and selective arterial calcium stimulation testing (SACST) was positive. Strict dietary modifications, maximal medical therapy, gastrostomy tube feeding, and stomal reduction failed to alleviate symptoms. Ultimately, he underwent laparoscopic reversal of RYGB. Now, 9 months after reversal, he has markedly reduced hypoglycemia burden. *Discussion.* Hyperfunctioning islets secondary to exaggerated incretin response and altered intestinal nutrient delivery are hypothesized to be causative in NIPHS. For refractory cases, there is increasing skepticism about the safety and efficacy of pancreatic resection. RYGB reversal may be successful.

1. Introduction

Roux-en-Y gastric bypass (RYGB) is frequently performed for the management of morbid obesity. While it offers significant and sustained weight reduction and favorably impacts several metabolic parameters, we are now encountering some unique and challenging postprocedure complications. One such long-term complication is postprandial hypoglycemia. A rare cause of postprandial hypoglycemia is noninsulinoma pancreatogenous hypoglycemia syndrome (NIPHS). NIPHS is characterized by endogenous hyperinsulinemic hypoglycemia (EHH) with positive selective arterial calcium stimulation testing (SACST) and negative imaging studies for insulinoma.

When first described, gastric bypass patients with NIPHS were noted to have diffuse hyperplasia of the beta cells of the pancreatic islets, akin to nesidioblastosis, resulting in inappropriately elevated levels of insulin [1]. Subsequent studies proposed that an exaggerated incretin hormonal response to meals stimulated this hyperplasia of the islet beta cells [2].

Historically, management of mild cases has included dietary modifications such as carbohydrate-restricted diets and medications such as acarbose, verapamil, octreotide, and diazoxide [3, 4]. For patients with severe or refractory symptoms, gradient-guided partial or total resection of the pancreas has been performed; however, hypoglycemic events persist in majority of the patients [2, 3]. Gastric bypass reversal for the treatment of refractory NIPHS has been sparsely described, with equivocal results [2, 5–7]. We report a case of severe refractory NIPHS successfully managed with gastric bypass reversal.

2. Case Report

A 58-year-old Caucasian male presented to our institution after suffering a generalized tonic-clonic seizure lasting five minutes, followed by a brief postictal state with complete amnesia to the event. A home glucometer read less than 70 mg/dL, so he was transported to our facility for further evaluation. His past medical history included coronary artery disease necessitating coronary artery bypass surgery, ischemic cardiomyopathy with biventricular intracardiac defibrillator placement, hypertension, type 2 diabetes, and RYGB 9 months earlier for morbid obesity. The patient had been a diabetic for 4 years prior to the RYGB and had been maintained on a relatively stable regimen of subcutaneous insulin with metformin, with hemoglobin A1c ranging between 8.5 and 10%. Following the procedure, he had continued to be on the same regimen with no reported side effects. Upon admission, he was hemodynamically stable and afebrile, with unremarkable physical examination and no focal neurological deficits. Complete cell count and metabolic panel were within normal limits except for blood glucose (BG) level of 69 mg/dL, notably after 25 gm of dextrose was administered intravenously, en route to the hospital. Electroencephalogram and computed tomography (CT) scan of his head were nonrevealing. Of note, in the month prior to RYGB, his weight was 287 pounds with body mass index (BMI) of 42 kg/m^2 and hemoglobin A1c (HbA1c) of 9.6%. At the time of admission, he reported a 75-pound weight loss, with decrease in BMI to 30 kg/m^2 and HbA1c to 5.5%. His insulin and oral antihypoglycemic regimen were discontinued after this episode of presumed hypoglycemic seizure.

Over the next 6 months, the patient had several more hypoglycemic seizures that occurred several hours after eating, with perievent BG ranging from 30 to 80 mg/dL. CT scan of the abdomen was notable for surgical changes and a 2.1 cm adrenal nodule. Laboratory testing revealed normal levels of urine and plasma metanephrines, random serum and 24-hour urine cortisol, and appropriate response to cortisol stimulation and low dose dexamethasone suppression test. Testing for insulin antibodies and oral hypoglycemics was negative and a 72-hour fast was completed without hypoglycemia. The patient was advised to eat small meals every 4 hours, rich in proteins and complex rather than simple carbohydrates, and educated on continuous blood glucose monitoring as well as the use of a glucagon kit. However, the hypoglycemic seizures persisted.

Upon further testing, induced hypoglycemia with 75% carbohydrate meal intake showed BG of 36 mg/dL three hours later, with inappropriately elevated C-peptide (7.8 ng/mL; normal [nr] <0.2 in hypoglycemia), proinsulin (11.5 pmol/L; nr: <5 pmol/L in hypoglycemia), and insulin levels (22.4 μIU/mL; nr < 3 in hypoglycemia), consistent with EHH. He was sequentially trialed on maximum doses of acarbose (50 mg TID), octreotide (100 mcg TID), and diazoxide (50 mg BID) without resolution of the hypoglycemic episodes. Subsequent SACST revealed a 2-, 3-, and 9-fold increase in insulin levels, 120 seconds after injection of calcium gluconate, in the gastroduodenal, midsplenic, and proper hepatic arteries, respectively, suggestive of hyperfunctioning islets or islet hypertrophy localized to the head or body of the pancreas.

Percutaneous gastrostomy tube placement to the remnant stomach with intermittent tube feeding was attempted; however, with one missed feeding, he again suffered a hypoglycemic seizure. Endoscopic gastrojejunal stomal reduction to delay transition of food was performed. Symptoms improved temporarily but with ultimate recurrence of hypoglycemic episodes. The patient had over 25 hospitalizations for hypoglycemia during a period of 2 years. In view of the life-threatening nature of his episodes, the patient underwent laparoscopic reversal of RYGB three years after original procedure, with resection of the roux limb and restoration of normal anatomy by creation of gastrogastrostomy. Currently, the patient is nine months after reversal, weighs 230 pounds with a BMI of 34 kg/m^2 and HbA1c of 5.5, and has had only episode of hypoglycemic seizure since the surgery. This occurred eight months after reversal when he was working outdoors after missing a meal. His blood glucose dropped to 50 mg/dL but he was unable to hear the alarm of the continuous glucose monitor due to a noisy environment. With the exception of this singular event, the patient has not had any other episodes of hypoglycemia or hospitalizations.

3. Discussion

Over the last decade, several studies have contributed to our understanding of the underlying pathologic mechanisms in NIPHS and influenced management strategies.

The most widely accepted hypothesis proposes increased levels of the incretin hormone glucagon-like peptide-1 (GLP-1) leading to islet cell hyperplasia, postprandial hyperinsulinemia, and subsequent hypoglycemia [8]. Based on this, recent trials have evaluated GLP-1 analogs [9] and GLP-1 receptor antagonists [4] for treatment of postprandial hypoglycemia with promising preliminary results. However, islet cell expansion is not consistently observed in pathological specimens of patients managed with pancreatectomy [1, 2]. Also, a retrospective assessment of 15 patients who had undergone pancreatic resection reported persistent hypoglycemic symptoms in 77% of patients after the procedure [3].

Refinement of the previously mentioned hypothesis proposes that the insulin dysregulation after RYGB is a result of rapid delivery of nutrients to the distal intestine, leading to an exaggerated response of the incretins GLP-1 and gastric inhibitory peptide (GIP), which causes postprandial hyperinsulinemia/hypoglycemia without necessarily leading to islet cell hyperplasia [10]. This was first suggested by McLaughlin et al. in 2010 when they noted that, by inserting a gastrostomy tube and directly feeding the remnant stomach, the hypoglycemic episodes were prevented, thus implicating altered nutrient delivery as a provocative factor [10]. This theory was further supported by an observation that, with laparoscopic reversal of gastric bypass to normal anatomy or with revision of bypass by performing modified sleeve gastrectomy, decrease in the frequency of hypoglycemic episodes and resolution of neuroglycopenia occurred in 4 patients with refractory post-RYGB NIPHS [6]. Notably, each of these patients had been successfully trialed with a gastrostomy tube to the remnant stomach prior to the reversal. Himpens et al. also reported success with bypass reversal in 1 patient [5].

Failure of resolution of symptoms with gastric bypass reversal was first described by Patti et al. in one patient whose symptoms persisted despite maximal medical therapy, takedown of bypass, and 80% distal pancreatectomy, and eventually Whipple's procedure was performed [2]. Furthermore, Lee et al. conducted mixed meal challenges in two patients who had undergone reversal of RYGB for NIPHS and noted no improvement in the hyperinsulinemic hypoglycemia, despite improvement in GLP-1 levels. Interestingly, they detected an increase in GIP levels after reversal, not observed in previous studies, which may have contributed to reversal failure [7].

In our patient, RYGB was followed by significant weight reduction and remission of diabetes but was complicated by development of NIPHS nine months postoperatively, refractory to dietary modification and medical therapy. In a prior case series, time to development of this complication ranged from 1 to 56 months and the cause for this variability is as yet unclear [3]. Gastrostomy tube feeding to the remnant stomach reduced the number of hypoglycemic episodes, but, without strict adherence, his symptoms recurred, which suggests possible alternate mechanisms which do not rely on food intake stimulated pathways and may merit further investigation. Use of continuous glucose monitor enabled him to identify and correct episodes of hypoglycemia and thus prevent seizures; however, multiple breakthrough seizures occurred. Endoscopic stomal reduction, with the objective of prolonging gastric emptying time, was successful for a short period of time; however, hypoglycemic episodes persisted. Surgical procedures such as gastric pouch reduction or adjustable band placement have been trialed; however, limited data exists on the mechanism and benefit of these measures. In our particular case, the roux limb was resected due to an intraoperative finding of severe adhesions and possible small bowel anastomosis in two different segments of the roux limb, which may have further hastened nutrient delivery to his distal intestine and thus exacerbated the hypoglycemia. Following bypass reversal, he has not required hospitalization and his overall burden of hypoglycemia has been dramatically reduced.

4. Conclusion

Our understanding of post-RYGB NIPHS, its etiology, and appropriate surgical procedures for its management is limited by the fact that this syndrome is rare and only recently recognized. There is now increasing skepticism about the rationale, effectiveness, and safety of pancreatic resection for this condition. Critical appraisal of the literature reveals few prior reports of gastric bypass reversal, each with variable results, which may be attributable to differences in underlying anatomy and variations in surgical techniques. Here, we report the successful treatment of a case of refractory NIPHS with reversal of RYGB. Further investigations to better elucidate the hormonal milieu before and after reversal are necessary to facilitate better management of this challenging condition.

Ethical Approval

All procedures performed in this study, involving a human participant, were in accordance with the standard of the international and/or national research committee and with the 1964 Helsinki declaration and its later amendments or comparable ethical standards.

Disclosure

This case was presented at the American College of Gastroenterology conference at Philadelphia on October 20, 2014.

References

[1] G. J. Service, G. B. Thompson, F. J. Service, J. C. Andrews, M. L. Collazo-Clavell, and R. V. Lloyd, "Hyperinsulinemic hypoglycemia with nesidioblastosis after gastric-bypass surgery," *The New England Journal of Medicine*, vol. 353, no. 3, pp. 249–254, 2005.

[2] M. E. Patti, G. McMahon, E. C. Mun et al., "Severe hypoglycaemia post-gastric bypass requiring partial pancreatectomy: evidence for inappropriate insulin secretion and pancreatic islet hyperplasia," *Diabetologia*, vol. 48, no. 11, pp. 2236–2240, 2005.

[3] V. K. Mathavan, M. Arregui, C. Davis, K. Singh, A. Patel, and J. Meacham, "Management of postgastric bypass noninsulinoma pancreatogenous hypoglycemia," *Surgical Endoscopy*, vol. 24, no. 10, pp. 2547–2555, 2010.

[4] M. Salehi, A. Gastaldelli, and D. A. D'Alessio, "Blockade of glucagon-like peptide 1 receptor corrects postprandial hypoglycemia after gastric bypass," *Gastroenterology*, vol. 146, no. 3, pp. 669.e2–680.e2, 2014.

[5] J. Himpens, A. Verbrugghe, G.-B. Cadière, W. Everaerts, and J.-W. Greve, "Long-term results of laparoscopic roux-en-y gastric bypass: evaluation after 9 years," *Obesity Surgery*, vol. 22, no. 10, pp. 1586–1593, 2012.

[6] G. M. Campos, M. Ziemelis, R. Paparodis, M. Ahmed, and D. Belt Davis, "Laparoscopic reversal of Roux-en-Y gastric bypass: technique and utility for treatment of endocrine complications," *Surgery for Obesity and Related Diseases*, vol. 10, no. 1, pp. 36–43, 2014.

[7] C. J. Lee, T. Brown, T. H. Magnuson, J. M. Egan, O. Carlson, and D. Elahi, "Hormonal response to a mixed-meal challenge after reversal of gastric bypass for hypoglycemia," *The Journal of Clinical Endocrinology & Metabolism*, vol. 98, no. 7, pp. E1208–E1212, 2013.

[8] M.-E. Patti and A. B. Goldfine, "Hypoglycemia after gastric bypass: the dark side of GLP-1," *Gastroenterology*, vol. 146, no. 3, pp. 605–608, 2014.

[9] N. Abrahamsson, B. E. Engström, M. Sundbom, and F. A. Karlsson, "GLP1 analogs as treatment of postprandial hypoglycemia following gastric bypass surgery: a potential new indication?" *European Journal of Endocrinology*, vol. 169, no. 6, pp. 885–889, 2013.

[10] T. McLaughlin, M. Peck, J. Holst, and C. Deacon, "Reversible hyperinsulinemic hypoglycemia after gastric bypass: a consequence of altered nutrient delivery," *The Journal of Clinical Endocrinology and Metabolism*, vol. 95, no. 4, pp. 1851–1855, 2010.

57

Adrenal Lymphangioma Masquerading as a Catecholamine Producing Tumor

Israel Hodish,[1] Lindsay Schmidt,[2] and Andreas G. Moraitis[3]

[1]Division of Internal Medicine, University of Michigan Medical Center, Ann Arbor, MI 48109, USA
[2]Department of Pathology, University of Michigan, Ann Arbor, MI 48109, USA
[3]Corcept Therapeutics, Menlo Park, CA 94025, USA

Correspondence should be addressed to Andreas G. Moraitis; andreas.moraitis@yahoo.com

Academic Editor: Takeshi Usui

Objective. To report the unusual case of an adrenal lymphangioma presenting in a patient with an adrenal cystic lesion and biochemical testing concerning for pheochromocytoma. The pertinent diagnostic and imaging features of adrenal lymphangiomas are reviewed. *Methods.* We describe a 59-year-old patient who presented with hyperhidrosis and a 2.2 by 2.2 cm left adrenal nodule. Biochemical evaluation revealed elevated plasma-free normetanephrine, urine normetanephrine, urine vanillylmandelic acid, and urine norepinephrine levels. Elevated plasma norepinephrine levels were not suppressed appropriately with clonidine administration. *Results.* Given persistent concern for pheochromocytoma, the patient underwent adrenalectomy. The final pathology was consistent with adrenal lymphangioma. *Conclusions.* Lymphangiomas are benign vascular lesions that can very rarely occur in the adrenal gland. Imaging findings are generally consistent with a cyst but are nonspecific. Excluding malignancy in patients presenting with adrenal cysts can be difficult. Despite its benign nature, the diagnosis of adrenal lymphangioma may ultimately require pathology.

1. Introduction

Lymphangiomas are benign vascular lesions that most commonly occur in the head, neck, and axilla [1]. Lymphangiomas of the adrenal gland are very rare, with an estimated incidence of 0.064 to 0.18 percent in autopsy series [2]. These lesions are generally asymptomatic but may be found incidentally on radiographic imaging during work-up for unrelated conditions. Therefore, it is important to distinguish these benign cysts from malignant adrenal lesions. Here, we present the diagnostic dilemma of a patient who presented with an adrenal cystic lesion and biochemical evaluation concerning for pheochromocytoma. The patient was ultimately found to have an adrenal lymphangioma.

2. Case Report

A 59-year-old male with past medical history of hypertension, obesity, hyperhidrosis, and secondary polycythemia presented to his outpatient hematologist in 2009 for evaluation of hyperhidrosis. The patient endorsed several-year history of profuse episodic sweating that interfered with his social interactions. He denied any headaches or palpitations. The patient had a known history of 1.7 by 1.4 cm adrenal nodule discovered incidentally on MR scan performed that same year. The nodule did not enhance, and imaging characteristics were most consistent with a cyst.

Biochemical evaluation in 2009 included an elevated 24-hour urine normetanephrine, norepinephrine, and vanillylmandelic acid as indicated in Table 1. Urine 24-hour metanephrine and epinephrine were both within normal limits. The patient was not taking any medications that could interfere with the measurement of catecholamines or metanephrines. In 2010, the patient underwent an I^{123} metaiodobenzylguanidine (MIBG) scan that was negative for pheochromocytoma.

Given continued symptoms of hyperhidrosis, the patient was referred to endocrinology in 2013. Repeat biochemical

TABLE 1: Patient's catecholamine levels before and after left adrenalectomy.

	2009 (Preoperative)	Reference range	2013 (Preoperative)	2013 (Postoperative)	Reference range
Plasma-free normetanephrine	nd	nd	**1.6 nmol/L**	0.53 nmol/L	<0.90 nmol/L
Plasma-free metanephrine	nd	nd	<0.20 nmol/L	<0.20 nmol/L	<0.50 nmol/L
Plasma norepinephrine	nd	nd	**891 pg/mL**	**659 pg/mL**	0–500 pg/mL
Plasma epinephrine	nd	nd	52 pg/mL	24 pg/mL	0–100 pg/mL
Urine normetanephrine	**1868 μg/24 hours**	110–1050 μg/24 hours	**1123 μg/24 hours**	nd	50–800 μg/24 hours
Urine metanephrines	254 μg/24 hours	35–460 μg/24 hours	123 μg/24 hours	nd	0–300 μg/24 hours
Urine norepinephrine	**414 μg/24 hours**	0–140 μg/24 hours	**257 μg/24 hours**	nd	0–100 μg/24 hours
Urine epinephrine	16 μg/24 hours	0–32 μg/24 hours	10.2 μg/24 hours	nd	0–20 μg/24 hours
Urine vanillylmandelic acid	**9.6 μg/24 hours**	0.0–7.5 μg/24 hours	nd	nd	nd

nd: not done.
Results outside the reference range are indicated in bold.

evaluation at that time was notable for an elevated plasma-free normetanephrine, plasma norepinephrine, 24-hour urine normetanephrine, and 24-hour urine norepinephrine as documented in Table 1. Plasma-free metanephrine, plasma epinephrine, urine 24-hour metanephrine, and urine 24-hour epinephrine were within normal limits. He was also diagnosed with new onset diabetes.

With regard to further imaging studies, adrenal protocol CT demonstrated a 2.1 by 2.2 cm left adrenal nodule which could not be classified as lipid rich adenoma. The density measurement of the nodule was 12 Hounsfield units before contrast and 22 Hounsfield units on the enhanced study. The absolute enhancement washout value was 20%, below the 60% threshold for an adenoma. Adrenal protocol MR demonstrated a 2.2 × 2.2 cm lesion with uniformly high signal intensity on T2-weighted sequences and low signal on T1-weighted images with no enhancement on contrast administration. MR findings were most consistent with a cyst (Figure 1).

Given the patient's modestly elevated normetanephrine and norepinephrine, confirmatory testing was performed with a clonidine suppression test. Norepinephrine was 891 pg/mL (normal reference range < 500 pg/mL) prior to 0.3 mg clonidine administration and 708 pg/mL 3 hours after clonidine administration. Normetanephrine was 0.95 nmol/L (normal reference range < 0.90 nmol/L) prior to clonidine administration and 0.94 nmol/L 3 hours after clonidine administration which is suggestive of pheochromocytoma.

Due to persistent concern for potential pheochromocytoma with cystic degeneration, he was started on phenoxybenzamine and underwent laparoscopic left adrenalectomy without complications. Surgical pathology demonstrated a benign vascular cyst consistent with lymphangioma (Figure 2).

Repeat plasma fractionated metanephrines performed after surgery were within normal limits. Incidentally, patient reported significant improvement in his hyperhidrosis after surgery and also significant weight loss and improvement of diabetes control. Polycythemia was most likely not related to the adrenal tumor, since no changes have been noticed up to 6-month postop follow-up.

3. Discussion

Adrenal cysts can be classified as pseudocysts, endothelial cysts, epithelial cysts, or parasitic cysts. The estimated frequency of each subtype varies by series, with approximately 39–78% classified as pseudocysts, 20–45% endothelial cysts, 2–9% epithelial cysts, and 0–7% parasitic cysts [3–5]. Endothelial cysts can be further divided into lymphangiomatous and angiomatous cysts. Lymphangiomas are believed to arise from faulty lymphatic development leading to either isolation of the lymphangioma from larger lymphatic channels or lack of fusion with the venous system [1, 4, 6].

An estimated 7–15% of adrenal cysts are associated with malignancy [3, 5, 7, 8]. Although lymphangiomas are benign lesions, aspiration or surgical removal becomes necessary when malignancy cannot be excluded based on imaging alone. On ultrasonography, lymphangiomas generally present as well-demarcated multiloculated cysts. Less commonly, they present as unicameral cysts [9, 10]. On CT scan, they display capsular enhancement with internal attenuation values generally in the range of water [9–11]. On MR, these cysts are hypointense and nonenhancing on T1-weighted images and hyperintense on T2-weighted images [11]. However, the sensitivity and specificity of these imaging modalities for excluding malignancy remain unknown. In our case the mild postcontrast enhancement reported on the adrenal CT scan was primarily enhancement of the rim of the cystic lesion specifically from the part of the lesion abutting the normal adrenal tissue. Including the entire surface of the lesion on HU density measurement is advisable when there is suspicion of pheochromocytoma with cystic degeneration. Postcontrast HU of the lesion excluding the rim of the lesion showed no enhancement.

Identification of surgically excised adrenal cysts can be confirmed histologically. Adrenal lymphangiomas are characterized by multicystic architecture with a simple endothelial lining. On immunohistochemistry, these lesions stain negative for keratin and positive for D2-40, a marker of lymphatic endothelium [4].

Diagnosis in this case was complicated by biochemical testing that was concerning for possible functional adrenal

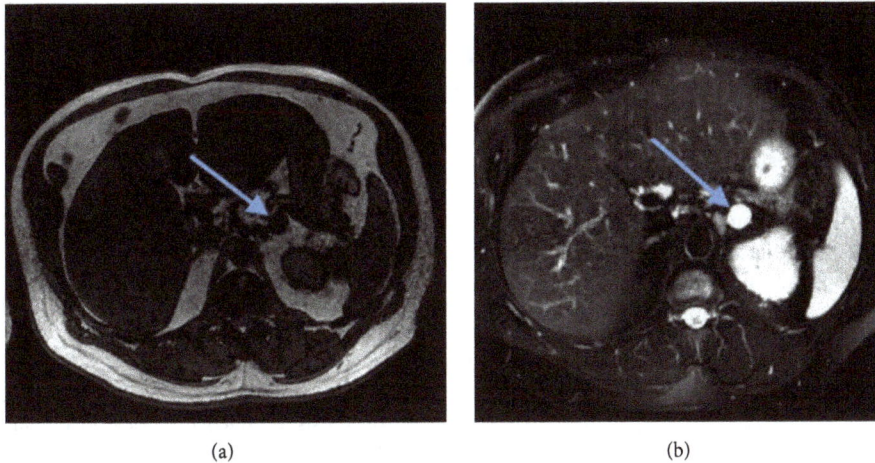

(a)

(b)

FIGURE 1: MRI of the adrenals. Within the lateral limb of the left adrenal gland, there is a 2.2 × 2.2 cm lesion (blue arrows) with uniformly high signal intensity on T2-weighted sequences (b) and low signal on T1-weighted images (a) with no significant loss of signal on opposed phase relative to in phase images.

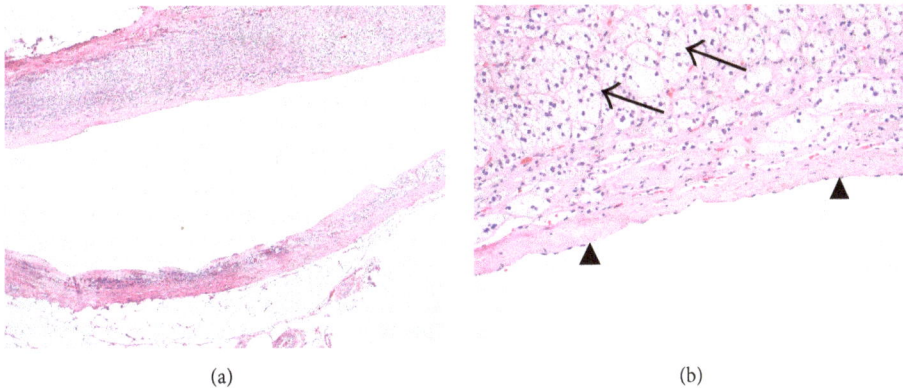

(a)

(b)

FIGURE 2: (a) Gross pathology demonstrated a 2 cm fluid-filled cyst. Hematoxylin and eosin stain at low magnification demonstrates a smooth-lined cyst. (b) Hematoxylin and eosin stain at high magnification shows endothelial cells lining the wall of the cystic lesion (black arrowheads). The stroma contains foamy cells (black arrows) with some mononuclear infiltrates. The entire picture is most consistent with benign vascular cyst.

tumor. Given the low prevalence of pheochromocytoma in the general population, even screening tests with high specificity will have more false-positive results than true-positive results [12, 13]. In cases where there is high clinical suspicion for pheochromocytoma, plasma-free metanephrines and normetanephrines are an appropriate first screening test given their high reported sensitivity of 96–99% [13, 14]. Large elevations in plasma metanephrines or normetanephrines several times the upper limit of normal are highly suggestive of pheochromocytoma and should prompt further investigation to localize the tumor [12–15]. In cases where plasma metanephrine or normetanephrine elevations are mild, further testing can be performed to help confirm or exclude the diagnosis including plasma catecholamines, urinary fractionated metanephrines, urinary catecholamines, and vanillylmandelic acid. Factors that can interfere with the diagnostic accuracy of these tests should also be addressed. Physiologic stress, obstructive sleep apnea, caffeine, nicotine, and several medications including many antihypertensives, antidepressants, stimulants, and sympathomimetics can all interfere with test results and lead to false-positive results [13].

In cases where biochemical test results are equivocal, a clonidine suppression test can be used to help clarify the diagnosis. Clonidine is a central alpha2-agonist that suppresses catecholamine release by the sympathetic nervous system. Release of catecholamines from a pheochromocytoma is thought to be autonomous and therefore would not be suppressed by clonidine [16]. Although several criteria have been proposed to define an appropriate clonidine response, a 3-hour postclonidine plasma norepinephrine level of less than 500 pg/mL with a decline of at least 50% has been used with a sensitivity and specificity of 97% and 74%, respectively [17]. The specificity of the test is significantly reduced in patients with a preclonidine plasma norepinephrine level in the normal range [18]. Yet, even using the much more specific criteria which define an abnormal test result simply as a plasma norepinephrine level of 500 pg/mL or less after clonidine administration (specificity of 96%) [17], our patient still had an abnormal clonidine response. Beta-blockers, tricyclic antidepressants, and thiazide diuretics have all been reported to produce false-positive results; however, none of these medications are applicable to our patient. This case illustrates the difficulty in ruling out pheochromocytoma in patients with benign adrenal lesions.

Adrenal cysts are usually asymptomatic, although local symptoms can vary with the size and position of the lesion. In one case series of 9 patients with adrenal lymphangioma 44% (4/9) presented with abdominal, flank, or back pain while an additional 44% (4/9) were asymptomatic and found incidentally [4]. In the same series one case was found on workup for labile hypertension that reportedly normalized after resection [19]. Interestingly, our patient reported resolution of his hyperhidrosis after surgery. However, given that adrenal lymphangiomas are nonfunctional cysts, the mechanism by which this could be tied to his hyperhidrosis remains unclear.

4. Conclusion

Here, we present the diagnostic dilemma of a patient with a cystic adrenal lesion in the setting of laboratory testing concerning for pheochromocytoma. Work-up included an elevated plasma norepinephrine level that was not not suppressed appropriately with clonidine administration. The patient ultimately underwent adrenalectomy that revealed an adrenal lymphangioma. This case illustrates the difficulty of definitely excluding pheochromocytoma in a patient with a rare benign adrenal cyst.

References

[1] S. Weiss and J. Goldblum, *Soft Tissue Tumors*, Mosby Elsevier, St. Louis, Mo, USA, 5th edition, 2001.

[2] H. R. Wahl, "Adrenal cysts," *The American Journal of Pathology*, vol. 27, no. 4, pp. 758–761, 1951.

[3] L. A. Erickson, R. V. Lloyd, R. Hartman, and G. Thompson, "Cystic adrenal neoplasms," *Cancer*, vol. 101, no. 7, pp. 1537–1544, 2004.

[4] D. G. Foster, "Adrenal cysts. Review of literature and report of case," *Archives of Surgery*, vol. 92, no. 1, pp. 131–143, 1966.

[5] L. M. Neri and F. C. Nance, "Management of adrenal cysts," *American Surgeon*, vol. 65, no. 2, pp. 151–163, 1999.

[6] S. Wiegand, B. Eivazi, P. J. Barth et al., "Pathogenesis of lymphangiomas," *Virchows Archiv*, vol. 453, no. 1, article 108, 2008.

[7] J. Khoda, Y. Hertzanu, G. Sebbag, L. Lantsberg, and Y. Barky, "Adrenal cysts: diagnosis and therapeutic approach," *International Surgery*, vol. 78, no. 3, pp. 239–242, 1993.

[8] A. Rozenblit, H. T. Morehouse, and E. S. Amis Jr., "Cystic adrenal lesions: CT features," *Radiology*, vol. 201, no. 2, pp. 541–548, 1996.

[9] B. Vargas-Serrano, N. Alegre-Bernal, B. Cortina-Moreno, R. Rodriguez-Romero, and F. Sanchez-Ortega, "Abdominal cystic lymphangiomas: US and CT findings," *European Journal of Radiology*, vol. 19, no. 3, pp. 183–187, 1995.

[10] A. J. Davidson and D. S. Hartman, "Lymphangioma of the retroperitoneum: CT and sonographic characteristics," *Radiology*, vol. 175, no. 2, pp. 507–510, 1990.

[11] Y.-K. Guo, Z.-G. Yang, Y. Li et al., "Uncommon adrenal masses: CT and MRI features with histopathologic correlation," *European Journal of Radiology*, vol. 62, no. 3, pp. 359–370, 2007.

[12] G. Eisenhofer, D. S. Goldstein, M. M. Walther et al., "Biochemical diagnosis of pheochromocytoma: how to distinguish true- from false-positive test results," *The Journal of Clinical Endocrinology & Metabolism*, vol. 88, no. 6, pp. 2656–2666, 2003.

[13] J. W. M. Lenders, K. Pacak, M. M. Walther et al., "Biochemical diagnosis of pheochromocytoma: which test is best?" *The Journal of the American Medical Association*, vol. 287, no. 11, pp. 1427–1434, 2002.

[14] Y. C. Kudva, A. M. Sawka, and W. F. Young Jr., "The laboratory diagnosis of adrenal pheochromocytoma: the Mayo Clinic experience," *The Journal of Clinical Endocrinology & Metabolism*, vol. 88, no. 10, pp. 4533–4539, 2003.

[15] J. W. M. Lenders, G. Eisenhofer, M. Mannelli, and K. Pacak, "Phaeochromocytoma," *The Lancet*, vol. 366, no. 9486, pp. 665–675, 2005.

[16] E. L. Bravo, R. C. Tarazi, F. M. Fouad, D. G. Vidt, and R. W. Gifford Jr., "Clonidine-suppression test: a useful aid in the diagnosis of pheochromocytoma," *The New England Journal of Medicine*, vol. 305, no. 11, pp. 623–626, 1981.

[17] R. J. Sjoberg, K. J. Simcic, and G. S. Kidd, "The clonidine suppression test for pheochromocytoma: a review of its utility and pitfalls," *Archives of Internal Medicine*, vol. 152, no. 6, pp. 1193–1197, 1992.

[18] W. J. Elliott and M. B. Murphy, "Reduced specificity of the clonidine suppression test in patients with normal plasma catecholamine levels," *The American Journal of Medicine*, vol. 84, no. 3, pp. 419–424, 1988.

[19] G.-R. Joliat, E. Melloul, R. Djafarrian et al., "Cystic lymphangioma of the adrenal gland: report of a case and review of the literature," *World Journal of Surgical Oncology*, vol. 13, article 58, 2015.

58

Nonclassical Congenital Adrenal Hyperplasia and Pregnancy

Neslihan Cuhaci,[1] **Cevdet Aydın,**[1] **Ahmet Yesilyurt,**[2] **Ferda Alpaslan Pınarlı,**[2] **Reyhan Ersoy,**[1] **and Bekir Cakir**[1]

[1]Department of Endocrinology and Metabolism, Faculty of Medicine, Yildirim Beyazit University, 06800 Ankara, Turkey
[2]Department of Genetics, Dıskapı Yildirim Beyazit Education and Research Hospital, Ankara, Turkey

Correspondence should be addressed to Neslihan Cuhaci; neslihan_cuhaci@yahoo.com

Academic Editor: Yuji Moriwaki

Objective. The most common form of congenital adrenal hyperplasia (CAH) is 21-hydroxylase (21-OH) deficiency due to mutation of the *CYP21A2* gene. Patients with nonclassical CAH (NC-CAH) are usually asymptomatic at birth and typically present in late childhood, adolescence, or adulthood with symptoms of excessive androgen secretion. Subfertility is relative in NC-CAH, but the incidence of spontaneous miscarriage is higher. Here, we report a previously undiagnosed female who gave birth to a normal male child and is planning to become pregnant again. *Case Report*. A 32-year-old female was referred to our clinic for obesity. Her medical history revealed that she had had three pregnancies. She was planning to become pregnant again. Her laboratory results revealed that she had NC-CAH. Since her husband is the son of her aunt and she had miscarriages and intrauterin exitus in her history, their genetic analyses were performed. *Conclusion*. Since most patients with NC-CAH have a severe mutation, these patients may give birth to a child with the classical CAH (C-CAH) if their partner is also carrying a severe mutation. Females with NC-CAH who desire pregnancy must be aware of the risk of having an infant with C-CAH.

1. Introduction

Congenital adrenal hyperplasia (CAH) is a group of autosomal recessive disorders that are characterized by impaired cortisol synthesis and adrenal androgen excess, caused by a deficiency in one of the enzymes necessary for cortisol production [1–3]. The most common form of CAH is 21-hydroxylase (21-OH) deficiency due to mutation of the *CYP21A2* gene, which encodes the adrenal steroid 21-OH enzyme and is located on chromosome 6p21.3 [1, 4–9].

It can be defined as classical CAH (C-CAH), or nonclassical or late-onset CAH (NC-CAH). C-CAH can be of either the salt wasting (SW) or simple virilizing (SV) type.

NC-CAH 21-OH deficiency is much more common than C-CAH [8], with a reported prevalence of 0.1–0.4% in the general population [10]. It is also more frequent in certain ethnicities such as Ashkenazi Jewish, Mediterranean, Middle-Eastern, and Indian populations [11].

Patients with NC-CAH are usually asymptomatic at birth [7] and typically present in late childhood, adolescence, or adulthood with symptoms of excessive androgen secretion [12]. In adolescent and adult females, the symptoms of hyperandrogenism include hirsutism, acne, menstrual irregularity, androgenic alopecia, and impaired fertility [2, 6].

Subfertility is relative in NC-CAH, but the incidence of spontaneous miscarriage is higher [2]. However, few data regarding the fertility of NC-CAH patients are available [13].

Many females with NC-CAH conceive spontaneously, whereas others have ovulatory infertility but respond to glucocorticoid (GCC) or GCC plus clomiphene citrate treatment. However, the risk of spontaneous miscarriage is higher in these females compared with normal females (>25 versus 10–15%, resp.) [13–18]. Approximately 70% of individuals with NC-CAH have a point mutation of Val281Leu at exon 7, which prevents 20–50% of enzyme activity [19]. Previous studies reported that 27–76% of patients with NC-CAH have a severe mutation [13]. If their partner also carries a severe mutation, these patients might conceive a child with C-CAH [13].

In this study, we report a previously undiagnosed female who gave birth to a normal male child and is planning to become pregnant again.

2. Case

A 32-year-old female was referred to our clinic for obesity. She had hypothyroidism and was using L-thyroxin replacement therapy. Her medical history revealed that she had had three pregnancies: one had resulted in a healthy boy, one had resulted in ectopic pregnancy with twins and intrauterine exitus, and the latest, which had occurred 4 months earlier, had been terminated by miscarriage. She was planning to become pregnant again.

A physical examination revealed that her body mass index (BMI) was 26 kg/m^2. She had no purple striae or a buffalo hump and no hirsutism: her Ferriman-Gallwey score was 5. Laboratory results related to obesity revealed normal thyroid function tests, insulin resistance calculated using the HOMA-index was 1.8, and her initial random serum cortisol level was 17.8 µg/dL. Because of the high cortisol level, 1 mg dexamethasone suppression test (DMST) was applied, which successfully suppressed her cortisol level to 0.6 µg/dL. A follicular phase hormonal evaluation identified elevated 17-OHP (12.8 ng/mL) and ACTH (56 pg/mL) levels. The other hormonal profiles were all normal, including follicle-stimulating hormone (FSH), luteinizing hormone (LH), estradiol (E2), progesterone, prolactin (PRL), dehydroepiandrosterone sulfate (DHEA-SO4), and testosterone. There was no pathology on pelvic ultrasonography. We next performed an ACTH stimulation test and found 17-OHP levels at basal, 30 and 60 minutes of 14, 21, and 26 ng/mL, respectively, which confirmed the diagnosis of NC-CAH.

During these processes, we learned that she was a carrier of the *MTHFRC677* mutation. Before admission to our hospital, karyotype analysis was performed due to the previous miscarriage and intrauterine exitus. The results revealed a normal constitutional karyotype of 46, XX. Her husband, who is the son of her aunt (in other words their mothers are sisters), also had a normal constitutional karyotype of 46, XY. Because we confirmed the diagnosis of CAH and she is related to her husband, we also studied his laboratory tests, but no pathology was found. Genetic analyses were then performed on both the patient and her husband. In the genetic test results the patient had revealed a compound heterogeneous mutation of Q318X and P453S in the *CYP21A2* gene, and her husband revealed a 453S heterogeneous mutation in the *CYP21A2* gene. They have the same P453S mutations in the *CYP21A2* gene. Because both parents were carriers of *CYP21A2* mutations, we recommended preconception genetic counseling to the couple. They were informed of the risks to the fetus and newborn child, and fetal sampling was recommended if she became pregnant. Many patients with NC-CAH are asymptomatic and current recommendations argue against treatment for those without symptoms [19]. Treatment with glucocorticoid therapy is typically only recommended for those individuals with symptomatic hyperandrogenism [19]. Nonpregnant adults may be treated with the longer-acting DM or prednisone, alone or in combination

with hydrocortisone [8]. Hydrocortisone is the preferred treatment of pregnant women affected with CAH, because unlike DM, it is metabolized by the placental enzyme 11-β OH steroid dehydrogenase II and does not affect the fetus [8]. We did not start treatment before pregnancy, as suggested by the Endocrine Society guidelines [3], but, instead, planned to begin treatment when pregnancy occurred.

3. Discussion

Unlike the situation with C-CAH, few studies have assessed fertility in females with NC-CAH [13]. Bidet et al. analyzed 190 females with NC-CAH, 95 of whom wanted to become pregnant [13]. They reported that 187 pregnancies occurred in 85 females, which resulted in 141 births from 82 individuals. A total of 99 pregnancies (52.9%) occurred before diagnosis with NC-CAH (96 spontaneous and three with ovulation inducers), and 88 occurred after diagnosis (11 spontaneously and 77 with hydrocortisone treatment). The miscarriage rate was 6.5% and 26.3% in the patients treated with GCC and untreated patients, respectively. The authors also reported that 1.5% of the infants were born with C-CAH [13]. Birnbaum and Rose [20] observed 12 pregnancies among 22 NC-CAH patients who desired pregnancy, whereas Feldman et al. [16] observed that, of 20 patients wanting pregnancy, 10 had conceived before diagnosis, and nine after NC-CAH diagnosis and hydrocortisone treatment. Some studies have also assessed fertility in males with NC-CAH [19]. Although oligospermia has been reported, gonadal functions and sperm counts are relatively normal in males with NC-CAH, which suggests that NC-CAH might be underdiagnosed [21, 22]. One study reported that affected males are usually asymptomatic, and they are commonly diagnosed after the diagnosis of a female family member [23], as seen in our patient's husband.

Females with NC-CAH who desire pregnancy must be aware of the risk of having an infant with C-CAH. The incidence of C-CAH is 1 : 10,000–1 : 20,000, and the incidence of carriers in the general population is 1 : 50–1 : 71 (median 1 : 60) [19]. As such, the chance of having a child with C-CAH in a patient with C-CAH is 1 : 120 [19, 24]. Since most patients with NC-CAH carry a severe *CYP21A2* mutation in one allele, they are at risk of having a child with C-CAH [19]. Therefore, parents with NC-CAH would be predicted to have a 1 : 240 chance of having a child with C-CAH $(1/60 \times 1/2) \times (1 \times 1/2)$ [3, 19, 24]. Furthermore, because two-thirds of patients with NC-CAH are compound heterozygotes, the predicted incidence is ~1 : 360 $(1/60 \times 1/2) \times (2/3 \times 1/2)$ [19]. One study that investigated the pregnancy outcomes of 101 females with NC-CAH determined that the risk of having a birth with C-CAH was much higher (2.5%) and that at least 15% of offspring would have NC-CAH [15]. In our case, both parents carried heterogeneous *CYP21A2* mutations: the female had Q318X and P453S mutations, whereas her husband carried a 453S mutation. Seventy percent of NC-CAH individuals carry a point mutation, Val281Leu, at exon 7 [19]. P453S and R339H are also associated with NC-CAH; also R369W and I230T are two novel mutations associated with NC-CAH [19]. Additionally, Q318X mutation has been reported in association with CAH [6]. Large deletions and a splicing mutation that ablate enzyme activity comprise about 50% of C-CAH alleles [3]. A nonconservative amino substitution in exon 4 is associated with simple virilizing C-CAH [3]. Because they have the chance of giving birth to a child with C-CAH, our parents were offered preconception genetic counseling.

Prenatal treatment for CAH is still experimental. The aims of treatment include the genital virilization of the fetus, reducing the anxiety of the parents who might have a child with ambiguous genitalia [24]. However, prenatal treatment does not prevent the need for lifelong GCC and mineralocorticoid (MCC) replacement therapy, and intensive medical monitoring during infancy and later life, or the potential life-threatening salt-wasting crises that occur when postnatal treatment is discontinued [24]. Dexamethasone (DM) is commonly used because it binds minimally to cortisol-binding globulin (CBG) in the maternal blood and, unlike hydrocortisol, it is not inactivated by placental 11-beta hydroxysteroid dehydrogenase type II [6, 8]. Consequently, it crosses the placenta and suppresses ACTH secretion [8]. If karyotype or DNA analyses reveal that the fetus is male or an unaffected female, respectively, treatment is discontinued [8]. Because fetal genital virilization begins 6-7 weeks after conception, treatment must be started as soon as the female learns she is pregnant [3, 24]. However, because chorionic villous biopsies can be obtained after 10–12 weeks for genetic diagnosis and the procedure takes additional time, all pregnancies deemed to be at risk for virilizing CAH are treated, even though only 1 in 4 is affected, and only 1 in 8 affected fetuses is female [3, 6, 24]. Therefore, it was suggested that DM exposure is undesirable and unethical in 7 out of 8 fetuses (males and unaffected females) [24]; this remains controversial [24]. Because of the methodological limitations and small sample sizes, evidence for the maternal and fetal sequelae of prenatal DM treatment to accurately assess the fetuses at risk for CAH is limited or is of poor quality [3, 25]. Endocrine Society guidelines suggest that prenatal treatment should be pursued using protocols approved by Institutional Review Boards at all centers that are capable of collecting outcome data from a sufficiently large number of patients, which will allow the risks and benefits of this treatment to be defined more precisely [3]. Therefore, we did not start treatment before pregnancy occurred, as suggested by Endocrine Society guidelines [3]. In the study of New and colleagues [26], they found that the average Prader score of the fetuses treated with DM was 1.7, which was much lower than the average Prader score of 3.73 in those not treated. Although their data demonstrated no significant abnormality in the long-term medical and cognitive outcomes in the patients treated with DM prenatally, the procedures such as chorionic villus sampling and amniocentesis were invasive and also all the fetuses treated unnecessarily before the sex and the affection status of the fetus is known. In a recent study of New et al. [27], they developed a noninvasive method for early prenatal diagnosis of fetuses at risk for CAH and found that cell-free fetal DNA obtained from maternal plasma could potentially provide the diagnosis of CAH, noninvasively, so, only the affected female fetuses will be treated before

the 9th week of gestation. Their study seems promising. But we decide to treat the patient when pregnancy occurs, obtain chorionic villous sampling 10–12 weeks into the pregnancy, and then manage the treatment appropriately.

References

[1] L. S. Levine, "Congenital adrenal hyperplasia," *Pediatrics in Review*, vol. 21, no. 5, pp. 159–171, 2000.

[2] I. N. Purwana, H. Kanasaki, A. Oride, and K. Miyazaki, "Successful pregnancy after the treatment of primary amenorrhea in a patient with non-classical congenital adrenal hyperplasia," *Journal of Obstetrics and Gynaecology Research*, vol. 39, no. 1, pp. 406–409, 2013.

[3] P. W. Speiser, R. Azziz, L. S. Baskin et al., "Congenital adrenal hyperplasia due to steroid 21-hydroxylase deficiency: an Endocrine Society clinical practice guideline," *Journal of Clinical Endocrinology and Metabolism*, vol. 95, no. 9, pp. 4133–4160, 2010.

[4] N. Krone, V. Dhir, H. E. Ivison, and W. Arlt, "Congenital adrenal hyperplasia and P450 oxidoreductase deficiency," *Clinical Endocrinology*, vol. 66, no. 2, pp. 162–172, 2007.

[5] P. C. White and P. W. Speiser, "Congenital adrenal hyperplasia due to 21-hydroxylase deficiency," *Endocrine Reviews*, vol. 21, no. 3, pp. 245–291, 2000.

[6] S. F. Witchel, "Non-classic congenital adrenal hyperplasia," *Steroids*, vol. 78, no. 8, pp. 747–750, 2013.

[7] K. Unluhizarci, M. Kula, M. Dundar et al., "The prevalence of non-classic adrenal hyperplasia among Turkish women with hyperandrogenism," *Gynecological Endocrinology*, vol. 26, no. 2, pp. 139–143, 2010.

[8] O. Lekarev and M. I. New, "Adrenal disease in pregnancy," *Best Practice and Research: Clinical Endocrinology and Metabolism*, vol. 25, no. 6, pp. 959–973, 2011.

[9] S. F. Witchel, "Management of CAH during pregnancy: optimizing outcomes," *Current Opinion in Endocrinology, Diabetes and Obesity*, vol. 19, no. 6, pp. 489–496, 2012.

[10] H. Pinkas, S. Fuchs, Y. Klipper-Aurbach et al., "Non-classical 21-hydroxylase deficiency: prevalence in males with unexplained abnormal sperm analysis," *Fertility and Sterility*, vol. 93, no. 6, pp. 1887–1891, 2010.

[11] R. C. Wilson, S. Nimkarn, M. Dumic et al., "Ethnic-specific distribution of mutations in 716 patients with congenital adrenal hyperplasia owing to 21-hydroxylase deficiency," *Molecular Genetics and Metabolism*, vol. 90, no. 4, pp. 414–421, 2007.

[12] S. F. Witchel, "Nonclassic congenital adrenal hyperplasia," *Current Opinion in Endocrinology, Diabetes and Obesity*, vol. 19, no. 3, pp. 151–158, 2012.

[13] M. Bidet, C. Bellanné-Chantelot, M.-B. Galand-Portier et al., "Fertility in women with nonclassical congenital adrenal hyperplasia due to 21-hydroxylase deficiency," *Journal of Clinical Endocrinology and Metabolism*, vol. 95, no. 3, pp. 1182–1190, 2010.

[14] N. M. M. L. Stikkelbroeck, A. R. M. M. Hermus, D. D. M. Braat, and B. J. Otten, "Fertility in women with congenital adrenal hyperplasia due to 21-hydroxylase deficiency," *Obstetrical and Gynecological Survey*, vol. 58, no. 4, pp. 275–284, 2003.

[15] C. Moran, R. Azziz, N. Weintrob et al., "Reproductive outcome of women with 21-hydroxylase-deficient nonclassic adrenal hyperplasia," *Journal of Clinical Endocrinology and Metabolism*, vol. 91, no. 9, pp. 3451–3456, 2006.

[16] S. Feldman, L. Billaud, J.-C. Thalabard et al., "Fertility in women with late-onset adrenal hyperplasia due to 21-hydroxylase deficiency," *Journal of Clinical Endocrinology and Metabolism*, vol. 74, no. 3, pp. 635–639, 1992.

[17] D. Dewailly, "Nonclassic 21-hydroxylase deficiency," *Seminars in Reproductive Medicine*, vol. 20, no. 3, pp. 243–248, 2002.

[18] M. J. Zinaman, E. D. Clegg, C. C. Brown, J. O'Connor, and S. G. Selevan, "Estimates of human fertility and pregnancy loss," *Fertility and Sterility*, vol. 65, no. 3, pp. 503–509, 1996.

[19] C. M. Trapp and S. E. Oberfield, "Recommendations for treatment of nonclassic congenital adrenal hyperplasia (NCCAH): an update," *Steroids*, vol. 77, no. 4, pp. 342–346, 2012.

[20] M. D. Birnbaum and L. I. Rose, "Late onset adrenocortical hydroxylase deficiencies associated with menstrual dysfunction," *Obstetrics and Gynecology*, vol. 63, no. 4, pp. 445–451, 1984.

[21] A. Augarten, R. Weissenberg, C. Pariente, and J. Sack, "Reversible male infertility in late onset congenital adrenal hyperplasia," *Journal of Endocrinological Investigation*, vol. 14, no. 3, pp. 237–240, 1991.

[22] I. Kalachanis, D. Rousso, A. Kourtis, F. Goutzioulis, G. Makedos, and D. Panidis, "Reversible infertility, pharmaceutical and spontaneous, in a male with late onset congenital adrenal hyperplasia, due to 21-hydroxylase deficiency," *Archives of Andrology*, vol. 48, no. 1, pp. 37–41, 2002.

[23] M. Bidet, C. Bellanné-Chantelot, M.-B. Galand-Portier et al., "Clinical and molecular characterization of a cohort of 161 unrelated women with nonclassical congenital adrenal hyperplasia due to 21-hydroxylase deficiency and 330 family members," *Journal of Clinical Endocrinology and Metabolism*, vol. 94, no. 5, pp. 1570–1578, 2009.

[24] W. L. Miller and S. F. Witchel, "Prenatal treatment of congenital adrenal hyperplasia: risks outweigh benefits," *American Journal of Obstetrics & Gynecology*, vol. 208, no. 5, pp. 354–359, 2013.

[25] M. Mercè Fernández-Balsells, K. Muthusamy, G. Smushkin et al., "Prenatal dexamethasone use for the prevention of virilization in pregnancies at risk for classical congenital adrenal hyperplasia because of 21-hydroxylase (CYP21A2) deficiency: a systematic review and meta-analyses," *Clinical Endocrinology*, vol. 73, no. 4, pp. 436–444, 2010.

[26] M. New, M. Abraham, T. Yuen, and O. Lekarev, "An update on prenatal diagnosis and treatment of congenital adrenal hyperplasia," *Seminars in Reproductive Medicine*, vol. 30, no. 5, pp. 396–399, 2012.

[27] M. I. New, Y. K. Tong, T. Yuen et al., "Noninvasive prenatal diagnosis of congenital adrenal hyperplasia using cell-free fetal DNA in maternal plasma," *Journal of Clinical Endocrinology and Metabolism*, vol. 99, no. 6, pp. E1022–E1030, 2014.

Permissions

List of Contributors

Nikos Sabanis and Sotirios Vasileiou
Department of Nephrology, General Hospital of Pella, 58200 Edessa, Greece

Eleni Gavriilaki and Asterios Kalaitzoglou
Medical School, Aristotle University ofThessaloniki, 54124Thessaloniki, Greece

Eleni Paschou
Department of General Practice and Family Medicine, General Hospital of Pella, 58200 Edessa, Greece

Dimitrios Papanikolaou and Pinelopi Ioannidou
Department of General Surgery, General Hospital of Pella, 58200 Edessa, Greece

Carmen Aresta, Giorgia Grassi, Livio Luzi and Stefano Benedini
Department of Biomedical Sciences for Health, Universit`a degli Studi di Milano, Milan, Italy

Antonietta Tufano
Endocrinology Unit, IRCCS Policlinico San Donato, San Donato M.se (MI), Italy

Gianfranco Butera
Department of Congenital Cardiology and Cardiac Surgery, IRCCS Policlinico San Donato, San Donato Milanese (MI), Italy

H. S. Villanueva-Alvarado and C. Higueruela-Mínguez
Service of Endocrinology and Nutrition, University Clinical Hospital of Salamanca, Paseo de San Vicente No. 58, 37007 Salamanca, Spain

A. Herrero-Ruiz and J. M. Recio-Cordova
Service of Endocrinology and Nutrition, University Clinical Hospital of Salamanca, Paseo de San Vicente No. 58, 37007 Salamanca, Spain
Department of Medicine, University of Salamanca, Campus Miguel de Unamuno, s/n, 37007 Salamanca, Spain

J. J. Corrales-Hernández
Service of Endocrinology and Nutrition, University Clinical Hospital of Salamanca, Paseo de San Vicente No. 58, 37007 Salamanca, Spain
Department of Medicine, University of Salamanca, Campus Miguel de Unamuno, s/n, 37007 Salamanca, Spain

Cancer Research Institute (IBMCC-CSIC/USAL) and Institute for Biomedical Research, University of Salamanca, Salamanca, Spain

J. Feito-Pérez
Service of Anatomic Pathology, University Clinical Hospital of Salamanca, Paseo de San Vicente No. 58, 37007 Salamanca, Spain

Preneet Cheema Brar, Elena Dingle and Manish Raisingani
Department of Pediatrics, Division of Pediatric Endocrinology and Diabetes, New York University School of Medicine, New York, NY, USA

John Pappas
Department of Pediatrics, Clinical Genetics Services, New York University School of Medicine, New York, NY, USA

S. S. C. Gunatilake and U. Bulugahapitiya
Department of Endocrinology, Colombo South Teaching Hospital, Kalubowila, Sri Lanka

V. Larouche
Adult Endocrinology and Metabolism Training Program, McGill University, Montréal, QC, Canada

N. Garfield
Division of Endocrinology, McGill University Health Centre, Montréal, QC, Canada

E. Mitmaker
Division of General Surgery, McGill University Health Centre,Montréal, QC, Canada

Pejman Cohan
Specialized Endocrine Care Center, 150 North Robertson Boulevard, Suite 210, Beverly Hills, CA 90211, USA

Rohan K. Henry
Division of Endocrinology, Department of Pediatrics, Nationwide Children's Hospital, The Ohio State University College of Medicine, Columbus, OH 43205, USA

Ram K. Menon
Division of Endocrinology, Department of Pediatrics, C. S. Mott Children's Hospital, Michigan Medicine, University of Michigan Medical School, Ann Arbor, MI 48109, USA

Meredith Wasserman
TheWarren Alpert Medical School, Brown University, Providence, RI, USA

Erin M. Mulvihill
College of Human Ecology, Cornell University, Ithaca, NY, USA

Angela Ganan-Soto
Alexian Brothers Women and Children's Hospital and Amita Health Medical Group, Hoffman Estates, IL, USA

Serife Uysal and Jose Bernardo Quintos
Division of Pediatric Endocrinology, Rhode Island Hospital and Hasbro Children's Hospital, TheWarren Alpert Medical School, Brown University, Providence, RI, USA

Ana Patricia Torga
Summer Intern, Division of Pediatric Endocrinology and Diabetes, Rhode Island Hospital/Hasbro Children's Hospital, 111 Plain St, 3rd Floor, Providence, RI 02903, USA

Juanita Hodax and Jose Bernardo Quintos
Division of Pediatric Endocrinology and Diabetes, Rhode Island Hospital/Hasbro Children's Hospital, TheWarren Alpert Medical School of Brown University, 111 Plain St, 3rd Floor, Providence, RI 02903, USA

Mari Mori and Jennifer Schwab
Division of Human Genetics, Hasbro Children's Hospital, The Warren Alpert Medical School of Brown University, 2 Dudley Street, Suite 460, Providence, RI 02903, USA

Alex Gonzalez-Bossolo, Alexis Gonzalez-Rivera and Santiago Coste-Sibilia
Internal Medicine Training Program, Department of Medicine, University District Hospital, University of Puerto Rico School of Medicine, San Juan, PR 00936-5067, USA

Makoto Daimon
Department of Endocrinology and Metabolism, Hirosaki University Graduate School of Medicine, 5 Zaifu-cho,Hirosaki, Aomori 036-8562, Japan

Kazunori Kageyama, Noriko Ishigame and Aya Sugiyama
Department of Endocrinology and Metabolism, Hirosaki University Graduate School of Medicine, 5 Zaifu-cho,Hirosaki, Aomori 036-8562, Japan

Department of Endocrinology and Metabolism, Odate Municipal General Hospital, 3-1 Yutaka-cho, Odate 017-8550, Japan

Akiko Igawa and Takashi Nishi
Department of Gastroenterological Surgery, Hirosaki University Graduate School of Medicine, 5 Zaifu-cho,Hirosaki, Aomori 036-8562, Japan

Satoko Morohashi and Hiroshi Kijima
Department of Pathology and Bioscience, Hirosaki University Graduate School of Medicine, 5 Zaifu-cho,Hirosaki, Aomori 036-8562, Japan

Sonali Sihindi Chapa Gunatilake and Uditha Bulugahapitiya
Endocrinology, Colombo South Teaching Hospital, Kalubowila, Sri Lanka

Ronak Ved, Neil Patel and Michael Stechman
University Hospital of Wales, Cardiff CF14 4XW, UK

Zaid Ammari, Stella C. Pak, Mohammed Ruzieh, Osama Dasa and Abhinav Tiwari
Department of Medicine, College of Medicine and Life Sciences, University of Toledo, Toledo, OH, USA

Juan C. Jaume
Department of Medicine, College of Medicine and Life Sciences, University of Toledo, Toledo, OH, USA
Division of Endocrinology, Diabetes and Metabolism, College of Medicine and Life Sciences, University of Toledo, Toledo, OH, USA
Center for Diabetes and Endocrine Research (CeDER), College of Medicine and Life Sciences, University of Toledo, Toledo, OH, USA

Maria A. Alfonso-Jaume
Department of Medicine, College of Medicine and Life Sciences, University of Toledo, Toledo, OH, USA
Center for Diabetes and Endocrine Research (CeDER), College of Medicine and Life Sciences, University of Toledo, Toledo, OH, USA
Division of Nephrology, College of Medicine and Life Sciences, University of Toledo, Toledo, OH, USA

S. Ali Imran
Division of Endocrinology and Metabolism, Department of Medicine, Dalhousie University, Halifax, NS, Canada

Adam Hinchey
Dalhousie Medical School, Halifax, NS, Canada

Rob Hart
Division of Otolaryngology, Department of Surgery, Dalhousie University, Halifax, NS, Canada

Martin Bullock
Department of Pathology, Dalhousie University, Halifax, NS, Canada

Andrew Ross and Steven Burrell
Division of Nuclear Medicine, Department of Diagnostic Radiology, Dalhousie University, Halifax, NS, Canada

Murray B. Gordon
Allegheny Neuroendocrinology Center, Departments of Medicine and Neurosurgery, Allegheny General Hospital, 320 East North Avenue, Pittsburgh, PA 15212, USA

Samer Nakhle
Palm Research Center, 9280 West Sunset Road, Suite 306, Las Vegas, NV 89148, USA

William H. Ludlam
Novartis Pharmaceuticals, 1 Health Plaza, East Hanover, NJ 07936, USA

Niranjan Tachamo, Bidhya Timilsina, Rashmi Dhital, and Theresa Lynn
Department of Internal Medicine, Reading Hospital, Reading, PA, 19611, USA

Vasudev Magaji and Ilan Gabriely
Section of Endocrinology, Reading Hospital, Reading, PA, 19611, USA

Se Won Kim and Sun Hee Park
Division of Endocrinology, Department of Internal Medicine, Sahmyook Medical Center, Seoul, Republic of Korea

Seung-Eun Lee and Jae Hyeon Kim
Department of Medicine, Samsung Medical Center, Sungkyunkwan University School of Medicine, Seoul, Republic of Korea

Young Lyun Oh
Department of Pathology, Samsung Medical Center, Sungkyunkwan University School of Medicine, Seoul, Republic of Korea

Seokhwi Kim
Graduate School of Medical Science and Engineering, Korea Advanced Institute of Science and Technology, Daejeon, Republic of Korea

Karl Lhotta, Emanuel Zitt and Hannelore Sprenger-Mähr
Department of Internal Medicine 3, Academic Teaching Hospital Feldkirch, Feldkirch, Austria

Lorin Loacker
Central Institute for Medical and Chemical Laboratory Diagnostics, Medical University Innsbruck, Innsbruck, Austria

Alexander Becherer
Department of NuclearMedicine, Academic Teaching Hospital Feldkirch, Feldkirch, Austria

Khaled Ahmed Baagar, Mashhood Ahmed Siddique, Shaimaa Ahmed Arroub and Amin Ahmed Jayyousi
Endocrine Department, Hamad Medical Corporation, Doha, Qatar

Ahmed Hamdi Ebrahim
Emergency Department, Hamad Medical Corporation, Doha, Qatar

Kirstie Lithgow and Christopher Symonds
Department of Medicine, Cumming School of Medicine, University of Calgary, Calgary, AB, Canada

Antonio Balestrieri
Endocrinology and Diabetology Unit, "M. Bufalini" Hospital, ASL of Romagna, Cesena, Italy

ElenaMagnani
Internal Medicine Unit, "M. Bufalini" Hospital, ASL of Romagna, Cesena, Italy

Fiorella Nuzzo
Pathology Unit, "M. Bufalini" Hospital, ASL of Romagna, Cesena, Italy

Suhaib Radi and Andrew C. Karaplis
Division of Endocrinology, Department of Medicine, Jewish General Hospital, McGill University, Montreal, QC, Canada H3T 1E2

Karun Badwal, Tooba Tariq, andDiane Peirce
Western Michigan University Homer Stryker M.D. School of Medicine, USA

Roberto Ruiz-Cordero
Department of Hematopathology, University of Texas MD Anderson Cancer Center, Houston, TX 77030, USA

Alia Gupta
Department of Pathology, Jackson Memorial Hospital/ University of Miami Miller School of Medicine, Miami, FL 33136, USA

Merce Jorda
Department of Pathology, Jackson Memorial Hospital/ University of Miami Miller School of Medicine, Miami, FL 33136, USA

Department of Urology, Jackson Memorial Hospital/ University of Miami Miller School of Medicine, Miami, FL 33136, USA

Arumugam R. Jayakumar
South Florida Foundation for Research and Education Inc., Veterans Affairs Medical Center, Miami, FL 33125, USA

Gaetano Ciancio
Department of Surgery, Jackson Memorial Hospital/ University of Miami Miller School of Medicine, Miami, FL 33136, USA

Gunnlaugur Petur Nielsen
Department of Pathology and Center for Cancer Research, Massachusetts General Hospital, Charlestown, MA 02129, USA

S. A. Ghaznavi and N. M. A. Saad
Department of Medicine, Division of Endocrinology and Metabolism, University of Calgary, Calgary, AB, Canada

L. E. Donovan
Department of Medicine, Division of Endocrinology and Metabolism, University of Calgary, Calgary, AB, Canada
Department of Obstetrics and Gynaecology, University of Calgary, Calgary, AB, Canada

Niranjan Tachamo
Department of Internal Medicine, Reading Health System, West Reading, PA 19611, USA

Brian Le
Department of Pathology, Reading Health System,West Reading, PA 19611, USA

Jeffrey Driben
ENT Head and Neck Specialists,Wyomissing, PA 19610, USA

Vasudev Magaji
Department of Endocrinology, Reading Health System, West Reading, PA 19611, USA

Nooshin Salehi
Department of Medicine, Riverside University Health System Medical Center, Moreno Valley, CA, USA

Anthony Firek and Iqbal Munir
Division of Endocrinology, Department of Medicine, Riverside University Health System Medical Center, Moreno Valley, CA, USA

Elizabeth S. Sandberg and Ali S. Calikoglu

Division of Endocrinology, Department of Pediatrics, University of North Carolina at Chapel Hill, Chapel Hill, NC, USA

Karen J. Loechner
Division of Pediatric Endocrinology, Department of Pediatrics, Children's Healthcare of Atlanta, Atlanta, GA, USA

Lydia L. Snyder
Division of Pediatric Endocrinology, Department of Pediatrics, Nemours Children's Health System, Jacksonville, FL, USA

RH Bishay and A. Suryawanshi
Department of Endocrinology and Metabolism, Concord Repatriation General Hospital, Concord, Sydney, NSW2139, Australia
Sydney Medical School, University of Sydney, Sydney, NSW2005, Australia

Anastasios Anyfantakis and Irene Vourliotaki
Department of Endocrinology, Venizeleio General Hospital, Heraklion, Crete, Greece

Dimitrios Anyfantakis
Primary Health Care Centre of Kissamos, Chania, Crete, Greece

Jin Sae Yoo
Department of Internal Medicine, Wonju Severance Christian Hospital, Yonsei University Wonju College of Medicine, Wonju, Republic of Korea

Jung Soo Lim
Department of Internal Medicine, Wonju Severance Christian Hospital, Yonsei University Wonju College of Medicine, Wonju, Republic of Korea
Institute of Evidence Based Medicine, Wonju Severance Christian Hospital, Yonsei University Wonju College of Medicine, Wonju, Republic of Korea

Juwon Kim
Department of Laboratory Medicine, Wonju Severance Christian Hospital, Yonsei University Wonju College of Medicine, Wonju, Republic of Korea

Hyeong Ju Kwon
Department of Pathology, Wonju Severance Christian Hospital, Yonsei University Wonju College of Medicine, Wonju, Republic of Korea

Edward J. Bellfield, Jacqueline Chan and Claudia Boucher-Berry
Division of Pediatric Endocrinology, University of Illinois College of Medicine, Chicago, IL 60612, USA

Sarah Durrin
University of Illinois College of Medicine, Chicago, IL 60612, USA

Valerie Lindgren
Department of Pathology, University of Illinois College of Medicine, Chicago, IL 60612, USA

Zohra Shad
Division of Genetics, University of Illinois College of Medicine, Chicago, IL 60612, USA

Jacqueline Chan, Fabiola D'Ambrosio Rodriguez, Deepank Sahni and Claudia Boucher-Berry
Department of Pediatric, Children's Hospital of the University of Illinois, Chicago, IL, USA

Sartaj Sandhu
Advocare DelGiorno Endocrinology, Sewell, New Jersey, USA

Akshata Desai, Manav Batra, Robin Girdhar, Kaushik Chatterjee, Antoine Makdissi and Ajay Chaudhuri
Department of Endocrinology, Diabetes and Metabolism, State University of New York, Buffalo, New York, USA

E. Helen Kemp
Department of Oncology andMetabolism, University of Sheffield, Sheffield, UK

Victoria Mendoza-Zubieta and Lourdes Josefina Balcázar-Hernández
Endocrinology Department, Hospital de Especialidades, Centro Médico Nacional Siglo XXI, IMSS, 06720 Mexico City, DF, Mexico

Mauricio Carvallo-Venegas, Jorge Alberto Vargas-Castilla, Nicolás Ducoing-Sisto and Alfredo Alejandro Páramo-Lovera
Faculty of Medicine, Universidad Nacional Autónoma de México (UNAM), 04510 Mexico City, DF, Mexico

JuliánMalcolm Mac Gregor-Gooch
Division of Medicine, Hospital de Especialidades, Centro Médico Nacional Siglo XXI, IMSS, 06720 Mexico City, DF, Mexico

Asma Deeb
Paediatric Endocrinology Department, Mafraq Hospital, Abu Dhabi, UAE

Alice Abraham, Mishaela Rubin, Domenico Accili, John P. Bilezikian and Utpal B. Pajvani
Division of Endocrinology, Department of Medicine, Columbia University College of Physicians and Surgeons, New York, NY 10032, USA

Alexander A. Leung, Jennifer Yamamoto and Julie McKeen
Division of Endocrinology and Metabolism, Department of Medicine, University of Calgary, Calgary, AB, Canada T2T 5C7

Paola Luca
Division of Endocrinology and Metabolism, Department of Pediatrics, University of Calgary, Calgary, AB, Canada T3B 6A9

Paul Beaudry
Division of Pediatric Surgery, Department of Surgery, University of Calgary, Calgary, AB, Canada T3B 6A9

Adriana Handra-Luca and Mouna Bendib
Service d'Anatomie Pathologique, APHP GHU Avicenne, UFR Médecine, Université Paris Nord Sorbonne Cité,125 rue Stalingrad, 93009 Bobigny, France

Marie-Laure Dumuis-Gimenez,
Service Medecine Nucleaire, APHP GHU Avicenne, 93009 Bobigny, France

Panagiotis Anagnostis
Division of Endocrinology, Police Medical Centre, Monastiriou 326, 54627 Thessaloniki, Greece

KevinM. Pantalone, Betul Hatipoglu and Laurence Kennedy
Endocrinology and Metabolism Institute, Cleveland Clinic, Desk F-20, 9500 Euclid Avenue, Cleveland, OH 44195, USA

Amir H. Hamrahian
Endocrinology and Metabolism Institute, Cleveland Clinic, Desk F-20, 9500 Euclid Avenue, Cleveland, OH 44195, USA
Department of Endocrinology, Cleveland Clinic Abu Dhabi, Abu Dhabi, UAE

Manjula K. Gupta
Pathology and Laboratory Medicine Institute, Cleveland Clinic, Desk LL3-140, 9500 Euclid Avenue, Cleveland, OH 44195, USA

Lima Lawrence, M. Cecilia Lansang, and Vinni Makin
1Cleveland Clinic, Department of Endocrinology andMetabolism, Cleveland, OH, USA

Oscar Tovar-Camargo
Cleveland Clinic, Department of Anesthesiology, Cleveland, OH, USA

Enzo Ragucci
Diabetes and Endocrinology Consultants, 2 Crosfield Ave, No. 204, West Nyack, NY 10994, USA

Dat Nguyen, Michele Lamerson and Andreas G. Moraitis
Corcept Therapeutics, 149 Commonwealth Drive, Menlo Park, CA 94025, USA

Pooja E. Mishra
St John's Medical College, Bangalore, India

Betsy L. Schwartz
Pediatric Endocrinology, Park Nicollet, Minneapolis, MN, USA

Kyriakie Sarafoglou and Anna Petryk
Pediatric Endocrinology, University of Minnesota, Minneapolis, MN, USA

Kristen Hook
Pediatric Dermatology, University of Minnesota, Minneapolis, MN, USA

Youngki Kim
Pediatric Nephrology, University of Minnesota, Minneapolis, MN, USA

Kunal Mehta, Irene Weiss and Michael D. Goldberg
Westchester Medical Center, Department of Medicine, Division of Endocrinology, Taylor Care Pavilion, Room D342, 100Woods Road, Valhalla, NY 10595, USA

Lama Alfaraidi, Abrar Alfaifi, and Rawan Alquaiz
College of Medicine, King Saud University, Riyadh, Saudi Arabia

Faten Almijmaj and Horia Mawlawi
Department of Pediatrics, Prince Sultan Military Medical City, Riyadh 11159, Saudi Arabia

D. Magalhães
Endocrinology, Diabetes and Metabolism Department, Centro Hospitalar São João, Porto, Portugal
Faculty of Medicine of University of Porto, Porto, Portugal
Instituto de Investigação e Inovação em Sa´ude, University of Porto, Porto, Portugal

C. Costa, M. J. Matos, A. P. Santos and I.Torres
Endocrinology Department, Instituto Português de Oncologia, Porto, Portugal

I. Furtado
Internal Medicine Department, Centro Hospitalar do Porto, Porto, Portugal

H. Duarte
Nuclear Medicine Department, Instituto Português de Oncologia, Porto, Portugal

M. Afonso
Pathology Department, Instituto Português de Oncologia, Porto, Portugal

J. Lobo
Pathology Department, Instituto Portugu^es de Oncologia, Porto, Portugal
Cancer Biology and Epigenetics Group, Research Center, Instituto Português de Oncologia, Porto, Portugal
Pathology and Molecular Immunology Department, Institute of Biomedical Sciences Abel Salazar (ICBAS), University of Porto, Porto, Portugal

Oscar R. Vázquez and Frieda Silva
Nuclear Medicine Section, Radiological Sciences Department, University of Puerto Rico, San Juan, Puerto Rico, USA

Eduardo Acosta-Pumarejo
Radiology Department, VA Caribbean Healthcare System, San Juan, Puerto Rico, USA

Maria L. Marín
Pathology Department, Isaac Gonzalez Oncologic Hospital, San Juan, Puerto Rico, USA

Olga Astapova, Anindita Biswas, Alessandra DiMauro, Jacob Moalem and Stephen R. Hammes
Division of Endocrinology and Metabolism, Department of Medicine, University of Rochester School of Medicine and Dentistry,Rochester, New York 14642, USA

Ibrahim Alali, Ghadeer Mardini, Nermeen Hijazi, Lama Hadid and Younes Kabalan
Endocrinology Department, Al-Assad University Hospital, Damascus University, Syria

Lilianne Haj Hassan
Endocrinology Department, Al-Mouwassat University Hospital, Damascus University, Syria

Marta Gonzalez Rozas
Internal Department, Hospital de Segovia, Segovia, Spain

Lidia Hernanz Roman and José Luis Pérez-Castrillón
Internal Department, Hospital Universitario R´io Hortega, Valladolid, Spain

Diego Gonzalez Gonzalez
Pathology Department, Hospital Universitario Río Hortega, Valladolid, Spain

Fatehi Elnour Elzein and Abdullah Aljaberi
Division of Infectious Diseases, Department of Medicine, Prince Sultan Military Medical City, Riyadh 11159, Saudi Arabia

Abdullah AlFiaar
Histopathology Department, Prince SultanMilitary Medical City, Riyadh 11159, Saudi Arabia

Abdullah Alghamdi
Urology Department, Prince Sultan Military Medical City, Riyadh 11159, Saudi Arabia

Sarah Pearlstein
Department of Surgery, Lenox Hill Hospital, New York, NY, USA

Arash H. Lahouti and Elana Opher
Department of Pathology, Lenox Hill Hospital, New York, NY, USA

Yuri E. Nikiforov
Department of Pathology, University of Pittsburgh Medical Center, Pittsburgh, PA, USA

Daniel B. Kuriloff
New York Head and Neck Institute, Lenox Hill Hospital, New York, NY, USA
Zucker School of Medicine at Hofstra/Northwell, New York, NY, USA

Tayane Muniz Fighera
Gynecological Endocrinology Unit, Division of Endocrinology, Hospital de Clinicas de Porto Alegre, Rua Ramiro Barcelos 2350, 90035-003 Porto Alegre, RS, Brazil

Poli Mara Spritzer
Gynecological Endocrinology Unit, Division of Endocrinology, Hospital de Clinicas de Porto Alegre, Rua Ramiro Barcelos 2350, 90035-003 Porto Alegre, RS, Brazil

Laboratory of Molecular Endocrinology, Department of Physiology, Federal University of Rio Grande do Sul, Rua Ramiro Barcelos 2350, 90035-003 Porto Alegre, RS, Brazil

Bhavana B. Rao and Benjamin Click
Department of Internal Medicine, University of Pittsburgh Medical Center, Pittsburgh, PA 15213, USA

George Eid
Division of Bariatric Surgery, Allegheny Health Network, Pittsburgh, PA 15212, USA

Ronald A. Codario
Division of Endocrinology, Department of Internal Medicine, VA Pittsburgh Healthcare System, Pittsburgh, PA 15240, USA

Israel Hodish
Division of Internal Medicine, University of Michigan Medical Center, Ann Arbor, MI 48109, USA

Lindsay Schmidt
Department of Pathology, University of Michigan, Ann Arbor, MI 48109, USA

Andreas G. Moraitis
CorceptTherapeutics, Menlo Park, CA 94025, USA

Neslihan Cuhaci, Cevdet Aydın, Reyhan Ersoy and Bekir Cakir
Department of Endocrinology and Metabolism, Faculty of Medicine, Yildirim Beyazit University, 06800 Ankara, Turkey

Ahmet Yesilyurt and Ferda Alpaslan Pınarlı
Department of Genetics, Dıskapı Yildirim Beyazit Education and Research Hospital, Ankara, Turkey

Index